Hearing Aids

Hearing Aids

Harvey Dillon, Ph.D.

Director of Research

National Acoustic Laboratories of Australia

Sydney, New South Wales

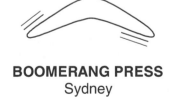

BOOMERANG PRESS
Sydney

2001

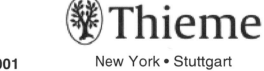

New York • Stuttgart

Boomerang Press

Box 7, 219 Kissing Point Road
Turramurra, 2074, Australia

Distributed exclusively

In the American continents by:	**In Australia and New Zealand by:**	**In the rest of the world by:**
Thieme	Boomerang Press	Thieme
333 Seventh Avenue	Box 7, 219 Kissing Point Road	14 Ruedigerstrasse
New York, NY 10001, USA	Turramurra, 2074, Australia	D-70469 Stuttgart
Phone: +1 212 760 0888	Phone: +61 (0)2 9440 2885	Germany
or 1 800 782 3488	Fax: +61 (0)2 94402583	Phone: +49 (0)711 893 1117
Fax: +1 212 947 1112	Email: publisher@BoomerangPress.com.a	Fax: +49 (0)711 893 1410
Email: custserv@thieme.com	Internet: www.BoomerangPress.com.au	Email: custserv@thieme.com
Internet: www.thieme.com		Internet: www.thieme.com

Typesetter: Jean Banning   Printer: Hamilton Printing Company   Cover design: Cyberdesign

Library of Congress Cataloging-in-Publication Data

Dillon, Harvey.
    Hearing aids / Harvey Dillon.
        p. cm.
    Includes bibliographical references and index.
    ISBN 1-58890-052-5
    1. Hearing aids. I. Title.

RF300 .D54 2000

617.8'9--dc21   00-069954

Important Note

This book is designed to educate, and be a reference tool for, students and professionals engaged in hearing rehabilitation through the use of hearing aids. While the book aims to have a wide scope, it is not the intention of author or publisher to present all the information that is available on this topic. The reader should obtain and read all the material that the reader considers necessary to competently perform hearing rehabilitation.

Audiology is an ever-changing science. Research and clinical experience are continually broadening and changing our knowledge, in particular our knowledge of proper treatment. Every effort has been made to make this book as complete and as accurate as possible. However, there may be mistakes both typographical and in content. This text should therefore be used only as a general guide and not as the ultimate source of information on hearing aids.

For these reasons the author, publisher and distributor shall have neither liability nor responsibility to any person or entity with respect to any loss or damage caused, or alleged to be caused, directly or indirectly by the information in this book. If you do not wish to be bound by the above, you may return this book to the point of sale for a full refund.

Some of the product names, patents and registered designs referred to in this book are in fact registered trademarks or proprietary names even though specific reference to this fact is not always made in the text. Therefore the appearance of a name without designation as proprietary is not to be construed as a representation by the publisher that it is in the public domain.

Printed in the United States of America

5   4

TNY ISBN 1-58890-052-5

GTV ISBN 3-13-128941-4

BRIEF CONTENTS

PREFACE XV

1   INTRODUCTORY CONCEPTS 1

2   HEARING AID COMPONENTS 18

3   HEARING AID SYSTEMS 48

4   ELECTROACOUSTIC PERFORMANCE AND MEASUREMENT 74

5   HEARING AID EARMOLDS, EAR SHELLS AND COUPLING SYSTEMS 117

6   COMPRESSION SYSTEMS IN HEARING AIDS 159

7   ADVANCED SIGNAL PROCESSING SCHEMES FOR HEARING AIDS 187

8   ASSESSING CANDIDACY FOR HEARING AIDS 209

9   PRESCRIBING HEARING AID PERFORMANCE 234

10   SELECTING AND ADJUSTING HEARING AIDS 281

11   PROBLEM SOLVING AND FINE-TUNING OF HEARING AIDS 302

12   COUNSELING THE NEW HEARING AID WEARER 322

13   ASSESSING THE OUTCOMES OF HEARING REHABILITATION 349

14   BINAURAL AND BILATERAL CONSIDERATIONS IN HEARING AID FITTING 370

15   SPECIAL HEARING AID ISSUES FOR CHILDREN 404

16   CROS, BONE-CONDUCTION, AND IMPLANTED HEARING AIDS 434

REFERENCES 451

INDEX 487

DETAILED CONTENTS

PREFACE xv

1   **INTRODUCTORY CONCEPTS** 1
    1.1   **Problems Faced by People with Hearing Impairment** 2
        1.1.1   Decreased audibility 2
        1.1.2   Decreased dynamic range 3
        1.1.3   Decreased frequency resolution 4
        1.1.4   Decreased temporal resolution 5
        1.1.5   Deficits in combination 6
    1.2   **Acoustic Measurements** 6
        1.2.1   Basic physical measures 6
        1.2.2   Linear amplifiers and gain 7
        1.2.3   Saturation sound pressure level 9
        1.2.4   Couplers and real ears 9
    1.3   **Types of Hearing Aids** 10
    1.4   **Historical Perspective** 12
        1.4.1   The acoustic era 13
        1.4.2   The carbon era 13
        1.4.3   The vacuum tube era 14
        1.4.4   The transistor and integrated circuit era 15
        1.4.5   The digital era 16

2   **HEARING AID COMPONENTS** 18
    2.1   **Block Diagrams** 19
    2.2   **Microphones** 21
        2.2.1   Principle of operation 21
        2.2.2   Frequency response of microphones 22
        2.2.3   Microphone imperfections 23
        2.2.4   Directional microphones 25
        2.2.5   Microphone location 28
    2.3   **Amplifiers** 28
        2.3.1   Amplifier technology 29
        2.3.2   Amplifier performance 29
        2.3.3   Peak clipping and distortion 30
        2.3.4   Output amplifiers 31
        2.3.5   Compression amplifiers 33
    2.4   **Digital Circuits** 34
        2.4.1   Analog-to-digital converters 34
        2.4.2   Digital signal processors 36
        2.4.3   Digital-to-analog converters 36
    2.5   **Tone Controls and Filters** 36
        2.5.1   Filter and tone control structures 37

	2.5.2	Passive, active, and digital tone controls	38
2.6		**Receivers**	**39**
	2.6.1	Principle of operation	39
	2.6.2	Frequency response of receivers	39
2.7		**Acoustic Dampers**	**41**
2.8		**Telecoils**	**42**
2.9		**Audio (Electrical) Input**	**42**
2.10		**Remote Controls**	**43**
2.11		**Bone Conductors**	**44**
2.12		**Batteries**	**45**
	2.12.1	Principle of operation	45
	2.12.2	Operating voltage	45
	2.12.3	Capacity and physical size	46
2.13		**Concluding Comments**	**47**
3		**HEARING AID SYSTEMS**	**48**
3.1		**Custom and Modular Construction**	**48**
	3.1.1	Custom hearing aids	49
	3.1.2	Modular hearing aids	49
	3.1.3	Semi-modular, semi-custom hearing aids	50
3.2		**Analog Hearing Aids**	**50**
3.3		**Digitally Programmable Analog Hearing Aid Systems**	**51**
	3.3.1	Programmers, interfaces, and software	52
	3.3.2	Multi-memory programmable hearing aids	53
	3.3.3	Paired comparisons	53
3.4		**Digital Hearing Aids**	**53**
	3.4.1	Digital hard-wired hearing aids	54
	3.4.2	Digital general arithmetic processor hearing aids	54
	3.4.3	Sequential processing versus block processing	55
	3.4.4	Specifications for digital hearing aids	56
	3.4.5	Advantages of digital hearing aids	58
3.5		**Remote Sensing and Transmitting Hearing Aid Systems**	**58**
3.6		**Induction Loops**	**59**
	3.6.1	Field uniformity and direction	59
	3.6.2	Magnetic field strength	61
	3.6.3	Loop frequency response	61
3.7		**Radio-frequency Transmission**	**64**
	3.7.1	Principles and FM capture effect	64
	3.7.2	Coupling to the hearing aid	66
	3.7.3	Combined FM and local microphones	68
3.8		**Infrared Transmission**	**69**
3.9		**Classroom Sound-field Amplification**	**69**
3.10		**Strengths and Weaknesses of Remote Transmission Systems**	**70**
3.11		**Assistive Listening Devices**	**72**
3.12		**Concluding remarks**	**73**

4   ELECTROACOUSTIC PERFORMANCE AND MEASUREMENT 74

4.1   Measuring Hearing Aids in Couplers and Ear Simulators 75

4.1.1   Couplers and ear simulators 75

4.1.2   Test boxes 79

4.1.3   Measurement signals 80

4.1.4   Gain-frequency response and OSPL90-frequency response 82

4.1.5   Input-output functions 84

4.1.6   Distortion 85

4.1.7   Internal noise 87

4.1.8   Magnetic response 88

4.1.9   ANSI and IEC standards 89

4.2   Real-Ear Aided Gain (REAG) 89

4.2.1   Positioning the probe for REAG measurement 91

4.2.2   Relationship between REAG, coupler gain and ear simulator gain 93

4.2.3   Detecting incorrect aided measurements 95

4.3   Insertion Gain 96

4.3.1   Positioning the probe for insertion gain measurement 98

4.3.2   Relationship between insertion gain, coupler gain and ear simulator gain ... 99

4.3.3   Control microphones and insertion gain 100

4.3.4   Detecting incorrect insertion gain measurements 101

4.3.5   Accuracy of insertion gain measurements 101

4.4   Practical issues in real-ear testing 101

4.4.1   Probe calibration 101

4.4.2   Effects of wax 102

4.4.3   Contamination by background noise 102

4.4.4   Hearing aid saturation 103

4.4.5   Loudspeaker orientation 104

4.4.6   Measurement signal characteristics 105

4.5   Aided Threshold Testing and Functional Gain 106

4.6   Feedback in Hearing Aids 107

4.6.1   The feedback mechanism 107

4.6.2   Effects of feedback on sound quality 109

4.6.3   Probe-tube measurements and feedback 110

4.7   Troubleshooting Faulty Hearing Aids 111

4.8   Concluding Comments 113

5   HEARING AID EARMOLDS, EARSHELLS AND COUPLING
**   SYSTEMS 117**

5.1   Earmold and earshell physical styles 120

5.1.1   BTE earmold styles 120

5.1.2   ITE, ITC, and CIC earshell styles 122

5.2   Overview of Earmold and Earshell Acoustics 123

5.3   Venting 123

5.3.1   Effects of vents on hearing aid gain and OSPL90 126

5.3.2   Venting and the occlusion effect 130

5.3.3   Effects of vents and leaks on feedback oscillation 134

5.3.4   Parallel versus Y (or diagonal) vents 136

5.4   The Sound Bore: Tubing, Horns and Constriction **137**
  5.4.1   Acoustic horns and constrictions 137
  5.4.2   Special-purpose earhooks 142
5.5   Dampers **143**
5.6   Specific Tubing, Damping and Venting Configurations **144**
5.7   Procedure for Selecting Earmold and Earshell Acoustics **144**
5.8   Ear Impressions **146**
  5.8.1   Standard ear impression techniques 146
  5.8.2   Ear impression techniques for CICs and high gain hearing aids 149
  5.8.3   Ear impression materials 151
5.9   Earmolds and Earshells **152**
  5.9.1   Earmold and earshell construction 152
  5.9.2   Materials for earmolds and earshells 152
  5.9.3   Instant earmolds and hearing aids 155
  5.9.4   Modifying and repairing earmolds and earshells 155
5.10   Concluding Comments **157**

6   COMPRESSION SYSTEMS IN HEARING AIDS **159**
6.1   Compression's Major Role: Reducing the Signal's Dynamic Range **160**
6.2   Basic characteristics of a compressor **161**
  6.2.1   Dynamic compression characteristics: attack and release times 161
  6.2.2   Static compression characteristics 164
  6.2.3   Input and output control 167
  6.2.4   Multichannel compression 169
6.3   Rationales for Use of Compression **169**
  6.3.1   Avoiding discomfort, distortion and damage 169
  6.3.2   Reducing inter-syllabic and inter-phonemic intensity differences 170
  6.3.3   Reducing differences in long-term level 172
  6.3.4   Increasing sound comfort 173
  6.3.5   Normalizing loudness 175
  6.3.6   Maximizing intelligibility 177
  6.3.7   Reducing noise 177
  6.3.8   Empirical approaches 180
6.4   Combinations of Compressors in Hearing Aids **180**
6.5   Benefits and Disadvantages of Different Compression Systems **181**
  6.5.1   Compression relative to linear amplification 182
  6.5.2   Benefits of multichannel relative to single-channel compression 184
6.6   Concluding Comments **186**

7   ADVANCED SIGNAL PROCESSING SCHEMES **187**
7.1   Multi-Microphone and Other Directional Hearing Aids **188**
  7.1.1   Fixed directional arrays 188
  7.1.2   Adaptive arrays 191
7.2   Single-Microphone Noise Reduction **195**
7.3   Feedback Reduction **198**
  7.3.1   Feedback reduction by gain-frequency response control 198
  7.3.2   Feedback reduction by phase control 200
  7.3.3   Feedback reduction by feedback path cancellation 201

7.3.4   Feedback reduction by frequency shifting 202
7.4   Frequency Transposition **202**
7.5   Speech Cue Enhancement **204**
7.6   Concluding Comments **207**

8   ASSESSING CANDIDACY FOR HEARING AIDS **209**
8.1   The Lower Limit of Aidable Hearing Loss **211**
8.1.1   Pure tone loss and audiogram configuration 213
8.1.2   Speech identification ability 215
8.1.3   Self reported disability and handicap 215
8.1.4   Listening environment, needs and expectations 216
8.1.5   Cosmetic concerns 219
8.1.6   Manipulation and management 220
8.1.7   Age 220
8.1.8   Personality 221
8.1.9   Central auditory processing disorder 221
8.1.10   Tinnitus 222
8.1.11   Factors in combination 222
8.1.12   Counseling the unwilling patient: some examples 223
8.2   The Upper Limit of Aidable Hearing Loss **226**
8.2.1   Poor speech identification ability 227
8.2.2   Hearing aids or cochlear implants? 228
8.2.3   Hearing aids or tactile aids? 232
8.3   Medically Related Contra-indications to Hearing Aid Fitting **233**
8.4   Concluding Comments **233**

9   PRESCRIBING HEARING AID PERFORMANCE **234**
9.1   General Concepts Behind Prescription and a Brief History **235**
9.2   Gain and Frequency Response Prescription for Linear Amplification **239**
9.2.1   POGO 239
9.2.2   NAL 239
9.2.3   DSL 242
9.2.4   Examples and comparisons: POGO II, NAL-RP and DSL 243
9.3   Gain, Frequency Response, and Input-Output Functions for Nonlinear
Amplification **249**
9.3.1   LGOB 249
9.3.2   IHAFF/Contour 250
9.3.3   Madsen Aurical method 251
9.3.4   ScalAdapt 252
9.3.5   FIG6 253
9.3.6   DSL[i/o] 254
9.3.7   NAL-NL1 255
9.3.8   Comparison of procedures 256
9.3.9   Prescribing compression thresholds 260
9.4   Allowing for Conductive and Mixed Hearing Losses **262**
9.5   Selecting Options for Multi-memory Hearing Aids **264**
9.5.1   Response alternatives for different environments and listening criteria 265
9.5.2   Candidates for multi-memory hearing aids 266

9.6   Prescribing OSPL90 ....**267**
   9.6.1   General principles: avoiding discomfort, damage and distortion 268
   9.6.2   Type of limiting: compression or peak clipping 268
   9.6.3   OSPL90 prescription 270
   9.6.4   Prescribing OSPL90 at different frequencies 272
   9.6.5   OSPL90 for nonlinear hearing aids 275
   9.6.6   OSPL90 for conductive and mixed losses 275
9.7   Excessive Amplification and Subsequent Hearing Loss **276**
9.8   Concluding Comments **278**

10   SELECTING AND ADJUSTING HEARING AIDS **281**
  **10.1   Selecting Hearing Aid Style: CIC, ITC, ITE, BTE, Spectacle Aid, or Body
        Aid** **282**
  10.2   Selecting Hearing Aid Features **284**
   10.2.1   Volume control 285
   10.2.2   Telecoil 285
   10.2.3   Direct audio input 285
   10.2.4   Directional microphones 286
  10.3   Selecting a Signal Processing Scheme and Prescription Method **286**
   10.3.1   Selecting a signal processing scheme 287
   10.3.2   Choosing a prescription procedure 288
  10.4   Overview of Hearing Aid Selection and Adjustment **289**
  10.5   Twelve Steps for Selecting and Adjusting Programmable Hearing Aids ...**290**
  10.6   Eleven Steps for Selecting and Adjusting Non-programmable Aids **293**
  10.7   Allowing for Individual Ear Size and Shape in the Coupler Prescription .**297**
  10.8   Allowing for Surgically Altered Ear Canals **300**
  10.9   Verifying and Achieving the Prescribed Real-ear Response **300**
  10.10 Verifying and Fine-tuning OSPL90 ....**300**
  10.11 Concluding Comments **301**

11   PROBLEM SOLVING AND FINE-TUNING OF HEARING AIDS **302**
  11.1   Solving Common Problems **303**
   11.1.1   Management difficulties 303
   11.1.2   Earmold or earshell discomfort 304
   11.1.3   Poor earmold or earshell retention 305
   11.1.4   Own voice quality and occlusion 305
   11.1.5   Feedback oscillation 307
   11.1.6   Tonal quality 308
   11.1.7   Noise, clarity, and loudness 308
  11.2   Systematic Fine-tuning Procedures **312**
   11.2.1   Paired comparisons 312
   11.2.2   Absolute rating of sound quality 314
   11.2.3   Systematic selection by paired comparisons 314
   11.2.4   Adaptive parameter adjustment by paired comparisons 316
   11.2.5   Adaptive fine-tuning by absolute rating of quality 318
   11.2.6   Fine-tuning at home with multi-memory hearing aids 320
  11.3   Concluding Comments: Fine-tuning in Perspective **320**

12   COUNSELING THE NEW HEARING AID WEARER 322

   12.1   Understanding Hearing Loss 323

   12.2   Acquiring a Hearing Aid 325

   12.3   Using Hearing Aids 327

   12.4   Adjusting to New Experiences with Sound and Hearing Aids 327

   12.5   Care of Hearing Aids 331

   12.6   Hearing Strategies 332

      12.6.1   Observing the talker and surroundings 332

      12.6.2   Manipulating social interactions 333

      12.6.3   Manipulating the environment 335

      12.6.4   Teaching hearing strategies 337

   12.7   Involving Families and Friends. 337

   12.8   Communication Training 338

   12.9   Avoiding Hearing Aid-Induced Hearing Loss 339

   12.10   Assistive Listening Devices 340

   12.11   Ongoing Support 340

   12.12   Counseling Styles 340

   12.13   Structuring Appointments 342

      12.13.1 The assessment appointment(s) 342

      12.13.2 The fitting appointment(s) 343

      12.13.3 The follow-up appointment(s) 343

      12.13.4 The power of groups 344

   12.14   Concluding Comments 347

13   ASSESSING THE OUTCOMES OF HEARING REHABILITATION 349

   13.1   Speech Identification Testing 351

      13.1.1   Limitations of speech tests to assess benefits 351

      13.1.2   Role of speech testing in evaluating benefit 352

   13.2   Self-report Questionnaires for Assessing Benefit 353

      13.2.1   Questionnaire methodology 353

      13.2.2   Practical self-report measures 356

   13.3   Meeting Needs and Goals 359

   13.4   Assessing Usage, Problems, and Satisfaction 363

   13.5   Changes in Outcomes with Time after Fitting 366

   13.6   Impact of Hearing Aids on General Health and Quality of Life ... 368

   13.7   Concluding Comments 369

14   BINAURAL AND BILATERAL CONSIDERATIONS IN HEARING AID
      FITTING 370

   14.1   Binaural Effects in Localization 372

      14.1.1   Localization cues in normal hearing 372

      14.1.2   Effects of hearing loss on localization 374

   14.2   Binaural Effects in Detection and Recognition 376

      14.2.1   Head diffraction effects 376

      14.2.2   Binaural squelch in noise 377

      14.2.3   Binaural redundancy 379

      14.2.4   Binaural loudness summation 380

   14.3   Advantages of Bilateral Fittings 380

14.3.1 Speech intelligibility 380
14.3.2 Sound quality 383
14.3.3 Avoiding late-onset auditory deprivation. 383
14.3.4 Localization 385
14.3.5 Suppression of tinnitus 387
14.3.6 Miscellaneous advantages 387
14.4 Disadvantages of Bilateral Fittings **388**
14.4.1 Cost 388
14.4.2 Binaural interference 388
14.4.3 Self-image 389
14.4.4 Miscellaneous disadvantages 389
14.5 Tests of Bilateral Advantage **390**
14.5.1 Bias in choosing the reference ear for the unilateral condition 390
14.5.2 The sensitivity of speech tests for assessing bilateral advantage 391
14.5.3 Role for speech tests in assessing bilateral advantage 392
14.5.4 Localization tests 394
14.6 Fitting Asymmetrical Hearing Losses **395**
14.6.1 Bilateral versus unilateral fittings for asymmetrical losses 395
14.6.2 Better ear versus poorer ear for unilateral fittings 396
14.6.3 Alternatives: FM and CROS 399
14.7 Deciding on Bilateral versus Unilateral Fittings **399**
14.8 Effect of Bilateral vs Unilateral Fitting on Electroacoustic Prescriptions . **402**
14.9 Concluding Comments **403**

15 SPECIAL HEARING AID ISSUES FOR CHILDREN **404**
15.1 Sensory Experience and Deprivation **405**
15.2 Assessment of Hearing Loss **406**
15.2.1 Frequency-specific and ear-specific assessment 406
15.2.2 Small ears and calibration issues 407
15.3 Hearing Aid and Earmold Features and Styles **408**
15.3.1 Hearing aids 409
15.3.2 Earmolds 410
15.3.3 FM wireless transmission systems 411
15.4 Prescribing Amplification for Children **412**
15.4.1 Speech identification ability and amplification requirements 412
15.4.2 Threshold-based versus loudness-based procedures 415
15.4.3 Allowing for small ear canals 416
15.5 Verifying Real-ear Performance **419**
15.6 Evaluating Aided Performance **419**
15.7 Helping Parents **425**
15.8 Hearing Habilitation Goals **428**
15.8.1 Goals and strategies for infants 429
15.8.2 Goals and strategies for toddlers 430
15.8.3 Goals and strategies for pre-schoolers 430
15.8.4 Goals and strategies for primary school children 430
15.9 Teenagers and Cosmetic Concerns **431**
15.10 Safety Issues **431**
15.11 Concluding Comments **433**

16   CROS, BONE-CONDUCTION, AND IMPLANTED HEARING AIDS 434

16.1   CROS Hearing Aids **434**

16.1.1   Simple CROS aids. 435

16.1.2   Bilateral CROS (BICROS) aids 439

16.1.3   Stereo CROS (CRIS-CROS) aids 440

16.1.4   Transcranial CROS aids 441

16.2   Bone-conduction Hearing Aids **442**

16.2.1   Applications of bone-conduction hearing aids 442

16.2.2   Bone-conduction hearing aid output capabilities 442

16.2.3   Prescribing electroacoustic characteristics for bone-conduction aids 444

16.2.4   Disadvantages of bone-conduction hearing aids 447

16.3   Implanted and Semi-implanted Hearing Aids **447**

16.3.1   Bone-anchored hearing aids 447

16.3.2   Middle-ear implants 449

16.4   Concluding Comments **450**

REFERENCES **451**

INDEX **487**

PREFACE

This book came into existence because there did not seem to be any single book that would be adequate as a text for courses on hearing aids or that could advise practicing clinicians on all aspects of hearing aids.

I have aimed to make the book both practically useful and theoretically sound. Issues are explained rather then described. Wherever possible, practical recommendations are based on empirical research, and where there is no research to draw upon, the tentative nature of the recommendation or conclusion is indicated. Readers who already know the field well will notice that the book contains some data and clinical procedures that are published for the first time, as well as hopefully some new insights and perspectives into older issues.

The book is designed to be read on a number of levels. For readers who need only an overview of a topic, the synopsis at the beginning of each chapter should suffice. Most readers will hopefully be enticed to read further; the essential information on each topic is marked with a shaded bar in the margin. These marked paragraphs are designed to be read, and to be understandable, without the intervening paragraphs. I think of the marked material as a thin book buried inside this thick book. Some academic courses may wish to restrict themselves to just this material, which includes approximately half the book. The remaining material provides a greater level of detail. Finally, the most detailed comments are tucked away as footnotes and as sections in small print. The material at all levels is further segmented by presenting the most theoretical material and the most practical material in the form of self-contained panels. These two types of panels are differentiated by their appearance and by the panel titles.

One of the difficult balancing acts was the extent to which I mention clinical tools developed by the research team at NAL. The major aim of the team is to produce scientifically defensible but practical tools that are useful to clinicians. I have tried to be objective about the advantages and limitations of procedures, no matter where they originated, and I hope the peer reviews that each chapter has been through will have over-ridden my biases.

Another difficulty was deciding what to call a person with a hearing impairment who is seeking help to overcome the difficulties caused by his or her hearing loss. Possible terms are *patient*, *client*, *consumer*, or even *customer*. Each of these terms seems to offend someone. At different parts of the encounter, different terms seem most appropriate. The person could be a patient when his or her hearing is being assessed, a consumer when he or she is deciding whether to buy an advanced (and expensive) hearing aid or a more basic one, and a client as he or she works through communication problems with the advice and guidance of the clinician. From the perspective of hearing impaired people, what the clinician says and does to help people is important, as is the attitude of the clinician towards people. The term used to describe them is much less important and probably only becomes important if it affects the attitude of the clinician. This book takes an extremely client-centered (or patient-centered!) approach to rehabilitation. In keeping with the most common usage, and in keeping with a recent survey of what most people attending a hospital outpatient hearing clinic expect to be called (Nair, 1998) (admittedly a biased sample), I have adopted the term "patient" throughout this book. Feel free to mentally replace it with your preferred term if you wish.

A big advantage of a single-authored book is that the material can be well integrated, so that new knowledge builds systematically upon old and the topic of hearing aids can be comprehensively covered. The big disadvantage is that no single author knows everything. I have been helped enormously by an army of colleagues around the world who have graciously given their time to review a section, a chapter, or more and to share their great expertise. Each section of the book has been critically reviewed by several people, mostly leading experts in that field. To all of the following I give my great thanks for their help and generosity in reviewing and/or providing information: Henning Anderson, Torburg Arvidsson, Herbie Baechler, Chris Barker, Lucille Beck, Greg Birtles, Arthur Boothroyd, Eric Burwood, Klaus-Dieter Butsch, Denis Byrne, Denis Carpenter, Teresa Ching, Laurel Christenson, Bob Cowan, Robyn Cox, Don Dirks, Richard Dowell, Wouter Dreschler, Claus Elberling, Todd Fortune, Stuart Gatehouse, Stan Gelfand, Gail Gudmundsen, David Hawkins, Louise Hickson, Karolina Smeds, Jeanette Jordt, Gitte Keidser, Juergen Keisling, Mead Killion, Pat Kricos, Dawna Lewis, Roger Lovegrove, Carl Ludvigsen, Phil McAlister, Hugh McDermott, Gus Meuller, Arlene Neuman, Philip Newall, Claus Nielsen, Bill Noble, Jerry Northern, Anna O'Brien, Sharon Page, Chester Pirzanski, Rick Pimentel, Jill Preminger, Suzanne Purdy, Larry Revit, Anders Ringdahl, Mark Ross, Susan Scollie, Richard Seewald, Joseph Smaldino, Greg Smith, Wayne Staab, Pat Stelmachowicz, Dafydd Stephens, Gerry Studebaker, Robert Sweetow, Richard Tyler, Dianne Van Tasell, Hans Verschuure, Barbara Weinstein, Søren Westermann, Sharan Westcott, and Helen Wortham. Readability of some of the material has been reviewed by audiology students at Macquarie University and the University of Iowa in the class of Ruth Bentler, and I would particularly like to thank them for their careful comments. Thanks also to Jean Banning for the painstaking layout and typesetting. Any faults in the final product are, of course, mine alone, and I would appreciate learning of them as soon as possible. Comments can be sent to: publisher@BoomerangPress.com.au.

Thanks are also due to my to employer (Australian Hearing, the National Acoustic Laboratories, and the Cooperative Research Centre for Cochlear Implant and Hearing Aid Innovations) and my work colleagues. For over twenty years I have been in an organization dedicated to effective habilitation and rehabilitation of people with hearing impairment using clinical methods founded on research-based evidence. Much of my knowledge and beliefs have been shaped by the talented people that have educated and inspired me concerning both research and practical clinical issues. Foremost among these people are the late Denis Byrne; there are many others.

Finally, and most importantly, I would like to thank my wife, Fiona Macaskill, without whom this book would never have come into existence. Fiona has kept our family intact and provided constant encouragement during the three years that my work on this book intruded most unreasonably into family life. Fiona's great clinical expertise has also provided me with many audiological insights that I would never have otherwise gained, and I hope that I have adequately reflected them in this book.

To Fiona, Louisa and Nicholas, for their patience and understanding.

In memory of Denis Byrne, his teaching, his wisdom and his example.

CHAPTER ONE

INTRODUCTORY CONCEPTS

Synopsis

Hearing aids partially overcome the deficits associated with a hearing loss. For a sensori-neural hearing loss, there are several deficits to be overcome. Some sounds are inaudible. Other sounds can be detected because part of their spectra is audible, but may not be correctly identified because other parts of their spectra (typically the high-frequency parts) remain inaudible. The range of levels between the weakest sound that can be heard and the most intense sound that can be tolerated is less for a person with sensorineural hearing loss than for a normal-hearing person. To compensate for this, a hearing aid has to amplify weak sounds more than it amplifies intense sounds. In addition, sensorineural impairment diminishes the ability of a person to detect and analyze energy at one frequency in the presence of energy at other frequencies. Similarly, a hearing-impaired person has decreased ability to hear a signal that rapidly follows, or is rapidly followed by, a different signal. This decreased frequency resolution and temporal resolution makes it more likely that noise will mask speech than would be the case for a normal-hearing person.

Taken together, all these auditory deficits mean that a person with a sensorineural hearing impairment needs a signal-to-noise ratio greater than normal in order to communicate effec-tively, even when sounds have been amplified by a hearing aid. By contrast, a conductive impairment simply attenuates sounds as they pass through the middle ear.

To understand how hearing aids work, the physical characteristics of signals must be under-stood. These characteristics include the rate at which sound fluctuates (frequency), the time taken for a repetitive fluctuation to repeat (period), the distance over which its waveform repeats (wavelength), the way sound bends around obstacles (diffraction), the strength of a sound wave (pressure and sound pressure level), the break-up of a complex sound into pure tone components at different frequencies (spectrum), or into several frequency bands (octave, one-third octave, or critical bands), and the degree to which a body of air vibrates when it is exposed to vibrating sound pressure (velocity and impedance).

The amplifiers inside hearing aids can be classified as linear or nonlinear. For sounds of a given frequency, linear amplifiers amplify by the same amount no matter what the level of the signal is, or what other sounds are simultaneously present. The degree of amplification can be represented as a graph of gain versus frequency (gain-frequency response), or as a graph of output level versus input level (I-O curve). The highest level produced by a hearing aid is known as the saturation sound pressure level (SSPL). The sound output by a hearing aid can be measured in the ear canal of an individual patient, or in a small coupler or ear simulator that has a volume similar to that of a real ear.

Hearing aids are described according to where they are worn. In order of decreasing size these categories are: body, spectacle, behind-the-ear, in-the-ear, in-the-canal and completely-in-the-canal.

Decreasing size has been a constant trend during the history of the development of the hearing aid. This history can be divided into five eras: acoustic, carbon, vacuum, transistor and digital. The last of these eras, which we are just entering, promises to hold advances at least as signifi-cant as the eras that preceded it.

Hearing aids are designed and fitted to lessen the problems faced by hearing-impaired people. To better appreciate what hearing aids can and cannot do, we will briefly review the ways in which hearing abilities deteriorate when hearing loss occurs.

1.1 Problems Faced by People with Hearing Impairment

Hearing loss involves a multifaceted loss of hearing ability. Except where noted, the following descriptions apply to the most common form of hearing loss, a *sensori-neural hearing loss*.

1.1.1 Decreased audibility

Hearing-impaired people do not hear some sounds at all. People with a severe or profound hearing loss may not hear any speech sounds, unless they are shouted at close range. People with a mild or moderate loss are more likely to hear some sounds and not others. In particular, the softer phonemes,[a] which are usually consonants, may simply not be heard. For example, the sequence of sounds *i e a ar*, might have originated as *pick the black harp*, but could be heard as *kick the cat hard*. To make sounds audible, hearing aids have to provide amplification, and this they do very well.

Hearing-impaired people also have trouble understanding speech because essential parts of some phonemes are not audible. Sounds are recognized by noting which frequencies contain the most energy. The vowel *oo* for example, is differentiated from the vowel *ee* by the location of the second intense region (the second *formant*), as shown in Figure 1.1. If, for example, a hearing loss caused all frequencies (and therefore all formants) above 700 Hz to be inaudible, as indicated by the shaded region, the two sounds could not be differentiated. Although both sounds could be detected, the similarity of their first formants would make them sound almost identical.

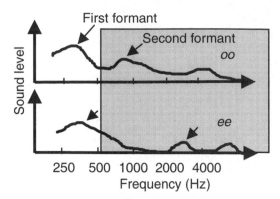

Figure 1.1 Similarity of the two vowels *oo* and *ee* when the second formant is inaudible because of hearing loss (grey area).

The high-frequency components of speech are weaker than the low-frequency components.[123] Furthermore, for approximately 90% of hearing-impaired adults and for 75% of hearing-impaired children, the degree of impairment worsens from 500 Hz to 4 kHz.[563] Most commonly, therefore, hearing-impaired people miss high-frequency information. Because the loudness of speech is dominated by low-frequency components, hearing-impaired people may not realize that they are hearing *less* of the speech signal, even when they cannot understand speech in many circumstances. Statements such as *speech is loud enough, but not clear enough* and *if only people would not mumble* are common.

To help overcome this difficulty, a hearing aid has to provide more amplification for frequencies where speech has the weakest components and where hearing loss is the greatest (i.e. usually the high frequencies). Hearing aids are very good at providing different amounts of gain in different frequency regions, and for many years, hearing aid selection consisted primarily of prescribing and adjusting the amount of gain provided at each frequency. This was achieved by selecting an appropriate model hearing aid and by varying the tone controls.

---

[a]   Phonemes are the basic sounds of speech, such as individual consonants or vowels.

1.1.2   Decreased dynamic range

As implied above, soft sounds can be made audible merely by amplifying them. Unfortunately, it is not appropriate to amplify everything by the amount needed to make soft sounds audible. A sensorineural hearing loss increases the threshold of hearing much more than it increases the threshold of loudness discomfort.[836] In fact, for mild and some moderate hearing losses, there is likely to be very little increase in loudness discomfort level, even though the threshold of hearing has increased by up to 50 dB.[431] Consequently, the *dynamic range* of an ear (i.e. the level difference between discomfort and the threshold of audibility) with a sensorineural impairment will be less than that of a normally hearing ear.

This problem of decreased dynamic range is shown pictorially in Figure 1.2. For normal-hearing Norm (a), a wide range of sounds in the environment can fit between Norm's threshold of hearing and the loudest level he can comfortably tolerate. For Sam, the range of sound levels in the environment exceeds his dynamic range from threshold to discomfort. Part (b) shows what happens without amplification: weak to moderate sounds are not heard. Part (c) shows what happens when there is enough amplification to make the weak sounds audible: the medium to intense sounds now become excessively loud. If the sounds in the environment are to fit within Sam's dynamic range, a hearing aid must give more amplification to weak sounds than it does to intense sounds. This squashing of a

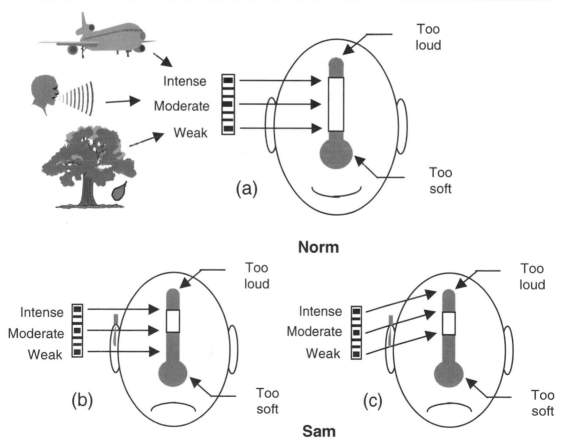

Figure 1.2 The relationship between the dynamic range of sounds in the environment and the dynamic range of hearing for: (a) normal hearing, (b) sensorineural hearing loss without amplification, and (c) sensorineural hearing loss with a constant amount of amplification for all input levels.

large dynamic range of levels in the environment into a smaller range of levels at the output of the hearing aid is called ***compression***. In essence, a compressor is nothing more than an amplifier that automatically turns itself down as the sound gets stronger.

Hearing aids are very good at reducing the dynamic range of the signal and compression can be applied to this task in a number of ways. As we shall see in Chapters 6 and 9, we are not yet certain of the best way to decrease dynamic range, but on the bright side, we have several good alternatives from which to choose.

1.1.3   Decreased frequency resolution

Another difficulty faced by people with sensorineural hearing loss is separating sounds of different frequencies. Different frequencies are represented most strongly at different places within the cochlea. In an unimpaired cochlea, a narrow band sound produces a clearly defined region of relatively strong vibration at one position on the basilar membrane. In turn, this produces a clearly defined region of activity within the auditory cortex. For a complex speech sound, concentrations of energy around a particular frequency also produce narrow, clearly defined regions of activity within the cochlea.

If a background noise contains some energy at a nearby frequency, the normal-hearing ear can do a good job of sending separate signals to the brain, one signal for each region of intense activity in the cochlea. The brain can then consider all the spectral information it is getting, as well as visual information (e.g. from lip-reading), information about the direction of arrival of the sounds (by comparing the sounds received by each ear), and information about the context of the message (especially if it is speech). Armed with all this information, the brain can then partly ignore the activity originated by the noise,

and decode the activity represented by the speech. That is, the ear has ***frequency resolution*** or ***frequency selectivity*** sufficiently precise to enable the brain to separate speech from noise, provided the speech component and the noise are sufficiently separated in frequency, given their relative levels.[b]

A person with sensorineural hearing loss has decreased frequency resolution. This occurs because the outer hair cells lose their ability to increase the sensitivity of the cochlea for frequencies to which the affected part of the cochlea is tuned. Psychoacoustically, this shows up as flatter ***masking curves*** and ***tuning curves***.[976] The significance of this is that even when a speech component and a noise component have different frequencies, if these frequencies are close enough, the cochlea will have a single broad region of activity rather than two finely tuned separate regions. Consequently, the brain is unable to untangle the signal from the noise.

The situation is represented pictorially in Figure 1.3. For the sound spectrum shown in (a), a normal-hearing cochlea would send a message to the brain that two separate bundles of energy existed in the region around 1000 Hz. One of these bundles may have

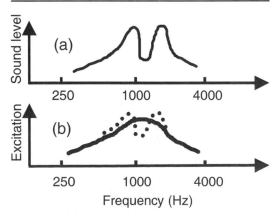

Figure 1.3 (a) Sound spectrum, and (b) representation in the auditory system for normal hearing (dotted line) and sensorineural hearing impairment (solid line).

---

[b]   As a minimum requirement, to be separately processed, the two frequencies have to be further apart than one critical band.

originated from a talker that the listener was trying to understand, while the other may have originated from some interfering sound. The impaired cochlea, by contrast, may send a message to the brain that there is just a broad concentration of energy around 1000 Hz. Consequently, the brain has no chance of being able to separate the signal from the noise.

There does not even need to be any noise for decreased frequency resolution to adversely affect speech understanding. If frequency resolution is sufficiently decreased, relatively intense low-frequency parts of speech (e.g. the first formant in voiced speech sounds) may mask the weaker higher frequency components (e.g. the second and higher formants, and high-frequency frication noise from the vocal tract). This is referred to as ***upward spread of masking***[195, 579] and is evident in the neural responses of cats with noise-induced hearing losses.[775] The potential to affect intelligibility is certainly present and the likelihood of it happening increases with the degree of loss. An appropriately prescribed hearing aid will minimize the amount of upward (and downward) spread of masking by making sure that there is no frequency region in which speech is much louder than for the remaining regions.

There is a second reason why decreased frequency resolution is a problem. Even normal-hearing people have poorer resolution at high intensity levels than at lower levels. Hearing-impaired people, especially those with severe and profound loss, have to listen at high levels if they are to achieve sufficient audibility. Consequently, their difficulty in separating sounds is partly caused by their damaged cochlea and partly caused by their need to listen at elevated levels.[247]

The extent to which inadequate frequency resolution affects speech understanding is still being debated. It is clear that frequency resolution gradually decreases as the amount of hearing loss increases. It seems highly probable that, for mild and some moderate hearing losses, decreased speech intelligibility is mostly caused by decreased audibility (i.e. some parts of speech lying below threshold). For people with severe and profound loss, and for some people with moderate loss, decreased frequency resolution is also likely to play a significant role.[325] Certainly it is true that speech intelligibility for such people is poorer than can be explained on the basis of decreased audibility alone.[147]

Once speech and noise in the same frequency region get mixed together inside the electronics of a hearing aid, there is as yet no way the hearing aid can separate these to enhance intelligibility. All hearing aids can do to minimize the problems caused by decreased frequency resolution is to:

- keep noise out of the hearing aid by picking up a signal remotely and transmitting it to the hearing aid (see Sections 3.5 to 3.9);

- use a directional microphone to emphasize wanted sounds coming from one direction and partially suppress unwanted sounds coming from other directions (see Section 2.2.4); and

- provide an appropriate variation of gain with frequency so that the low-frequency parts of speech or noise do not mask the high-frequency parts of speech (see Sections 9.2 and 9.3).

1.1.4   Decreased temporal resolution

Intense sounds can mask weaker sounds that immediately precede them or immediately follow them. This happens to a greater extent for people with sensorineural hearing impairment than for people with normal hearing.[196, 977] This adversely affects speech intelligibility.[325] Many real-life background noises fluctuate rapidly, and normal-hearing people extract useful snippets of information during the weaker moments of the background noise. Hearing-impaired people partially lose this ability to hear during the gaps in a masking noise, particularly if they are elderly.[249, 410, 699] The ability to hear weak sounds during brief gaps in a more intense masker gradually decreases as hearing loss gets worse.[147]

Hearing aids can help a little in compensating for decreased temporal resolution ability. Fast-acting compression, where the gain is rapidly increased during weak sounds and rapidly decreased during intense sounds, will make the weaker sounds more audible in the presence of preceding stronger sounds, and so will make them *slightly* more intelligible.[621] Unfortunately, it will make unwanted weak background noises more audible.

1.1.5   Deficits in combination

Each of the above aspects of a hearing loss (decreased audibility, dynamic range, frequency resolution and temporal resolution) can cause a reduction in intelligibility. In combination, they can cause a hearing-impaired person to understand much less than a normal-hearing person in the same situation, even when the hearing-impaired person is wearing a hearing aid. Looked at another way, the hearing-impaired person needs a better *signal-to-noise ratio* (*SNR*) than does a normal-hearing person, if both people are to understand the same amount of speech.[719]

On average, the SNR required for a given level of speech intelligibility increases as the amount of sensorineural hearing loss increases: The average SNR deficit associated with a mild hearing loss is estimated to be about 4 dB, and the average deficit associated with a severe hearing loss is estimated to be about 10 dB.[460] The loss in SNR, compared to normal, will be more marked than this if the noise fluctuates greatly in amplitude, such as occurs for a single competing speaker.[699] Despite these average trends, some individuals require a far higher or lower SNR than others with the same pure-tone hearing loss.

The situation is far simpler with conductive losses. These appear to cause a simple attenu-ation of sound, so that provided the hearing aid can adequately amplify sound, the normal cochlea can resolve sounds entering it just as well as the cochlea of someone with normal hearing.

1.2   Acoustic Measurements

1.2.1   Basic physical measures

The acoustic quantities of frequency, period, wavelength, diffraction, pressure, sound pressure level (SPL), waveform and spectrum must be understood before some parts of this book will make much sense.

Frequency describes how many times per second a sound wave alternates from positive pressure to negative pressure and back to the starting value. Frequency is measured in cycles per second, or, more usually, hertz (Hz) or kilohertz (kHz).

Period is the time taken for a repetitive sound wave to complete one cycle. Period is measured in seconds (s) or milliseconds (ms) and is equal to one divided by the frequency.

Wavelength describes the distance a sound wave travels during one period of the wave. It is measured in meters (m) and is equal to the speed of sound (which in air is 345 m/s) divided by the frequency of the sound. Low-frequency sounds therefore have large wavelengths (several meters) and high-frequency sounds have small wavelengths (a few centimeters).

Diffraction describes the way in which a sound wave is altered by an obstacle. When a sound meets an obstacle, like a head, the size of the wavelength compared to the size of the obstacle determines what happens. Obstacles much larger than a wavelength will cause a sound shadow to occur on the side of the obstacle away from the sound source (i.e. the sound is attenuated). Such obstacles will also cause the sound pressure to increase on the side closest to the source. Sounds with wavelengths much larger than an obstacle will flow smoothly, without attenuation, around the obstacle.

Pressure describes how much force per unit area a sound wave exerts on anything that gets in its way, such as an eardrum. It is measured in Pascals (Pa), mPa or µPa.

Sound pressure level (SPL) is the number of decibels (dB) by which any sound pressure exceeds the arbitrary, but universally agreed reference sound pressure of $2 \cdot 10^{-5}$ Pa. It is equal to 20 times the logarithm of the ratio of the actual sound pressure to the reference sound pressure. When pressure doubles, the SPL increases by 6 dB; when pressure increases ten times, the SPL increases by 20 dB.

rms stands for the root-mean-square value of a signal. It is a way of averaging a fluctuating signal so that a single number can represent its amplitude over a certain time.

Waveform describes how the pressure of a sound wave varies from moment to moment in time. The waveform of a pure tone, for example, is a sinusoid.

Spectrum describes the mixture of pure tones that, when added together, produce a particular complex sound over a specific portion of time. A complete spectrum specifies the amplitude and phase of every pure tone component in the complex sound, but often we are interested in only the amplitude spectrum. When the complex tone is *periodic* (i.e. each cycle looks like the preceding cycle), the pure tone components are called *harmonics.* These harmonics occur at integer multiples of the *fundamental frequency*, which is the frequency at which the complex wave itself repeats. A *Fourier transform* is a mathematical operation that enables the spectrum to be calculated if the waveform is known. Conversely, an inverse Fourier transform enables the waveform to be calculated if the spectrum is known. A spectrum and a waveform are thus two different ways of describing the same sound.

Octave bands and *one-third octave bands* are frequency regions one octave and one-third octave wide respectively. The spectrum of acoustic signals is often analyzed by filtering the signals into adjacent octave or one-third octave bands and measuring the rms level of the components that fall into each of the bands. An *octave* corresponds to a doubling of frequency. The origin of *octave* is that in music the eighth note in the scale has a frequency twice that of the first note in the scale.

Critical bands are frequency regions within which the ear groups together sounds of different frequency.[772] Sounds spaced apart by more than a critical band can be separately recognized by the brain, at least by normal-hearing people. Above 500 Hz, critical bands are a little narrower than a 1/3-octave band, and below 500 Hz they become progressively wider than a 1/3-octave band.

Impedance describes how easily a medium (e.g. air) vibrates when a sound pressure is applied to it. In free air, impedance is equal to the ratio of sound pressure to *particle velocity*, and always has the same value for any particular medium. In tubes, impedance is defined differently, and is equal to the ratio of sound pressure to *volume velocity*. Volume velocity is defined as particle velocity multiplied by the cross sectional area of the tube. Volume velocity can be thought of as the total quantity of sound flowing back and forth through any plane perpendicular to the length of the tube.

1.2.2   Linear amplifiers and gain

The gain of any device relates the amplitude of the signal coming out of the device to the amplitude of the signal going into the device. Gain is calculated as the output amplitude divided by the input amplitude. This applies whether the input and output signals are electrical signals, with their amplitudes measured in volts, or whether they are acoustical signals measured in Pascals. If an input signal of 20 mPa were amplified to become an output signal of 200 mPa, the gain of the hearing aid would be ten times. Expressing gain in this way best reflects what a *linear ampli-*

fier does: it makes everything bigger by multiplying the input signal by a fixed amount. This same amplifier system would multiply an input signal of 1 mPa up to an output signal of 10 mPa.

More commonly, and more conveniently, the input and output amplitudes are expressed as a level in decibels (e.g. dB SPL). Gain is then calculated as the output level minus the input level and is expressed in decibels. In the first example above, the input signal would have a level of 60 dB SPL, the output signal would have a level of 80 dB SPL so the gain would be 20 dB. Over a wide range of input signal levels, this same linear amplifier will always cause the output signal level to be 20 dB greater than the input signal level.

The relationship between input and output SPL of a particular frequency is often shown in an *input-output (I-O)* diagram. Figure 1.4 shows the I-O diagram for a hearing aid that is linear for all input levels up to 85 dB SPL. The linear portions of I-O diagrams are straight lines at an angle of 45°, because any increase in input level results in the same increase in output level.

The behavior of a linear amplifier is not affected by how many signals it is amplifying

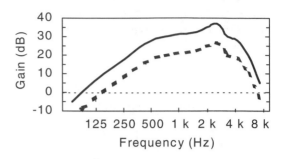

Figure 1.5 Gain-frequency response of an in-the-ear hearing aid at maximum volume control position (solid line) and reduced volume control position (broken line).

at the same time. If signal A is amplified by, say, 30 dB when it is the only signal present at the input, then it will still be amplified by 30 dB even when several other signals are simultaneously being amplified by the device.

The gain of electrical amplifiers often depends on frequency, and the gain of a hearing aid always does. To fully describe the gain of a linear amplifier it is thus necessary to state its gain at every frequency within the frequency range of interest. This is referred to as the *gain-frequency response* of the device, and is usually shown graphically. The solid line in Figure 1.5 shows an example of the gain-frequency response of an in-the-ear hearing aid. This is sometimes just called the *gain curve*.

Sometimes people will say things like *the gain of the hearing aid is 30 dB*. Such a statement is ambiguous and therefore of little value. It may refer to the gain at the frequency at which the gain is the greatest, the gain averaged across some (unspecified) particular frequencies, or the gain at some (unspecified) reference frequency. People will also shorten the term *gain-frequency response* to *frequency response*. This also is ambiguous, but usually what is meant is the manner in which gain varies with frequency, irrespective of what the actual gain is at any frequency. For example, the broken line in Figure 1.5 could be said to have the same

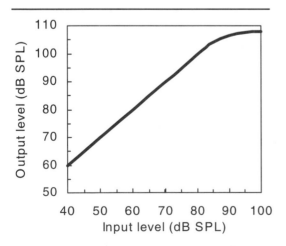

Figure 1.4 Input-output diagram for a hearing aid with 20 dB gain, showing how the output SPL depends on the input SPL, for a particular signal or frequency.

frequency response as the solid curve, because both curves have the same shape, even though they have different gains at every frequency. As a practical issue, the two curves shown in Figure 1.5 could be produced from the same hearing aid just by varying its volume control. For a gain-frequency response to convey useful information, it is important that the measurement conditions, especially the position of the volume control, be stated.

1.2.3   Saturation sound pressure level

All amplifiers become nonlinear when the input or output signals exceed a certain level. This happens because amplifiers are unable to handle signals larger than the voltage of the battery that powers the amplifier. For many reasons it is often desirable to limit the maximum output of the hearing aid to be even less than the limit imposed by the battery voltage and below the limit imposed by the receiver. The highest value of SPL that a hearing aid can produce is called the *saturation sound pressure level* (*SSPL*). As with gain, the SSPL varies with frequency, and a useful measure is the SSPL response curve. Figure 1.6 shows the SSPL response curve of an in-the-ear hearing aid.

Terms closely related to SSPL are *output sound pressure level for a 90 dB SPL input level* (*OSPL90*) and *maximum power output* (*MPO*). The term MPO, although often used, is not an appropriate term, because the quantity being measured is SPL, not power. The term OSPL90 is the most precise term as it states how the maximum output level of the

hearing aid is measured: a signal of 90 dB SPL is input to the hearing aid. This level is chosen as the standard input level because it is nearly always large enough to saturate the hearing aid (unless the volume control is set to a very low level). Devices that amplify in a nonlinear manner are considered in detail in several later chapters.

1.2.4   Couplers and real ears

The discussion of gain and SSPL has referred to the SPL at the output of the hearing aid without saying where or how the SPL is measured. There are two choices. Hearing aids are meant for ears, so the first important place to measure the output of a hearing aid is in the ear canal of a hearing aid wearer. The only practical way to measure this is with a soft, thin *probe-tube* attached to a microphone. Two different types of *real-ear measurement,* performed with such a probe-tube, are discussed in some detail in Sections 4.2 and 4.3.

It is also desirable to be able to measure a hearing aid in a standard way that does not require it to be mounted in a person's ear. It is inconvenient to enlist a human assistant every time a hearing aid has to be checked, and the response measured will vary from person to person. (This variation, due to differences in ear canal geometry and the way the hearing aid is coupled to the ear, is the reason why the hearing aid's performance should be measured in the ear of each individual hearing-impaired person.)

Hearing aids can be measured in a standard way by coupling them to a *coupler*. Couplers are small cavities. The hearing aid connects to one end of the cavity, and the other end of the cavity contains a microphone, which in turn is connected to a sound level meter. The cavity in the most commonly used coupler has a volume of 2 cm^3, so the coupler is called a 2-cc coupler. Couplers, and their more complex cousins, *ear simulators*, are described more fully in Section 4.1.1.

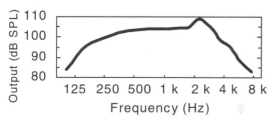

Figure 1.6 Saturated sound pressure level frequency response of an in-the-ear hearing aid.

1.3   Types of Hearing Aids

A hearing aid is basically a miniature public-address system. Its key components are:

- a microphone to convert sound into electricity;

- an amplifier to increase the strength of the electrical signal; in the process it will also alter the balance of the sound, usually giving more emphasis to high-frequency sounds and weak sounds than it does to low-frequency sounds and intense sounds;

- a miniature loudspeaker, called a receiver,[c] to turn electricity back into sound;

- a means of coupling the amplified sound into the ear canal; and

- a battery to provide the power needed by the amplifier.

Microphones and receivers are jointly referred to as *transducers* because they convert one form of energy into another.

Hearing aids can be categorized in many ways. The simplest way to categorize them is by the place in which they are worn, which also implies what the size of the hearing aid must be. The largest type of hearing aid is the *body aid*. These aids are typically about 60 x 40 x 15 mm (very approximately 2 x 2 x 0.5 inches). As implied by their name, they are worn somewhere on the body: in a pocket, in a pouch around the neck, or on the belt. They are connected, via a cable containing two or three wires, to a receiver, from which the amplified sound emerges. The receiver usually plugs into an earmold custom-made for the individual's ear canal and concha.

The next smallest type of hearing aid is the *behind-the-ear (BTE)* hearing aid. These are also two-piece hearing aids. The microphone, electronics, and receiver are mounted in the characteristic banana-shaped case, and the

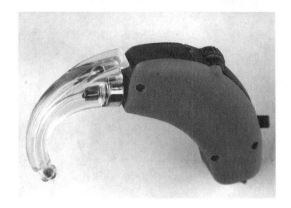

Figure 1.7 A BTE hearing aid.

sound is conveyed acoustically via a tube to a custom earmold. A BTE aid is shown in Figure 1.7.

The next smallest type is the *in-the-ear (ITE)* hearing aid. These vary in size from full concha styles that, as their name implies, fill the entire concha as well as about half the length of the ear canal. A smaller variation of the ITE hearing aid is the *half-concha* or *half-shell* ITE, which fills only the lower half of the concha (the cavum) up to the crus-helias. Another smaller variation is the *low-profile* ITE, which does not extend outwards from the ear canal sufficiently to fill the concha. The various features of the ear are defined in Figure 5.2.

When an ITE hearing aid occupies a sufficiently small portion of the cavum concha, it is referred to as an *in-the-canal* (ITC) hearing aid. (One would expect from the name that an ITC hearing aid would fit entirely within the ear canal, but the name is more a reflection of marketing-inspired optimism than an accurate description of where the hearing aid is located.)

Hearing aids that *do* fit entirely within the ear canal are known as *completely-in-the-canal (CIC)* hearing aids. These hearing aids use components small enough that none of the hearing aid need protrude into the concha.

---

[c]   Microphones used to be called transmitters, which explains why something that emits sound should be called a receiver.

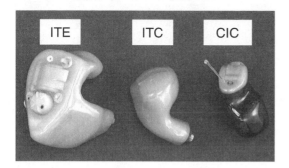

Figure 1.8 An ITE, an ITC and a CIC hearing aid.

Removing these hearing aids from the ear can be difficult, so often a small handle, similar to nylon fishing line with a small knob on the end, is attached to the hearing aid and this does extend into the concha. When the medial end of a CIC hearing aid is within a few millimeters of the eardrum, the CIC is referred to as a *peri-tympanic CIC*.

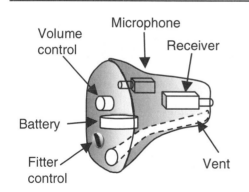

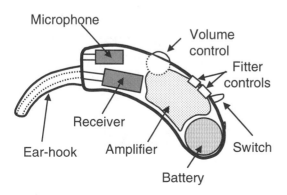

Figure 1.9 The typical location of components in an ITC and a BTE hearing aid.

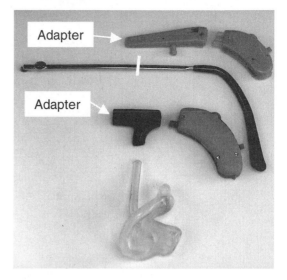

Figure 1.10 Spectacle adapter system showing two different adapters and BTE hearing aids, an earmold, and a spectacle bow. The bow would be cut at the white line and the left half inserted in the adapter.

Figure 1.8 shows an ITE, an ITC, and a CIC hearing aid. The typical locations of the major components within a BTE and ITC hearing aid are shown in Figure 1.9.

The last type of hearing aid is the *spectacle* or *eyeglass* aid. As the name suggests, these are a combination of spectacles and one or two hearing aids. There are actually two types of spectacle aids. In the first type, the side frame of the spectacles (the *bow*) contains all the hearing aid components. These were the first type produced and were bulky in appearance. In current models, the part of the bow that fits behind the ear on a conventional pair of spectacles is sawn off, and a short adapter is glued on in its place, as shown in Figure 1.10. The spectacle hearing aid (essentially a BTE) attaches to this adapter and a tube leads from the adapter to the ear. These are less conspicuous, and the frontal appearance is little different from the appearance of the spectacles alone. This is particularly true when the hearing aid couples into the ear without an earmold, using only tubing.[928]

1.4   Historical Perspective

By far the biggest change to hearing aids this century is that they have become smaller. The quest to make them smaller and less conspicuous has been a constant driving force behind technological progress. Sometimes size reductions have been achieved at the expense of performance, but over time performance has increased despite, and sometimes because of, the size reductions. Current hearing aids have better fidelity (wide bandwidth and low distortion) and greater adjustment flexibility, than has been possible at any time in the past.

The following brief historical review of hearing aid technology is heavily based on an excellent and authoritative chapter by Sam Lybarger (1988), who created many of the innovations in hearing aids during the past 50 years. The reader is referred to Lybarger (1988) and Berger (1984) for a more detailed history and more extensive references. Fitting procedures for hearing aids are not covered here because they are reviewed in Section 9.1.

The history of hearing aids may be divided into five eras: acoustic, carbon, vacuum tube, transistor, and digital. The last of these eras, which has emerged since the historical reviews referred to above, is bringing in changes as significant as those that occurred during each of the preceding eras.

Most of the technological features mentioned in this section are described in later chapters, and so may have limited meaning to some readers at this stage.

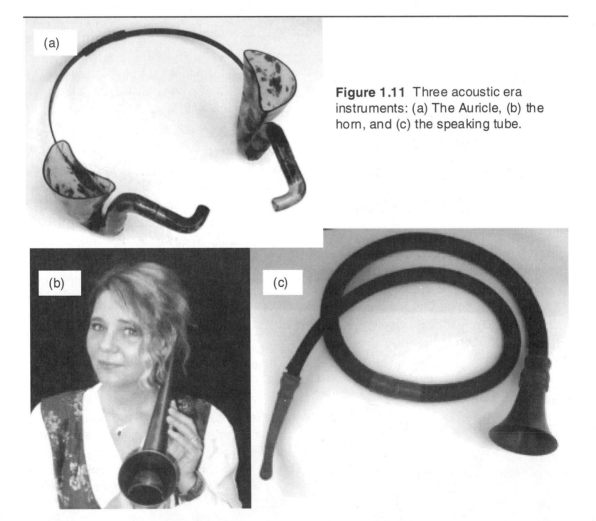

Figure 1.11 Three acoustic era instruments: (a) The Auricle, (b) the horn, and (c) the speaking tube.

1.4.1   The acoustic era

The acoustic era began the first time some-one cupped a hand (or a possibly a paw) behind an ear. This produces 5 to 10 dB of gain at mid- and high-frequencies by collecting sound from an area larger than the ear can by itself.[207] It also shields the ear from sounds coming from the rear, thus working as a very effective noise reduction system, at least for mid- and high-frequency sounds.

A more effective acoustic aid is formed by anything with a shape like a *trumpet, horn,* or *funnel*. Illustrations of horns appeared in 1673 and in 1650.[54, 409] The principle is to have a large open end to collect as much sound as possible. This energy is transferred to the ear via a gradual reduction in area along the length of the trumpet or funnel. (If the area decreases too quickly, most of the sound just reflects back out again instead of travel-ling into the ear.) Ear trumpets therefore have to be both wide and long to be effective.

The quest to make hearing aids smaller has been around a long time. Lybarger (1988) reports that the idea of coiling the trumpet to make it smaller dates from at least 1692. The desire to conceal the hearing aid also has a long history. Ear trumpets have been "hid-den" inside top hats, armchairs, fans and beards.[328]

If the open end of an acoustic hearing aid is moved closer to a talker, it picks up more intense sound as well as a greater area of sound. The *speaking tube*, as shown in Figure 1.11, is designed to do this and consists of a horn-shaped end attached to a long tube that terminates in an earpiece. If the talker speaks directly into the horn end, the signal-to-noise ratio at the input to the device is much better than that which the listener would receive naturally. As well as amplifying, the device thus improves signal-to-noise ratio, and by an amount not possible with even the most

sophisticated one-piece hearing aids now available.

Given that people, even those with normal hearing, still cup their hands behind their ears in adverse listening situations, one cannot say that the acoustic era ever ended.

1.4.2   The carbon era

A carbon hearing aid, in its simplest form, consists of a *carbon microphone*, a *battery* of 3 to 6 Volts and a *magnetic receiver*, all connected in series. The carbon microphone contained carbon dust, granules, or spherical globules.[d] When sound hit the microphone diaphragm, movement of the diaphragm pushed the bits of carbon closer together, or pulled them further apart, thus changing the electrical resistance of the microphone. This fluctuating resistance caused the electrical current to fluctuate in a similar way, and when this passed through a coil inside the receiver, it created a fluctuating magnetic field inside the receiver. This fluctuating magnetic field pushed and pulled against a permanent magnet, thus making the receiver diaphragm move in and out, in synchronism with the sound hitting the microphone. The sound level out of the receiver (when coupled into a small cavity) was, however, 20 to 30 dB greater than the input to the microphone.[552]

To achieve greater gain, a *carbon amplifier* was invented. If one microphone and receiver pair could increase the sound level, it was reasoned, then a second pair (but with only a single diaphragm in common) could increase it more. The carbon amplifier thus consisted of a coil, which vibrated a diaphragm, which moved some carbon granules or globules to produce a bigger fluctuating current.

The first carbon hearing aid, a large table model called the Akoulallion, appeared in 1899[54, 317], and the first wearable model (vari-ously called the Akouphone and the

---

[d]   The replacement of dust by granules and then by globules in 1901 is a good example of the technological refinements that inevitably follow each major change of technology.

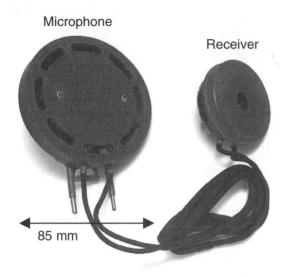

Figure 1.12 A carbon aid (The Acousticon) without its battery.

Acousticon[427]) appeared shortly after in 1902. Carbon hearing aids continued to be used through to the 1940s, but were satisfactory only for people with mild or moderate losses.

During the carbon era, the idea of amplifying different frequencies by different amounts (to suit the hearing loss) emerged. This was achieved by selecting different combinations of microphones, receivers, and amplifiers. Couplers, initially with a volume of 0.5 cc, first emerged during the carbon era, as did high-quality condenser measurement microphones.

Assistive listening devices, which are hearing aids that are not worn entirely on the hearing-impaired person, also emerged during the carbon era. Johnstone (1997) recalls seeing a microphone in a church pulpit wired to several hand-held receivers in selected pews around 1916, but were probably in use ten years before this.[650]

1.4.3   The vacuum tube era

The vacuum tube electronic amplifier was invented in 1907 and applied to hearing aids in 1920.[552] The vacuum tube allowed a small voltage, which came from the microphone,

to control the fluctuations in a large current. By combining several vacuum tubes in succession, very powerful amplifiers (70 dB gain and 130 dB SPL output) could be made, thus increasing the range of hearing losses that could be helped. The increasing sophistication of electronics also allowed the gain-frequency response shape to be better controlled than for carbon aids.

The biggest problem with vacuum tube hearing aids was their total size. Driven by military requirements, the size of the vacuum tubes themselves reduced enormously over time, but two batteries were needed to make them work. A low voltage *A* battery was needed to heat the filament of the tubes, and a high voltage *B* battery was needed to power the amplifier circuits. Vacuum tube hearing aids became practical during the 1930s, but until 1944, their batteries were so large that the batteries had to be housed separately from the microphone and amplifier. In 1944, vacuum tube and battery technology had advanced sufficiently to make possible a one-piece hearing aid. Batteries, microphone, and amplifier were combined into a single body-worn package, which connected to an ear-level receiver via a cable. There were further creative attempts to conceal the hearing aid during the vacuum tube era. This included enclosing the electronics, except for the trans-

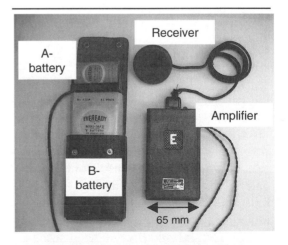

Figure 1.13 A relatively late vacuum tube hearing aid, with its two separate batteries.

ducers, inside a large pen-shaped case (the Penphone).[318] Microphones were concealed inside broaches and wristwatches, and receiver cords were enclosed within strings of pearls.[318]

Earmold venting, magnetic microphones, piezoelectric microphones and compression amplification were also devised during the vacuum tube era.[552] Piezoelectric substances have a crystal structure that generates a voltage when twisted or bent. In a microphone, the bending happens because a diaphragm is connected to one corner or end of the piezoelectric crystal. The early origin of compression amplification is surprising; compression seems to have rapidly become largely forgotten until the 1980s, but then became the dominant type of advanced amplification in the late 1990s.

1.4.4   The transistor and integrated circuit era

The transistor became commercially available in 1952.[812] So dramatic was the reduction in battery power required, that all new hearing aids used transistors rather than valves by 1953.[317] The reduction in battery size, and the small size of transistors relative to valves, meant that from 1954 the bits of the hearing aid could be moved up to the head. Head mounting had several advantages: clothing did not create noise as it rubbed the microphone, the body did not have such adverse effects on the tonal balance of sound coming from different directions, cables were no longer required, and true binaural hearing aids were possible.

First amongst the head-mounted aids were barrette hearing aids and spectacle or eyeglass aids. The barrettes, which had an external receiver like a body aid, came in a variety of shapes and were worn on or under the hair (or on the body on ties, lapels, or collars). Several were made to resemble jewelry.[812] Spectacle aids had all the hearing aid components built into the temple pieces (the bow) of spectacles. With a rapid and

continual reduction in the size of all the components, they could soon all be moved behind the ear, either as part of the spectacle bow, as a self-contained curved package that attached to a sawn-off standard spectacle bow, or finally as a stand-alone BTE hearing aid. During the following ten years, the BTE took over from the eyeglass aid as the dominant style, and remained so until the mid-1980s in the USA, and until the 1990s in much of Europe.

With further decreases in the size of components, ITE aids started to appear in the mid and late 1950s.[812] The first ITEs were so large by today's standards that Lybarger (1988) referred to them as *out-of-the-ear* hearing aids.

Two big leaps in the performance and size of components occurred during the 1960s. First, in 1964, the integrated circuit (IC) was applied to hearing aids. This meant that multiple transistors and resistors could be combined into a single component that was similar in size to any one of the individual transistors that it replaced. Second, in 1968, a piezoelectric microphone was combined with a relatively new type of transistor (the *field effect transistor*, or *FET*) inside a small metal can. For the first time, a small rugged microphone with a reasonably smooth, reasonably wide frequency response could be used in hearing aids.[469] A few years later, directional microphones emerged, using the same technology.

Microphone technology further improved in 1971 when the electret/FET microphone (described in Section 2.2) was developed.[470] These brought about even better responses and even smaller sizes. During the transistor era, receiver volume decreased from 1800 mm³ to 39 mm³ (Knowles model FS), whereas microphone volume decreased from 5000 mm³ to 23 mm³ (Knowles model TM). Egolf et al (1989) point out that most of the shrinkage in receiver volume occurred prior to 1970, so perhaps there may not be huge reductions in receiver size in the future.

By the early 1980s, ITE aids had become small enough for most of the components to fit within the ear canal portion of the aid, thus creating the ITC hearing aid.[335] With further improvements in battery chemistry, amplifier efficiency and transducer size, the entire hearing aid could finally be located inside the ear canal by the early 1990s. The CIC had arrived, and at last the hearing aid was invisible! This placement of the hearing aid also carried some acoustic advantages, as the useful sound-collecting and shielding properties of the pinna could be used when wearing a hearing aid. Also, wind noise was decreased.

Some of the advances during the transistor era include:

- zinc-air batteries, that allowed a halving of battery volume for the same electrical capacity (see Section 2.12);

- improved filtering, that led to more flexible response shaping and multi-channel processing of sound (see Section 2.5);

- miniature potentiometers, that allowed the clinician to adjust the amplification characteristics of even very small hearing aids (see Section 3.3);

- wireless transmission hearing aids, in which the hearing aid contains a wireless receiver that is tuned to a transmitter worn by a talker some distance away (see Section 3.8);

- class D amplifiers, that decreased the battery drain required to achieve a given output level with minimal distortion (see Section 2.3.4);

- improved understanding of the acoustics of earmolds and ear shells, that allowed more appropriate gain-frequency responses to be achieved,[467] and occlusion and feedback problems to be decreased, but not solved (see Chapter 5); and

- use of two microphones within a hearing aid, so that the user can select directional or omni-directional performance as needed (see Section 2.1.4).

A further very significant advance, which could arguably be placed in the next era, was the application in 1986 of digital control circuits and digital memories to hearing aids. These circuits replaced potentiometers, and because they occupied little space inside the hearing aid, many "controls" could be included in a hearing aid. These circuits thus enabled the amplification characteristics of hearing aids to be adjusted by the clinician with greatly increased flexibility and precision. A by-product of digital control circuits was that the user could also conveniently change the hearing aid's characteristics, usually with a remote control, which made multi-memory hearing aids practical, even in ITC or CIC hearing aids.

1.4.5   The digital era

As just mentioned, digital electronics first met hearing aids when the digital circuits acted as the controls for an otherwise conventional hearing aid. The real revolution came when the sound waveform itself was converted to a series of numbers and manipulated using digital circuits.

Research into digital processing began in the 1960s within Bell Laboratories.[525] Because of the slow speed of computers then, however, the necessary calculations could not be performed quickly enough for the signal to come out of the laboratory hearing aid as rapidly as a signal was put into it! It was not until the late 1970s that computers were fast enough for the output to be synchronized with (but delayed slightly behind) the input, and it was not until the 1980s that power consumption and size were decreased sufficiently to make a wearable hearing aid.

Because the first digital aid was a body aid and did essentially the same things to sound as ear-level analog hearing aids, it was not a commercial success and quickly ceased to be available. Finally, in 1996, fully digital BTE,

ITE and ITC hearing aids became commercially available, although several years previous to that, an analog hearing aid with a digital feedback reduction system was available.[254] Some excellent reviews of the development (and future!) of digital hearing aids have been written by Levitt (1987, 1997).

Advantages already seen for digital technology include:

- further increases in the flexibility with which response shaping and compression characteristics can be controlled;

- intelligent automatic manipulation of the gain and frequency response of the hearing aid, depending on how much signal and noise the hearing aid estimates is present in each frequency region;

- intelligent manipulation of the way gain varies for sounds coming from different directions, so that noise is minimized;

- increased gain without feedback oscillations occurring;

- reduction in size and required power from the battery, relative to an analog aid that manipulates sound in the same way; and

- intelligent automatic control of the gain of the hearing aid for sounds coming from different directions.

It is extremely likely that digital signal processing will confer many more advantages in the near future. Likely candidates include further improvement to feedback control, and better methods for reducing the effects of background noise, at least in certain circumstances. The impact of digital processing will be discussed in many places throughout this book.

Although hearing aid usage rates and satisfaction did not improve significantly from the late 1980s to the mid 1990s,[385, 482] the performance improvements that are now possible make it likely that marked improvements in both will be achieved over the next five years.

CHAPTER TWO

HEARING AID COMPONENTS

Synopsis

Hearing aids are best understood as a collection of functional building blocks. The manner in which a signal passes through these blocks in any particular hearing aid is indicated in a block diagram. The first block encountered by an acoustic signal is a microphone, which converts sound to electricity. Modern miniature electret microphones provide a very high sound quality, with only very minor imperfections associated with internal noise and sensitivity to vibration. Directional microphones, which have two entry ports, are more sensitive to frontal sound than to sound arriving from other directions. These enable hearing aids to improve the signal-to-noise ratio by 3 to 5 dB relative to omni-directional microphones, and hence improve the intelligibility of speech in noise. Dual-microphone hearing aids can be switched by the user to be either directional, or omni-directional, as required in different listening situations.

The small signals produced by microphones are made more powerful by the hearing aid amplifier. There are four types of output amplifiers used in hearing aids: Class A, Class B, Class D and Class H. The most efficient of these is the Class D amplifier. All amplifiers will distort the signal, by peak clipping it, if they attempt to amplify the signal to too great a level. Excessive distortion decreases the quality and intelligibility of sounds. To avoid distortion, compression amplifiers are used in many hearing aids. These amplifiers decrease their gain as the level of the signal put into them increases, in much the same way that a person will turn down a volume control when the level becomes too great.

Amplifiers can represent sound in an analog or a digital manner. The signals within analog amplifiers have waveforms that mimic the acoustic waveforms they represent. Digital systems represent signals as a string of numbers. Performing arithmetic on the string of numbers alters the size and nature of the signals these numbers represent. Filtering a signal is a common way in which hearing aids alter sound – whether this filtering is done in an analog or digital amplifier. Filters can be used to change the relative amplitude of the low-, mid- and high-frequency components in a signal. When the filters are made with variable, controllable characteristics, they function as tone controls operated by the user or the clinician. Filters can also be used to break the signal into different frequency ranges, so that different types of amplification can be used in each range, as required by the hearing loss of the hearing-impaired person.

Receivers are miniature headphones that use electromagnetism to convert the amplified, modified electrical signals back into sound. Their frequency response is characterized by multiple peaks and troughs, which are partly caused by resonances within the receivers, and partly caused by acoustic resonances within the tubing that connects a receiver to the ear canal. Inserting an acoustic resistor, called a damper, inside the receiver or tubing will smooth these peaks and troughs. A damper absorbs energy at the frequencies corresponding to the peaks, and this improves sound quality and listening comfort.

There are several other ways to put signals into hearing aids. A telecoil senses magnetic signals and converts them to a voltage. A direct audio input connector enables an electrical audio signal to be plugged straight into the hearing aid.

Users operate hearing aids via electromechanical switches on the case of the hearing aid, or by using a remote control. The hearing aid performs all its functions by taking electrical power from a battery. These batteries come in a range of physical sizes and capacities, depending on the power needed by each hearing aid, and the space available.

This chapter will describe the bits and pieces that make up a modern hearing aid. These pieces comprise the transducers that convert sound to and from electricity, and the things that alter sound while it is represented in electrical form. These electronic parts will be considered as functional boxes, rather than as electrical circuits. As we will see, the function of these boxes can be discussed irrespective of whether they are implemented as analog or digital circuits, but some of the special considerations of analog and digital circuits will also be considered. Combinations of these functional boxes are represented by block diagrams.

2.1 Block Diagrams

A decade ago, the operation of most hearing aids, for any setting of an aid's controls, could be understood just by looking at a few graphs of gain versus frequency and maximum output versus frequency. Most hearing aids are now more complicated, and the only way to understand how a more complex hearing aid changes a signal is to understand its *block diagram*.

A block diagram shows what operations a device carries out on signals within the hearing aid, and in what order each of these operations is carried out. Block diagrams also usually

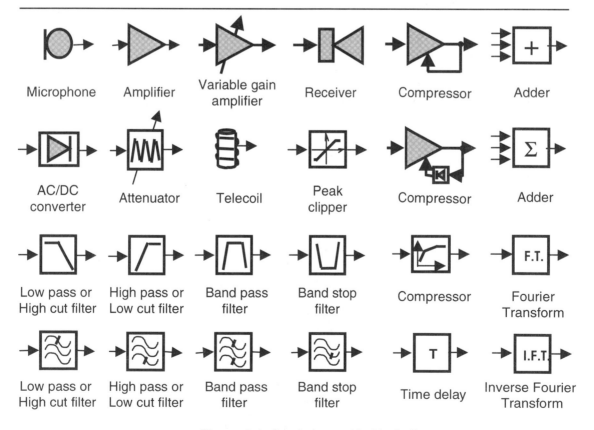

Figure 2.1 Symbols used in block diagrams.

show the location of fitter and user controls within the processing chain. This helps the clinician understand what effect varying a control will have, and, just as importantly, what effects it will not have.

Figure 2.1 shows the symbols used in this book for each of a number of blocks. Most of these blocks will be more fully described later in this chapter. Some of the blocks have synonyms. The *AC/DC converter*, used in conjunction with compression amplifiers, is sometimes called a *level detector*, or an *averaging circuit*. The *adder* is sometimes called a *summer*.

An arrow drawn diagonally through a block indicates that some characteristic of the block can be altered, usually by a fitter or user control, but sometimes by the output of another block. Figure 2.1 shows an example for a variable gain amplifier, but any of the blocks except for the microphone or the receiver can be made variable in this manner. Most of the blocks have an input (or several inputs) and an output.

Unfortunately, there is no absolute standardization for block diagram symbols. The symbols and alternative symbols shown in Figure 2.1 are most common, but further alternatives exist. The origins of some symbols are easy to see. The filters and the compression amplifier shown in the third row

simply show the graph that results when the electroacoustic performance of the block is measured in the most meaningful way. This is a gain-frequency response in the case of a filter and an input-output diagram in the case of a compression amplifier.

In more advanced hearing aids, the signal may be altered in ways that would be too complex to represent as a combination of simple blocks. In this case, the appropriate symbol is a box with a short description of the process written inside the box.

Some conventions and rules govern how block diagrams are drawn. Arrows on the lines connecting blocks show that a signal is being passed *from* one block *to* another. A convention is that signals usually flow from left to right, though it is often necessary to make exceptions in complex diagrams, and the arrows on the connecting lines make this clear. A rule is that when the output of a device is fed simultaneously to the input of several other blocks, the entire output signal goes to each of the blocks to which it is connected. Another rule is that an input cannot be driven by more than one output. Connecting two outputs to one input would produce a logical conflict as both devices try to tell another device what its input signal should be. Where possible, block diagrams are drawn so that there are no crossing lines connecting the various

Figure 2.2 A three channel compression hearing aid.

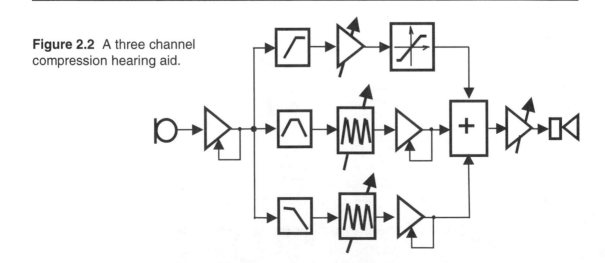

blocks, although sometimes this cannot be avoided. Lines that cross and connect to each other usually have the connection indicated by a dot at the point of intersection. Figure 2.2 shows a block diagram of a three-channel hearing aid with a compressor in each channel.

Let us consider the following examples of what can be learned from a block diagram like the one shown in Figure 2.2. You may like to re-read this final paragraph after learning more about the individual blocks, and particularly about the effects of compressors, later in this chapter and in Chapter 6. The microphone converts input signals to electricity and these electrical signals are amplified by a compression amplifier of some type. The resulting signal is split into its low-frequency, mid-frequency and high-frequency components. The low- and mid-frequency bands of signal are attenuated by a selectable amount and each band is amplified by a compression amplifier. The high-frequency band is amplified by a selectable amount, and then peak clipped. The three parts of the modified signal are recombined and amplified by a user- or fitter-controlled amount, before being delivered to the receiver. The effects of the controls on the operation of the aid can also be deduced, but the preceding description illustrates the information that can be easily read from a block diagram.

2.2   Microphones

The function of the microphone is to convert sound into electricity. Because it changes energy from one form to another it is known as a *transducer*. For a perfect microphone (and microphones *are* close to perfect), the waveform of the electrical signal coming out of the microphone is identical to the waveform of the acoustical signal going into the microphone. Microphones act in a linear fashion, so every time the pressure of the input signal doubles, for instance, the output voltage also doubles. The relationship between the size of the output voltage and the size of the

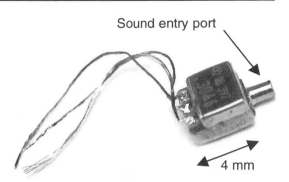

Figure 2.3 An electret microphone.

input sound pressure is known as the *sensitivity* of the microphone. Typical hearing aid microphones have a sensitivity of about 16 mV per Pascal, which means that sounds of 70 dB SPL produce a voltage of around 1mV.

2.2.1   Principle of operation

Microphones can be made using several fundamentally different types of technology, but since the early 1980s, hearing aids have used only one type of microphone: the electret microphone.[470, 794] Figure 2.3 shows a picture of an electret microphone, and Figure 2.4 shows a cross-section to illustrate the operating principle. Sound waves enter through the inlet port and reach one side of a very thin, very flexible plate with a metal-lized surface, called the *diaphragm.* Pressure fluctuations within the sound wave cause the diaphragm to move up and down (by an extremely small amount). A small air space separates the diaphragm from a rigid metal

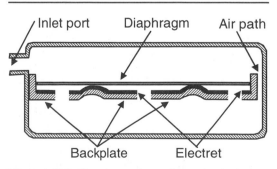

Figure 2.4 Cross section of an electret microphone.

plate, called the **back-plate.** Coated onto the back-plate is some thin teflon material called an **electret**. The diaphragm is held away from the back-plate by some bumps in the back-plate. The back-plate has holes in it to allow movement of air through it.

The electret material gets its name from the fact that it has a permanent electric charge comprising an excess of electrons on one side of it, and a shortage of electrons on the other. These electrical charges attract opposite electrical charges onto the diaphragm and the back-plate. When sound pressure forces the diaphragm downward towards the electret, the closer distance between the diaphragm and the electret induces an even greater charge on the diaphragm. This charge gets there by leaving the back-plate, flowing through the input circuit of an amplifier to which the microphone is connected, and thence on to the diaphragm. This, of course, is the point of the exercise, because in so doing, the microphone has turned a sound wave into an electrical voltage and current. An amplifier is built into the same container as the rest of the microphone. Its job is to turn the minute electrical currents flowing to and from the diaphragm into larger currents that can be passed on to the main hearing aid amplifier.

The microphone amplifier is sometimes referred to as a **FET,** because it is made using a type of transistor known as a field effect transistor. Alternatively, it is referred to as a **buffer amplifier** (because it stops the main amplifier from loading down the microphone), or as a **follower** (because the voltage out of the microphone amplifier follows or equals the voltage between the diaphragm and the back plate).

A new type of microphone is currently under development. The **silicon microphone** (also referred to as the **solid state** or **integrated** microphone) is made by etching away parts of a block of silicon, and depositing layers of other materials onto it, using techniques similar to those used to make an integrated circuit. Microphone manufacturers expect that when problems of low sensitivity and high internal noise are solved, it will eventually replace the electret microphone and should be smaller as well as being more reliable and reproducible. The silicon microphone should also eventually be cheaper as it can be made in a more automated fashion, and can potentially be made from the same block of silicon as the integrated circuit used for the main hearing aid amplifier.

2.2.2 Frequency response of microphones

Electret microphones have frequency responses that are essentially flat, although variations from a flat response occur both by design and by accident. A low cut is intentionally introduced into electret microphones used in hearing aids. The low cut makes the hearing aid less sensitive to the intense low-frequency sounds that often surround us. These may not be perceived, even by normal-hearing people, but they can cause a hearing aid to overload unless the microphone attenuates them.

Achieving the low cut is simple: a small passage-way between the front and back of the diaphragm allows low-frequency sounds to impact almost simultaneously on both sides of the diaphragm, thus reducing their effectiveness in moving the diaphragm. The larger the opening, the greater the attenuation, and the greater the frequency range over which attenuation occurs. The opening also equalizes the static air pressure between the front and back of the diaphragm, just as the Eustachian tube does for the ear. Microphones with different degrees of low cut are often used in custom hearing aids to help achieve a desired gain-frequency response for the hearing aid as a whole.

The second variation from a flat response is the result of an acoustic resonance within the microphone mounting. A resonance occurs between the air in the inlet port (an **acoustic**

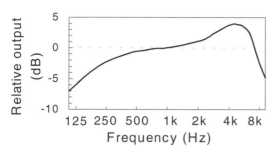

Figure 2.5 Frequency response of a typical electret microphone.

---

mass), and the volume of air next to the front of the diaphragm (an *acoustic compliance*, or spring). The mechanical compliance of the diaphragm itself, and of the air behind the diaphragm, also contribute to the resonance, which is called a *Helmholtz resonance*.[a] This resonance causes a peak in the gain-frequency response, typically about 5 dB high and centered at 4 or 5 kHz, as shown in Figure 2.5. Above the resonant frequency, and because of the resonance, the sensitivity of the microphone decreases as frequency increases. Some newer microphones are cylindrical in shape and have such a wide inlet port that the Helmholtz resonance frequency is moved up to a much higher frequency. The microphone consequently has a totally flat response within the hearing aid bandwidth.

2.2.3   Microphone imperfections

The major imperfection with microphones is that they eventually break down if they are exposed to adverse chemical agents, like perspiration.

Less dramatically, all electronic components generate small amounts of *random electrical noise*, and microphones are no exception. The noise is partly the result of random motion of air molecules against the diaphragm, and partly the result of random electrical activity within the internal microphone amplifier. This noise, when sufficiently amplified by the main hearing aid amplifier, is sometimes audible to the hearing aid user in quiet environments, particularly if the user has near-normal hearing at any frequency. Microphone noise is greatest in those microphones that use an internal acoustic path to steeply roll-off the low-frequency response of the microphone.

Another imperfection of microphones is that as well as being sensitive to sound, they are sensitive to *vibrations*. This occurs because if the microphone is shaken, the inertia of the diaphragm causes it to move less than the outer case of the microphone. Consequently, the diaphragm and the case move relative to each other, just as they do for a sound wave, so the microphone generates a voltage reflecting the magnitude and frequency of the vibration. Why does this matter?

The first consequence of a microphone's sensitivity to vibration is that any vibrations will be amplified into an annoying sound. For example, rubbing of the hearing aid case (e.g. by clothing next to a body aid) will be audible. Direct vibration of the body, such as occurs when running on a hard surface, may also be audible as an unwanted thumping noise.

The second consequence is that when the hearing aid receiver operates it creates vibrations as well as sound. The microphone picks up some of these vibrations, converts them to an electrical signal, and they are then amplified by the hearing aid and passed to the receiver, which creates further vibrations. If the mechanical transmission of the vibrations from the receiver to the microphone is strong enough, and/or if the gain of the hearing aid is high enough, then this feedback loop may cause an audible oscillation, usually at a low frequency. Hearing aid designers avoid this by careful mounting and placement of the microphone and receiver, but if either of these become displaced, the hearing aid can become unstable due to this internal feedback loop.

---

[a]   At the Helmholtz resonant frequency, the air in a tube and volume to which it is connected vibrates freely, just as a mass on a spring vibrates easily at its resonant frequency.

Displacement of the transducers from their proper position is more likely to occur for in-the-ear (ITE), in-the-canal (ITC) or completely-in-the-canal (CIC) hearing aids because of their small size and custom manner of construction. A repair consists of repositioning either or both transducers. *Internal feedback* that is not sufficiently strong to cause an audible oscillation can be detected from the coupler response of the hearing aid. It is indicated by bumps in the frequency response that are present at high volume control or gain settings, but which disappear at lower volume control or gain settings.

Another possible imperfection can occur with bad design or construction of a hearing aid. If the microphone is mounted with a long thin tube on its inlet port, the Helmholtz resonance referred to in the preceding section is moved downward in frequency. This causes a larger peak in the gain-frequency response, and a rapid decrease in gain for frequencies above this peak frequency.

The last imperfection is that microphones are subject to *wind noise*. When wind hits an obstacle like a head, a pinna, or a hearing aid, turbulence is created. Turbulence consists of pressure fluctuations, so the microphone indiscriminately converts these to electrical fluctuations: in this case an audible low- and mid-frequency noise. Keeping the microphone inlet away from the wind flow can minimize the amount of wind noise. A cosmetically unacceptable, but very effective way to do this is to place some plastic foam over the microphone port. A better way to achieve it is to

---

How directional microphones work

Microphones can be made to have a sensitivity that depends on direction of arrival by feeding sounds to both sides of the diaphragm from two separate inlet ports (the open ends of the microphone tubing), as shown in Figure 2.6. The directional properties of the microphone depend on two delays:

- The external time delay is the time taken for sounds outside the hearing aid to get from one inlet port to the other, and is approximately equal to the distance between the ports divided by the speed of sound in the vicinity of the head.*

- The internal time delay arises because the rear port contains an acoustic damper or resistor (see Section 2.7). This combines with the cavity at the back of the diaphragm to create a low-pass filter that passes most of the amplified frequencies without attenuation, but with some delay that is inherent to all filters (Carlson & Killion, 1974).

Sound coming from the rear direction hits the front port later than the rear port. However, the sound entering the rear port is delayed when it gets to the internal low-pass filter. If the internal and external delays are equal, then sound from the rear will reach both sides of the diaphragm at the same time, and there will be no net force on the diaphragm. Such a microphone is insensitive to sounds from the rear. If the internal delay is less than the external delay, the microphone will be insensitive to sounds coming from other directions.

* The effective speed of sound is lower than usual near the surface of the head because of waves that diffract around the head in both directions (Madaffari, 1983).

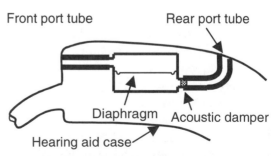

Front port tube   Rear port tube

Diaphragm   Acoustic damper

Hearing aid case

Figure 2.6 Diagram showing the sound paths in a directional microphone.

place the microphone port deep inside the ear canal, as occurs for deeply seated CIC hearing aids. A third, but less effective option is for the manufacturer to place a mesh screen over the microphone port opening so that less turbulence enters the microphone port. A more effective option that is suitable for some people is to wear a light scarf.[94] This will prevent wind from hitting the hearing aid and the pinna, and will prevent turbulence created by the head from directly flowing past the microphone port.

2.2.4   Directional microphones

Directional microphones suppress noise coming from some directions, while retaining good sensitivity to sounds arriving from one direction.

The directional sensitivity of microphones is usually indicated on a ***polar diagram***. Figure 2.7(a) shows the polar diagram for a microphone like the one described in the accompanying panel. This particular response shape is called a ***cardioid***, because of its heart shape. By changing the ratio of the internal delay to the external delay, a whole family of response shapes can be generated as shown in Figure 2.7. As the shape moves from a cardioid to a ***super-cardioid*** to a ***hyper-cardioid***, the sensitivity to sounds from the back grows, but the sensitivity to sounds from the sides diminish. In the extreme case, which is referred to as a ***figure-8*** or ***bi-directional*** pattern, the front and rear have the same sensitivity, but the microphone is completely insensitive to sounds coming from the sides.

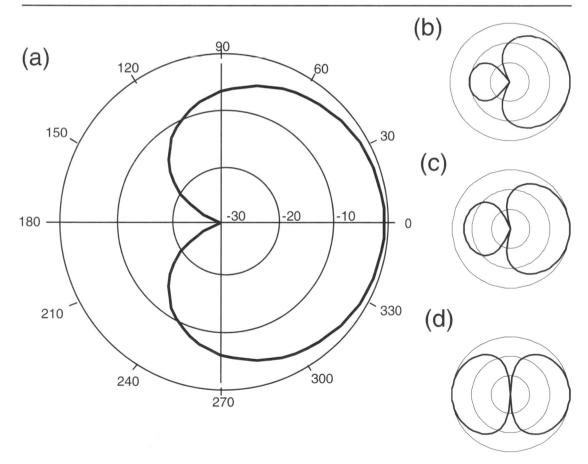

Figure 2.7 Directional sensitivity (in dB) of a microphone with (a) a cardioid response, (b) a super-cardioid response, (c) a hypercardioid response, and (d) a figure-8 response, all measured in an unobstructed sound field.

The other extreme is an ***omni-directional*** (i.e., non-directional) microphone, which has a single port and a polar diagram in the shape of a circle.

What response shape is most desirable? In many real life situations, unwanted noise arrives more or less equally from all directions, because even if the noise originates from only one or two sources, room reflections cause the energy to arrive at the aid wearer from all directions. By contrast, if the aid user is standing close to the person he or she wants to hear, the wanted signal will arrive mostly from directly in front. A good directional microphone should therefore have maximum sensitivity for sounds arriving from directly ahead, but the sensitivity averaged across all other possible directions should be as low as possible, if intelligibility in noisy environments is to be maximized.

This ratio of sensitivity for frontal sounds relative to sensitivity averaged across all other directions is referred to as the ***directivity index (DI).***[b] It is expressed in dB. The "other directions" included in the average may include all directions in a two dimensional horizontal plane (i.e. around a circle), or may include all directions in three-dimensional space (i.e. around a sphere). The latter calculation method usually leads to larger directivity indexes for highly directional microphones, although there may not be much difference for simple directional microphones like those discussed in this section. Sometimes, the ratio of frontal sensitivity to rearward sensitivity is quoted in hearing aid specifications. This ***front-to-back ratio*** is a misleading measure because it says nothing about the effectiveness of the hearing aid in suppressing noise arriving from directions other than precisely behind the aid wearer. For cardioids of different shapes, the highest three-dimensional directivity index (equal to 5.9 dB) is actually obtained with the hyper-cardioid (Figure 2.7c),

which has a rather poor front-to-back ratio. The highest two-dimensional directivity index (equal to 4.8 dB) is obtained for a super-cardioid (Figure 2.7b).

Neat polar responses like those shown in Figure 2.7 occur only for hearing aids suspended in free space, because when hearing aids are worn, the head introduces a polar pattern of its own. In fact, all microphones act as though they are somewhat directional when they are placed on the head. Directionality occurs because the head and pinna attenuate the sound when they come between the source and the microphone, and boost the sound when the microphone is positioned between them and the source. These boosting and attenuating effects of head diffraction increase in magnitude as frequency rises (see Figure 14.4).

Figure 2.8(a) shows a polar response for an omni-directional microphone mounted in a behind-the-ear (BTE) hearing aid when it is being worn. As expected from head diffraction effects, the maximum sensitivity occurs for

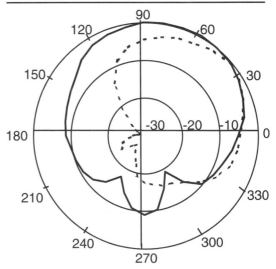

Figure 2.8 Directional sensitivity of (a) an omnidirectional (solid line) and (b) a directional (dotted line) microphone, mounted on the head at 2 kHz. Data adapted from Knowles, TB21.

---

[b]   More precisely, the ***directivity factor*** is the ratio of power out of the microphone for a frontal source, to the power out of the microphone when sound comes equally from all directions. The ***directivity index*** is the decibel equivalent of this directivity factor.

sounds coming from the aided side of the person wearing the hearing aid, about 80 degrees from the front. Figure 2.8(b) shows the result when a microphone with a cardioid pattern is mounted on the head. The result reflects both the directivity of the microphone (Figure 2.7a) and the directivity of the head (Figure 2.8a). The most sensitive direction is now about 30 degrees from the front.

Directional microphones have been available for decades, in both BTE and ITE hearing aids, but have most commonly been used in BTE hearing aids.[727] Many early hearing aids appear to have had poorly designed directional microphones, such that they were barely more directional than an omni-directional microphone when mounted on the head.[43]

One problem is that the microphone is directional only for frequencies less than the cut-off frequency of the internal, acoustic low-pass filter. This limits performance if the cut-off frequency is too low.[c]

A second problem is that directional microphones create a low-frequency cut in the gain-frequency response. This cut occurs because for low-frequency sounds, the time delay between the sounds reaching the front and back of the diaphragm is small compared to a period no matter which direction sound arrives from. The two waves are therefore almost in phase and have only a small net effect on the diaphragm. An electronic filter can be used to boost the low-frequency gain and so partially compensate for this, but such a filter also boosts the internal microphone noise, which may then become excessive. Either for this reason or because of the extra complexity involved, such low boost filters are only sometimes incorporated in hearing aids. If the gain is sufficiently low, the user may not receive *any* amplified low-frequency sound, thus removing all directivity at low frequencies (see Section 5.3.1). The low-cut characteristic of an uncompensated directional microphone makes it difficult to attain

a desired frequency response shape for hearing aid users who need a lot of low-frequency gain.

A final problem is that the hearing aid user may not want the microphone response to be directional in all situations (see Section 10.2.4).

Using a *dual-microphone* hearing aid can solve this last problem. Two separate omnidirectional microphones, each with one inlet port, are used instead of a single microphone with two ports. The output from the second microphone is electronically delayed and subtracted from the first microphone output. When ambient noise is not a problem, the user can switch off one of the microphones, thus reverting to omni-directional mode, and retain a flat low-frequency response if that is desired. The ability to switch between directional and omni-directional modes also enables the user to appreciate the advantages of the directional mode.[729] Figure 2.9 shows the two-dimensional directivity index versus frequency for various representative hearing aids. Note, however, that depending on the design (primarily the port spacing and internal low-pass filter or delay used), particular

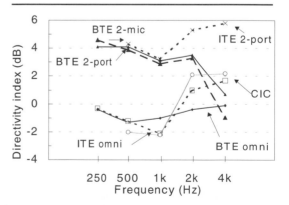

Figure 2.9 Directivity index, measured in the horizontal plane, for an omnidirectional BTE and a two-port BTE (Dillon & Macrae, 1984), a two-microphone BTE (Raicevich, 1997), a two-port ITE (Killion et al., 1998), and a CIC or the unaided ear (Dillon and Macrae, 1984).

---

[c]   A low cut-off frequency occurs if the internal delay is too large. A large internal delay is needed to achieve good low- and mid-frequency directivity if the microphone ports are placed too far apart.

hearing aids can have directivity indexes larger or smaller than those shown.

Directional microphones are particularly important to hearing aids because they are the only form of signal processing that can improve the *signal-to-noise ratio* (*SNR*) in a way that leads to improved intelligibility. The benefits are well established.[368, 472, 519, 903] The benefit decreases, however, as the environment becomes more reverberant, unless the signal source is very close to the listener.

The degree to which a conventional directional microphone improves speech understanding (when expressed as the SNR at which a 50% intelligibility score is obtained) is independent of the type of speech material or background noise.[962,d] The extent to which a conventional directional microphone improves the ability to understand non-reverberant speech in noise can be estimated by averaging the directivity across frequency. Because some frequencies contribute more to intelligibility than others, it is necessary to weight the DI at each frequency according to the importance of that frequency to intelligibility. A suitable set of weighting values is the importance function used in the *Articulation Index* (*AI*) method (which is also known as *Speech Intelligibility Index*).[331]

The weighted-average directivity index is thus known as the *AI-DI*. It tells us how much the noise level would have to be decreased if performance were to remain the same when an omni-directional microphone replaced a directional microphone. Every dB improvement in AI-DI results in an increase of speech understanding (for sentence material) of approximately 10 percentage points.

AI-DI values are close to 0 dB for omni-directional hearing aids, and range from 2 to 5 dB for two-port and two-microphone directional hearing aids. Because of this

variation across hearing aids, it is important to examine the specifications of a directional hearing aid to find out how effective its directional microphone is when mounted on a head. When noises come from a single direction, directional microphones can suppress noise to a much greater, or lesser, extent than indicated by the AI-DI value.

The interfering effect of background noise is the single greatest problem reported by hearing aid wearers. Directivity indexes even larger than those shown in Figure 2.9 can be obtained with hand-held or chest-worn microphone arrays. These accessories connect to hearing aids via a cable, wireless link, or magnetic loop/telecoil. These and other more complex (and effective) forms of directional microphones are covered in Section 7.1.1.

2.2.5   Microphone location

Hearing aid microphones are usually located within the hearing aid, but can be located in an accessory such as a hand-held microphone, a wireless transmitter, or a satellite microphone located on the opposite side of the head. These devices will be covered in Chapters 3 and 16, and the acoustic effects of different microphone locations will be covered in Section 4.2.2.

2.3   Amplifiers

The basic function of an amplifier is simply to make a small electrical signal into a larger electrical signal. Because the microphone has already converted the sound to electrical voltages and currents, the amplifiers can do three things. First, they can make the voltage larger, but not affect the current. Second, they can make the current larger, but not affect the voltage. (We have already met one of these inside the microphone case.) Third and most commonly, they can make both the voltage and the current larger.[e] All three options re-

---

d   This would not necessarily be true for hearing with a DI that varies markedly with frequency, especially if there were also marked differences between the noise spectra, or between the speech spectra.

e   For readers not familiar with voltage and current, a water analogy might be useful: Voltage is the equivalent of water *pressure*, whereas current is the equivalent of water *flow*.

sult in the signal having more power when it comes out of the amplifier than when it entered. Of course, this additional power must come from somewhere. The job of the amplifier is to take power from the battery and transfer it to the amplifier output in a manner controlled by the input signal. Thus, the output waveform (either voltage or current or both) is simply a larger version of the input waveform.

2.3.1   Amplifier technology

The key element in an amplifier that allows a current to be controlled by a smaller current (or by a small voltage) is the *transistor*. Although a single transistor will provide amplification, amplifiers usually are made up of several transistors and resistors connected together to provide better performance than is achievable with a single transistor. These multiple transistors and resistors are made, using photographic and chemical techniques, into an *integrated circuit (IC)*. Transistors can be made using one of two broadly different types of technology: bipolar and CMOS (Complementary Metal Oxide Semiconductor), each of which has advantages. Bipolar transistors tend to have lower internal noise, and CMOS transistors tend to use less battery power. Both types are used in hearing aids, and both can have acceptably low noise and power consumption. For hearing aid applications, an IC amplifier can contain from a few dozen to a few thousand transistors, depending on the complexity of the hearing aid.

Complete amplifiers also need other electrical components. *Diodes*, which allow current to flow one way but not the other, are used to sense the size of signals, and are built into the IC. *Capacitors* are needed for various purposes, including the making of filters. If they are small enough, these are also built into the IC. If not, separate, discrete capacitors have to be used.

In most hearing aids, the ICs are mounted onto *circuit boards* with electrical

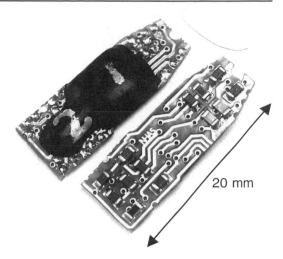

20 mm

Figure 2.10   An amplifier board from a high-power BTE hearing aid. Integrated circuits are mounted on one side (under the protective coating) and individual components are mounted on the other, The protective coating protects the ICs against physical damage and the ingress of moisture and contaminants.

connections already printed on them. These circuit boards can be made of fiberglass (which is rigid), or plastic (which is flexible). Alternatively, they can be made of rigid ceramic, in which case they are referred to as *substrates*. The boards fill two functions. First, they provide the electrical connections between discrete components (like capacitors) and the IC. Second, they make it easier for the person (or machine) assembling the hearing aid to connect other devices (like battery terminals and volume controls) to the amplifier than if the connection had to be made directly to the IC. The circuit boards with their IC(s) and other components are often referred to as *hybrids* (because they contain different types of electronic devices), though sometimes this term is reserved for boards made of ceramic material.

2.3.2   Amplifier performance

While the construction details of amplifiers are sometimes used in the marketing of hearing aids, it is the performance of amplifiers that really matters. An ideal amplifier would have the gain-frequency response required, would generate no noise internally, and would not distort the signal, no matter how large the input signal was. Real amplifiers live up to this ideal to varying degrees. The most noticeable deviation from ideal occurs when signals get too large for an amplifier to handle properly.

2.3.3   Peak clipping and distortion

Amplifiers cannot produce signals larger in voltage than some specified maximum. This maximum is usually equal to, or related to, the battery voltage. If the biggest signal in the amplifier (usually the output signal) is near this maximum, and either the input signal level or the gain of the amplifier is increased, then the amplifier will clip (remove) the peaks of the signal. An exception to this occurs for amplifiers containing compression limiting, as discussed in Section 2.3.5.

Figure 2.11 shows the output waveform that results from *peak clipping* when the input signal is a sine wave. The thin line shows what the output signal would be if no peak clipping occurred. Because the output is no longer a sine wave, it contains components at frequencies not in the input signal. These additional components are called *distortion*

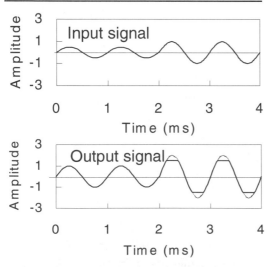

Figure 2.11 A linearly amplified and a peak clipped signal.

products. When the input is a sine wave, the distortion products occur at frequencies that are harmonics (i.e. integer multiples) of the input frequency. Consequently, the process is called *harmonic distortion*. All amplifiers create some distortion, and all amplifiers create large amounts of distortion if the signal is sufficiently peak clipped. If the peak clipping is symmetrical, the distortion products occur only at odd harmonics of the input frequency. If it is asymmetrical, then even and odd harmonics are likely to be produced. Usually, the low-order harmonics (the second and the third) are the most powerful. Consequently, distortion is sometimes quantified by expressing the power of each of these two components relative to the power of the wanted signal. More commonly, the power of all the distortion products is summed and expressed relative to the power of the wanted output signal component. This ratio is referred to as *total harmonic distortion (THD)*.

Distortion degrades the quality of speech and other signals when present in moderate amounts.[8, 185, 364, 438, 856] When present in larger amounts it also degrades intelligibility.[184, 185, 323, 423] Even when the distortion represents only 10% of the total signal power, speech quality is adversely affected.[516] Section 9.6.2 will discuss under what circumstances peak clipping is acceptable, and sometimes even recommended, for use in hearing aids.

When a more complex signal is peak clipped, the distortion products occur at frequencies that are harmonics of all the frequencies in the input signal, and at frequencies that are combinations of all the harmonics. If two tones, with frequencies f_1 and f_2 are input, for example, distortion components will occur at $2f_1$, $3f_1$, $4f_1$, $2f_2$, $3f_2$, $4f_2$, f_2-f_1, $2f_2$-f_1, $2f_1$-f_2, $3f_1$-f_2, to name but a few frequencies. Although the mechanism causing the distortion is exactly the same as for harmonic distortion (peak clipping is the most common cause), the result is called *intermodulation distortion*, because the distortion products arise from the modulation (mixing) of all the components in the input signal with each other.

Although peak clipping has been discussed here in the context of amplifier performance, hearing aid microphones (uncommonly) and receivers (more commonly) can also peak clip a signal.

2.3.4   Output amplifiers

Although a hearing aid may contain many amplifiers, the final amplifier, called the output amplifier, is especially important. This amplifier has to output more powerful signals than any of the other amplifiers, and so it uses more of the battery current than any of the others. Also, its output signal usually has a voltage larger than any of the others, so if peak clipping occurs anywhere, it is most likely to occur in the output amplifier. Peak clipping does, however, sometimes occur in earlier amplifiers, particularly in badly designed hearing aids. There are four varieties of amplifiers used in hearing aids, referred to as Class A, Class B, Class D, and Class H.

Class A Amplifiers

Class A amplifiers are the simplest type of amplifier. The final transistor is arranged (the technical term is **biased**) so that a steady amount of current flows through it to the receiver when the amplifier is not receiving any audio signal. This steady current causes a steady deflection of the receiver diaphragm, which does not cause an audible sound, except for a click when the amplifier is first turned on. When a signal is input to the Class A amplifier, positive parts of the input waveform cause the output current to increase, while negative parts of the input waveform cause the output current to decrease. Figure 2.12 shows an example.

A little thought will show that because the output current cannot decrease below zero, the largest negative signal that the amplifier can output is equal to the original steady current, which is known as the **quiescent**

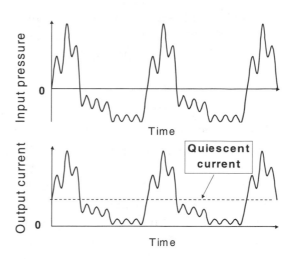

Figure 2.12 Output current of a Class A amplifier in response to an input audio voltage.

current. This creates a dilemma for the hearing aid designer. On the one hand, this quiescent current should be made as small as possible so that battery life is as long as possible. On the other hand, the quiescent current should be as large as possible so that the negative peaks of the waveform are not clipped. This no-win situation has led many hearing aids to be designed so that peak clipping occurs even for moderate level output signals. These hearing aids have been referred to as "crummy-peak-clipping" or "starved Class A" hearing aids. The terms are useful, because they illustrate that Class A amplifiers do not intrinsically have high distortion, just when their operating current is limited. In fact, Class A amplifiers have extremely low distortion when operating current is not a concern.

Class A amplifiers are, however, inherently inefficient. They consume output current even when the hearing aid is not amplifying a signal. That is, their operating current is equal to their quiescent current. Even when a (pure tone) signal is present, the Class A amplifier can, at best, transfer 50% of the power it uses to the receiver; the remaining power only heats up the amplifier. Efficiency decreases markedly as the signal waveform becomes more peaky, as is the case for speech waveforms. The usage of Class A amplifiers is decreasing. They are suitable only for very low-power hearing aids, and even for these, they will probably not be optimal.

Class B amplifiers

Class B amplifiers are the traditional way to decrease the power wasted in the output amplifier. The Class B amplifier comprises two separate amplifiers, shown as X and Y in Figure 2.13, each with zero (or a very small) quiescent current. One of the amplifiers (amplifier Y in Figure 2.13) is fed with an inverted version of the input signal (i.e. the waveform multiplied by -1). Each amplifier handles one half of the waveform: amplifier X pushes the receiver diaphragm in one direction and amplifier Y pulls it in the other.[f] Not surprisingly, Class B amplifiers are also called ***push-pull amplifiers***.

Because their output power is not limited by their quiescent power, Class B amplifiers are particularly suitable for high-power amplifiers (and hence high-power hearing aids). They are still not ideal amplifiers: Their theoretical maximum efficiency for a sine wave at maximum power is only 79% (i.e., 21% of the power drawn from the battery never makes it to the receiver). Again, their efficiency is further decreased for peaky signals with larger crest factors (like speech) and for smaller signals. Another disadvantage is that Class B

amplifiers often must have large capacitors connected to them, and this makes it harder to construct a very small hearing aid.

Class D amplifiers

Class D amplifiers were introduced to hearing aids in the late 1980s when they were incorporated into the same metal can that contained the receiver. Instead of directly amplifying the audio signal, a Class D amplifier uses the audio signal to modulate (i.e. vary) the width of each pulse within a high-frequency (e.g. 100 kHz) train of pulses. Although each pulse always has the maximum possible voltage (the battery voltage), the strength of the pulse also depends on the pulse length. An intense signal can thus be generated by a series of long pulses separated by brief gaps, and a weak signal by a series of short pulses separated by long gaps. Negative signals are handled by switching the pulses through the receiver coil in the opposite direction, or by using two coils, as for Class B amplifiers. Because at any instant the maximum possible voltage is applied to the receiver, the Class D amplifier has a theoretical maximum efficiency of 100%, no matter what type or strength of signal is being amplified. Although the signal delivered to the receiver is being switched on and off at the pulse rate (e.g. 100,000 times a second), the receiver is unable to respond to this rate, partly because the coil smoothes out the current, and partly because the diaphragm cannot vibrate this rapidly. Consequently, the receiver outputs a smooth audio signal, as required. Because of the switching action they employ, Class D amplifiers are also called ***switching amplifiers***.

Class D amplifiers, because of their greater efficiency, will probably completely replace Class A and B devices, though Class B may remain the best choice for very high-powered amplifiers for some time. Even digital hearing aids use a principle similar to the class D amplifier for their output stage, as discussed in Section 2.4.3.

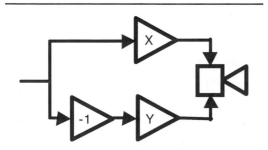

Figure 2.13 Block diagram of the Class B or push-pull amplifier.

---

[f]   This is achieved either by using a receiver with two coils wound in opposite directions, or by making one of the amplifiers deliver current and the other amplifier accept current.

Class H amplifiers

A Class H amplifier is a Class A amplifier that has a variable bias current. It is also called a sliding Class A amplifier. When a strong signal is being amplified, the bias current is increased, and when a weak signal is being amplified, the bias current is decreased. This enables the amplifier to operate at the maximum efficiency possible for a Class A device, but this is still less than the efficiency possible with Class D devices. Class H amplifiers inevitably add some distortion to the signal. They cannot slide slowly, or peak clipping will occur while they are adjusting, but if they slide too fast, the changing bias current will itself be audible.

2.3.5   Compression amplifiers

Section 1.1.2 discussed how people with sensorineural hearing impairment have dynamic ranges smaller than normal, so that less amplification is required for intense input sounds than for weak input sounds. Chapter 6 and Section 9.3 will further elaborate on how the amount of amplification could and should decrease as input level increases. It is the job of the compression amplifier to achieve this change of amplification when input level changes. The concept is simple and dates back to 1937: [836] *a compressor is nothing more than an amplifier that turns down its own gain as the input to (or the output from) the amplifier increases.*

Figure 2.14 shows the block diagram of a *feedback compressor*. The signal at the feedback point, *F*, is fed to the level-detecting device, which converts the rapidly varying audio signal into a more slowly varying control signal. The size of the control signal represents the level of the signal at *F* averaged in some desired way over some appropriate period. The control signal is fed back into the control input, *C*, of the compression amplifier and tells the compression amplifier how much gain should be applied to the input signal. We can immediately see why the waveform at *F* cannot be applied directly to the control input of the compression amplifier: If the

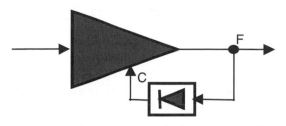

Figure 2.14 Basic feedback type compression amplifier block diagram.

compressor gain decreased every time the instantaneous waveform increased in size, the compressor would distort the detailed shape of the waveform. The compressor is meant to leave the fine detail in the waveform unchanged, while it more gradually varies the gain applied to the waveform. A compression amplifier is also called an *automatic gain control* (*AGC*) or *automatic volume control* (*AVC*). The last term is used only when the compressor varies the gain very slowly.

Figure 2.15 shows the effect that a compressor might have on an input signal that varies in level. Notice that the difference in level between the low and high intensity parts of the signal has been decreased, but the detail of the waveform has not been significantly affected. The compressor functions just as if a human finger inside the hearing aid had rapidly, but smoothly, turned down the volume control as soon as the output signal increased in level.

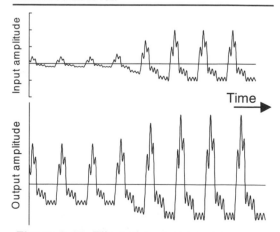

Figure 2.15 Effect of a compressor on a waveform varying in level.

2.4 Digital Circuits

The amplifiers and signals discussed in the preceding sections all strictly relate to *analog* technology. In analog technology, which has been around since the invention of the telephone, an electrical voltage (or current) is *analogous* to the acoustic sound pressure, hence the name. When the sound pressure increases from one moment to the next, so too does the electrical signal. A newer technology, which has been used in research for twenty years, became available in head-worn hearing aids in the mid-1990s. This, of course is *digital* technology. The advantages of digital technology include greater precision, less internal noise, and the ability to do complex operations in small ICs that consume little power. The special application of digital circuits to hearing aids will be covered in Section 3.4 and throughout Chapter 7, but the basic components of digital technology are described in the following sections. As in analog hearing aids, digital hearing aids use a microphone to convert sound to an analog voltage.

2.4.1 Analog-to-digital converters

In digital technology, sound is represented as an ever-changing string of numbers. It is the job of the *analog-to-digital converter* (*ADC*) to change the analog electrical voltage coming from the microphone into these numbers. *Sampling* is the first step in this process. A signal is sampled by first noting the size of the signal at regular intervals in time, and totally ignoring the value of the signal at other times between these sampling points. If we want the sampled signal to be a good representation of the original signal, these samples must be obtained very often. They must follow each other more quickly than the signal waveform can make marked changes of course. It can be shown mathematically that no information about the original signal is lost provided the *sampling frequency* (also called

sampling rate) is greater than twice the highest frequency component present in a complex signal. Thus, if a hearing aid is to faithfully amplify signals up to, say, 10 kHz, the sampling frequency has to be at least 20 kHz. This means the waveform is sampled every 1/20,000 of a second, or every 50 μs. In practice the sampling frequency has to be about 20% higher than the theoretical minimum frequency (e.g. 22 kHz in the above example).

A hearing aid has to contain a low-pass filter to make sure that signals going into the analog-to-digital converter are indeed lower in frequency than half the sampling frequency.[g] This filter is called the *anti-aliasing filter*. It gets this name because if a signal component with a frequency *greater* than half the sampling frequency gets into the analog-to-digital converter, the hearing aid will amplify this signal as though it has a frequency *lower* than half the sampling frequency. That is, signals with excessive frequency *alias* themselves down to lower frequencies. The anti-aliasing filter, which may be an intrinsic part of the analog-to-digital conversion process, prevents this undesirable aliasing from occurring.

Having sampled the waveform, each of these samples then has to be represented as a number. The designer of a digital system decides how many different numbers are going to be allowed. Suppose, for simplicity, only the eight integers from 0 to 7 were to be allowed. The waveform shown at the top of Figure 2.16 would be represented by the numbers (called the *code*) shown at the bottom of the figure, because these numbers are the allowable code values closest to the actual sample values. The sampled waveform has now been *digitized*.

One more step remains. The digitized code values are broken up into *bits*. The word *bit* is a contraction of the words *binary digit*. The numerals we use in everyday life are allowed

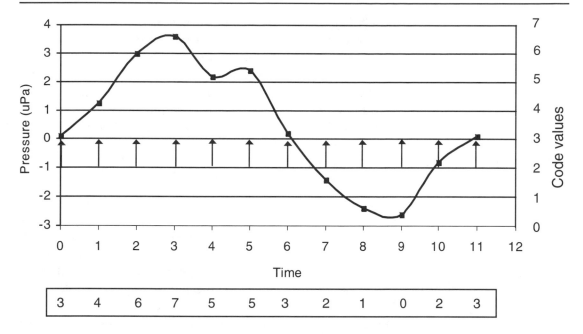

Figure 2.16 An analog waveform, the sampled values (shown by the dots on the waveform), the sampling signal (represented by the regular series of arrows), and the digitized codes that approximate and represent the sampled values (enclosed in the rectangle).

to have only one of ten values (from 0 to 9), and we make up bigger numbers by combining them using multipliers of ten or a hundred, and so on. Binary digits are allowed to have only two values (0 or 1), and we make up bigger numbers by combining them using multipliers of 2, 4, 8, 16, and so on. The numbers shown at the bottom of Figure 2.16 are repeated in Table 2.1, and the corresponding bits are shown there.

Table 2.1 Break-up of the digitized code values of Figure 2.16 into three-bit words.

Digitized code		Fours	Twos	Ones
3	=	0	1	1
4	=	1	0	0
6	=	1	1	0
7	=	1	1	1
5	=	1	0	1
5	=	1	0	1
3	=	0	1	1
2	=	0	1	0
1	=	0	0	1
0	=	0	0	0
2	=	0	1	0
3	=	0	1	1

A little thought will show that just as we can represent eight numbers (0 to 7 inclusive) with a three-bit word, we can represent 16 numbers with a four-bit word, 32 numbers with a five-bit word, and so on. Home compact disk players use a 16-bit word to represent sounds, and this word length means that 65,536 different numbers can be represented. Hearing aids use a similar number or slightly lower number of bits. Eight bits comprise the *byte* that computer enthusiasts talk about when bragging about how much memory their computer or hard disk has. The memory capacity of these devices is usually measured in Megabytes (a million bytes) and Gigabytes (a billion bytes) respectively.

Digital hearing aids also require memory, so that their electroacoustic performance can be programmed to suit particular aid wearers. The memory size of hearing aids, measured in Kilobytes and eventually Megabytes will soon be part of the specification sheet of hearing aids as well.

Why is it necessary to break the sampled values up into bits? First, it is convenient for computers, because they can most efficiently represent signals as either *on* or *off* and these can easily be thought of as the two values of a binary digit. More importantly, having only two allowable values makes a signal almost incorruptible when it is stored, transmitted, or used in any way. Suppose that inside a hearing aid, a "0" corresponds to 0 Volts, and a "1" corresponds to 1 Volt. What will happen if electrical noise inside a hearing aid causes the 0 V signal to be turned into, say 0.1 V as the signal is passed from one part of the hearing aid to the next? Nothing! The next stage of the hearing aid knows that signals are allowed only to be 0 V or 1 V, so it treats the corrupted signal as if it was the closest allowable value, which is 0 V. The internal hearing aid noise has caused no error whatsoever, whereas in an analog signal the noise would be inextricably mixed up with the signal and would eventually get passed to the hearing aid wearer. Note that this advantage applies only to noise generated internally after the microphone, not noise picked up by the hearing aid or created within the microphone.

2.4.2   Digital signal processors

Apart from adding little or no noise, conversion to digital form carries a second advantage. Once sound has been represented as a series of numbers, we can modify the sound just by doing arithmetic with the numbers. For example, if we wished to amplify a sound by 6 dB, then we must double the amplitude of the sound. Simply multiplying each number by 2 will do this. For greater amplification, we multiply each sample of the sound by a larger number. Suitable combinations of arithmetic operations accomplish other changes to the sound. For example, to make a low-pass filter, we can take each sample of the sound and add to it some fraction of the preceding sample. We can think of this as averaging or smoothing a series of numbers, which decreases the size of any rapid fluctuations that are present (i.e., the high-frequency components). Using

arithmetic, we can modify the sound in just about any way that we can with analog electronics. Fortunately, digital electronics can do more than simply mimic analog electronics. General digital processing techniques and some specific signal processing algorithms will be discussed in detail in Section 3.4 and Chapter 7.

2.4.3   Digital-to-analog converters

After the digital signal processor has altered the sound in some desired manner, the hearing aid must present the modified and amplified sound to the aid wearer. As there is no use presenting the aid wearer with a string of numbers, the modified numbers must be converted into an acoustical signal. This conversion is the job of the *digital-to-analog converter* (*DAC*) combined with the hearing aid receiver. Digital devices have traditionally done this by having a digital-to-analog converter that outputs an analog voltage, which in turn is fed to a receiver of some type to make the final conversion to sound.

To minimize power consumption, digital hearing aids use a different solution. The multiple bits that comprise each sample are converted into a single bit that changes at a rate many times higher than the sample rate. This principle is very similar to the Class D operating principle discussed in Section 2.3.4. The converter is referred to as a *digital-to-digital converter*. The high-speed serial output from this converter is fed to the receiver, which averages out the high-speed variations in the digital signal to produce a smooth analog signal. The receiver thus forms part of the overall digital-to-analog converter. The electronic part of the digital-to-analog converter can be located either with all the other amplifier parts or inside the metal can that houses the receiver.

2.5   Tone Controls and Filters

Tone controls in hearing aids have the same function as tone controls in home stereos: they cause the gain of the amplifier to vary with

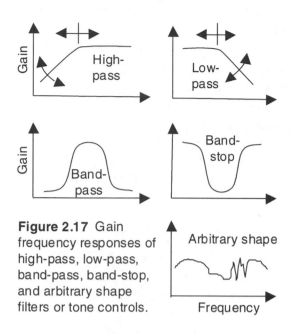

Figure 2.17 Gain frequency responses of high-pass, low-pass, band-pass, band-stop, and arbitrary shape filters or tone controls.

frequency. Tone controls get their name because they affect the *tonal quality*, or *timbre*, of sounds passing through them. The basic electronic structure that causes gain to vary with frequency is the *filter*. Filters are known by their effect on signals: *high-pass filters* provide more gain to high-frequency sounds than to low-frequency sounds, which gives the sound a treble, or shrill quality. Similarly, *band-pass filters* provide more gain to frequencies in a certain band than they do to either higher or lower frequencies, and *low-pass filters* provide more gain to low-frequency sounds than they do to high-frequency sounds. Most filters used in hearing aids in the past have been high-pass, low-pass, or band-pass. Digital circuits make it more easily possible to achieve an arbitrary response shape, such as that shown in Figure 2.17.

A tone control is constructed by making one or more of the electronic components within a filter controllable by a screwdriver control, or by a computer used to program the hearing aid. A high-pass filter, for example, can have its response varied by changing the *corner frequency* (also called the *cut-off frequency*)

of the filter, or by changing the *slope* of the filter, as indicated by the arrows in Figure 2.17. Slopes of filters are commonly integer multiples of 6 dB per octave (e.g. 6, 12, 18, 24 dB per octave).

2.5.1 Filter and tone control structures

For many years, hearing aids had one, or at most two, tone controls. Many hearing aids had a high-pass tone control (usually referred to as a *low-tone cut*), and some had a low-pass filter as well (usually referred to as a *high-tone cut*). Figure 2.18 shows a block diagram of a hearing aid comprising one low-pass, and one high-pass filter, and also shows the range of frequency responses that such a hearing aid can typically provide. The structure shown in Figure 2.18 is referred to as a serial structure, because all the sound passes through all the blocks, one after the other. Although combinations of high- and low-pass filters in a serial structure allows reasonable flexibility of response shape, flexibility is not ideal unless one of the filters can be made to have an arbitrary response shape.

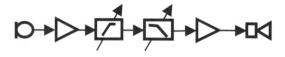

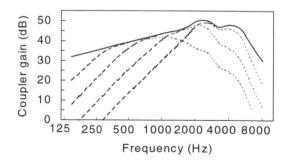

Figure 2.18 Block diagram of a serial structure, single-band hearing aid, and a range of low cut (dashed curves) and high cut (dotted curves) variations that might be made to the basic response (solid line).

Terminology: Multi-band or multi-channel?

The terms *multi-band* and *multi-channel* are usually used interchangeably, although some authors and hearing aid companies differentiate between them. Many hearing aids selectively filter those parts of a signal that lie within a certain frequency range, and process these parts differently from those parts of the signal at other frequencies. It is extremely important what this processing is (e.g. amplification or compression) but there is no form of processing that would dictate whether the group of signal components be called a *channel* rather than a *band* or vice versa. It could perhaps be helpful to use *band* to mean the components or frequency range in question, and to use *channel* to mean the physical chain of devices through which this band of signal components pass.

Parallel structures, such as shown earlier in the block diagram in Figure 2.2, generally allow more flexibility, even with simple filters. The filters divide the sound into adjacent frequency regions. These are variously called **bands** or **channels**. Sound in each region can then be amplified (or whatever) more or less independently of sound in other regions.[h] After the parts of the signal falling within each band have been amplified to the required degree, the parts are recombined in the adder.

2.5.2 Passive, active, and digital tone controls

Tone controls and filters can be divided into three broad types, depending on the technology used to implement them. The simplest type of tone control is based on a **passive** filter. These filters usually comprise very few components and consume no power from the battery. They are very simple to make, but unfortunately do not vary the gain-frequency response very effectively. Passive filters usually cause cuts of only 6 dB per octave, though cuts of 12 dB per octave are also possible. Even then, there is a very gradual transition from the frequencies that are cut to the frequencies that are passed without significant attenuation.

Using an amplifier at the heart of the filter can make better filters and tone controls.

These **active** filters consume a small amount of power from the battery. However, steeper cuts and boosts are achievable, and the response can go from significant attenuation to no attenuation over a very small frequency range, as shown in Figure 2.19.

The third type of filter is used mainly in digital circuits and is based on mathematical operations. If a signal is sampled in time, as discussed in Section 2.4.1, an output sample can be calculated by combining a fraction of the current input sample with fractions of each of the previous n samples, where n is the **length** of the filter. (To gain access to the previous input samples, they are temporarily

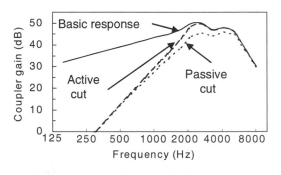

Figure 2.19 High pass responses achievable with passive and active tone controls, both having a cut of 12 dB per octave for the lowest frequencies.

---

[h]   Control of gain in each frequency region will be independent of gain in the other frequency regions provided each of the filters has a slope sufficiently steep to prevent sound from leaking to adjacent frequency bands.

stored and then discarded.) Filters made in this way can generate arbitrarily shaped responses. That is, we are not limited to simple low-pass, high-pass or band-pass filters. These filters are said to have a *finite impulse response (FIR)* because once the input signal ceases, the output completely dies away a short time later.

If the output sample at a given time is also made to depend on the output samples at previous times, then every input signal will have an effect on the output that lasts for ever (though its effect continuously gets smaller with time). These filters are said to have an *infinite impulse response (IIR)*. Their advantage is that even more complex filter shapes can be generated with few computations. Their disadvantage is that they are harder to design and can become unstable and oscillate. The terms FIR and IIR are likely to become part of hearing aid terminology as hearing aids increasingly become digital, because the filters are easy to implement in digital systems. These filters can also be made in devices in which the waveforms have been sampled, but left as analog voltages rather than converted to numbers. These analog voltages are switched from one capacitor to another in a suitable circuit so the filters are called *switched-capacitor filters*.

2.6   Receivers

The receiver, which externally looks just like the microphone shown earlier in Figure 2.3, converts the amplified and modified electrical signal into an acoustic output signal.

2.6.1   Principle of operation

The receiver operates by magnetic forces. Figure 2.20 shows the receiver's operating principle and the basis of construction.[256] Current passes through a coil that encloses a piece of metal, temporarily turning it into a magnet. As the current alternates in direction, this piece of metal, called an *armature*, is alternately attracted and repelled by two

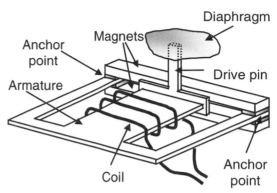

Figure 2.20 Principle of operation of the moving coil receiver.

permanent magnets. The armature is very thin and can bend, so the end of the middle arm of the armature is free to move up and down between the magnets. The free end of the armature is linked by a drive-pin to the diaphragm, so that the *diaphragm* also vibrates backwards and forwards, and this produces the sound. Only a portion of the diaphragm is shown in Figure 2.20. This transducer seems simple, but making all this in such a way that it has a wide frequency response, consumes little power, leaks little magnetic field outside the case, and occupies almost no volume is a major technological feat.

An important implication of the construction is that the receiver will peak-clip, and hence not operate linearly, once the armature travels sufficiently far that it touches either of the magnets. Greater output can be obtained only by using a receiver with a bigger diaphragm, which increases the size of the receiver, or with the magnets further apart, which then requires greater electrical power for the receiver to operate.

2.6.2   Frequency response of receivers

Figure 2.21 shows the frequency response of a receiver connected to the tubing used in a BTE hearing aid and earmold. What causes

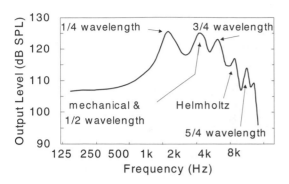

Figure 2.21 Frequency response of a receiver in a BTE hearing aid.

all these bumps and dips? Mostly, it is the tubing. This tubing comprises a short length of tubing inside the hearing aid, the earhook, and finally the flexible tubing terminating at the tip of the earmold. The combined length of these tubes typically has a length of 3 inches, or 75 mm. The earmold end of the tubing opens out into the ear canal, which, being wider than the tube, has an acoustic impedance less than that of the tube. The hearing aid end of the tubing system connects, eventually, to the receiver. Because the receiver is so small, it has a high acoustic output impedance (compared to the impedance of air in the tube). This means that acoustically, the tube has one end almost open and one end almost closed.

Such tubes have **wavelength resonances** at odd multiples of the speed of sound divided by four times the length of the tube.[i] This produces resonances at around 1 kHz, 3 kHz, and 5 kHz. The resonance at 4 kHz appears to be a **Helmholtz resonance** between the mass of air in the tube and the volume (and hence compliance) of air inside the receiver.[165] The bump at 2 kHz is primarily caused by the **mechanical resonance** of the receiver:

the mass of the diaphragm and springiness, or compliance, of the diaphragm combined with the compliance of the air inside the receiver. Even this resonance, however, is affected by the tubing. At its resonant frequency, the receiver actually has a low acoustic impedance, so at this frequency, the tube acts as though it is acoustically open at both ends. It then has a resonance at multiples of the speed of sound divided by twice the length of the tube. This occurs at about 2 kHz, so the second bump in Figure 2.21 is actually a resonance of both the receiver and the tubing.[165]

Figure 2.22 shows the frequency response typical in a receiver for an ITE or ITC hearing aid. There are only two peaks, one somewhere in the range 2.2 to 3 kHz, and one around 5 kHz. The first of these is the mechanical resonance in the receiver. It is often at a frequency higher than occurs in BTE hearing aids because ITE and ITC aids usually have a smaller receiver with a lighter, stiffer diaphragm. It is desirable for receivers to have a peak in the 2.5 to 3 kHz range because the unaided adult ear has a natural resonance in this frequency range (again the result of a quarter wave resonance, this time of the ear

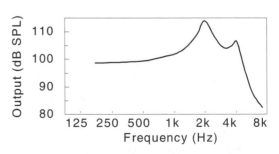

Figure 2.22 Frequency response of a receiver in an ITE or ITC hearing aid, connected to a 2 cc coupler via a tube 10 mm long and 1 mm in inner diameter.

---

[i]   Wavelength resonances are created by the sound wave reflecting backwards whenever the tube they are travelling in changes its diameter, and hence its impedance. An open end and a closed end are extreme examples of a change in impedance. The tube with one open and one closed end is said to have a quarter wave resonance, because at the resonant frequency, the length of the tube equals one quarter of a wavelength.

canal). Consequently, a receiver resonance at this frequency helps the hearing aid restore the natural resonance and gain that is lost when the hearing aid is inserted in the ear. Different resonant frequencies in the hearing aid can be achieved by using different model receivers. Once a particular receiver is chosen, the hearing aid manufacturer can alter the resonant frequency a little by changing the electrical output impedance of the hearing aid amplifier, though only some brands and models of hearing aids have this flexibility. The higher frequency peak in ITE, ITC and CIC hearing aids is predominantly caused by a quarter-wave resonance of the receiver tubing.

When coupled with suitable tubing (see Chapter 5) and dampers (next section), receivers can have a smooth, wide frequency response to 8 kHz or more that allows a very good sound quality to be achieved.[474] It is not yet possible, however, to achieve a flat response out to 8 kHz in a very high power receiver.

2.7   Acoustic Dampers

Does it matter whether the receiver response has bumps and dips, and does it matter what causes them? The answer to both questions is yes! Peaks and troughs (especially peaks) in the gain-frequency response adversely affect speech intelligibility[421] and quality[517] of the amplified sound. Peaks become objectionable if they rise by more than 6 dB above the smooth curve joining the dips.[232] Peaks caused by the receiver and tubing affect the shape of the maximum output curve of the hearing aid just as much as they affect the shape of the gain-frequency response. Such peaks make it harder to get all sounds loud enough without some sounds becoming excessively loud (see Section 9.6).

Understanding the cause of the peaks and troughs is important because the cause of a peak determines how its size can be decreased. Placing an acoustic resistor, also

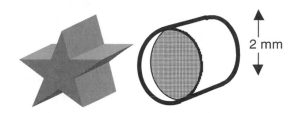

Figure 2.23 A star damper and a fused-mesh damper that can be inserted inside #13 tubing of internal diameter 1.93 mm.

called a damper in the tubing at an appropriate place decreases the peaks. One type of damper consists of a fine mesh (like a fly screen designed to stop *extremely* small insects) inserted across a small metal cylinder or ferrule, as shown in Figure 2.23. As the particles of air move backwards and forwards, in response to the sound wave in the tube, they lose energy when they have to change course slightly to avoid the wires in the mesh so that they can flow through the holes in the mesh. The more quickly the particles are flowing, the more energy they will lose when the mesh is added. In a tube, the particles flow most quickly at the resonant frequencies, and they flow most quickly at the open end of the tube, and at any location a half-wavelength away from an open end. Thus, a damper will decrease the receiver output most at the resonant frequencies, but only if the damper is placed in an appropriate place (see Section 5.5).

Apart from the fused-mesh dampers just described, dampers are also made from sintered stainless steel (fine particles of metal). Another variety, made of plastic, looks like a star-shaped prism, and is known as a star damper. Dampers are also made from lamb's wool and from plastic foam. The degree to which a damper decreases resonant peaks depends on the impedance of the damper, which is determined by the fineness, length, and number of air paths through the damper. Fused-mesh dampers and sintered-steel dampers are available in a range of standard impedances. The impedance of star dampers, lamb's wool dampers, and foam dampers is varied by using different lengths of material.

Dampers can be placed in the tubing connected to a receiver or in the inlet port of the microphone. Some receivers have dampers built-in when they are manufactured. Damping in different places to achieve specific effects will be covered in Section 5.5.

2.8   Telecoils

A *telecoil* is a small coil of wire that produces a voltage when an alternating magnetic field flows through it. The magnetic field to be picked up by the telecoil is generated by an electrical current that has the same waveform as the original audio signal. This magnetic field may occur as a by-product of some device, such as from a loudspeaker or a receiver in a telephone, or may be generated intentionally by a loop of wire around a room or other small area. The process of an electrical current inducing a voltage in a coil some distance away is called *induction*. Induction loop systems are discussed in more detail in Section 3.6.

To increase the effectiveness of a telecoil, the wire is coiled around a rod made of *ferrite* material. Like iron, but even more so, ferrite provides an easy path for magnetic fields to flow through. It thus attracts and concentrates the magnetic flux. If more flux flows through the coil, then more voltage is generated by the coil, which is desirable so that the audio signal is large compared to the internal noise generated by the hearing aid. The other ways to make coils more sensitive are to increase their area, and number of turns, but both of these increase the physical size of the coil.

Not all hearing aids include a telecoil, although most behind-the-ear hearing aids and many ITE hearing aids do so. The hearing aid user can select the coil, instead of the microphone, for amplification by switching the hearing aid to the *T* (for Telecoil) position. In

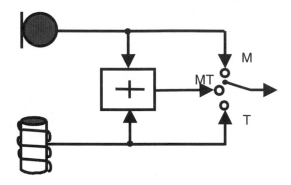

Figure 2.24 Block diagram of the input stage of a hearing aid with M, T, and MT selector switch.

the *M* position, only the microphone is connected to the hearing aid amplifier. Some hearing aids also include an *MT* position in which the outputs from the coil and microphone are combined. Figure 2.24 shows the block diagram of the input stage of such a hearing aid. The MT combination is useful if the aid wearer wants to receive both the acoustic and magnetic signals simultaneously or in quick succession, but has the disadvantage that any acoustic noise present will be amplified even if the aid wearer is trying to listen only to the magnetic signal.

2.9   Audio (Electrical) Input

An alternative way to get an audio signal into a hearing aid is to connect it via an electrical cable. This is referred to as *direct audio input*. The electrical audio signal may have originated from equipment such as a tape recorder, a hand-held microphone, or an FM wireless receiver (see Section 3.7.2). If the device producing the signal is itself receiving a clear signal (i.e., with little added noise or reverberation) the device should also be able to output a clear signal to the hearing aid. Provided the signal put into the hearing aid is not so large that it overloads the hearing aid, and not so small that it is obscured by noise generated within the hearing aid, then the hearing aid too will be able to output a clear signal. Furthermore, the hearing aid will be able to shape the signal in the right way for the individual aid wearer: The frequency response, maximum output, and other amplification characteristics applied to the signal will be just as if the hearing aid microphone picked up the sound directly.

In fact, the direct audio input connector is normally connected into the same part of the hearing aid (the input amplifier) to which the hearing aid microphone is connected. This means that the size of the signal should be about the same as for signals sent by the microphone, which is about 1 mV for typical input levels. In some hearing aids, the input connector and the microphone are simply connected together. In other hearing aids, they are connected via a switch, so that the user can select either the microphone input, the audio input, or a mixture of both.

When the hearing aid does not contain such a switch, what happens when the microphone sends one signal to the hearing aid amplifier while the external device sends another signal to the amplifier via the direct audio input? The answer depends on the *output impedance* of the external device connected to the hearing aid. Hearing aid microphones have an output impedance of about 3000 ohms. If the output impedance of the external device is much less than 3000 ohms, the external device wins the struggle to control the hearing aid, so the internal microphone output is greatly attenuated. Conversely, if the output impedance of the external device is much greater than that of the microphone, the microphone wins the struggle. When the two devices have about the same impedance, each causes the other to be attenuated by 6 dB, and the aid wearer hears the two signals evenly mixed together.

Some FM wireless systems use this dependence on output impedance to automatically attenuate the hearing aid microphone when they wish to send a signal to the hearing aid, without needing the user to make any adjustments (see Section 3.7.3).

2.10 Remote Controls

Remote controls serve the same function for hearing aids that they do for televisions or video players: they allow the user to vary the way a device works without having to actually touch it. The advantage of a remote control for hearing aids is primarily one of size. Because hearing aids are so small, it is difficult to fit many, or sometimes any, user controls on them. Also, because a hearing aid is located in or behind the ear, the user cannot see the controls, and so may have trouble locating a control, particularly if the hearing aid does indeed have more than one.

Buttons on the remote control are easier to operate than those on the hearing aid partly because they are larger, and partly because the user can look directly at the controls while they are being operated. Alternatively, some users like to operate the remote control while it is in their pocket because it does not draw attention to the hearing aid, as can occur when the aid itself is manipulated.

A remote control usually has a volume control. It may also enable the user to select an alternative program or programs (see Section 3.3.2). Other features that are commonly provided on remote controls include selection of telecoil, electrical audio input, directional versus omni-directional microphone response, tone control, and on-off switch.

Remote controls work by transmitting electrical signals to the hearing aid. These signals can have any effect on the aid that a switch actually located on the hearing aid could have. Various methods of transmission are used in hearing aids currently available. Some of these are explained in more detail (in the context of transmitting audio signals) in Chapter 3.

Infrared. This uses the same technology as used for television remote controls, and transmits an infrared light wave. The remote control must be within "sight" of the hearing aid and pointed towards it. The hearing aid contains an infrared detector on its exterior.

Ultrasonic. The remote control transmits an acoustic wave too high in frequency to be heard (by humans), but which can be received by the hearing aid microphone. It also requires line of sight operation.

Radio wave. An electromagnetic radio wave is transmitted by the remote and received by a small aerial within the hearing aid.

Magnetic induction. The control signals are transmitted from the remote to the hearing aid by creating a magnetic field at a frequency above the audible range. The hearing aid receives this using either a special purpose coil or the same telecoil that receives audio magnetic signals.

Each of these methods has its advantages and disadvantages,[928] as summarized in Table 2.2. A concern that is sometimes raised about the use of remote controls is their potential to interfere with *pacemakers*. Because pacemakers are designed to sense small voltages, it is very sensible to be concerned about interference from sources of electrical or magnetic energy. Although remote controls put out only a small amount of power, they could be operated in extremely close proximity to the pacemaker. Because there are multiple brands of pacemakers and multiple brands of remote controls, it is difficult for manufacturers of either type of device to give any guarantees about freedom from interference.

On physical grounds, it is difficult to see how a remote control using either ultrasonic sound

waves or infrared electromagnetic waves could interfere with a pacemaker. Both forms of energy are greatly attenuated as they enter the body, and neither form of energy is readily transferred to a wire sensor. By contrast, magnetic induction is not attenuated at all by the body, and radio waves are somewhat attenuated. The degree of attenuation of radio waves changes with frequency. In summary, if a remote control has to be used for someone with a pacemaker, it should operate using infrared or ultrasonic transmission, unless the manufacturer of the specific pacemaker or the manufacturer of the specific remote control can provide an assurance that interference to the pacemaker is not possible.

2.11 Bone Conductors

Bone conductors are alternative output transducers intended for people who, for various reasons, cannot wear a receiver coupled to the ear canal. Bone conductor transducers directly vibrate the skull, which in turn transmits these vibrations to the cochlea. The bone conductor works on the same principle as the receiver, except that instead of a light diaphragm, it has a heavy mass that is shaken by the audio current passing through a coil. The inertia of this mass causes it to resist being shaken, so the case of the vibrator shakes as well as the mass. This vibration of the case is transferred to the skull. For efficient transfer of power, the transducer has to be held firmly against the skull by means of a tight headband or spectacle frame. Bone conductor transducers require considerable power, so they are usually driven by high-powered hearing aids. The hearing aid

Table 2.2 Advantages of different remote control technologies. *Interference* refers to interference of the remote control by other devices.

	Ultrasonic	Infrared	Radio waves	Magnetic induction
Freedom from interference		✓		
Operated from any position			✓	✓
Simultaneous bilateral operation			✓	✓
Simple technology	✓	✓		✓

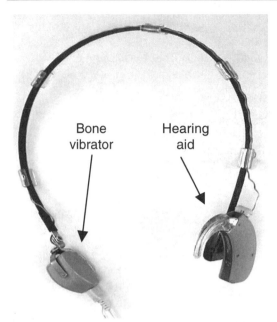

Figure 2.25 A bone conductor hearing aid

amplifier output is connected to the bone conductor transducer, instead of its usual receiver, by wires emerging from the hearing aid or by a plug and socket arrangement, as shown in Figure 2.25.

2.12 Batteries

The battery provides the increased signal power that the hearing aid delivers to the aid wearer. The important characteristics of the battery are its *voltage*, its *capacity*, the *maximum current* it can supply, its *electrical impedance* and its *physical size*.

2.12.1 Principle of operation

Batteries (which are really called cells)[j] generate electricity by putting two different materials (called the *electrodes*) in close proximity in a medium (called the *electrolyte*) that conducts electricity in the form of ions. Charged particles are attracted from one of the materials to the other via the electrolyte, and this can continue only if electrons can

get from one electrode to the other via an external electrical circuit. This external current of electrons is, of course, the current that the hearing aid amplifier makes use of. The process continues until one of the electrodes is used up in that it can no longer supply charged particles and electrons.

2.12.2 Operating voltage

The voltage generated by a battery depends solely on the type of materials used for the electrodes. The batteries most commonly used for hearing aids use Zinc and Oxygen as their negative and positive electrodes, respectively, so the batteries are known as *Zinc-air* batteries. These batteries, whatever their physical size, generate approximately 1.4 Volts when not connected to anything and approximately 1.25 V when in use. When the zinc is close to being depleted, the battery voltage drops suddenly, and the hearing aid gets weaker, more distorted, and eventually ceases to operate once the voltage becomes too low. Few hearing aids will operate well once the battery voltage drops below 1.1 V. Some hearing aids become unstable when the battery is near the end of its life, and the hearing aid generates and emits a low-frequency tone. This can sound like a motor-boat, and the phenomenon is called motor-boating. Such sounds can be thought of either as a fault, or as a useful indicator that the battery is nearly dead!

Other combinations of materials that are sometimes used in hearing aids are Mercuric Oxide and Zinc, which generate 1.35 Volts. Still available, but rarely used, are batteries comprising Silver Oxide and Zinc which generate 1.5 Volts. Body-level hearing aids use larger batteries, such as AA or AAA size. These have Manganese dioxide and Zinc as their electrode materials and also generate 1.5 V. Alternatively, they can use Nickel and Cadmium as their electrodes, in which case

---

[j]   Formally, a battery is a number of cells connected together to give a higher voltage, though the terms are used interchangeably in everyday use.

Batteries: practical tips

- The sticky tabs on zinc air batteries restrict air from getting in to the zinc electrodes. The battery will not operate until the tab is removed, but once it is removed, the battery has a shelf life of only a few weeks.

- If the sticky tab was *too* well sealed to the battery, the battery will not be useable until the air has had time to percolate into the battery. This can be speeded up by leaving the battery a few minutes before putting it into the hearing aid.

- If a new battery appears to be dead, leave it for a few minutes after removing the tab - it may make a miraculous recovery!

- If a hearing aid is left unused for a period, the battery should be removed, to protect the hearing aid (especially the battery contacts) from potential battery leakage and corrosion.

- For a high-powered hearing aid, it is worth investigating the battery life and sound quality obtainable with an HP battery

---

they are rechargeable and generate 1.3 V. Another range of batteries sometimes used in body aids use Lithium instead of Zinc as their negative electrode and one of several materials as the positive electrode. These are more expensive and generate 3 V.

2.12.3 Capacity and physical size

Batteries last longer the more electrode material they contain. Bigger batteries therefore last longer than smaller batteries with the same chemistry. The electrical capacity of a battery is measured in *milliamp hours (mAh)*. A battery with a capacity of 100 mAh, for example, can supply 0.5 mA for 200 hours, 1 mA for 100 hours, or 2 mA for 50 hours. There is an upper limit to how much current a battery can supply at any instant. If the current gets too high, even for a fraction of a

second, the battery voltage will drop excessively because of the internal resistance of the battery. Momentary intense noises will therefore cause the voltage to momentarily decrease, perhaps so much that the hearing aid temporarily ceases to operate, giving a very distorted sound. Bigger batteries can generally supply bigger maximum currents, as well as having a larger mAh capacity.

High-powered hearing aids need the greatest current, and some batteries are advertised as being more able to supply the high currents these hearing aids need without losing too much voltage. These are referred to as **HP** (*High Performance* or *High Power*) batteries, and may have the prefix *H* in their type number. These are also Zinc-air cells, but have bigger holes to allow oxygen in at a faster rate and use an electrolyte that causes

---

Table 2.3 Names and typical capacities of zinc air batteries of various sizes.

Type	Standard Label	Capacity (mAh)	Hearing aid types
675	PR44	575	BTE
13	PR48	260	BTE, ITE
312	PR41	140	ITE, ITC
A10 (or 10A, or 230)	PR70	70	ITC, CIC
A5		35	CIC

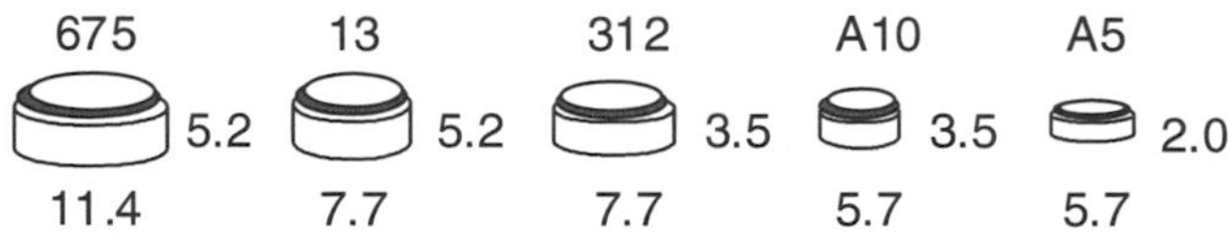

675	13	312	A10	A5
5.2	5.2	3.5	3.5	2.0
11.4	7.7	7.7	5.7	5.7

Figure 2.26 Hearing aid batteries of various types drawn full size, with typical dimensions shown in mm. Minimum and maximum allowable dimensions are 0.1 to 0.2 mm smaller and larger than these dimensions.

less voltage drop during high current demand. HP batteries should give a longer life than a standard battery if the hearing aid has a high peak-current demand, but will give a shorter life if the hearing aid has a low peak-current demand. HP batteries should be used if a hearing aid draws more than about 8 mA (for a size 13 or 312 battery) or more than about 18 mA (for a size 675 battery) when it is saturated.[582] Peak-current demand can be assessed in a test box equipped with a battery pill, by applying a 500 Hz signal at 90 dB SPL with a high volume control setting. Read the current as soon as you switch on the sound.

Table 2.3 shows the capacity of good Zinc-air batteries of various sizes. Some brands claim greater capacity than those shown, and some have less capacity. Mercury batteries have capacities about half that of Zinc-air batteries of the same size. Two labeling systems are used: the labels in the first column are most common, while those in the second column are specified in international standards.[411] Figure 2.26 shows each of the batteries drawn full size.

Zinc-air batteries are currently the preferred battery type because they are the cheapest (per mAh), they do not have to be changed as often as Mercury or Silver batteries, and they have less adverse environmental consequences than Mercury batteries when they are discarded. Mercury batteries can provide higher currents and provide better performance for some high-powered hearing aids, but only for the first few hours of their life.

2.13 Concluding Comments

Although the major components in hearing aids (transducers, amplifiers, and batteries) have existed in some form for a century, there has been a dramatic improvement in their quality and a dramatic reduction in their size over this time. These technological advances have enabled hearing aids to provide amplification in increasingly sophisticated and effective ways. In the following chapter, we will see how the individual components are combined to provide complete hearing aids and amplification systems.

CHAPTER THREE

HEARING AID SYSTEMS

Synopsis

Components can be combined into hearing aids in an extremely customized manner, such that individual components are selected for each patient and are located in the position that best suits each ear. The other extreme is a modular aid, which is prefabricated in a totally standard manner. Many hearing aids fall somewhere between these extremes.

Hearing aids can be classified by their technology into analog, digitally programmable analog, and fully digital types. Digitally programmable hearing aids employ conventional analog circuits for changing the sound, but use a digital control circuit to alter the characteristics of the analog circuit. This enables the circuit, and hence the sound, to be more flexibly altered than is possible with fully analog devices. The digital programming circuit also enables the user to switch between listening programs in different situations. Fully digital circuits may be constructed so that they process sounds in ways specific to each device, or may be able to perform any arithmetic operation, in which case the type of processing they do depends on the software that is loaded into them. Some manipulations of sound are performed more efficiently with digital processing, and some complex operations are only feasible with digital processing.

The most effective way to make speech more intelligible is to put the microphone near the lips of the person talking. This markedly decreases noise and reverberation, but requires a means of transmitting the signal from the microphone to the hearing aid wearer some distance away. Methods to do this currently include magnetic induction from a loop of wire to a small telecoil inside the hearing aid, radio transmission of a frequency-modulated electromagnetic wave, infrared transmission of an amplitude-modulated electromagnetic wave, and acoustic transmission of an amplified sound wave. Each of these systems has strengths and weaknesses compared to the others.

Hearing aids that are not worn entirely on the head or body of the hearing-impaired person are referred to as assistive listening devices. These include the remote transmission systems just described, as well as devices that alter sound (such as a telephone amplifier), and devices that convert sound to other sensory modalities (such as smoke detectors and doorbells that cause a light to flash or that provide a vibratory sensation).

Chapter 2 described all the bits and pieces that go to make up a hearing aid. This chapter will describe how these bits and pieces are combined to make complete hearing aids, including hearing aid systems that transmit and receive signals across a distance.

3.1 Custom and Modular Construction

The basic styles of hearing aids (body, BTE, ITE, ITC, and CIC) have already been intro-duced in Section 1.3. The ITE, ITC and CIC styles can be completely **custom-made** for the individual hearing aid wearer. Alternatively, any of the styles can be manufactured in totally standardized shapes and sizes, which is referred to as **modular** construction. Hearing aids can also be constructed in an intermediate way, which is referred to as **semi-custom** or **semi-modular** construction. The following sections will describe the differences between each of these construction techniques.

3.1.1   Custom hearing aids

Custom hearing aids (ITEs, ITCs, and CICs) take full advantage of the size and shape of an individual aid wearer's ear. Construction begins when the clinician makes an *ear impression* and sends it to the hearing aid manufacturer. The manufacturer, through a casting technique, uses the impression to make a hollow ear shell that fits snugly within the ear canal and (if appropriate) the concha of the aid wearer.

Customization of the hearing aid components happens to different degrees. Most commonly, the manufacturer will have a number of standard amplifier boards from which to choose, and the selected one will be combined with a suitable microphone and receiver. These will be soldered to the other major components: the battery compartment, the volume control, any fitter controls, and if appropriate, the telecoil and switch. Usually, the battery compartment will have been manufactured as an integral part of the hearing aid *faceplate.* This is a flat or contoured sheet of plastic that is trimmed to size and becomes the outer surface of the hearing aid.

In hearing aids that have very adjustable amplification characteristics, identical electronics may be used for people with a variety of hearing losses, in which case all the components may be pre-assembled to be loosely attached to the faceplate. For hearing aids that are not highly adjustable, even some of the components on the amplifier board may be selected to suit the expected requirements for a particular aid wearer. Figure 3.1 shows a faceplate with all the other components attached, next to the ear shell to which it is about to be fitted.

The next stage of construction is positioning the components within the ear shell and on the faceplate. These positions are chosen so that as much material as possible can be cut from the outer part of the shell before the faceplate is attached. (This makes the aid as small as possible for the components chosen.)

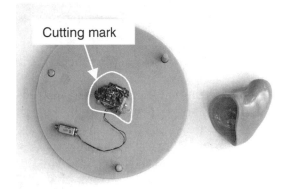

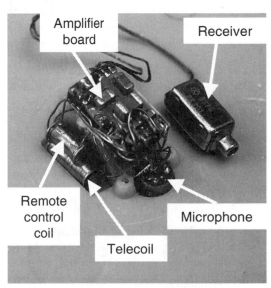

Figure 3.1 (a) A faceplate with components mounted, next to a shell far an ITC hearing aid. After gluing the two parts together, all material outside the cutting mark is removed. (b) A close-up of the components mounted on the faceplate.

Finally, the faceplate is glued to the shell and any excess trimmed off. This raises the obvious problem of how repairs are carried out on these aids. Most repairs require the faceplate to be prized away from the shell, which can usually (but not always) be done without damage to either part.

3.1.2   Modular hearing aids

Modular ITE/ITC/CIC hearing aids are those in which the hearing aid components are manufactured as a standard package. ITC hearing aids, in particular, have been made in a variety of cases having standard shapes.

These can be thought of as *ready-to-wear* hearing aids, and physically fitting these aids to the ear merely comprises selecting the case with the shape that best matches the person's ear canal and concha.

Modular hearing aids have several advantages and disadvantages. First, the module can be manufactured and tested in a more automated manner, which lowers cost and increases reliability. Second, it can be attractive for the client and the clinician to be able to fit a hearing aid as soon as a hearing assessment has been carried out, rather than at a later appointment. The disadvantages can be severe. For many ears, there may be no standard case that fits in a cosmetically or functionally acceptable manner. The aid may fall out too easily, or there may be so much leakage that the hearing aid whistles at gain settings lower than those needed by the aid wearer for adequate audibility. Low-cost mail-order hearing aids are, by necessity, modular devices.

Some modular hearing aids have a foam sleeve or silicon flange around the canal section of the aid, which solves the problem of a loose fit and feedback oscillation. The disadvantage is that the soft material deteriorates. Either the soft material, or the complete hearing aid, has to be disposable.

BTE and body-level hearing aids could also be called modular hearing aids, as the electrical and mechanical components have a fixed size and shape, which are then connected to an individual earmold. They are not usually referred to as modular aids, because no one has yet invented any way to make a custom BTE aid.

3.1.3   Semi-modular, semi-custom hearing aids

ITE or ITC hearing aids that combine a standard module with a custom-made ear shell can be referred to as semi-custom or semi-modular hearing aids. The modules are usually clipped, rather than glued, to the individual ear shell, which makes repairs

faster, cheaper and unlikely to damage the earshell or faceplate, as can occur in a custom aid. The disadvantage is that because the components can not be rearranged to take advantage of the individual ear's geometry, a semi-modular hearing aid will generally be larger than a custom hearing aid with the same components.

There is a continuum from fully custom to fully modular aids. At the fully custom extreme, the position of any component relative to any other component can be varied, and the manufacturer individually selects many of the components for each hearing aid wearer. At the fully modular extreme, the entire hearing aid is manufactured in a totally standardized manner (such as the ready-to-wear aids mentioned in the preceding section).

Most CIC/ITC/ITE hearing aids sold lie closer to the fully custom extreme. They typically combine a glued-on faceplate with the battery compartment, volume control, and programming socket (if any) in a fixed position relative to each other. The microphone and integrated circuit are often also fixed in position relative to the faceplate. The receiver is individually positioned within a custom shell.

3.2   Analog Hearing Aids

Hearing aids can be classified according to whether they are fully analog, analog with digital control circuits for programming the aid, or fully digital. At the time of writing (2000) most hearing aids are still fully analog, but the proportion of digital aids is growing rapidly.

As introduced in Section 2.4, within an analog hearing aid, different voltages represent sounds of different strengths (i.e. different pressures). The voltage representing the signal can be any voltage between 0 V and the battery voltage. Electronic components, most of which are within integrated circuits, are wired together to make signal processing blocks that modify the sound in various ways.

Because each hearing-impaired person has different hearing characteristics, each hearing aid must be manufactured and/or adjusted to suit the person. Adjustments, made with a small screwdriver, alter the characteristics of one of the signal processing blocks by adjusting the value of a small variable resistor, called a *potentiometer*. This is often abbreviated to *pot* or *trimpot*. In some hearing aids, a small screwdriver-operated switch, to which a group of resistors is connected, is used instead of a pot. This provides a more reproducible setting, with greater long-term reliability, but is more expensive to manufacture.

The top half of Figure 3.2 shows a simplified block diagram for an analog hearing aid: all the individual signal processing blocks are contained within the large block called *signal path*. Three controls (indicated by screw slots) vary the characteristics of blocks within the analog signal path.

Unfortunately, because of the small size of hearing aids, it is rarely possible to fit more than three controls on a hearing aid. (The world record, achieved in one BTE hearing aid, is six controls). The controls can be labeled in terms of:

- the electroacoustic parameters they vary (e.g. the SSPL values that can be obtained), or,
- a mnemonic for the operations they perform (e.g. *H* for high-frequency emphasis), or,
- the degree of hearing loss that is believed to match each position of the control.

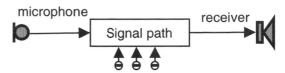

Analog hearing aid

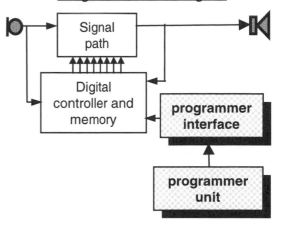

Programmable hearing aid

Figure 3.2 Block diagram of an analog hearing aid (top) and a digitally programmable hearing aid (bottom).

Again, the small size of hearing aids often makes it difficult to put meaningful, legible labels on controls. This is not a problem to the clinician that specializes in only a few models (or families) of hearing aids, but can provide difficulties to clinicians who fit a wide range of aids.

3.3   Digitally Programmable Analog Hearing Aid Systems

The second type of construction, shown in the bottom half of Figure 3.2, overcomes the

Parameters that are commonly adjustable in hearing aids	
Frequency response filtering	**Gain and Power**
Low-cut slope or corner frequency	SSPL90 (Peak clipping or AGC_o)
High-cut slope or corner frequency	Gain
Cross-over frequency (between channels)	**Compression**
Low-frequency gain	Compression ratio
High-frequency gain	Compression threshold
Low-high balance	Gain for low input levels
	Gain for high input levels

difficulties arising from trying to fit a large number of controls onto a small hearing aid. The *digitally programmed analog hearing aid* contains an analog sound path very similar to that of fully analog hearing aids. The difference lies in how these sound paths are adjusted. A digitally programmable analog aid uses digital control circuits, contained within the hearing aid, to control the characteristics of each of the analog signal processing blocks. These digital control circuits are in turn controlled by an external device that plugs into the hearing aid when the aid is being programmed. Because there need not be any fitter controls on the hearing aid, it becomes possible to include many more controls, and hence to have much greater flexibility in how the signal path is altered. Consequently, it is more easily possible to tailor the hearing aid to the requirements of each aid wearer.

Digitally programmable hearing aids are sometimes provided with a remote control, as it is technologically easy to add a remote control once digital control circuits have been added to the hearing aid (see Section 2.10).

3.3.1   Programmers, interfaces, and software

The clinician changes the contents of the digital control circuits using a programming device. Most commonly now, this device is a computer. There are, however, a number of smaller special-purpose programming devices that can be used with particular brands of hearing aids.

During the early 1990s this situation looked like getting out of hand: most hearing aid brands had to be used with their own specific programming device, although a few companies combined to use a common device called the PMC programmer. To be used with a particular brand of hearing aid, a module from that hearing aid manufacturer first had to be plugged into the back of the PMC programmer. A clinician using several brands of digitally programmable hearing aids needed an array of modules and/or programming devices, and connecting cords, all of them doing a job that was previously done (admittedly in a less flexible manner) by one small screwdriver. This situation has improved.

As computers became smaller, cheaper, more portable, and more powerful, virtually all manufacturers adopted a common standard for storing data and sending information from computers to hearing aids. That standard is called *NOAH* (as in: "we are all in the same boat"). The NOAH standard specifies how common data (like the audiogram and age of the client) should be stored, and how information should be sent to and received from the hearing aid.[752] Because the hearing aid has

---

Advantages of digitally programmable hearing aids

- Greater electroacoustic flexibility resulting in greater sound comfort and quality, without needing to send the hearing aid back to the manufacturer.

- Remote controls possible, enabling easier operation of the volume control, multiple programs for different listening needs, and simultaneous operation of two volume controls (for bilateral fittings).

- Fewer mechanical parts, resulting in fewer breakdowns.

- Hearing aid performance can be preset by the programming computer, resulting in faster fitting (compared to a non-programmable aid of the same complexity).

- Paired comparisons of different settings can be used to fine-tune the fitting.

- Lower manufacturing costs (eventually)

to be sent electrical signals different from those that computers can provide, an interface between the computer and the hearing aid is required. This interface, a small box with suitable sockets, is called the *HiPro* (**h**earing **i**nstrument **pro**grammer) interface.

To program hearing aids from different manufacturers, specific software provided by that manufacturer is needed. However, once the client's data has been entered, those data can be accessed from any manufacturer's program, so that potential fittings from different manufacturers can be compared. Alternatives include replacement of the HiPro interface with either a PCMCIA interface card plugged into a laptop computer or a wireless connection.[28] Hopefully, manufacturers will also standardize the sockets in the hearing aids so that clinics do not need a wall full of leads if they use a variety of hearing aid brands and models.

3.3.2   Multi-memory programmable hearing aids

Another advantage of using a digital controller within the hearing aid is that the controller can contain more than one *memory*, so the user can have access to different *programs*. Why does the hearing aid wearer need to change programs? It is not as if a drama can be heard on one program and a comedy on another. The first reason is that sounds entering the hearing aid can have acoustic properties that differ vastly from one environment to another. For optimal listening, the hearing aid should have different amplification characteristics in each environment. Of course, the hearing aid could sense the acoustic environment and automatically change the amplification characteristics (and many hearing aids do). It is possible, however, that the user can do a better job of selecting the optimal characteristics than an automatic circuit.

There is a second reason for needing more than one program, and an automatic circuit can not satisfy this need. Depending on the circumstances (such as interest in a particular talker), listeners sometimes wish to optimize intelligibility, and sometimes wish to optimize comfort. These goals can require different amplification characteristics.[934] An automatic circuit, no matter how smart, can not know which of these (or other) listening criteria is most important at any given time.

In most digitally-programmable hearing aids, all of the parameters that can be adjusted in one program can be independently adjusted in the other program or programs. The user, at the press of a button, can thus access the sound qualities of two or more entirely different hearing aids if that is how the clinician programs the aid. Most commonly the listening programs are adjusted to be identical except for one or two key parameters, or may be the means of selecting different inputs, such as a telecoil, FM system, or directional microphone. Methods for prescribing multiple memory hearing aids are covered in Section 9.5.

3.3.3   Paired comparisons

A final advantage of digitally controlled hearing aids is that if they have multiple memories, the hearing aid can be rapidly switched between two programs during the fitting process. This enables the hearing aid wearer to compare two responses in quick succession and state which is preferable. The clinician can use these preferences to fine-tune the response when the hearing aid is initially programmed and at any follow-up appointments. Procedures for doing *paired comparisons* are covered in Section 11.2.

3.4   Digital Hearing Aids

The third type of hearing aid, which has become commercially available only in the last few years, is the fully digital hearing aid. In these hearing aids, an analog-to-digital converter changes sound to a series of numbers, as outlined in Section 2.4.1. The hearing aid's digital signal processor then performs arithmetic on these numbers to manipulate the sound (see Section 2.4.2), before the numbers are turned back into an analog signal by the digital-to-analog converter (Section 2.4.3). There are two types of digital signal processors in the hearing aids now on the market. These could be referred to as **hard wired** and **general arithmetic processor** hearing aids, though the terminology to describe these hearing aids is being developed along with the aids themselves. General arithmetic processor hearing aids are sometimes described as **open platform,**[695] although this may convey an ambiguous impression. In the computing world, this term means that the internal structure is standardized in some way and able to be used by a variety of manufacturers, which is not yet the case with hearing aids.

3.4.1   Digital hard-wired hearing aids

In hard-wired digital hearing aids, the parts of the processor that do the arithmetic are connected together in a particular configuration. That is, the samples of the sound wave are passed through the various blocks of the processing in a particular order, and each block can do only the function (e.g. filtering, compression) that is has been designed to do.

Another way of thinking about this is that if the digital hearing aid is represented as a block diagram (just as with an analog aid), it can process sounds in *only* the way represented by that particular block diagram. Like digitally programmable hearing aids, however, the amounts by which digital hearing aids amplify and filter can be programmed in a very flexible manner. Thus there is no disadvantage in a digital aid being hard-wired, provided the block diagram is appropriate for the aid wearer's hearing loss, and provided the parameters of each block (e.g. compression ratio, filter corner frequency) can also be adjusted to values appropriate to the aid wearer. Digital hard-wired aids currently on the market have amplification characteristics that can be adjusted very flexibly.

3.4.2   Digital general arithmetic processor hearing aids

An alternative to the hard-wired digital aid is an aid that simply has an arithmetic processor at its heart. What would such an aid do? As with a computer, it would do whatever its software told it to do! If its software told it to filter the signal into three parallel bands, compress the signals in each band, and add these signals together, then the general arithmetic processor would function just as if it was a three-channel compression hearing aid. If some different software was loaded into the hearing aid, then the aid could function as a single-channel peak-clipping hearing aid.

There is no real limit to what hearing aids of this type *could* do. Unfortunately, other than the usual operations of amplification, filtering and compression, and some newer operations like feedback suppression, we are still not too sure what we would *like* them to do. (Of course, we would *like* them to amplify sound so that the output is always comfortable, always intelligible, and never has any noise in it. Unfortunately this is not a very productive wish unless we are able to say exactly what operations the digital signal processor should perform on the sound to achieve this delightful state of affairs.)

If a hearing aid incorporating a general arithmetic processor has to be configured to a particular block diagram before it can function, is it useful to have a general processor of this type? Yes, and the extreme flexibility will probably be useful in three ways. First, such an aid can truthfully, and usefully, be marketed as several different types of hearing aid, depending on the software loaded into the aid by the manufacturer, after the aid has been assembled.[695] The resulting cost saving to the manufacturer should eventually be passed on to the aid purchaser. Second, the manufacturer may market the aid as a super-flexible aid, in which the aid wearer can switch between different signal processing schemes (each with its own block diagram) using a remote control. This would be a straightforward extension of the multiple memory feature that is available in many digitally programmable analog aids. Third, as new and improved processing schemes are developed (and hopefully proven), aid wearers could purchase new software that enabled their existing hearing aid to perform the new type of processing, provided the hearing aid has adequate processing power. Thus, we will have to view hearing aids as we now view computers: there is a hardware component and a software component (in addition to the software in the fitting system), and either can be upgraded without necessarily changing the other. It is even possible that some manufacturers will sell only the hardware, and others will sell only the software.

These advantages come at a price, however. Any particular set of calculations requires more processing power (and hence battery current) to perform than if the calculations were to be done in a purpose-designed, hard-wired digital circuit.[503] Alternatively, for the same battery current, hard-wired processors can do more complex operations than general arithmetic processors.

Although hard-wired and general arithmetic processors have been presented as the only two alternatives, they are actually just the two extremes of a continuum. General arithmetic processors can contain dedicated hard-wired circuits to handle frequently repeated calculations in an efficient manner. Conversely, hard-wired processors can contain a small general arithmetic processor that can control how parts of a hard-wired circuit are configured.[a] For some time, most digital hearing aids are likely to be a hybrid of hard-wired circuits and general arithmetic processors.

The implication of all this is that the clinician should pay little attention to what manufac-

turers say about *how* the signal processing is performed. The clinician should simply ask what processing features are included that benefit patients and how flexibly that processing can be tailored to the needs of the patient. Whether the hearing aid is made out of digital hard-wired circuits, digital general-purpose circuits, analog circuits, or for that matter play-dough, is irrelevant.

3.4.3   Sequential processing versus block processing

The way that hearing aids amplify sounds invariably depends on frequency. To achieve frequency-dependent amplification, digital hearing aids process sounds in two broadly different ways. The first way, which is analogous to how analog hearing aids operate, is to process the incoming signal *sequentially*. At any given time, the computer is processing the current sample of the input signal, although the processing it does to that sample often will depend on what the values of the preceding samples were. For a slow-acting compressor, for example, the gain given to the current sample may depend on the value of many thousands of previous samples.

An alternative to this is *block processing* (also known as *frame processing*, or *windowing* the signal). In this approach a number of input samples (typically 64, 128, 256, 512, or 1024) are taken in by the hearing aid before *any* computations on them are performed. Processing a complete block of input data at one time enables a *Fourier transform* to be calculated, with the result that the complete block is now represented by an amplitude and phase at every frequency, rather than as the instantaneous value of the waveform at each point in time. The greater the number of input samples processed at once, the more finely the individual frequencies can be specified within the hearing aid. We say that the signal is now represented in the *frequency domain.* Fourier Transforms require a lot of arithmetic

---

[a]   Even some digitally programmable analog hearing aids can have their arrangement of processing blocks rearranged by the digital control circuit.

to be calculated, so efficient calculation methods must be used. The most common method is known as the *fast Fourier transform (FFT)*. After the complete block of data has been processed (i.e. altered in the desired way), an *inverse FFT* is used to convert the block back into the time domain. Each sample in the block is then output by the hearing aid, one sample at a time.

What the hearing aid does with this information depends on what we are trying to accomplish. It may monitor the spectrum from block-to-block to deduce when the hearing aid is whistling because of feedback, and then automatically change the amplification conditions until the whistle disappears. Alternatively, it may provide one frequency response characteristic when sound has dominant high-frequency components and a different characteristic when sound has dominant low-frequency components. We may note the way the spectrum changes from block-to-block, deduce whether the signal is predominantly noise or predominantly speech, and alter the amplification characteristics in an appropriate manner.

When sounds are processed in blocks of samples, the output samples are delayed with respect to the input samples by at least the length of the block. As the delay increases beyond about 10 ms, the combined effect of the delayed sound plus non-amplified sound increasingly affects the user's perception of his or her own voice.[851] Even longer delays of 40 ms or more put the auditory information out of synchronization with visual information and so may disturb lip-reading.[589, 863]

Any delay, including the very short delay found in analog hearing aids, can disrupt the gain-frequency response for people with mild or moderate losses because part of the sound received is not passed through the hearing aid and is therefore not subject to additional delay. The two sound paths can partially cancel at particular frequencies (see Section 5.3.1). The greater the delay, the greater is the likelihood

that this cancellation will occur. Sound quality is adversely affected if part of the frequency range is delayed by more than about 5 ms with respect to the remainder of the frequency range.[608] Even if samples are processed sequentially, filters will delay the signal in a complex manner. This is best characterized by the *group delay* at each frequency, which describes the delay applied to the envelope of signal components in each frequency region.[161]

3.4.4 Specifications for digital hearing aids

Digital and analog hearing aids have the same types of specifications, such as gain, maximum output, range of tone control adjustment, compression characteristics, internal noise, and current consumption. With digital hearing aids, however, some additional specifications indicate the likely audio quality and processing capabilities of the hearing aid. The following five specifications are justifiably likely to feature in the advertising of digital hearing aids.

Sampling rate: The sampling rate, or sampling frequency (see Section 2.4.1), describes how many times per second the hearing aid samples the input signal. The major impact of the specification is that the hearing aid can amplify sounds only up to about 40% of the sampling frequency, with the absolute theoretical maximum being 50%. A second impact is that if the sampling rate is unnecessarily high, the complexity of the processing that the hearing aid can perform will be unnecessarily limited. This occurs simply because the hearing aid is having to do each of the operations on more speech samples every second than may be justified by, say the upper frequency limit of the hearing aid receiver. Consequently, fewer operations can be performed on each sample. Just as with analog hearing aids, the bandwidth of a digital hearing aid is limited by the component that has the most restricted bandwidth, so there is no advantage in other components having an excessively high bandwidth.

Instructions per second: Digital processors are characterized by the number of instructions or operations (such as multiplication or addition) that they can do in a second. A particular processor, for example, may be able to do 40 ***MIPS***, which stands for 40 million instructions per second. Complex signal processing schemes generally require a greater number of instructions per second than less complex schemes. As examples, compression is more complex than peak clipping, multi-band processing is more complex than single band processing, and the more effective varieties of automatic feedback suppression are more complex than tone controls. For a given integrated circuit, increasing the number of instructions per second, to perform more complex processing, will increase current consumption and thus decrease battery life. Unfortunately, one cannot assume that a hearing aid that is calculating 40 MIPS is performing more complex processing than one that is calculating 10 MIPS, because each "instruction" in the lower-speed hearing aid may be more complex than in the higher-speed hearing aid.

Number of bits: Section 2.4.1 showed that we can represent each sample of the audio waveform by a number, which in turn is represented as a string of bits. The greater the number of bits, the greater the number of analog voltage levels that we can represent. If there are too few levels, the digital approximation of the original signal is too coarse. The errors made by selecting the nearest allowable level are equivalent to adding noise to the signal, and this is referred to as ***quantization noise***. Thus, the greater the number of bits, the better the digital approximation of the signal, and the less the quantization noise. The amount of quantization noise, compared to the biggest signal that can be represented without overload, can easily be estimated. The noise is approximately $6b$ dB below the biggest signal, where b is the number of bits. A 12-bit system will therefore have quantization noise 72 dB below the highest signal. When the largest possible signal was input to the hearing aid, the SNR would thus be 72 dB. While this sounds like a very high signal to noise ratio, if the input level were to be decreased by 70 dB (say from 110 dB SPL to 40 dB SPL), the SNR would be only 2 dB, which does not seem so acceptable! Hearing aids may use different numbers of bits in different parts of the aid, depending on the dynamic range needed in each part. Also, clever coding schemes can be used to make a smaller number of bits sound as good as simple coding schemes with a greater number of bits. When comparing the performance of different digital hearing aids, specifications for the number of bits should thus be interpreted warily. In general though, the more bits, the better, as the hearing aid will be able to handle a greater dynamic range of signals without adding excessive noise of its own.

Current consumption: The current consumption, and hence battery life and feasible battery size, depends on the instruction rate, the voltage at which the integrated circuit operates, and the technology used to make the integrated circuit. None of this is under the control of the clinician, or need be understood by the clinician, but the consumption directly affects the size and hence appearance of the finished hearing aid. Current consumption, for a given number of instructions per second, is spiraling steadily downward and should continue doing so for as long as general computer technology continues to improve.

Physical size: Complex circuits, especially when they contain a lot of computer memory of the type needed by programmable hearing aids, can require an integrated circuit several mm by several mm (or approaching a quarter inch by a quarter inch). Because transducers have been shrinking continuously in size for the last forty years, the size of the integrated circuit can have a big effect on the finished size of the hearing aid.

3.4.5 Advantages of digital hearing aids

There are many current and potential advantages of fully digital hearing aids. The biggest advantage is that they can perform more complex processing than is possible in analog hearing aids. Some operations just cannot realistically be done in analog aids (e.g. block processing to finely represent signals in the frequency domain), and many operations can be done with less power and circuit size if done digitally. Digital hearing aids are also able to make decisions about how to process the sound, depending on what they sense the overall acoustic environment to be. Further, provided they have enough processing capacity, digital circuits containing a general arithmetic processor can potentially be updated with new processing schemes as knowledge advances or hearing loss changes.[b]

Another advantage of digital processing is that with advances in technology, the physical size and power consumption of digital circuits is reducing at a faster rate than is the case for analog circuits. By 1998, digital hearing aids had advanced sufficiently that they required slightly less power and volume than analog hearing aids performing operations of similar moderate complexity. The power and size advantage of digital aids will grow rapidly with time. The hearing aid can be made smaller if the integrated circuit is smaller. If the integrated circuit consumes less power, a smaller battery can be used for the same battery life. Consequently, the hearing aid can again be made smaller. Because of all these advantages, digital hearing aids will fully replace analog aids. Several major manufacturers have already ceased developing new analog hearing aids.

It is also worth stating what digital aids cannot do. Digital hearing aids are sometimes referred to as *providing CD sound quality*. This analogy is only partly true: they use the same type of technology as compact disk players. Once a sound is converted into digital form, it is possible for the sound to be manipulated without the hearing aid adding any significant noise of its own. Unfortunately, by the time digital hearing aids get to manipulate the sound, it has noise mixed in with it, because background noise enters the hearing aid along with the wanted sound. Also, the hearing aid microphone will add noise to the signal before the sound is converted to digital form. By contrast, compact discs are usually recorded in very quiet studios under ideal conditions. Consequently, there is no chance for noise to be added anywhere along the way, and the result, for CDs, is a virtual lack of background noise. *This is never likely to be true for hearing aids.*

3.5 Remote Sensing and Transmitting Hearing Aid Systems

When a sound wave travels away from its source its power spreads out over an ever-increasing area and so it gets weaker. This causes two types of sound quality degradation. First, the decreased level is more easily masked by background noise. Second, reflected sounds, in the form of *reverberation*, add delayed versions of the original sound to the direct sound. Reverberant sound is smeared out in time and not surprisingly is much less intelligible than direct sound, particularly when the room has a long reverberation time. The *critical distance* is defined as the distance from the source beyond which the level of the reverberant sound exceeds the level of the direct sound. Noise and reverberation thus both cause intelligibility to diminish as the listener gets further from the source.

---

[b]   As with computers, the latest software may need the capabilities of the latest hardware to operate properly.

A solution to this problem is to pick up the signal where it is strongest and clearest (next to the talker's mouth), and transmit this strong, clear signal to a hearing aid wearer either as an electromagnetic wave or as a magnetic field, rather than as a sound wave. Provided the hearing aid wearer has the equipment necessary to turn the electromagnetic wave or magnetic field back into a sound wave, the wearer can hear the signal as clearly as though his or her ear was right next to the talker's mouth. There are three types of electromagnetic transmission systems used to get the signal from the talker to the listener, and these are covered in the following three sections.

3.6   Induction Loops

There is an intimate connection between electricity and magnetism. *Induction loops* take advantage of this by converting an audio signal into an electrical current that flows through a loop of wire, and hence into a magnetic field that can travel through space. This field is sensed by a coil of wire, and *induces* an electrical voltage in the coil (see Section 2.8). This voltage is then amplified and converted by a receiver back into sound. Figure 3.3 shows the complete path from talker to listener. The loop that emits the magnetic field can be as large as a length of wire around the perimeter of an auditorium or as small as a device that can fit behind the ear, alongside the usual hearing aid. In-between are loops that surround an individual

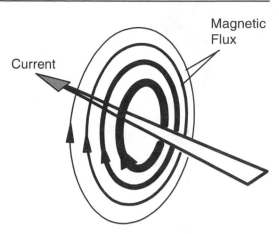

Figure 3.4 Lines of magnetic flux flowing around a conductor carrying a current.

listener (on the floor or attached to a favorite chair) and loops that are worn around the neck of the listener. The coil that picks up the magnetic signal is invariably mounted inside the listener's hearing aid.

3.6.1   Field uniformity and direction

Although magnetic fields emerge outwards from the wire and current that cause them, the *magnetic lines of force,* and the resulting *magnetic flux*, which can be thought of as the flow of magnetism, actually flow in circles *around* the current that causes the field, as shown in Figure 3.4. As the circles become more distant from the current, the magnetic force and the magnetic flux become weaker. To visualize the flow of magnetism, angle your right thumb at right angles to the finger on your right hand, and then curl your fingers. If your thumb points in the direction of the electrical current, the curled fingers will show the circular path taken by the magnetic field around the line of the thumb. (In fact, engineers call this the *right-hand rule* and use it to deduce which way around the circle the magnetism is flowing.)

Let us apply this to an imaginary loop on the floor in the room in which you are now sitting. Suppose the loop is hidden away in the corner where the floor meets the walls (as it often is in practice). Suppose the current is flowing

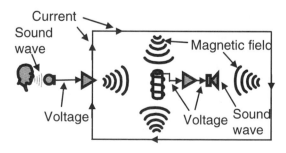

Figure 3.3 The complete chain, from sound wave in to sound wave out, for a magnetic loop induction system.

Practical Tips: Room loops

- Immediately above (or below) the wire forming a loop, the magnetic field flows almost horizontally. A vertical coil, as in a hearing aid, will not pick up much signal. Room loops therefore have to be a little larger than the area over which the loop has to work.

- Building steel near the loop can greatly weaken the strength of the magnetic field and change its direction.

- Purpose-designed loop amplifiers should include a compressor so that the magnetic field is always close to the optimum strength, even for soft talkers.

- Magnetic fields spill over outside the loop, so two loops with different audio signals in the one building should be well separated.

- Many home audio appliances have sufficient power to drive a small loop directly, but an additional, high-wattage volume control (and electronics expertise) will be needed if they are to drive the loop and a loudspeaker with an appropriate balance.

- Loops at floor level can be run over doorways without adversely affecting performance.

---

clockwise around the room when you look down on the floor, as shown in Figure 3.5. Now put your thumb next to the imaginary wire next to one of the walls in the room. Notice where your curled fingers are pointing, and imagine the complete circles of magnetism (of various diameters) around each wire. Immediately above each wire, your fingers, and hence the magnetic field, should be pointing horizontally into the room. Within the room, at floor level, the magnetic field should be pointing straight down, no matter

which section of the wire you think of as the source of the magnetism.

This last fact is very fortunate. Recall that as the circles get further from the wire, the magnetism gets weaker. As you move away from one section of wire, however, you are always moving closer to another section of wire. Also, if the wire is at floor level and the aid wearer is seated or standing, the magnetic field just inside the loop is more horizontal than vertical. (Use your right hand to see this for yourself.) The result is that at head height, the vertical part of the magnetic field has a nearly constant strength over most of the room, except for just inside the loop, where the total field is strong, but the vertical part is weak. This is important because if the receiving coil in the hearing aid is mounted vertically, it will pick up only the vertical part of the magnetic field.[c]

Although we have talked about the current going around the loop in one direction, if the source is an audio signal, the direction will reverse many times per second, corresponding to the positive and negative pressure variations in the original acoustic wave.

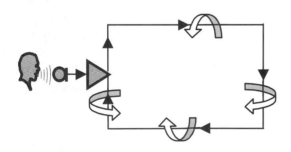

Figure 3.5 A complete induction loop system, showing how lines of magnetism from all parts of the loop add constructively within the region enclosed by the loop.

---

[c]   A magnetic field at some intermediate angle, such as 30° from the vertical, can be considered to have a vertical component added to a horizontal component, in the right mix of strengths to produce the actual angle of the field.

Consequently, the circular magnetic fields will also reverse their direction many times per second. It is actually this constantly changing magnetic flux that enables a coil to sense the magnetism and produce an audio voltage. (The earth's magnetic field does not affect a coil, because the earth's field has a constant strength and direction.)

3.6.2   Magnetic field strength

The strength of the magnetic field near the center of the room is directly proportional to the magnitude of the current in the loop and to the number of turns in the loop, and is inversely proportional to the diameter of the loop. International standards (IEC 118-4, BS7594) specify that the long-term rms value of the magnetic field, should be 100 mA/m (that is, milliamps per meter). The actual strength of the field at the center of a circular loop of diameter a meters, with n turns around the loop, can be calculated using Equation 3.1:

$$H = \frac{nI}{a} \qquad ..... 3.1,$$

where H is the magnetic field strength, in Amps per meter, and I is the rms value of the current, in Amps. For a square loop, of size a by a meters, the magnetic field strength is 10% less than the value calculated by Equation 3.1. If the long-term rms strength of the loop has to be 100 mA/m, the loop must be able to output an rms level of at least 400 mA/m (and preferably 560 mA/m), so that excessive peak clipping can be avoided during the more intense sounds in speech.

It is important that the magnetic output of loops not be much weaker than this. The loop will not be the only electrical wire in a building producing a magnetic field. All the building wiring will also be producing magnetic fields with a frequency of the electricity power supply (50 or 60 Hz, depending on the country) and at harmonics of that frequency. This constitutes magnetic interference or background noise (which actually sounds like a hum or a buzz). If the audio magnetic field is too weak, the SNR will not be adequate. A hearing aid wearer can conveniently switch from microphone to telecoil mode without changing the volume control if the hearing aid produces the same output for a magnetic field strength of 100 mA/m as it does for an acoustic input of around 70 dB SPL.

In small hearing aids, with small coils, this telecoil sensitivity is achieved by using a separate pre-amplifier for the coil signal. While the user could compensate for a weaker field by turning up the volume control, this is inconvenient, particularly if the user needs to switch frequently between the telecoil and microphone positions. Also, compensation is possible only if the hearing aid has adequate reserve in the volume control, and if the gain can be sufficiently increased without causing feedback. Even on telecoil position, feedback oscillations can occur if the gain is too great. Just as acoustic waves cause feedback by leaking back from the receiver to the microphone, so too magnetic fields can cause feedback in the T position by leaking back from the receiver to the telecoil.

Ideally, telephones would also emit a magnetic field strength of 100 mA/m. Unfortunately, few do. Very old telephones generally produce a satisfactory magnetic field strength, because they accidentally leak a strong magnetic field. Very new telephones and public telephones have been designed to emit a magnetic field specifically for use by hearing-impaired people. These telephones are often satisfactory (see panel). The problem lies in the telephones in-between which were designed to be efficient for their acoustic output, a consequence of which was that only a very weak magnetic signal leaked out.

3.6.3   Loop frequency response

The frequency response of a loop and telecoil system can sometimes be unsatisfactory, although this need not be so. Because the

---

Practical tips: Telephones that emit weak magnetic signals.

International telephone standards require phones to emit magnetic fields with strengths between 32 and 141 mA/m. Phones designed near the bottom of this range (and most are), when combined with a weak talker or a poor line will emit an unusably small signal. Potential solutions to this problem, not all of which are practical in all circumstances, are:

- Have the telephone supplier add a sending coil (i.e., a small loop) in parallel to the receiver.

- Have the telephone supplier add an amplifier to the telephone (and then use the hearing aid on *T* if the magnetic field is now strong enough, or without the hearing aid if not).

- Change the telephone!

- Purchase a ***telephone coupler*** that slips over the telephone receiver. This will pick up the acoustic signal, amplify it, and output it as a magnetic signal via a sending coil.

- Use a hearing aid that is seated in the ear sufficiently deeply (i.e., a CIC or possibly an ITC) that it can be used acoustically, with the telephone placed over the ear, or angled partly over the ear, without causing feedback.

The last two solutions are portable: they will work with any telephone.

---

hearing aid acoustic response will have been carefully adjusted to suit the aid wearer, it is important that the combined response of the loop and hearing aid telecoil not be too different from the acoustic response. One exception to this is that some additional cut for frequencies below about 500 Hz *may* be beneficial (for some people in some situations), as this is the frequency region where magnetic interference is most likely to occur. Unfortunately, this may also be the most important frequency region for people with profound hearing losses. Fortunately, multi-memory hearing aids (see Section 3.3.2) often make it possible to adjust the response separately for the telecoil and microphone operation, so that the best telecoil response for an individual aid user can be selected. Some remote controls even allow the user to select a low-tone cut when needed, such as in rooms with a lot of magnetic interference. (Fluorescent lights, and lights with dimmers operating are particularly troublesome.)

There are two reasons why a user might experience a different frequency response in the telecoil position than in the microphone position. First, the loop may emit a weaker magnetic signal for high-frequency sounds than it does for low-frequency sounds. This can happen because the electrical impedance of the loop comprises an ***inductance*** as well as a ***resistance***. An inductance has an impedance that increases with frequency, so the total impedance of the loop starts to rise once the frequency exceeds a certain frequency known as the ***corner frequency***. (At the corner frequency, the impedance of the inductance equals the impedance of the resistance.) If the loop is powered by a conventional audio power amplifier, the current, and hence the magnetic signal, will both decrease as frequency rises above the corner frequency. The solution is to make sure the corner frequency is 5 kHz or higher. This can be achieved by using either:

- wire with a small diameter (provided it does not overheat);

- a special current-drive power amplifier (with a high output impedance);

- very few turns, or one turn, in the loop;

- a graphic equalizer; or

- an external series resistor.

Practical tips: Installing or improving a loop

- Make the loop as small as you can get away with.

- The resistance of the loop (which can be measured with a multimeter, or calculated with the equation below) should not be less than the amplifier is able to safely drive. Four ohms or more is usually safe, but wherever possible, read the amplifier specifications!

- A room of size 5 m by 5 m can be looped with two turns of 0.4 mm diameter wire, powered by an amplifier of 10 Watts (or more). Alternatively, thicker wire could be used for convenience with a 10 Watt, 3 to 5 ohm resistor added in series to provide the necessary minimum total resistance. Figure 3.6 shows how a twin-core cable can be connected to provide the the two turns required.

If you do not like equations, read no further!

- For a loop of n turns, each turn having a perimeter of p meters, made of wire with a diameter d mm (excluding the insulation), and producing a maximum rms field strength of 0.4 A/m, the following can be calculated to design a loop or to check an existing loop:

$$\text{Minimum amplifier power} = \frac{p^3}{2800n\,d^2} Watts$$

$$\text{Minimum wire diameter to avoid overheating} = \sqrt{\frac{p}{62n}}\text{mm}$$

$$\text{Corner frequency} = \frac{7610}{nd^2 \log_{10}(446\,p/d)} Hz$$

$$\text{Loop resistance} = 0.022\frac{np}{d^2}\text{Ohms}$$

These equations, which are in part derived from Philbrick (1982) and from British Standard 7594, assume that no external resistor is used to increase the total resistance. If one is used, the minimum amplifier power and the corner frequency are both increased by the ratio of total resistance to resistance of the loop itself. An amplifier power of twice the minimum power calculated above is desirable to minimize peak clipping.

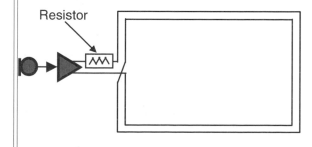

Resistor

Figure 3.6 The connections needed to make a loop of two turns using a single run of cable that has two separate wires. The location of an optional series resistor is also shown.

The last three options all may require a more powerful amplifier. Simultaneously achieving the right resistance, field strength, and frequency response, without overheating the wire in the loop, is easy for small loops, and difficult (or rather, more expensive) for large loops. An alternative solution is to use a grid of small loops, which must be placed under the carpet or mat, rather than around the perimeter of the room. This also minimizes spillover from the loop to adjacent rooms. Such systems should be purchased commercially, rather than being assembled from commonly available components.

The second reason why the telecoil frequency response might be different from the acoustic response lies in the hearing aid itself. Coils inherently produce a voltage that rises with frequency. The hearing aid designer can compensate for this, either partially or completely, by the way in which the telecoil connects to the hearing aid amplifier. The shape of the telecoil response, relative to the microphone response, is evident from the specification sheet for the hearing aid, or by measuring each response in a test box (see Section 4.1.8).

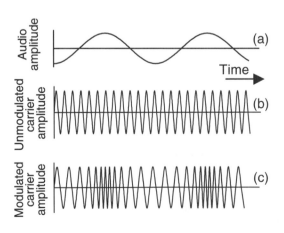

Figure 3.7 The waveform of a carrier before (b), and after (c), it has been frequency modulated by a sinusoidal audio signal (a).

3.7 Radio-frequency Transmission

Radio-frequency transmission provides a more portable way to get a signal from a talker to a listener without corrupting the signal by noise or reverberation. The talker wears a small *transmitter,* usually clipped to a belt or worn in a pocket. A microphone, clipped to the lapel or worn on the head, is attached to the transmitter by a cable, and this wire also serves as an aerial for the transmitter.

The *receiver* is worn by the hearing-impaired person. It can be coupled to the hearing aid by a cable or by a loop worn around the neck. Alternatively, the whole receiver can be incorporated in the hearing aid or clipped onto the hearing aid, as discussed further below.

3.7.1 Principles and FM capture effect

In radio-frequency transmission, the audio electrical signal is not directly converted to another form of energy (as it is with loops and telecoils), but instead modifies or - *modulates* the characteristics of an electromagnetic wave. This electromagnetic wave is called the *carrier*. In the absence of an audio signal, the carrier is a sinusoidal wave. It can convey information only when the audio signal alters some aspect of the carrier. In the hearing aid field, it is the carrier frequency that is most commonly altered, so we refer to this as *frequency modulation* or *FM*.

Figure 3.7 shows an audio wave, an unmodulated carrier, and the resulting modulated carrier. The job of the receiver is to detect the carrier and then produce a voltage that is proportional to the original audio signal. This extraction of the modulating waveform is called *demodulation*. There are other forms of modulation that could be used, the most common of which is *amplitude modulation*, in which the audio signal modulates the amplitude, rather than the frequency of the carrier. The advantage of

---

Practical tips: Wearing a transmitter

- Wearing the microphone on a head-mounted boom just below the mouth will result in a SNR about 10 dB better than clipping it to the lapel, and the signal transmitted will not be affected by extreme head turns away from the microphone.

- Clipping the transmitter microphone to the lapel will result in a SNR about 10 dB better than clipping it at waist level. (Many people clip it too low, especially if the waist is the most obvious feature when looking down!)

---

using modulation (of either sort) is that the strength of the audio signal coming out of the receiver does not depend on the strength of the carrier wave, and hence does not depend on the distance between the transmitter and the receiver. As the carrier wave becomes weaker, however, the transmission process will progressively add noise to the audio signal. When the carrier becomes extremely weak, reception will cease entirely.

There are probably many hundreds of electromagnetic waves, coming from many hundreds of transmitters, passing through the room in which you are now sitting. How does the receiver select just one of these before it demodulates the audio signal it contains? The receiver is tuned to be most sensitive to a particular carrier frequency. Only when the receiver frequency matches the frequency sent out by the transmitter will the receiver pick up the transmitted signal. What happens if two transmitters are sending out signals at the same frequency? There is certainly the potential for much confusion in the receiver. Licensing authorities minimize the problem by designating different parts of the electromagnetic spectrum (i.e., different carrier frequencies) for different types of transmitters. In various countries, the frequency bands available for hearing aid devices are 37, 43, 72-76, 173, 183, and 216 MHz. Within each of these bands, a number of different transmission frequencies are allowed, and the narrow frequency region around each is referred to as a *transmission channel*.

With FM transmission and reception, an additional phenomenon helps when a receiver is exposed to two different transmissions at the same carrier frequency, or to two carrier frequencies that are only slightly different. Because the demodulator works by "locking on" to the carrier, and then measuring how much its frequency varies with time, it can lock on to a strong carrier even if a weaker carrier is simultaneously present. This phenomenon of demodulating only the stronger signal is known as the *FM capture effect* because the receiver is captured by the strongest signal. If two transmitters of the same output power are generating the two signals, then the stronger of the two signals at the receiver will be the one originating from the closer of the two transmitters. The field intensity coming from a transmitter decreases in inverse proportion to the square of the distance from the transmitter (known as the *inverse square law*), just as for acoustic waves.

The FM capture effect can be used to advantage in schools. Two classrooms can use the same transmission channel provided the classrooms are sufficiently far apart for all children in each class to receive their own teacher's signal much more strongly than they receive a signal from teachers in any other classroom operating at the same frequency. Unfortunately, it is not always clear just how far this should be. The inverse square law does not apply exactly if there are large metal objects nearby, which there invariably are indoors. Long metal objects can cause signals from

Practical Tips: Fixing unreliable reception

- Check that the transmitter and receiver batteries are fresh.
- Make sure that the problem is not a faulty connecting cord or plug (try a new one, or for intermittent operation, wiggle the cords).
- Check that the transmitter and receiver aerial wires are not cut off or curled up.
- Rearrange the room so that the teacher and/or children are usually in different locations, preferably closer together and away from large metal objects.
- Choose a different transmitter (and receiver) channel.

distant transmitters to be received with stronger than expected intensity. Metal objects can also cause reflections of the electromagnetic wave. These reflections can cancel the signal coming directly from the transmitter, thus causing the signal strength to be very low at certain places in the room. A receiver at these positions will not be able to adequately detect the carrier and a ***dropout*** occurs. The listener will then hear only noise. More sophisticated receivers will detect that a dropout has occurred and will ***mute*** or ***squelch*** the output signal, so that silence occurs when the receiver detects that it is not receiving a carrier wave.

Radio-frequency waves pass through non-conductive obstacles (such as brick walls) extremely well. They are attenuated by large conductors such as sheet metal walls, and, to a lesser extent, by the human body.

3.7.2　Coupling to the hearing aid

The signal coming from the receiver is useful only if it can be delivered to the ears of the hearing-impaired user. The simplest form of output is for the receiver to directly drive an earphone, usually a button-style earphone connected to an individual earmold. The major disadvantage is that receivers do not usually contain sophisticated (or sometimes any) tone controls or adjustable forms of compression. It is thus not possible to adjust the amplification characteristics to suit the requirements of the individual aid wearer.

Individual amplification needs can be met more accurately if the FM receiver output is coupled to the person's own hearing aid. This coupling can be achieved via a cable to the hearing aid's electrical (audio) input connector, assuming it has one. Alternatively, the FM receiver can drive a loop worn around the user's neck, which then sends a magnetic signal to the hearing aid telecoil. A third alternative is for the FM receiver to drive a small coil mounted in a thin plastic case that is positioned behind the wearer's ear, right beside the wearer's own BTE hearing aid. This coil is known as a ***silhouette*** coil, because its case has the same profile as that of a BTE hearing aid.

Each of these methods has its advantages and disadvantages, and is likely to produce a different frequency response for the combined amplification system.[366] The direct electrical connection provides a well-defined signal, although the cable is inconvenient, cosmetically undesirable, and often breaks.[426] The connectors at each end can also become unreliable after much use. An important advantage is that speech-operated switching systems (see next section) are most easily possible with direct connection. The neck loop is cosmetically superior (particularly important to teenagers) and there are no cables outside the clothing to interfere with an active lifestyle or to be grabbed by small hands. Disadvantages are that the low frequencies can be attenuated, and the strength of the magnetic coupling (and hence of the audio

Adjusting the FM receiver output controls

The first aim in coupling an FM receiver to a hearing aid is for the receiver to output the same signal level and spectrum when the transmitter is used as when the hearing aid alone is used.

- With the hearing aid volume control in the position normally used for hearing aid alone, and the hearing aid coupled to a 2 cc coupler, input a test signal at 70 dB SPL, and record the output response. The test signal should have a speech-like spectrum, and ideally should have speech-like amplitude fluctuations. Such signals are now available in some real-ear gain analyzers.

- Connect the FM receiver to the hearing aid and input the same type of test signal to the FM transmitter, but at a level of 85 dB SPL. (This level assumes that the transmitter microphone is to be worn on the lapel. For a head-mounted microphone, use a level of 95 dB SPL.) Adjust any gain (and tone controls if any) on the FM receiver until the response out of the hearing aid matches the response obtained for hearing aid alone.

Note that the adjustment obtained with the above procedure is only applicable when the FM and hearing aid are to be used in an *FM-only* mode, or in a *speech-operated switching* mode. The two test levels recommended here are slightly higher than those suggested by Hawkins (1987) and by ASHA (1994), but are considered more typical of real life. The absolute levels chosen, as well as the difference between the two levels, will affect the final adjustment because FM transmitters include a compression limiter to prevent over-modulation of the carrier.

When the system is operated in a *combined* mode, such that the transmitter microphone and hearing aid or receiver microphone are *simultaneously* operating, the output from the FM path has to be increased relative to the output from the local microphone path by 5 to 15 dB. How large this differential should be, and whether it should be achieved by increasing the FM output, or by decreasing the local microphone output, or by both, is difficult to say. There is undoubtedly no single correct answer. If the hearing aid user has poor communication ability in the hearing aid alone condition (because of either the degree of loss or the noisiness of the room), a relatively large differential should be used. If the wearer has a frequent need to hear people other than the person using the transmitter, a relatively small differential should be used. Lewis (2000) recommends increasing the transmitter microphone sensitivity by 5 dB and decreasing the local microphone sensitivity by 5 dB. Be aware that with some FM systems, switching from *FM-only* to *combined* mode will automatically lower the hearing aid microphone sensitivity. The desired 5 to 15 dB FM advantage should thus be confirmed with the FM system and the hearing aid connected together and operating.

The difficulty inherent in achieving a good compromise between the sensitivity of the two microphone paths in the combined mode reinforces the value of having a system that can operate in speech-operated switching mode. Both the FM microphone and the hearing aid microphone can individually be optimally set and the speech-operated switching provides the desired precedence for the FM microphone.

The description in this box assumes that the FM receiver and the personal hearing aid are separate units that must be connected together. For self-contained FM systems, the principles involved and steps required are identical. The term *hearing aid* should be interpreted to mean those components in the unit that provide local reception of acoustic signals independently of the FM transmission system.

signal) can be decreased when the head is inclined to either side. (Boring school lessons can produce a 90-degree bend of the neck, by which angle none of the magnetic signal is picked up by the telecoil, possibly making the lesson even less interesting!) Also, magnetic signals are prone to interference from nearby electrical apparatus. The silhouette coil has all the disadvantages associated with the presence of a cable, and the potential for interference, and is thus a poor choice for a coupling method.

The method that has the best combination of reliability and cosmetic acceptability is when the FM receiver is mounted *inside* the BTE hearing aid, or is mounted in a small boot that plugs onto the bottom of the hearing aid and connects to the direct electrical input. Both of these options have become available in recent years.

If the patient has near-normal hearing in any frequency region, the FM receiver should be coupled to the ear with an open earmold or earshell. Open coupling enables the aid wearer to hear nearby sounds in the good ear via the unaided sound path.[490] This applies whether the FM is coupled directly to the ear or is coupled via a hearing aid.

3.7.3 Combined FM and local microphones

When children are working in small groups, or otherwise need to hear other children talking, it is not satisfactory for the hearing aid to receive only the signal coming from the FM transmitter, because the transmitter may be far away from the person talking. FM systems overcome this problem in a number of ways. One solution is to switch the receiver and hearing aid to a *combined* position. In the combined position the wearer hears a mixture of sound coming from the transmitter, and sound being picked up by the hearing aid microphone (see also Section 2.9). While this allows a nearby talker to be heard (though possibly with decreased volume), the hearing aid microphone continues to pick up noise

and reverberation even when the teacher is talking into the transmitter, thus removing most of the advantage provided by the FM system.[77, 160, 362] In some FM systems, this *local* microphone (also called an *environmental* microphone) is mounted in the FM receiver, but the combined position has the same advantages and problems as when it is in the hearing aid.

There is a great dilemma with using such systems: the clearest signal from the teacher is received in the FM-alone condition, the worst signal from the teacher is obtained using the local microphone, and a signal of intermediate clarity is obtained in the combined position.[160, 362] The dilemma is that when children are asked which operating mode they prefer, the order is exactly reversed,[160] presumably because the children feel increasingly detached from their immediate environment as their local microphone becomes less dominant.

The solution to this dilemma lies in an automatic switch within the FM system that selects FM alone when an audio signal is coming from the transmitter, but which selects the local microphone alone when there is no such audio signal coming from the transmitter. (Alternatively, one of the operating modes selected by the automatic switch could be the combined position referred to in the previous paragraph.) These systems are referred to by a variety of names: *speech-operated switching (SOX), voice-operated switching (VOX), FM priority,* or *FM precedence*. Figure 3.8 shows the block diagram of one such system. If the local microphone is in the hearing aid, rather than in the receiver, the receiver can attenuate the output of the microphone (rather than switch it off altogether) by lowering the output impedance of the receiver, or by injecting a voltage that turns the microphone off. For this to work, any hearing aid used with the FM system must have its direct electrical input connector wired in parallel with its microphone (see Section 2.9).

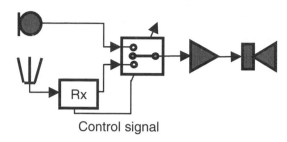

Figure 3.8 An FM system with Speech Operated Switching (SOX) in the receiver to select either the local microphone signal or the FM signal (from the aerial) for amplification by the hearing aid.

3.8   Infrared Transmission

Infrared radiation is the same type of electromagnetic energy as radio waves, except that it occurs at a much, much higher frequency (approximately 10^{14} Hz). For frequencies slightly higher than this, electromagnetic radiation is perceived by humans as a red light, hence the term *infra-* (meaning *below*) *red*. Transmission of audio signals via infrared electromagnetic waves also requires that the carrier (the infrared wave) be modulated by the audio wave. In this case, it is more convenient to use amplitude modulation. In particular, the infrared wave is pulsed on and off, with the audio signal directly or indirectly controlling the timing of the pulses. The infrared receiver first detects the pulsing infrared carrier, and then demodulates the pulses to recover the audio signal. Just as for FM radio-frequency signals, the output can directly drive a headphone, or can be coupled to a hearing aid. It is more common for infrared systems to be used directly with an earphone or earphones, though there is no fundamental reason why this should be so.

Because infrared operates at almost the same frequency as light waves, infrared radiation behaves in the same way as light waves. It travels in straight lines, is easily blocked by opaque obstacles, and reflects (with some attenuation) off flat, light colored surfaces, like ceilings. You can experiment (but not now!) with how well infrared systems work in the presence of obstacles by noting the conditions in which your TV or video remote control works or does not work.

3.9   Classroom Sound-field Amplification

Unlike the three systems just described, sound-field amplification systems get sound to the listener using acoustic waves. They work on the premise that if SNR is adversely affected by background noises and distance from the talker, both of these problems can be minimized by amplifying the wanted sound and positioning a loudspeaker near the listener. The most common application is a classroom, and because children are likely to be located throughout the classroom, several loudspeakers must be positioned around the walls of the room. The most basic systems thus consist of a microphone, an amplifier, and one or more loudspeakers. An obvious limitation of this basic system is that the teacher has to either remain next to a fixed microphone, or carry round a microphone with a long cable. A useful addition is therefore an FM (or potentially infrared) link between the teacher and the amplifier, which enables the teacher to move freely around the room. Figure 3.9 shows the block diagram of such a system.

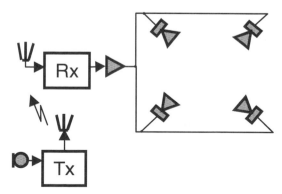

Figure 3.9 Block diagram of a sound-field amplification system comprising a transmitter worn by the teacher, a receiver and amplifier mounted somewhere convenient in the room, and four loudspeakers distributed around the room.

Sound-field amplification systems have several advantages over the three other types of transmission systems already discussed. First, they do not require the listeners to wear any special equipment. This simplifies supply logistics, and increases system reliability because there is nothing for the children to break! Second, the improved sound clarity is available to all children in the classroom, not just those with hearing aids, and there is some evidence that many children with normal hearing thresholds will benefit educationally from receiving a clearer signal.[186, 969] Third, the advantages will therefore be available to those who have a temporary conductive hearing loss. This is particularly advantageous for some indigenous populations where the incidence of conductive loss can be high. The fluctuating nature of the loss makes it difficult for children to be fitted with individual hearing aids at all times when they need it. In some cases, cultural factors can lead to rejection of individual devices. An initially unexpected advantage of sound field systems is that teachers report considerably less voice fatigue, and decreased incidence of voice nodules when they use these systems.[287]

Of course, there are also disadvantages. Sound-field amplification systems can increase the sound level in typical classrooms only by about 10 dB before feedback oscillation occurs.[d] Consequently, the improvement in SNR is also limited to around 10 dB if nothing else changes. The increase in SNR may be less if background noise levels also rise when the system is used, or may be greater if background noise levels fall. The latter is anecdotally reported to occur. The increase in SNR achieved is greatest if the teacher wears a microphone on the head, positioned on a boom so that the microphone is close to the lips but not directly in front of them.[288]

Although sound field systems can increase the ratio of direct to reverberant sound received

by each child, the magnitude of the increase depends on the distance between the child and the closest loudspeaker and on the distance between the child and the teacher. Unfortunately, each loudspeaker adds to the reverberant sound as well as to the direct sound. Loudspeakers should be positioned so that each child is as close as possible to a loudspeaker. There is potential for these systems to provide even better performance if they were to incorporate advanced processing schemes that allowed additional gain to be achieved without feedback (see Section 7.3).

As with other remote transmission systems, the basic system is suitable for only a single talker. Team teaching, or interactive work between the teacher and the children, requires that two transmitters be used, and that the outputs of their corresponding receivers be summed prior to being amplified. Equipment to do this is available, but the second transmitter must be passed around if the advantages are to be achieved whenever a child is the talker. Children generally react well to having control of the microphone when reading or making presentations to the rest of the class.

3.10 Comparative Strengths and Weaknesses of Magnetic Loops, Radio-frequency (FM), Infrared, and Sound-field Amplification Systems

The four remote transmission hearing aid systems can be compared in a number of ways: effectiveness in improving SNR, effectiveness in increasing the ratio of direct signal to reverberant signal, convenience, reliability, and cost. We will assume that the sound field system has been implemented with an FM link between the teacher and the amplifier. We will also assume that the application is a classroom containing several hearing-impaired children, each of whom

---

[d]   The maximum gain achievable without feedback whistling depends on the amount of sound absorbing material in the room. Adding soft furnishings will allow higher gains to be achieved (and will also improve sound quality in the absence of the system).

Table 3.1   Relative advantages of each of the remote transmission systems, for application in a classroom containing several hearing-impaired children. For each criterion, a greater number of check marks indicates a greater relative advantage.

	Magnetic Loops	FM transmission	Infrared transmission	Sound-field amplification
SNR improvement	✓✓	✓✓	✓✓	✓
Reverberation decrease	✓✓	✓✓	✓✓	✓
Convenience		✓	✓	✓
Consistency and reliability	✓			✓
Privacy			✓✓	✓
Low cost	✓			✓

already has an individually fitted hearing aid with direct electrical input connections and/or telecoils, as appropriate. Table 3.1 shows which of the systems have advantages over the others in each of these areas.

Each of the first three systems, because they transmit energy in a non-acoustic form, are able to deliver large increases in SNR, and large decreases in reverberant energy, provided the microphone is placed sufficiently close to the teacher's mouth. These improvements can be 20 dB or more, and are therefore much more substantial than can be achieved with a sound-field amplification system.

The sound-field amplification system, however, is probably the most convenient to use. The receiver, amplifier and loudspeaker components do not have to be touched, and there is therefore only one transmitter to be handled. Convenience rapidly decreases, however, once there are two or more talkers to be amplified, unless the system has been designed to work with two transmitters simultaneously.[684, 685] The magnetic loop system is the least convenient. With a conventional implementation, the teacher has to stay near a fixed microphone or carry a microphone with a long lead. Of course, an FM system could be used to get the signal from the teacher to the loop amplifier. Furthermore, all children have to switch to the T position of their hearing aids to receive the loop signal,

and they will then be detached from their local acoustic environments. If their hearing aids have a combined MT position, they can receive both the loop signal and acoustic signals, but the same disadvantages apply as for FM systems in the combined position.

The sound-field amplification system provides the most consistent performance, partly because there is only one mobile component, and partly because it is immediately apparent to the teacher if the system fails, so corrective action can be taken immediately. Magnetic loops are the next most consistent, again because there are few mobile components, and provided the system has been installed so that it produces a sufficiently strong magnetic signal. While magnetic interference can occur, the sources of interference do not usually come and go, so systems can remain interference-free if they are initially so.

FM systems are less consistent in operation, partly because of *dropouts*, partly because of *interference* (which can come from distant places at unpredictable times), but mainly because there may be several receivers and even transmitters, each with their own cables, connectors and batteries to be maintained. In the classroom, infrared systems are less prone to interference, but may have numerous dropouts whenever the transmitter and the receiver are not directly facing each other. Infrared systems are particularly well suited to applications where the listeners are all facing in the same direction and where the transmitter always directly faces the listeners. In indoor situations where this is true, infrared systems are free from interference and drop-outs.

Infrared systems are the clear winner when it comes to privacy: there is virtually no spillover outside the room in which the transmitter is located. Apart from any confidentiality issues, the lack of spill-over means that many rooms in a building can have identical systems installed, without any interference between adjacent rooms. The other three systems radiate signals outside the room in which they are being used, with the extent of radiation being greatest for FM systems, although eaves-dropping requires access to a receiver with the correct carrier frequency. If confidentiality is not an issue, then electromagnetic spillover is not a problem provided that the equipment used in different classrooms operates at different frequencies. It is advantageous to have a choice of frequencies so that interference can be avoided.

Finally, magnetic loops and sound-field amplification systems are the cheapest to install and maintain, as only one device per classroom is needed, rather than one device per child. Only sound field systems provide an improved signal to children who are not wearing any individual hearing device.

3.11 Assistive Listening Devices

Any devices that help hearing-impaired people detect sounds or understand speech, but which are not worn totally on the head or body are referred to as *assistive listening devices* or *ALDs*. The various wireless systems described in Sections 3.6 to 3.9 are all ALDs, but there are other types. Many of these comprise a sensor of some type (e.g. smoke, clock, ringing phone, doorbell button) linked to an output that can be easily detected by the hearing-impaired person (flashing

light, vibrator, or intense low-frequency sound). Devices comprising a microphone, amplifier, and stereo headphones (on a headband or as individual lightweight ear buds) are sometimes referred to as assistive listening devices, although these would be better classified as body aids.

Assistive listening devices, including those already discussed in more detail, can be considered under three categories:

Devices to improve speech intelligibility

- A personal wireless system (infrared or FM) with the receiver coupled to a hearing aid or coupled to headphones and used without a hearing aid.

- A personal wireless system with the transmitter coupled electrically to the TV sound circuit, or the transmitter microphone positioned in close proximity to the TV loudspeaker.

- An induction coil (room-sized, chair-sized, or ear-sized) connected to an amplifier and microphone or auxiliary input jack.

- An amplified telephone.

- A telephone amplifier that is inserted between a regular telephone and its wall socket, or installed within the telephone itself.

- A telephone coupler/amplifier that straps onto the telephone receiver. Its microphone picks up the acoustic signal coming from the receiver and amplifies it. It may produce a stronger acoustic output and/ or may produce a stronger magnetic output for use with telecoils. These devices are more portable than the preceding three telephone amplification devices.

- A classroom sound-field amplification system with FM radio input.

- A telephone, answering machine, or any audio product that can be safely coupled to the audio input socket of a hearing aid. It can be dangerous to connect a mains-operated (i.e. 110 to 240 V) device to the audio input connector of a hearing aid. A fault within the mains-operated device could enable the full mains voltage to be applied to the hearing aid, almost certainly destroying the hearing aid, and potentially electrocuting the hearing aid wearer. This danger is avoided if the mains-operated device has an *optically isolated* output circuit.

Devices to detect environmental sounds

- An alarm clock with a vibrating alarm that can be placed in the bed.

- A doorbell that emits a loud low-pitched sound or a flashing light.

- A telephone extension that emits a loud low-pitched sound or a flashing light or a vibrator within a bed.

- An alarm clock that emits a loud low-pitched sound or a flashing light or a vibrator within a bed.

- A baby alarm that emits a flashing light.

Miscellaneous devices

- A sound absorbing pad that fits onto a telephone receiver to allow the receiver to be brought in close proximity to the hearing aid without feedback occurring.

3.12 Concluding remarks

The advent of digital technology has revolutionized the *methods* hearing aids use to change sounds. In many respects, however, the *result* (the sound coming out of the hearing aid) is no different from the sound emerging from analog hearing aids. Fortunately, there are already a few examples, as we will see in Chapters 6 and 7, of how digital hearing aids can modify sounds in ways that have never been possible with analog hearing aids. Basic digital hearing aids should decrease in cost as they become the standard hearing aid technology. High-performing devices will continue to have a premium price.

Hearing aid amplification systems involving remote transmission can provide a much higher level of performance than individual devices worn on the head. Remote transmission devices such as radio-frequency FM, infrared, induction loop, and sound field systems should be used whenever good intelligibility is critical, such as in school systems. High performance does not always require high expense. The telecoil, a low-cost device that has been available in hearing aids for decades, is capable of being used much more often than is now the case.

A high level of innovation in hearing aid systems is likely in the next decade. Hearing aid, mobile telephone, and computer technologies now have much in common, so hearing aids will benefit from advances made in the other higher volume fields. For example:

- hearing aids on each side of the head may be able to communicate with each other to achieve more dramatic noise reduction than has so far been possible;

- a hearing aid wearer may be able to position several miniature remote microphone-transmitters in his or her immediate vicinity, and a hearing aid with in-built wireless receivers may be able to combine the outputs to produce even more dramatic noise reduction.

A more immediate problem for audiology is to find the place for low-cost, mail-order modular hearing aids that best helps hearing-impaired people. These devices, including disposable hearing aids, have the potential to give an increased proportion of the hearing-impaired population a first-hand experience of amplification. In all those cases where the physical fit or electroacoustic performance is not well suited to the hearing-impaired person, however, they have the potential to reinforce negative and outdated beliefs about the limited effectiveness of hearing aids.

CHAPTER FOUR

ELECTROACOUSTIC PERFORMANCE AND MEASUREMENT

Synopsis

The performance of hearing aids is most conveniently measured when the hearing aid is connected to a coupler. A coupler is a small cavity that connects the hearing aid sound outlet to a measurement microphone. Unfortunately, the standard 2-cc coupler is larger than the average adult ear canal with a hearing aid in place, so the hearing aid generates lower SPL in this coupler than in the average ear. This difference is called the real ear to coupler difference (RECD). A more complex measurement device, which better simulates the acoustic of the human ear, is called an ear simulator.

Test boxes provide a convenient way to get sound into the hearing aid in a controlled manner. These sounds can be pure tones that sweep in frequency, or can be complex, broadband sounds that, like speech, contain many frequencies simultaneously. Broadband sounds are necessary to perform meaningful measurements on many nonlinear hearing aids. The measurements most commonly performed using these sounds are curves of gain or output versus frequency at different input levels, and curves of output versus input at different frequencies. The curve of output versus frequency when measured with a 90 dB SPL pure tone input level is usually taken to represent the highest levels that a hearing aid can create.

Some other test box measurements that are less commonly performed are measures of distortion, internal noise, and response to magnetic fields. These measurements are used to check that the hearing aid is operating properly.

Test box measurements are but a means to an end. That end is the performance of the hearing aid in an individual patient's ear. This performance can be directly measured using a soft, thin probe-tube inserted in the ear canal. Real-ear gain can be expressed as real-ear aided gain (REAG) which equals the level of sound in the ear canal minus the level in the air near the patient. Alternatively, real-ear gain can be expressed as real-ear insertion gain (REIG) which equals the level of sound in the ear canal when aided minus the level in the same place when no hearing aid is worn. Each of these measures requires the probe to be carefully located, and the requirements for probe placement are a little different for the two types of gain.

Both types of real-ear gain are different from coupler gain, partly because of the real ear to coupler difference already mentioned, and partly because the input to the hearing aid microphone is affected by sound diffraction patterns around the head and ear. The changes in SPL caused by diffraction are referred to as microphone location effects. Insertion gain is further different from coupler gain because resonance effects in the unaided ear form a baseline for the insertion gain measurement. This baseline, referred to as the real-ear unaided gain, provides the link between the REAG and the REIG.

Many factors can lead to incorrect measurement of real-ear gain. These factors include incorrect positioning of the probe, squashing of the probe, blockage of the probe by cerumen, background noise, and hearing aid saturation. Fortunately, there are some simple checks one can do to verify measurement accuracy.

Feedback is a major problem in hearing aids. It happens when the amplification from the microphone to the receiver is greater than the attenuation of sound leaking from the output back to the input. Clinicians must be able to diagnose the source of excess leakage. Other problems that often have simple solutions include no sound output, weak output, distorted output, and excessive noise.

We cannot know what a hearing aid does unless its performance is measured. The block diagram shows us what *types* of things a hearing aid does, but it requires a measurement to determine the *extent* to which it does these things to the sound.

4.1   Measuring Hearing Aids in Couplers and Ear Simulators

Hearing aids are most conveniently measured in **couplers** and **ear simulators**. The availability of standard couplers and simulators allows measurements to be made in different places and at different times under identical conditions.

4.1.1   Couplers and ear simulators

A coupler is simply a cavity. It has a hearing aid connected to one end and a microphone connected to the other. The coupler provides a repeatable way for the hearing aid to be connected to the microphone, and hence to a sound level meter, without sounds leaking out to other places. The standard coupler used for hearing aids has been around for over 50 years and has a volume of 2 cubic centimeters.[757] This volume was chosen because it was an approximation of the volume of the adult ear canal past the earmold (i.e. the **residual ear canal volume**) when a hearing aid is worn. Unfortunately, it is not a good approximation of the average adult ear canal volume, and is an even worse approximation of the acoustic impedance of the ear at high frequencies.

The SPL generated in any cavity by a hearing aid depends directly on the impedance of the cavity, which in turns depends on the vol-ume of the cavity, and on the nature of anything connected to the cavity. In the average adult ear, the residual ear canal has a physical volume of about 0.5 cc.[424] This volume acts as an acoustic spring, or more formally, an **acoustic compliance.** The ear canal, of course, terminates in the eardrum, on the other side of which is the middle ear cavity. The compliance of the middle ear cavity and eardrum together act as if they have a volume of about 0.8 cc.[978] The combined 1.3 cc volume determines the impedance for low-frequency sounds.[514] As frequency rises, the mass of the eardrum and ossicles causes their impedance to rise, while the impedance of the residual ear canal volume falls. Consequently, for increasing frequency, the total impedance does not decrease as much as would be expected for a simple cavity.

An ear simulator mimics this variation of impedance with frequency. Figure 4.1 shows the concept behind one ear simulator. As well as the main cavity, with a volume of 0.6 cc, the simulator shown has four side cavities, each with volumes from 0.10 to 0.22 cc, connected to the main cavity by small tubes,

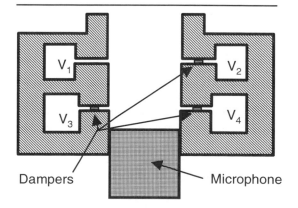

Dampers   Microphone

Figure 4.1 Simplified internal structure of a four-branch ear simulator.

three of which also contain dampers (ANSI S3.25, 1979). As frequency rises, the impedance of these tubes rise and they effectively close off, thus causing the effective total volume to gradually fall from 1.3 cc to 0.6 cc. One ear simulator with four cavities is known as the Zwislocki coupler and is sold commercially as the Knowles DB100 ear simulator. Another ear simulator in common use is the Bruel & Kjaer 4138 ear simulator. It operates on the same principles, except that it has two side cavities instead of four. The two simulators have a very similar variation of impedance with frequency.

Several standards published by the American National Standards Institute (ANSI) and International Electroacoustical Commission (IEC) specify how hearing aids should be tested (see Section 4.1.9). The two sets of standards have many things in common and a few differences. A key difference is that ANSI S3.22 specifies that hearing aids be measured in a 2-cc coupler, whereas IEC 118-0 specifies that hearing aids be measured in an ear simulator, though it allows a 2-cc coupler to be substituted. To correctly interpret a hearing aid specification sheet, it is essential to determine whether the data refer to coupler or ear simulator performance,[a] and whether the hearing aid has been measured in a test box or on an *acoustic manikin.* An acoustic manikin comprises a head and torso, with an ear simulator incorporated inside each ear. As we shall see, the choices of coupler versus ear simulator, and test box versus manikin make a big difference to the numbers quoted.

Couplers and ear simulators have to connect to any type of hearing aid, and to achieve this, a range of adapters is used. Figure 4.2 shows several couplers, simulators and adapters, and Figure 4.3 shows some details and dimensions of 2-cc couplers. An essential concept is that of the *reference plane.* This is a plane, at right angles to the longitudinal axis of the

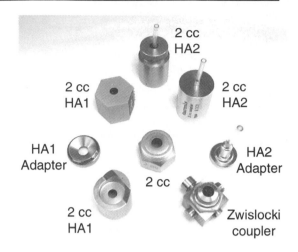

Figure 4.2 Several couplers and their adapters, and an ear simulator.

ear canal, located at the point in the ear canal where the earmold or ear shell usually terminates (defined in the standards to be approximately 13 mm from the eardrum). An ear simulator (and very approximately, a coupler) represents the acoustic impedance of the residual ear canal volume and middle ear from this point inward. ITE and ITC hearing aids usually terminate at this point, so these hearing aids are directly connected to a coupler or ear simulator. BTE and body aids, however, connect to the real ear via an earmold, so an *earmold simulator* is added between the coupler or ear simulator and the hearing aid. In addition, BTE hearing aids use tubing when connecting to a real ear, so they also require tubing when connecting to the coupler or simulator.

ANSI S3.3 describes a 2-cc coupler as being used in several different applications, the most important of which are:

- the *HA1 coupler* has no earmold simulator and is used for ITE and ITC aids, which are connected to the coupler via putty;

- the *HA2 coupler* includes an earmold simulator, which is connected to the BTE hearing aid via tubing, or into which a receiver for a body aid snaps.

---

a   On a hearing aid specification sheet, the use of a 2-cc coupler may be signified just by mention of ANSI S3.7, IEC 126, or IEC 60 126. Use of an ear simulator may be signified by ANSI S3.25, IEC 711, or IEC 60 711.

Figure 4.3 The internal dimensions and coupling methods for several 2-cc couplers.

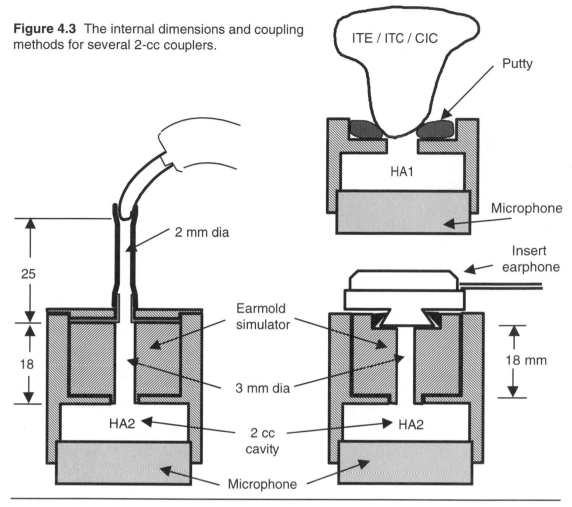

Connection methods for ear simulators are similar to those used for 2-cc couplers. CIC hearing aids are measured in the same way as ITE and ITC hearing aids, though in actual use, many are inserted beyond the reference plane.

Because an ear simulator accurately reflects the variation of impedance with frequency of the average ear, a hearing aid will generate the same SPL in an ear simulator as it does when inserted to the reference plane in an average adult ear.[b] This is not true of a 2-cc coupler. Figure 4.4 shows the difference in SPL generated by a hearing aid receiver connected via an earmold to a 2-cc coupler and the average real ear.[767] Table 4.1 shows these data at the audiometric frequencies. These data are extremely useful, as the gain and OSPL90 of hearing aids is sometimes quoted based on 2-cc coupler measurements, and sometimes quoted based on ear simulator measurements. For both gain and OSPL90, the data in Figure 4.4 and Table 4.1 (first row) can be subtracted from ear simulator responses to give the expected 2-cc coupler response.[c] This difference is known

---

[b]   The simulator response matches the average real ear response only over the frequency range for which leakage around the earmold or ear shell is insignificant in the real ear.

[c]   Strictly speaking, the 2-cc response can be predicted from the ear simulator response, and vice-versa, only if the receiver and tubing connected to the coupler and simulator has an acoustic impedance much higher than that of the ear simulator. Fortunately, hearing aid receivers have an output impedance 20 to 30 dB greater than that of an ear simulator (Olafson, private communication).

Table 4.1 RECD: SPL generated in the average real ear minus the SPL generated in a 2-cc coupler (dB). The BTE values assume that the BTE earmold has a constant diameter #13 tubing when in the real ear. These values for the BTE have been derived from those in the first row by applying the HA2 to HA1 coupler differences.[219] All values assume no venting and no leakage around the earmold (see Section 5.3.1).

	Frequency (Hz)								
	125	250	500	1 k	2 k	3 k	4 k	6 k	8 k
ITE or ITC: insertion to reference plane in real ear relative to HA1 coupler.	3	3	4	5	8	10	12	14	15
BTE: insertion to reference plane in real ear relative to HA2 coupler.	3	3	5	6	8	8	7	7	13
CIC: deep placement in real ear, relative to HA1 coupler (e.g. CIC).	6	6	8	10	15	19	20	23	25

as the average *real ear to coupler difference*, or **RECD**. Table 4.1 also shows RECD data reported for CIC hearing aids, which terminate well beyond the reference plane.[49, 339] Note that these "CIC" values would equally apply to any hearing aid or earmold with a deeply seated medial end. Similarly, the values shown for ITE or ITC hearing aids would apply to a CIC hearing aid if its medial end were 13 mm from the eardrum.

The advantage of the ear simulator over the 2-cc coupler is that the ear simulator directly

indicates the SPL that a hearing aid would generate in the average adult ear canal. This equivalency assumes that the hearing aid is coupled to the ear simulator in the same way that it is coupled to the ear canal. (The effect of different coupling methods on hearing aid response is covered in Chapter 5.) Even the ear simulator, however, cannot show the SPL that would be present in an individual ear, which is our ultimate interest.

The disadvantages of the ear simulator compared to the 2-cc coupler are its higher cost and the potential for the small openings inside the simulator to become blocked. Both 2-cc couplers and ear simulators will produce inaccurate results if:

- the sound bore of an ITE/ITC/CIC hearing aid is poorly sealed to the coupler or simulator;
- the tubing connecting to a BTE hearing aid becomes stiff and does not properly seal at either end;
- the o-ring connecting a button receiver wears out; or
- the pressure equalization hole becomes blocked or excessively open.[d]

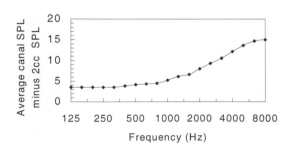

Figure 4.4 RECD: SPL generated in the average adult real ear canal minus SPL generated in an HA1 2-cc coupler.

---

d   Both 2-cc couplers and ear simulators create a very fine pressure equalization hole by drilling a hole and then partially filling it with a fine wire. With some designs it is possible for the fine wire to be removed by someone fiddling with the device.

Except for the blocked pressure equalization hole, the remaining faults will all decrease the apparent low-frequency gain and power of the hearing aid being measured, and may also create a spurious mid-frequency resonance (see *Vent-associated resonance* within Section 5.3.1).

4.1.2   Test boxes

The coupler and ear simulator provide a way for the *output* from the hearing aid to be measured. Just as important is the means to put a controlled sound *into* the hearing aid. A *test box* generates sounds of a required SPL at the hearing aid microphone. A test box includes a tone and/or noise generator, an amplifier, a loudspeaker, and a control microphone. The *control microphone* (also called a *reference microphone*) is placed next to the hearing aid microphone, as shown in Figure 4.5. The control microphone monitors the SPL reaching the hearing aid from the loudspeaker. If the input level is higher or lower than the desired level, the control microphone circuit automatically turns the volume of the sound coming from the test box speaker down or up, respectively, until the required level is obtained.

The control microphone works in one of two ways. With the *pressure method*, the control microphone is placed as close as possible to the hearing aid microphone while the measurement is taking place. The control microphone does its job of correcting the field during every measurement. With the *substitution method*, the control microphone is placed in the test position *prior* to the actual measurement. During a calibration measurement, the control microphone measures the

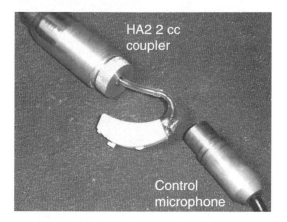

Figure 4.5 A hearing aid connected to a coupler, with a control microphone positioned next to the hearing aid microphone.

SPL present at each frequency, and stores any discrepancy between the actual and desired SPLs. During all subsequent measurements, the test box adjusts its outputs to compensate for these discrepancies.[e]

As well as providing a connection and a home for all the bits and pieces needed to measure a coupler or simulator response, the test box performs two other important functions. First, it attenuates ambient noise by having a lid that seals well to the box, by being constructed with solid, dense walls, and by containing absorbent material inside. Second, the absorbent material decreases internal sound reflections so that most of the sound reaching the hearing aid microphone comes directly from the loudspeaker. The resulting decrease in reflections, and hence in standing waves (see panel in Section 4.2.1) makes it easier for the control microphone to achieve the desired SPL at the hearing aid input.

---

e   Because the pressure method removes any diffraction effects caused by the hearing aid, but the substitution method does not, the two methods can give different results for high-frequency sounds. If the substitution method has to be used, then the results can be made to agree by performing both calibration and measurement with the control microphone and the hearing aid next to each other, as with the pressure method. A complication is that with some equipment, there is only one microphone, and it is used as both the control microphone and as the coupler microphone. In such cases, when the microphone is moved from the control position to the coupler to measure the hearing aid's output, a dummy microphone that matches the size of the real microphone has to be positioned at the place just vacated by the real microphone. ANSI S3.22 gives a full description.

For omni-directional microphones, when using the pressure method of calibration, it is important only that the control microphone and the hearing aid microphone be close to each other and the same distance away from the loudspeaker. (This arrangement makes sure that neither of them acts as an acoustical barrier that could cast an acoustic shadow over the other one.)

For directional microphones, it is important that the sound from the loudspeaker hits the hearing aid at the same angle that it would when the hearing aid is being worn and the source is directly in front of the person wearing the hearing aid. Often, this will mean that the line joining the two inlet ports of the directional microphone will pass through the center of the loudspeaker, with the front port closest to the loudspeaker. Make sure you know whether the loudspeaker is in the lid or in the base of the test box, and whether it is in the center or off to the side! Directional hearing aids should be measured with the lid of the test box open. (An open lid decreases the strength of any reflections arriving at the hearing aid from the wrong direction.) Directional hearing aids will usually have to be supported in the desired orientation by a piece of putty or absorbing foam, whereas omni-directional hearing aids can just lie flat on the surface of the test box.

As with all measurements, the measurements are useless unless the microphone(s) in the test box have been calibrated, and the calibration checked at regular intervals. Opinions vary about what those regular intervals should be, but a full calibration once every two years, plus a one-minute calibration check (see adjoining panel) once a week may be reasonable.

4.1.3 Measurement signals

Test boxes use one (or both) of two different types of measurement signals. The traditional measurement signal has been a **pure tone** that automatically sweeps in frequency over the desired frequency range (typically from 125 Hz to 8 kHz). More recently, test boxes

---

Practical tip: quick calibration check

A full calibration of a test box will check that the correct input levels are generated and that the SPL at the coupler or simulator microphone is correctly displayed. The following is *not* a substitution for a full calibration, but is a valuable quick and simple check:

- If possible, take the coupler or simulator off the microphone. Otherwise, take any earmold simulator off the coupler or ear simulator.

- With test boxes that use a separate control microphone, place the control microphone next to the coupler microphone and measure the frequency response with an input level of 90 dB SPL. With test boxes that use the substitution method, *Calibrate* or *Level* first, and then measure the frequency response for a 90 dB SPL input level with the measuring microphone at the calibration or leveling position.

- If the coupler/simulator could be removed, the output measured by the coupler/simulator microphone should be 90 ± 2 dB SPL at all frequencies.

- If the coupler/simulator could not be removed, then the output should be 90 ± 2 dB up to 500 Hz.

This quick procedure will *not* reveal an improperly calibrated test box if the control microphone and the coupler/simulator microphone are both out of calibration by the same amount, and in the same direction. With two-microphone systems, this is less likely to happen than just one of the microphones becoming out of calibration.

Terms used to summarize the gain-frequency response

High-frequency average (HFA) gain: Average of the gains at 1000, 1600 and 2500 Hz (ANSI S3.22).

Special purpose average gain: Average of the gains at three frequencies, each separated by 2/3 octaves. This is used for hearing aids with unusual frequency responses (ANSI S3.22).

Frequency range: This is the range of frequencies between the lowest and highest frequencies whose gains are 20 dB below the HFA gain (ANSI S3.22).

---

incorporating **broadband** noise-like signals have become available. These signals have all frequencies present simultaneously. The test box uses a Fourier Transform (See Sections 1.2 and 3.4.3) or a swept filter to determine the level in each frequency region of the signal coming out of the hearing aid. Because the analyzer stores the level of each frequency component at the input to the hearing aid, it can hence calculate the gain at each frequency. If the hearing aid is operating linearly, measurement with pure tones will give exactly the same gain-frequency response as measurement with broadband noise, no matter what the spectral shape of the broadband signal. Why then is it worth using the more complex measurement stimulus?

The main answer is that many hearing aids intentionally do not amplify linearly over a wide range of input levels. In hearing aids currently available, the most common cause of nonlinearity is compression, which as we have seen in Section 2.3.5 involves an amplifier whose gain depends on the input signal. Suppose a hearing aid amplifier includes a high-pass filter (i.e. a low tone cut) followed by a compressor. If such a hearing aid were to be measured with a swept pure-tone signal, then as frequency increases, the signal level passed by the filter to the compressor would increase. Consequently,

the compressor would increasingly turn down the gain, thus partially (or even wholly) undoing the effect of the filter. However, if a broadband signal of any fixed spectral shape[f] were to be input to the aid, the compressor would settle down to a particular gain. Analysis of the output spectrum would reveal that the filter had its full effect on the spectrum of the input signal. Swept pure tones and broadband noises would thus reveal very different response shapes.

Which is the *real* response of the hearing aid? Neither! Real input signals, such as speech sounds, are not narrowband signals like swept pure tones, nor are they signals whose spectra remain fixed with time. Rather they are signals whose spectrum varies from moment to moment. The broadband noise will accurately represent how the hearing aid changes the spectral shape of speech signals. If the compressor changes gain rapidly compared to the duration of speech syllables, the response measured with the broadband input signal will not show how the levels of two succeeding sounds with different spectral shapes are affected. Neither measurement thus tells the full story, but overall, the measurement made with the broadband stimulus seems more realistic.

If we imagine a more complex hearing aid, such as the three-channel compression aid shown in Figure 2.2, the gain-frequency

---

[f]   Signals that have a spectral shape that does not vary with time (other than the random fluctuations that occur in noise signals) are referred to as *stationary* signals.

response measured will also depend on the shape of the input spectrum. Imagine that two different signals are used: Signal A with intense components in the low frequencies and Signal B with intense components in the high frequencies. For Signal A, the compressor in the low-frequency channel will turn its gain down greatly, but for Signal B, the peak clipper in the high-frequency channel will clip heavily. The most realistic assessment of the effect of the hearing aid on speech will occur when the input spectrum has a spectrum similar to that of speech. Broadband signals used in test boxes thus usually have such a spectrum. They are comprised of either spectrally shaped random noise, or a repetitive waveform with appropriate spectral shape and even *crest factor* (the ratio of a waveform's peak value to its rms value).

Some advanced hearing aids attempt to distinguish speech from background noise, and to alter their amplification characteristics according to how much of each they detect in each frequency region. Such hearing aids may treat swept pure tones and stationary noise test signals as though they were background noise and decrease their amplification accordingly. Advanced test boxes contain signals that will cause such hearing aids to amplify the test signals as if they were

speech. These special test signals invariably have amplitude fluctuations similar to those in real speech.

4.1.4 Gain-frequency response and OSPL90-frequency response

The measurements most commonly performed on hearing aids are the gain-frequency response and OSPL90-frequency response. Figure 4.6 shows an example of each, obtained with a BTE hearing aid in an HA2 style 2-cc coupler and measured with a swept pure-tone signal. The gain-frequency response was obtained with an input signal level of 60 dB SPL. The results can be shown with either of two different, but related, vertical axes. The left-hand axis shows the output in dB SPL. The gain at any frequency can be calculated as the output SPL at that frequency minus the input SPL, which in this case is 60 dB SPL. This gain can is shown directly on the right-hand axis in Figure 4.6.

Both the IEC and ANSI standards specify that hearing aid maximum output should be measured using a 90 dB SPL input signal, and both standards now use the term OSPL90 to describe the measurement.[728] This level is high enough to cause many hearing aids to reach their highest possible output level at each frequency. When the hearing aid output

Figure 4.6 Gain-frequency response (measured with a 60 dB SPL input level) and OSPL90-frequency response of a BTE measured in a 2-cc coupler with a swept pure tone. The 60 dB curve can be read against either axis; the OSPL90 curve must be read against the left hand axis.

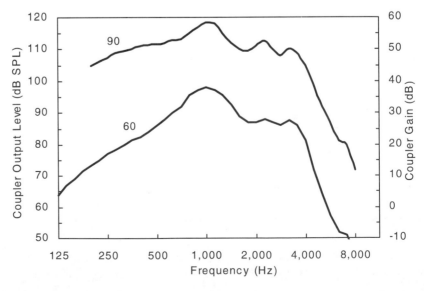

has not be saturated at low frequencies, so in such instances, the measurement will underestimate the true maximum output of the hearing aid at low frequencies. At mid and high frequencies, for many hearing aids, there will be an increase in output level as the input rises from 90 to 100 or 110 dB SPL, but this is nearly always small enough to be of no consequence. The vertical axis of the OSPL90-frequency response graph is always shown in dB SPL.

When a broadband measurement signal is used, the results are more meaningful if the vertical axis shows gain rather than output level. The problem is that broadband signals have a relatively small amount of energy at every frequency, so SPL can be measured only by combining all the energy within some finite analysis bandwidth.[g] The bigger the analysis bandwidth, the greater will be the SPL measured. The actual SPL thus depends on whatever analysis bandwidth is arbitrarily chosen by the designer of the test equipment. One solution is to show the level as the SPL that exists in each band of frequencies 1 Hz wide.[h] These complications do not arise if the vertical axis displays gain, because the same analysis bandwidth is used to measure the input signal and the output signal. Consequently, the gain is largely independent of the analysis bandwidth chosen.

There is a further problem if the maximum output of a hearing aid is measured with a broadband measurement signal. The OSPL90 measured with a swept pure-tone indicates how large a signal the hearing aid can produce when all the power of the hearing aid is concentrated into one narrow frequency region at a time. The output measured with a broadband signal, by contrast, indicates how large a signal the hearing aid can produce in *each* frequency region when it is simultaneously producing signals in *all* frequency regions. Because the total power that the hearing aid can produce has to be divided among all the signal frequencies, the power available for any particular frequency region is less than for the swept pure-tone measurement.[842] A broadband output curve therefore underestimates the true maximum output of the hearing aid for narrowband sounds (which do occasionally occur in the real world). Furthermore, the broadband output at any frequency depends on the spectral shape of the test signal. Hearing aid maximum output is therefore most meaningfully measured with swept pure-tones.[741]

The amount of gain measured with a hearing aid depends on where the volume control and all the fitter controls are set. The volume control should either be in the full-on position, in which case the **full-on gain** is obtained, or else should be in the **reference-test gain-control position**, in which case the resulting gain curve is referred to as the **basic frequency response** (IEC 118-0) or the **frequency response curve** (ANSI S3.22). The purpose of reducing the volume control to a reference position is to set the hearing aid so that it is not saturated for mid-level input signals.

In the IEC 118 standard, the volume control is adjusted so that at 1.6 kHz (the **reference frequency**) a 60 dB SPL input signal results in the output being 15 dB less than the OSPL90 at the same frequency. For high-frequency emphasis hearing aids, the reference test frequency is instead chosen to

---

g   In fact, for random noise, sound pressure exists at every frequency, so there is an infinitesimal amount of sound pressure at any particular frequency.

h   This is sometimes expressed as *SPL per* $\sqrt{Hz}$, but this is a misleading expression as it is the underlying pressure density ($Pa/\sqrt{Hz}$) that must be multiplied by the square root of bandwidth to obtain SPL. To convert an *SPL per* $\sqrt{Hz}$ value to SPL in a wider band (such as might correspond to one channel in a multichannel hearing aid), add *10 log(B)*, where *B* is the bandwidth in Hz of the channel concerned. The situation is even more complex if the level in each 1 Hz band changes significantly within the channel.

be 2.5 kHz. The ANSI standard is similar, except that instead of a single reference frequency, the procedure is based on the high-frequency average gain and high-frequency average OSPL90, such that the HFA output has to be 17 dB below the HFA OSPL90. With some hearing aids, it is not possible to achieve an output level as high as 15 or 17 dB below OSPL90, and in such cases, the gain is measured at the full-on setting. In all cases, OSPL90 is measured at the full-on gain setting. For measurement of both gain and OSPL90, all other controls are usually set to the position that gives the widest frequency response with the greatest average gain. These settings must be recorded on the measurement; otherwise, the measurement is meaningless.

The two standards emphasize measurement of the gain-frequency response for an input level of 60 dB SPL, although both standards specify that the input level should be decreased if the hearing aid is not in its linear operating region when the full-on gain is measured. (Linear operation can be checked by decreasing the input level by 10 dB and ensuring that at all frequencies of interest, the output decreases by 10 ± 1 dB. This is equivalent to the gain not changing).

Of course, many hearing aids are now intentionally nonlinear over a wide range of input levels. For such hearing aids, it is more meaningful to display the gain for each of a range of input levels. Two commonly chosen sets of levels are 50, 60, 70 80 and 90 dB SPL (ANSI S3.42), and 50, 65, and 80 dB SPL.

4.1.5   Input-output functions

Whereas a gain-frequency response shows the gain (or output level) versus frequency for one input level, an ***input-output function*** shows the output level versus input level, for one frequency or for one broadband test signal. It is thus the same type of data, but is displayed in a different manner. Because all hearing aids become nonlinear at high input levels, and because many are nonlinear at most input levels, the input-output (I-O) function is an invaluable tool for understanding how a hearing aid modifies sound. Let us examine what can be learned from an I-O function.

Figure 4.7 shows the I-O diagram for a hearing aid with two compressors. Also shown are some lines that would correspond to the I-O function for a linear hearing aid with different amounts of gain. Note that all of these dotted lines are at an angle of 45°. Look in particular at the dotted line labeled *30*. For every point on the line, the output is 30 dB more than the corresponding input. The line thus represents the I-O function for a hearing aid with a fixed gain of 30 dB. Notice that the upper (or left-most) lines have the greater gain. Lines below the 0-dB gain diagonal have negative gains, and thus represent attenuation by the hearing aid. As a general principle, gain increases for movements vertically upwards or horizontally to the left, or both simultaneously, on an I-O diagram. Gain remains constant for movement simultaneously upwards and to the right at 45°.

Now turn your attention to the hearing aid's I-O curve in Figure 4.7. It comprises three sections. For input levels below 50 dB SPL,

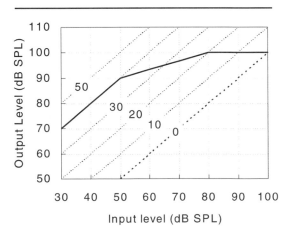

Figure 4.7 Input-output diagram of a compression hearing aid at 2 kHz (bold line) and lines of constant gain (dotted lines).

Understanding gain, attenuation, compression, and expansion on the I-O diagram

Make sure that you really understand the four terms gain, attenuation, compression, and expansion.

- Gain and attenuation each describe how large the output signal is compared to the input signal. They correspond to different regions on the I-O diagram: above and below the 0-dB gain diagonal, respectively.

- Compression and expansion each describe the effect of the amplifier on the dynamic range of a signal that varies in amplitude over time. They correspond to different slopes on the I-O diagram: less than and greater than 45° respectively. Linear operation corresponds to a slope of exactly 45°.

A compressor makes the signal's dynamic range smaller, whether the output level is smaller or larger than the input level. By contrast, an expander increases dynamic range.

For a small range of levels around a given input level, a hearing aid can, in principle, simultaneously amplify and compress, or amplify and expand, or attenuate and compress, or attenuate and expand. In practice, amplification combined with either compression or linear operation is most common.

---

the hearing aid behaves in a linear fashion, with a constant gain of 40 dB. In the second section of the curve, for input levels between 50 and 80 dB, the line still slopes upwards, but with a slope of less than 45°. Any increase in input level thus results in a smaller increase in output level. This effect, of course, is compression. For an input level of 50 dB SPL, the output is 90 dB SPL and the gain is therefore 40 dB. As the input level increases, the I-O function crosses several lines of constant gain. The hearing aid gain is thus decreasing (as one would expect for a compressor) and when the input level reaches 80 dB SPL, the gain has decreased to 20 dB.

The third section of the curve is horizontal, which is referred to as *limiting* because the output cannot rise above a certain limit, in this case 100 dB SPL. From the I-O diagram alone, we cannot tell whether this limit is set by peak clipping or by compression limiting. As the input level increases beyond 80 dB SPL, the gain decreases further. In fact, the gain decreases by 1 dB for every 1 dB increase in input level. The hearing aid begins to act as an attenuator (i.e. an earplug)

at this frequency for input levels greater than 100 dB SPL, where the output level becomes smaller than the input level.

The opposite of compression is *expansion*, in which the gain decreases as the input level decreases. Expansion, which is also called *squelch* and *noise-gating*, is used in some hearing aids, and is useful for decreasing the audibility of very low-level sounds, including hearing aid internal noise. Such a reduction in audibility is good as long as all the noises made inaudible really are unwanted noises.

Measuring the I-O curves for two different settings of the volume control will reveal how the volume control affects the operation of the compressor, as we will return to in Section 6.2.3.

4.1.6   Distortion

The concepts of harmonic distortion and intermodulation distortion have already been introduced in Section 2.3.3 in the context of peak clipping. Mechanisms other than peak clipping can give rise to distortion within hearing aids, but peak clipping is the most common cause and produces the largest amounts of distortion. **Harmonic distortion** is measured by putting a pure tone into the hearing aid, and then analyzing the output waveform to measure the distortion components relative to the total power of the signal.

The relative size of the distortion components can be expressed in a few ways. First, it can be expressed in dB or it can be expressed as a percentage.[i] Second, the distortion can be expressed separately for each harmonic (usually just the second and third), or it can be expressed for all the harmonics summed together. When the power in all the harmonics is summed, the final number is referred to as **total harmonic distortion (THD)**:

$$THD = 100 \sqrt{\frac{p_2^2 + p_3^2 + p_4^2 + ...}{p_1^2 + p_2^2 + p_3^2 + p_4^2 + ...}} \%$$

.... 4.1

$$THD = 10 \log_{10} \left(\frac{p_2^2 + p_3^2 + p_4^2 + ..}{p_1^2 + p_2^2 + p_3^2 + p_4^2 + ..} \right) dB$$

.... 4.2,

where p_n is the pressure of the n'th harmonic. The first harmonic (of amplitude p_1) is the fundamental (the frequency of the input signal), which represents the undistorted part of the signal. The clinician will never have to use Equations 4.1 and 4.2; test boxes do these calculations automatically and display the results.[j] A distortion of 1% is equivalent to -40 dB, 3% is equivalent to -30 dB, 10% to -20 dB, and 30% to -10 dB.

The standards specify that distortion be measured with a 70 dB SPL input signal with the volume control set to the reference test position. It is just as relevant however, to know what distortion occurs at lower and, particularly, higher input levels. The distortion results may be displayed as distortion versus frequency at a particular input level, or distortion versus level at a particular frequency.

Harmonic distortion measurement can be a misleading indicator of hearing aid distortion for low and high input frequencies. For high input frequencies, the harmonics will fall above the response range of the receiver, and so will not be discernable in the acoustic output, although the hearing aid amplifier may be clipping heavily. The distortion will, however, be audible and objectionable when a more complex (broadband) input signal is used. (See intermodulation distortion in Section 2.3.3.) For low frequencies, a hearing aid with a steeply rising response will emphasize the harmonics of a low-frequency signal if the peak clipping in the hearing aid precedes the filter that causes the steeply rising response. In this case, the distortion for broadband signals will not be as bad as one would expect based on the harmonic distortion measures.

A method of measuring distortion applicable to broadband signals is the **coherence** between the input signal and the output signal. Coherence quantifies the proportion of the output signal at each frequency that is linearly related to the input signal at the same frequency. It ranges from 1, when there is no noise or distortion, down to 0, when the output is not at all linearly related to the input. A measure similar to THD can be deduced from coherence as follows.[730]

$$THD = 100 \sqrt{\frac{1 - \text{coherence}}{\text{coherence}}} \%$$

..... 4.3

---

[i]   A square root is taken before calculating the percentage so that the final ratio refers to sound pressures, or voltages, rather than intensities or powers.

[j]   ANSI S3.22 allows an alternative and preferred distortion formula, in which the power of only the fundamental component appears in the denominator. The two versions give almost identical results for THD less than 20%.

Distortion can be measured for the following purposes:

- Ensuring that a hearing aid continues to meet its published specifications. Measurements may be made following a repair on the hearing aid, or in response to adverse comments by the aid wearer about the sound quality.

- Comparing the fidelity of two different hearing aids.

- Establishing whether a hearing aid uses compression limiting or peak clipping, (because it cannot be deduced from the I-O function). The THD of compression limiting hearing aids should always be less than 10%, whereas the THD of peak clipping hearing aids will rise rapidly above this once peak clipping commences.

4.1.7   Internal noise

As mentioned in Chapter 2, microphones and amplifiers generate noise. The internal noise of a hearing aid is quantified by expressing it as the *equivalent input noise (EIN)*. The EIN is the amount of noise that would have to be applied to the input of a noiseless hearing aid with the same gain-frequency response, if the noise coming out of this noiseless hearing aid were to be the same as that coming from the hearing aid under test. It is sensible to express noise relative to the input of the hearing aid for three reasons. First, most of the noise in a well-designed hearing aid originates from the microphone, and most of the remaining noise originates from the input amplifier.

Second, and because of this, the output-referred noise will vary markedly with the position of the volume control, whereas input-referred noise will be less affected by the position of the volume control and other fitter controls. Third, if the noise were expressed as the output noise, high-gain hearing aids would always be noisier than low-gain aids, even though the wearers of these aids (people with severe or profound hearing loss) may be less aware of the internal noise than the wearers of low-gain aids.

The EIN is determined by measuring the magnitude of the noise at the output of the hearing aid and then subtracting the gain of the hearing aid. Two types of measurement can be performed. In the simpler type of measurement, the total output noise SPL (usually A-weighted) is measured, and the gain at the reference test frequency (IEC) or the HFA gain (ANSI) is subtracted. This measurement does not reveal how much noise is present in each frequency range. Also, the magnitude of the equivalent input noise will depend on whether the reference frequency or frequencies happen to coincide with a peak or a trough in the gain-frequency response of the hearing aid. (When the reference test frequency coincides with a peak, the gain will be high, and the equivalent input noise will consequently appear to be unrealistically low.) The method therefore cannot be used to compare the noisiness of two aids with different gain-frequency responses. It is, however, suitable for ensuring that a hearing aid is operating within its specifications.

Practical tip: Measuring internal noise

- To ensure that ambient noise does not affect the measurement of output noise, close the test box lid, and if necessary, place putty over the microphone inlet port. (It *is* necessary if adding the putty causes the output noise to decrease.)

- When the gain is measured for the purposes of the noise measurement, the input level must be low enough for the hearing aid to be in its linear operating mode. (This makes internal noise measurement difficult for hearing aids with a very low compression threshold.)

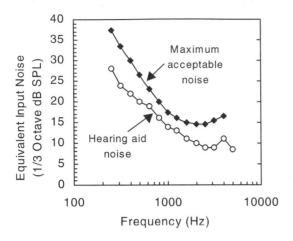

Figure 4.8 Equivalent 1/3-octave input noise of a typical hearing aid as a function of frequency, and maximum acceptable 1/3-octave noise.

A more thorough method of measuring internal noise is to filter the output signal into bands (usually 1/3 octave, or one octave) and so measure the level of output noise that falls within each band. The equivalent input noise at each frequency is then calculated by subtracting from these output levels the gain at the center frequency of each band. The result is a graph of equivalent input noise (for the measurement bandwidth used) as a function of frequency. The input-referred noise for a typical hearing aid is shown in Figure 4.8, along with the maximum equivalent input noise considered acceptable.[562]

4.1.8   Magnetic response

The principles of magnetic induction have been explained in Sections 2.8 and 3.6. Measurement of the magnetic response is straightforward if the test box contains a loop to generate a magnetic field and impossible if it does not. The only precautions are:

- Make sure that the volume control is full-on (ANSI S3.22, IEC 118-1) or at its reference position (IEC 118-1 when measuring magnetic frequency response);

- Orient the hearing aid so that maximum possible output SPL is obtained (IEC), or orient it as it would be oriented in regular use (ANSI).

The standards specify that the magnetic response of a hearing aid be measured with a field strength of 10 mA/m (IEC) or 31.6 mA/m (ANSI). ANSI S3.22 refers to the hearing aid output as the SPL for a vertical inductive field (SLPIV). The shape of the magnetic frequency response should be similar to the shape of the acoustic frequency response. There will, however, be some differences, because the coil probably will not have a resonance to match the microphone Helmholtz resonance, and because the coil response may have been given an additional low cut by the aid designer (see Section 3.6.3). The result of the magnetic response is displayed as a graph of output SPL versus frequency for the specified input magnetic field strength. The concept of *gain* does not strictly apply because the input and output quantities are different. An equivalent gain can, however, be deduced if a magnetic field strength of 100 mA/m is considered to be equivalent to an acoustical input signal of 70 dB SPL (see Section 3.6.2). Provided the aid amplifies linearly for input levels from 10 mA/m to 100 mA/m, the equivalent acoustic gain equals the output SPL for a 10 mA/m input minus 50 dB SPL (IEC) or the output SPL for a 31.6 mA/m input minus 60 dB SPL (ANSI).[k]

Because telephones are such an important source of magnetic signals, ANSI S3.22 specifies a telephone magnetic field simulator that generates magnetic signals similar in level and field shape pattern to those generated by a telephone. The output of the hearing aid is referred to as the SPL for an inductive telephone simulator (SPLITS).

ANSI S3.22 specifies another method to compare acoustic and telecoil sensitivity. It

---

k   The 50 and 60 dB SPL figures come from the assumption that a magnetic input of 100 mA/m is equivalent to an acoustic input of 70 dB SPL input level.

Table 4.2 ANSI standards relevant to hearing aids.

Number	Year	Title	Comment
S3.13	1977	An artificial headbone for the calibration of audiometer bone vibrators	Specifies the artificial mastoid
S3.22	1996	Specification of hearing aid characteristics	Test conditions, procedures and tolerances
S3.25	1979	An occluded ear simulator	Matches the Zwislocki coupler
S3.3	1990	Methods for measurement of electroacoustical characteristics of hearing aids	Specifies that a 2-cc coupler be used
3.35	1997	Methods of measurement of performance characteristics of hearing aids under simulated in-situ working conditions	Uses a manikin and ear-simulator
S3.42	1997	Testing hearing aids with a broadband noise signal	
S3.46	1997	Methods of measurement of real ear performance of hearing aids	
S3.7	1995	Methods for coupler calibration of earphones	Defines the 2-cc coupler
504-1	1994	Magnetic field intensity criteria for telephone compatibility with hearing aids	

defines two terms called *simulated telephone sensitivity (STS)*, and *test loop sensitivity (TLS)*. These are the equal to the output signal (SPLITS or SPLIV respectively) minus an input level of 60 dB SPL. They are intended to describe how much the user would have to increase the volume control so that the acoustic output will be the same when listening via the telecoil as when listening via the microphone. The first term applies to telephone use; the second term applies to room-loop use. Values of SLS and TLS close to 0 dB (i.e. the volume control does not have to be adjusted) are most desirable.[728]

4.1.9   ANSI and IEC standards

Frequent references have already been made to the IEC and ANSI standards, and some of their similarities and differences have been outlined. Table 4.2 lists several standards that are directly relevant to hearing aids. There are further standards in the IEC 118 series, dealing with issues such as hand-held microphones and wireless systems (part 3), insert earphone nipples (part 5), electrical input circuits (part 6), symbols and markings (part 11), electrical connectors (part 12), electromagnetic interference (part 13), and digital interfaces (part 14).

4.2   Real-Ear Aided Gain (REAG)

It is the response of a hearing aid in the individual's ear that matters. For the past 15 years, it has been possible to measure hearing aids in individual ears with commercially available probe-tube measurement equipment that is suitable for the clinic. There are two fundamentally different types of real-ear gain. The first of these is called the real-ear aided gain, described in this section. The second is called real-ear insertion gain, described in the next section. Some prescription procedures prescribe in terms of real-ear aided gain, and some prescribe in terms of insertion gain.

Measurement of real-ear aided gain is a necessary step in the measurement of insertion gain, so much of the information in this section is also relevant to insertion gain. The term *real-ear gain* will be used in a general sense; it will apply to both real-ear aided gain and insertion gain.

Table 4.3 IEC standards relevant to hearing aids

Number	Year	Title	Comment
60 118-0	1983	Hearing aids - Part 0: Measurement of electroacoustical characteristics	Specifies that an ear simulator be used
60 118-1	1995	Hearing aids - Part 1: Hearing aids with induction pick-up coil input	How to test telecoil response
60 118-2	1983	Hearing aids - Part 2: Hearing aids with automatic gain control circuits	How to measure I-O curves and attack and release times
60 118-4	1981	Hearing aids - Part 4: Magnetic field strength in audio-frequency induction loops for hearing aid purposes	Specifies 100 mA/m long-term level
60 118-7	1983	Hearing aids - Part 7: Measurement of the performance characteristics of hearing aids for quality inspection for delivery purposes	Test conditions and procedures
60 118-8	1983	Hearing aids - Part 8: Methods of measurement of performance characteristics of hearing aids under simulated in situ working conditions	How to measure a hearing aid mounted on a manikin
60 118-9	1985	Hearing aids - Part 9: Methods of measurement of characteristics of hearing aids with bone vibrator output	How to measure bone conductor hearing aids
60 118-10	1986	Hearing aids - Part 10: Guide to hearing aid standards	A glossary of terms and a guide to use
60 126	1973	IEC reference coupler for the measurement of hearing aids using earphones coupled to the ear by means of ear inserts	Defines the 2-cc coupler
60 373	1990	Mechanical coupler for measurements on bone vibrators	Specifies the artificial mastoid
60 711	1981	Occluded-ear simulator for the measurement of earphones coupled to the ear by ear inserts	Matches the B&K 4138 ear simulator
60 959	1990	Provisional head and torso simulator for acoustic measurements of air conduction hearing aids	Specifies a standard manikin

The *real-ear aided gain (REAG)*, expressed in dB, is defined as the SPL near the eardrum, *A*, minus the SPL at some reference point outside the head. This reference point is variously defined as the level in the undisturbed field, *F*, or the level at a *control microphone* mounted on the surface of the head, *C*, as shown in Figure 4.9. ANSI S3.46 specifies the level at the control microphone as the reference and refers to it as the *field reference point*. The control microphone, which is also referred to as a *reference microphone,* is mounted either just above or just below the ear. The real-ear measurement equipment uses the signal from the control microphone to regulate the sound level near the ear to the required level. This concept is the same as applied to control the level in test boxes (see Section 4.1.2). The control microphone thus removes diffraction effects from the free field to the surface of the head. These diffraction effects are minimal when the sound source is located directly in front of the aid wearer. At 45°, the maximum effect is only about 4 dB, and this occurs in the 500 to 1000 Hz range.[854] Measurement equipment thus actually displays the SPL at location *A* minus the SPL at location *C,* but for sounds from the front, this is approximately equal to *A-F*.

Synonyms for real-ear aided gain (REAG) are *real-ear aided response (REAR)*, *in-situ*

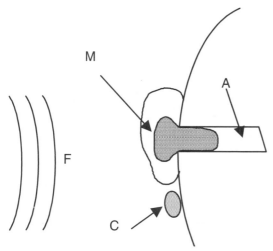

Figure 4.9 Location of SPLs involved in the measurement of real-ear aided gain. *F* is located in the undisturbed sound field (e.g. with the head absent), *C* is at the control microphone location on the surface of the head, *M* is at the hearing aid microphone port, and *A* is within the residual ear canal close to the eardrum.

gain, and ***real-ear transmission gain***. Some authors have used the word *response* instead of *gain* when they refer to a complete graph of gain versus frequency, rather than the gain at a specific frequency. Other authors and a recent standard (ANSI S3.46, 1997) use *response* when the measurement result is expressed as the absolute level of sound in the ear canal (i.e. in dB SPL), and use *gain* when it is expressed as the difference between the ear canal SPL and the input SPL (i.e. in dB). Fortunately, context usually makes the meaning clear.

4.2.1   Positioning the probe for REAG measurement

Measurement of REAG is straightforward. The precise details depend on the particular equipment used, but in all cases a flexible probe tube is inserted into the ear canal so that the SPL in the residual canal is sensed while the hearing aid is in place and operating. The probe is usually inserted first, and then the hearing aid or earmold. The only tricky part of the measurement is obtaining the correct depth of insertion. Provided the

probe tube is past the tip of the aid or mold, its position does not matter for frequencies up to 2 kHz. Up to 2 kHz, the wavelength is much bigger than ear canal dimensions, so the same SPL exists at all locations within the residual ear canal. As frequency increases above 2 kHz, however, placement becomes more critical because of standing waves in the residual ear canal.

Figure 4.10 shows the SPL in the ear canal for a frequency of 6 kHz, for example. Because we are interested in the sound pressure at the eardrum, we cannot afford to have the microphone more than 6 mm, which corresponds to 0.1 wavelengths, from the eardrum if we are to limit the error caused by the standing wave phenomenon to, say, 2 dB. As frequency increases (and wavelength decreases) it becomes necessary to have the probe-tube tip closer and closer to the eardrum. (The maximum distance in wavelengths stays the same). Table 4.4 shows how close the probe tube must be to the eardrum if the error due to standing waves is to be kept to within 1, 2, 3, 4 or 5 dB. As a further

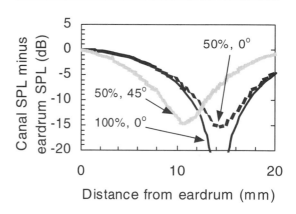

Figure 4.10 Calculated pattern of SPL in the ear canal versus distance from the eardrum at a frequency of 6 kHz. The solid curve is for total reflection from the eardrum with no phase shift at the drum, the dashed line is for 50% power reflected from the drum with no phase shift, and the speckled line is for 50% reflected with a 45 degree phases shift at the drum.

Theoretical explanation: Standing waves in the ear canal

Because some of the power transmitted down the ear canal is reflected back by the eardrum, SPL can vary markedly along the length of the ear canal. A probe tube in the residual cavity actually senses the addition of the inwards-going and outwards-going waves. At the eardrum, these waves add almost in phase, so the pressure is a maximum at this point. As the reflected wave travels back from the eardrum, a phase shift develops between the incident and reflected waves (because the reflected wave has traveled further). Consequently, the two waves add less constructively. At a distance back from the eardrum approximately equal to one quarter of the sound's wavelength, the two waves are half a cycle out of phase, and partially cancel. Because this distance depends on wavelength, it therefore depends on frequency, as shown in Figure 4.11. A probe microphone placed at this position (called a *node*) would misleadingly indicate that there was very little sound travelling along the ear canal at this frequency.

The position of the node will not precisely be one quarter of a wavelength back from the eardrum because some phase shift occurs as the wave is reflected from the eardrum (Voss & Allen, 1994).

Because the pattern of SPL versus distance looks like a wave that is always in the same place, the pattern is called a standing wave. For positions between the eardrum and the node of the standing wave, the waves partially cancel, or partially add, but the total sound pressure is always less than that at the eardrum.

Note that the discussion about how the incident and reflected waves combine near the eardrum did not require any assumptions about where the incident sound wave started. *Consequently, the variation of SPL with distance near the eardrum is exactly the same when a hearing aid is inserted in the ear as when the person is listening unaided.* Of course the actual SPL will be affected by the input level, by the hearing aid gain, and in the case of unaided listening, by the frequency of the sound relative to the resonant frequency of the ear canal.

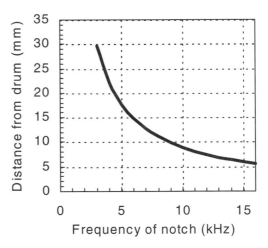

Figure 4.11 Distance from the eardrum at which SPL in the ear canal will be a minimum.

example, if we wished to measure the REAG up to 8 kHz, and were willing to tolerate an error of only 1 dB, the probe tube would have to be within 3 mm of the eardrum. At the other extreme, if we were concerned about REAG only up to 3 kHz, and were willing to toler-

ate 5 dB error, the probe tube could be up to 18 mm away from the eardrum, which means that any location within the residual ear canal would be acceptable.

Where the final distance from the eardrum can be estimated (see panel), and one is

Table 4.4 Maximum distance from the eardrum (in mm) if the error induced by standing waves is not to exceed the values shown in the first column. These values are based on calculations that assume complete reflection from the eardrum. The distances increase insignifiuly for partial, but strong, reflections, but decrease by 25 to 50% for a phase shift of 45° at the eardrum.

Standing wave error (dB)	Frequency (Hz)						
	2 k	3 k	4 k	5 k	6 k	8 k	10 k
1	13	9	6	5	4	3	3
2	18	12	9	7	6	4	4
3	22	14	11	9	7	5	4
4	24	16	12	10	8	6	5
5	27	18	13	11	9	7	5

particularly interested in accurate high-frequency measurements, but is unwilling to further insert the probe tube, then Table 4.4 can be used in reverse. The left-hand column shows the correction that should be added for each frequency at each of the distances included in the body of the table. The correction allows us to estimate the SPL present at the eardrum based on the SPL measured some distance from it.

The theory in this section assumes that the incident sound wave is a plane wave[1] progressing smoothly down the canal. This is not likely to be true in the 3 to 5 mm immediately past the tip of the mold or aid,

because the sound wave has to make a transition from the narrow sound bore to the wider canal.[100] The probe tube should never be positioned in this region, unless the hearing aid itself terminates within about 6 mm of the eardrum.

4.2.2   Relationship between REAG, coupler gain and ear simulator gain

There are several reasons why the REAG will differ from the 2-cc coupler response of the hearing aid, both on average, and for individual aid wearers.

First, for a given test stimulus level, the actual input to the hearing aid will be greater for

Table 4.5 Microphone location effects (MLE) due to body, head, pinna, concha, and canal diffraction and resonance: SPL at the hearing aid microphone port minus SPL in the undisturbed sound field, for two directions of the incoming signal. Body aid data are based on Kuhn & Guernsey (1983) and the remainder are based on Storey & Dillon (in preparation).

Aid type	Source	Frequency								
		125	250	500	1 k	2 k	3 k	4 k	6 k	8 k
Body	0°	2	3	5	3	2	1	0	0	0
BTE	0°	-1	0	0	0	3	2	1	1	2
ITE	0°	-1	0	1	1	3	5	7	3	2
ITC	0°	0	1	1	1	5	8	10	2	-2
CIC	0°	0	1	1	1	5	8	10	2	-2
BTE	45°	0	1	1	2	5	5	4	4	3
ITE	45°	0	2	3	3	5	7	9	7	5
ITC	45°	0	2	3	3	6	10	13	8	1
CIC	45°	0	2	3	4	6	11	14	8	2

---

[1]   A plane wave has uniform pressure across the wave front, which, over the area of interest, forms a flat plane.

Practical tip: Positioning the probe tube for REAG measurements

- Position a marker on the probe tube approximately 30 mm from the open end.

- Generate a continuous tone at 6 kHz, and move the probe inwards, smoothly and continuously, starting at the entrance to the ear canal, while monitoring the SPL sensed by the probe microphone. Find the position at which the SPL is a minimum by moving the probe past the minimum a few times. When the probe is positioned at the SPL minimum, the probe tip should be 15 mm from the acoustic center of the eardrum (compare to Figures 4.10 and 4.11). Be aware that movements of your hand or the client's head can affect the amount of sound entering the ear canal, and hence give a misleading impression of which position corresponds to the node (Sullivan, 1988).

- Move the probe tube in by the amount necessary to position it the desired distance from the eardrum. For example, to position the tip 6 mm from the eardrum, insert it a further 9 mm. The extent of extra insertion is monitored by noting the movement of the marker.

- Some real ear gain analyzers have a probe insertion section of the menu that facilitates probe placement using the notch in the frequency response created by the standing wave. The 6 kHz method described here can, however, be easily used with any real-ear gain analyzer. Also, the 6 kHz method avoids the problem of spurious notches in the frequency spectrum being created by loudspeaker or room acoustics, because all measurements are done at a single frequency.

- If the tip of a flexible probe tube gently touches the eardrum, physical damage and pain from mechanical force are unlikely, but loudness discomfort or pain from the acoustic sensation is possible.

- The skin near the eardrum in the final section of the canal can be very sensitive. The probe can cause pain if it is pushed into the canal wall in this area.

- In the ***average adult*** ear, 6 mm from the eardrum umbo corresponds to 18 mm past the ear canal entrance (1.5 mm more for males and 1.5 mm less for females), or 29 mm from the inter-tragal notch (Burkhard & Sachs, 1978; Salvinelli et al., 1991). If you rely on these dimensions instead of the acoustic technique described above, view the location of the probe tip relative to the eardrum otoscopically during insertion and use a smaller insertion depth if appropriate.

---

the REAG measurement than for the coupler measurement, at least for CIC, ITC and low profile ITE hearing aids. This occurs because for these aids, the diffraction effects from the free field to the microphone inlet port (*M-F* in Figure 4.9) are greater than the diffraction effects to the head surface (*C-F* in Figure 4.9) that are removed by the control microphone.

Table 4.5 shows the ***microphone location effects (MLE)*** from the undisturbed sound field to the microphone inlet port for each type of hearing aid, for two directions of

sound waves. With the exception of body aids, microphone location effects are limited to the high frequencies, where the wavelength of sound is comparable in size to the obstacles creating the diffraction effects: the head and pinna. Microphone location effects are greater the more the concha remains unfilled by the hearing aid.

The second reason why REAG will differ from coupler gain is that the hearing aid terminates in a smaller volume in the real ear than when it is connected to a 2-cc coupler,

---

Practical tip: Checking the aided measurement

If the hearing aid has a vent larger in diameter than the probe tube, then a REAG measurement can be checked as follows:

- Withdraw the probe tube from the ear, leaving the hearing aid in place.
- Inspect the tip of the probe for blockage by wax.
- Re-insert the probe tube, but via the vent hole this time, to the same depth as previously.
- Repeat the measurement.
- Withdraw the aid or mold and the probe tube together and make sure that the probe is extending beyond the aid or mold.

---

as discussed in Section 4.1.1. Thus, the real-ear to coupler difference (RECD) directly affects the relationship.

The third reason is that the hearing aid may use different coupling in the individual ear than when it is measured in the coupler. In particular, the sound bore may be different (for BTE and body aids), and the vent will not be included in the coupler measurement (and should not be, as discussed in the next chapter).

These differences are summarized in Equation 4.4, which assumes that the coupler gain and the REAG are obtained with the same volume control setting. The equation also assumes that the hearing aid is linear.[m]

$$REAG = \text{coupler gain} + RECD + MLE + \text{sound bore effects} + \text{vent effects} \quad ..... \ 4.4.$$

Sound bore effects and vent effects will be explained and quantified in Chapter 5. If an average value of RECD is assumed (Table 4.1), then Equation 4.4 can be used to predict REAG on the basis of coupler gain. Alternatively, if the RECD is measured for an individual aid user, then a more accurate prediction of REAG can be made. RECD is most worth measuring when it is most different from average. This occurs for infants[954] and for ears with middle-ear

pathology.[283] This topic is further discussed in Sections 10.8 and 15.4.3. If the volume of the residual ear canal were to halve, then for high-frequency sounds, RECD will increase by nearly 6 dB. For low-frequency sounds, the increase will be less because of the contribution of the eardrum and middle ear to the impedance.

We can write a similar equation to relate REAG to ear simulator gain:

$$REAG = \text{ear simulator gain} + MLE + \text{sound bore effects} + \text{vent effects} \quad ..... \ 4.5.$$

Note that the RECD term is missing, although REAG can still bc prcdictcd most accurately from ear simulator gain if the individual variation of RECD from average is taken into account (Section 10.7).

4.2.3   Detecting incorrect aided measurements

No physical measurement should be believed just because some buttons are pressed and a number or graph is obtained! Measurement of REAG is no exception, because several factors (discussed in Section 4.4) can affect the validity of the measurement. How can one know whether a measurement is correct? Fortunately, we can have some strong expectations of what the REAG should be, and for

---

[m]   For nonlinear hearing aids measured with pure tones, MLE must be divided by the compression ratio (see Section 6.2.2) applicable to that frequency and level, because sound diffraction affects the level of sound at the *input* to the hearing aid. For broadband sounds, the situation is more complex. These considerations apply wherever MLE appears in this chapter.

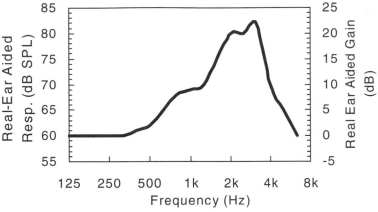

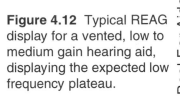

Figure 4.12 Typical REAG display for a vented, low to medium gain hearing aid, displaying the expected low frequency plateau.

vented aids there are some additional quick checks that can be done.

First, if the hearing aid is vented or not especially tight, low-frequency sounds will enter the residual ear canal directly via these air paths. As discussed in detail in Section 5.3.1, the SPL of these sounds in the canal will equal the SPL of the test stimulus outside the head. Consequently, if the gain is not too high, the aided response should show a low-frequency plateau (a horizontal line), as shown in Figure 4.12. If the REAG display is expressed in ear canal dB SPL, the amplitude of the line should equal the test stimulus level. If the display is expressed as dB of gain, then the plateau should be at 0 dB gain. (Figure 4.12 shows both of these vertical axes, though measurement equipment usually shows only one of these axes at a time.)

Second, the measurement can be repeated through the vent as described in the accompanying panel. If the probe fills most of the vent (i.e. their diameters are similar), the low-frequency response may change in a manner consistent with a reduction of vent size (see Section 5.3.1). If the mold or aid has a lot of leakage around it, or if the vent diameter is more than 50% larger than the probe diameter, then the two responses should be extremely similar. If not, something is wrong with one of the two measurements.

Finally, but less practically, Equation 4.4 or 4.5 can be applied at one or two frequencies

and the result compared to the measurements. The discrepancy should never be more than 15 dB, should rarely be more than 10 dB, and will often be less than 5 dB.[221]

The most common causes of inaccurate measurements are wax blockage, probe tips pushed into the ear canal wall, probes excessively squashed by a tight earmold,[882] and analyzer buttons pushed in the wrong sequence. If the hearing aid is accidentally left turned off, the result is instantly recognizable: one sees the REAG of the vent and leakage paths alone - typically 0 dB gain at low frequencies and attenuation at higher frequencies (see Section 5.3.1). This measurement is called the *real-ear occluded gain (REOG)*.

4.3   Insertion Gain

The second type of real-ear gain is called *real-ear insertion gain (REIG)*. This gain tells us how much extra sound is presented to the eardrum as a result of inserting the hearing aid in the ear. Figure 4.13 shows the ear in its unaided and aided states. Insertion gain is defined as the SPL at the eardrum when aided, A, minus the SPL at the eardrum when unaided, U. The key distinction between insertion gain and REAG is that insertion gain takes into account the amount of "amplification" the person was getting from the resonances in his or her concha and ear canal, prior to inserting the hearing aid. This

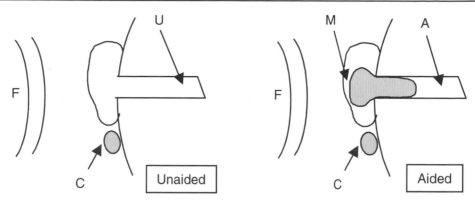

Figure 4.13 Location of SPLs involved in the measurement of insertion gain. F is located in the undisturbed sound field (with the head absent), C is at the control microphone location on the surface of the head, M is at the hearing aid microphone port, A is at the eardrum when aided, and U is at the eardrum when unaided.

Theoretical summary: real-ear gains

With reference to Figure 4.13, the following four equations summarize the relationships between the two types of real-ear gains.

REUG = U - C 4.6

REAG = A - C 4.7

Insertion gain = REAG – REUG 4.8

Consequently, for the same test level at position C in the aided and unaided measurements:

Insertion gain = A-U 4.9

Note that equations 4.8 and 4.9 are unchanged if the reference points for REUG and REAG are chosen to be F rather than C.

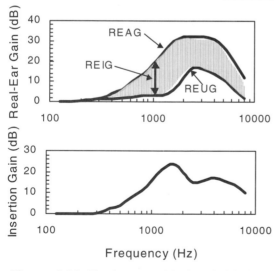

Figure 4.14 Real ear unaided and aided gains (top half). The difference between these curves is the insertion gain, shown as the shaded region in the top half and as the curve in the lower half.

natural amplification, called the *real-ear unaided gain (REUG),* is lost (mostly or totally) when a hearing aid is inserted. Before a hearing aid can provide additional signal, it must first provide at least this much gain. Insertion gain can be thought of as the net result: the REAG provided by the hearing aid minus the REUG provided by the unobstructed ear.

The top half of Figure 4.14 shows a typical REUG for an adult person for sounds incident from 45° and with a head-mounted control microphone in place (thus removing some of the head diffraction effects). It also shows the REAG for a hypothetical hearing aid. How much "gain" does the hearing aid provide at, say 3 kHz? The question is, of course, ambiguous. The SPL at the eardrum is 30 dB more than the SPL outside the head, so the

---

Practical tip: Positioning the probe for insertion gain measurement

- Inspect the ear canal for excessive wax or abnormalities.

- Insert the aid or mold in the ear and note where its lateral surface lies with respect to some landmark on the ear: the ear canal entrance for a CIC, or the inter-tragal notch or tragus for larger hearing aids – see Figure 4.15(a).

- Remove the aid or mold and lay the probe alongside the inferior surface (the part that touches the floor of the ear canal and concha). The tip of the probe should extend 5 mm or more past the tip of the aid or mold.

- Mark the probe, or position a sliding marker on the probe, at the position where the selected ear landmark would be when the mold or aid is inserted – see Figure 4.15(b).

- Insert the probe tube until the marker lines up with the selected landmark on the ear, and measure the REUG – see Figure 4.15(c).

- Insert the hearing aid, leaving the probe tip in the same position, and measure the REAG – see Figure 4.15(d). To leave the probe tip in the same position, the marker should be inserted 1 to 3 mm more for the aided measurement than for the unaided measurement, because of the more tortuous path followed by the probe in the aided condition (Revit, 1993).

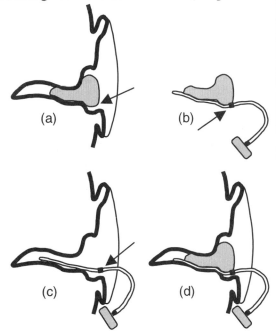

Figure 4.15 Probe positioning for measuring insertion gain: (a) noting a landmark on the ear; (b) marking the probe; (c) measuring the unaided response; (d) measuring the aided response.

REAG is 30 dB. However, the person's unaided concha and ear canal provide 18 dB of gain (the REUG) at this frequency, so the net effect of the hearing aid, that is, the insertion gain, is only 12 dB.

Consistent with its definition, insertion gain measurement is a two-step process. In the first step, the unaided response is obtained. This is the baseline for the second step: measurement of the aided response. The insertion gain finally displayed is then the difference between these two measures, though real-ear gain analyzers often show either or both of the two intermediate results as well.

4.3.1 Positioning the probe for insertion gain measurement

The position of the probe for insertion gain measurement is much less critical than it is for REAG measurement. Although we are interested in the increase in SPL at the eardrum caused by inserting the hearing aid, the same increase will occur at other points within the ear canal medial to the tip of the mold or aid. As explained in the panel *Standing waves in the ear canal* (Section 4.2.1), the increase in SPL from a mid-canal position to the eardrum does not depend on the source of the sound. *Consequently, the increase in SPL at the eardrum can be measured at a mid-canal point provided the probe tube is in the same place for the unaided and aided measurements.* As explained in Section 4.2.1, however, the probe tube must extend 5 mm or more past the end of the mold or aid, to avoid the transition region near the sound outlet.

4.3.2 Relationship between insertion gain, coupler gain and ear simulator gain

Insertion gain will differ from coupler gain for several reasons. As with REAG, insertion gain should exceed coupler gain because it is affected by head, pinna, and concha diffraction (i.e. the microphone location effects), and because the volume of the residual ear canal is smaller than a 2-cc coupler (i.e. the RECD effect). However, insertion gain should be less than coupler gain because the measurement of insertion gain involves subtracting REUG. These opposing adjustments to coupler gain approximately, but coincidentally, cancel each other for ITE and ITC aids up to 3 kHz. Consequently, for ITE and ITC aids, up to 3 kHz, insertion gain approximately equals coupler gain for the average adult. For other types of aids, there is a net difference between insertion gain and coupler gain, even on average. These factors are summarized in the following equations:

$$\text{Insertion gain} = \text{coupler gain} + \text{RECD} + \text{MLE} - \text{REUG} + \text{sound bore effects} + \text{vent effects} \quad \text{.....4.10.}$$

The difference between coupler gain and insertion gain, measured with no venting and with the same sound bore in each measurement is often referred to as **CORFIG**, which stands for **co**upler **r**esponse for a **f**lat **i**nsertion gain.[463] That is:

$$\text{CORFIG} = \text{coupler gain} - \text{insertion gain}$$
$$\text{.... 4.11.}$$

Comparison of equations 4.10 and 4.11, shows that:

$$\text{CORFIG} = \text{REUG} - \text{RECD} - \text{MLE}$$
$$\text{..... 4.12.}$$

This equation clearly shows the three factors that cause insertion gain to be different from coupler gain: the gain of the unaided ear, the difference in effective volume between the ear canal and the coupler, and head diffraction effects to the microphone. Average values for RECD and microphone location effects have already been given in Tables 4.1 and 4.5 respectively. Table 4.6 gives average values for REUG for two different directions of the incident sound.

Average values for CORFIG for each type of hearing aid, consistent with these separate values of RECD, diffraction, and REUG are

Table 4.6 Average real-ear unaided gain (REUG) for adults.[854] Measurements are given for two sound-field directions, and with and without the use of a head-mounted control microphone. Use of this microphone removes head diffraction effects but leaves ear diffraction and canal resonance effects in place. 0° corresponds to frontal incidence and 45° is towards the ear being tested.

Source angle	Control microphone present	Frequency (Hz)								
		125	250	500	1 k	2 k	3 k	4 k	6 k	8 k
0°	No	0	1	2	3	12	16	14	4	2
45°	No	0	1	3	5	13	20	18	9	3
0°	Yes	0	0	0	1	12	14	12	3	1
45°	Yes	0	0	0	1	12	17	15	7	2

Table 4.7 CORFIG factors for each type of hearing aid when measured in a 2-cc coupler.[854] The body and BTE data are relative to a HA2 coupler whereas the ITE/ITC/CIC data are relative to a HA1 coupler. All values assume no leakage around the earmold or shell, and the CIC is assumed to be very deeply seated at its medial end. CICs that extend 10 mm or less into the canal will have CORFIG values similar to those shown for an ITC.

Hearing aid type	Frequency (Hz)								
	125	250	500	1 k	2 k	3 k	4 k	6 k	8 k
Body aid	0	1	2	3	12	16	14	4	2
BTE	-2	-2	-3	-3	1	6	6	-4	-13
ITE	-3	-3	-4	-3	1	1	-5	-13	-15
ITC	-3	-3	-4	-4	-1	-2	-8	-13	-11
CIC	-7	-9	-11	-11	-9	-12	-20	-30	-28

given in Table 4.7. We can summarize the two uses of CORFIG by writing:

$$\text{Insertion gain} = \text{coupler gain} - \text{CORFIG} + \text{sound bore effects} + \text{vent effects} \quad ...... 4.13,$$

$$\text{Coupler gain} = \text{insertion gain} + \text{CORFIG} - \text{sound bore effects} - \text{vent effects} \quad ...... 4.14.$$

CORFIG values relate insertion gain to coupler gain at the same position of the volume control. CORFIG values are most often used to find the coupler gain that is equivalent to a certain insertion gain. In turn, these coupler gains are used to select an appropriate hearing aid and/or to adjust the hearing aid in a test box. Because hearing aids are often specified at their maximum volume control setting, but used at a mid volume control setting, it is appropriate to add some *reserve gain* to the coupler gain. This reserve gain is the amount by which the user can turn up the volume control from the position at which the target real-ear gain is achieved. Big aids, like BTEs, tend to have big volume controls, which tend to have big adjustment ranges, compared to small aids like ITCs. Consequently, BTEs are often fitted with a reserve gain of 15 dB, ITEs with a reserve gain of 10 dB, and ITCs with a reserve gain of 7 dB. To summarize this:

$$\text{Coupler gain}_{max\ v/c} = \text{Insertion gain}_{used\ v/c} + \text{CORFIG} - \text{sound bore effects} - \text{vent effects} + \text{reserve gain} \quad ...... 4.15$$

This section has not dealt specifically with ear simulator gain. Ear simulator gain can always be calculated from 2-cc coupler gain simply by adding RECD to the coupler gain.

4.3.3 Control microphones and insertion gain

Just as for REAG, and for measurements in a test box, the stimulus level is established using a control microphone. Most commonly, the pressure method of calibration is used, in which the control microphone does its job while the actual measurement is taking place. If the hearing aid wearer moves between the aided and unaided measurement, the control microphone compensates for the movement, thus avoiding the measurement error that would otherwise occur. For a linear hearing aid and a perfectly stationary patient, the control microphone does not affect the insertion gain values obtained. One of the advantages of insertion gain is that it is a difference measurement. This means that, at any frequency, provided everything is the same for the aided as for the unaided measurement (e.g. head position, stimulus level, and probe calibration), none of those factors will affect the final result, even if the probe microphone is totally uncalibrated. This makes insertion gain measurement resistant to errors. Despite this advantage, it is best to use the control microphone, in the pressure calibration mode, because of the protection it gives against errors created by the movements of the person being tested.

4.3.4   Detecting incorrect insertion gain measurements

Despite the in-built resistance to errors of insertion gain measurement, one still must be able to detect incorrect measurements. Because the measurement is done in two stages (unaided and aided) this involves being able to spot errors in either stage. We can legitimately have very strong expectations about what the first unaided measurement should look like. For an adult, it should look like the unaided curve in Figure 4.14. Of course, it would ordinarily not look exactly like this, or else there would be little point in measuring it for each person. It must however, have certain features in common:

a)   There **must** be a low-frequency plateau at the level of the test stimulus (if expressed in dB SPL) or at 0 dB (if expressed as a gain).

b)   There should be a peak somewhere between 2.2 kHz and 3.2 kHz with an elevation above the low-frequency plateau of between 12 and 22 dB.

The ranges in point (b) comprise plus or minus three standard deviations around the mean values of a sample of 20 adults.[855] There will be an occasional person (probably with observably very long or very short ear canals) where REUG goes outside this range. There will also be people who have had surgery to their ear canals (e.g. a mastoidectomy) that alters the shape of the ear canal. Fitting procedures for such people are covered in Sections 9.2.4, 10.8, and 15.4.3.

The second half of the insertion gain measurement is obtaining the aided response. Methods for checking the validity of this measurement have already been covered in Section 4.2.3.

4.3.5   Accuracy of insertion gain measurements

If an insertion gain measurement is not simply wrong, then how accurate can one expect it to be? This can be deduced from repeated measurements made with a variety of measurement methods.[233, 471] Over most of the frequency range, the difference between a single measurement and the average of many measurements (i.e. the true value) has a standard deviation of 3 dB. This means that 95% of measurements would be within 6 dB (two standard deviations) of the true value. In the high frequencies, because of the effects of standing waves and the impossibility of ensuring that the probe is in *exactly* the same place for the aided and unaided measurements, the standard deviation rises to 5 dB. There is a slight tendency for some probe-tube systems to underestimate high-frequency gain. This underestimation may occur as a result of constriction of the probe tube by the mold or aid in the unaided condition, or may occur because of inaccurate placement of the probe in the aided condition.[233, 882]

4.4   Practical Issues in Real-Ear Testing

The following practical issues affect the measurement of both REAG and insertion gain, though not necessarily to the same degree.

4.4.1   Probe calibration

Probe microphones have an inherently non-flat frequency response, because of the effect of the long thin probe tube. Real-ear gain equipment corrects for the response by including a calibration step in the measurement or by applying a correction stored in memory. Often, the probe microphone is

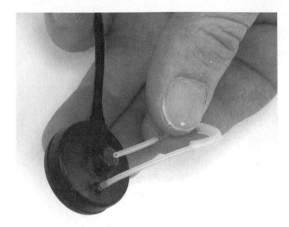

Figure 4.16 Positioning of the probe microphone against the control microphone during calibration.

calibrated against the control microphone, which does have a flat response. In this calibration step, the clinician should hold the tip of the probe tube closely against the control microphone inlet port, but without blocking the inlet port of either microphone. If the measurement system does not include a special clip to hold the two microphones together, it can be done with putty or with the fingers. The fingers and hand should be kept out of the way: that is, they should not be in a direct line between the speaker and the two microphones. Figure 4.16 shows the probe being held against the control microphone for one commercial analyzer.

4.4.2   Effects of wax

The most dramatic effect that wax can have on real-ear gain measurement is when it fills the tip of the probe tube. The equipment then incorrectly indicates that the signal level in the ear canal is very low. Apart from ingress of wax into the probe tube, real-ear gain measurement should not be greatly affected by cerumen in the canal. Cerumen should not have much effect on low-frequency real-ear gain until there is enough of it to fill a significant proportion of the residual ear canal volume. Cerumen should not have much effect on high-frequency real-ear gain until

there is enough of it to fill a significant proportion (e.g. one-third) of the cross sectional area of the canal at any point. There are, however, no empirical data on this issue.

4.4.3   Contamination by background noise

Real-ear gain measurement equipment employs a filter in the measurement chain to help discriminate against background noise. For swept pure tone measurement, the filter tracks the stimulus frequency. For broadband stimuli, the analysis process (usually a Fourier Transform) is in essence a large set of very narrowband filters. Some equipment also employs signal averaging to improve measurement accuracy. Because of these techniques, real-ear gain measurement systems are resistant to ambient noise, but are by no means immune to it. Swept pure tones or warble tones are much more resistant to background noise than broadband test signals. This is because all the signal energy is concentrated in one narrow region rather than being spread over the entire frequency range.

Some equipment monitors the consistency of repeated measurements at each frequency and rejects measurements that it considers are corrupted by background noise. Such equipment may give a warning message when background noise levels are excessive, or it may just lengthen the measurement time indefinitely. Other equipment gives no specific indication of noise corruption (see accompanying panel). Place the real-ear gain equipment in the quietest place available (the test booth is ideal if it is large enough). It is not, however, essential to have noise levels as low as those needed for audiological assessments, so locations other than the sound booth are likely to be suitable, especially for swept pure or warble tone measurement.

Wherever the equipment is located, you should identify the lowest signal level at which measurement is possible and avoid testing at lower levels. The quieter the place,

---

Practical tip: Checking for corruption by background noise

Any one of the following tests is probably enough to ensure that noise is not unduly affecting measurement accuracy. The first test alone may, however, misleadingly inspire confidence in the results, for steady background noises when the hearing aid is measured using equipment that employs signal averaging.

- Repeat the measurement and ensure that all the fine bumps and dips also appear in the second response.

- Using an aid operating in its linear region, decrease the signal level by 5 dB. If the two responses are 5 dB apart (or equal if expressed in dB gain) and equally smooth in appearance, then background noise is not a problem at either test level. For nonlinear hearing aids the output should decrease by 5 dB divided by the compression ratio (CR). This is equivalent to the gain increasing by 5(CR-1)/CR dB.

- With an aid operating in its linear region, and the display set to indicate output level (dB SPL), rather than gain, turn the signal level down by 15 dB or more and repeat the measurement. If the output level drops by 10 dB or more at all frequencies, then noise is not a problem at the higher test level.

---

the lower the levels at which you will be able to test, which is especially useful for nonlinear aids. Testing at 65 dB SPL is the bare minimum that is acceptable, even for linear aids. Being able to test down to 40 dB SPL is useful for some nonlinear aids, but will not be possible in most settings. If you cannot test at 65 dB SPL with broadband test signals, you either have to get a quieter location, test only with warble tones (see panel), or test only at higher levels and infer the response at lower levels from coupler measurements. The last two options greatly complicate testing nonlinear hearing aids.

4.4.4   Hearing aid saturation

Nothing is simple. Contamination by background noise could always be avoided by using a sufficiently high level for testing. Unfortunately, if too high a test level is used, a hearing aid will saturate (i.e. limit in some way), and the result obtained will not be indicative of the performance of the hearing aid at lower input levels. The problem is even greater for nonlinear aids. To find out how a nonlinear hearing aid performs at several input levels it is necessary to actually measure the aid at these levels.[n] Nonlinear operation of the hearing aid is most easily detected by increasing or decreasing the input level by 10 dB and repeating the measurement. If the two measured curves are not parallel and are not exactly 10 dB apart, then the aid is not operating in its linear region. (If the graph displays gain rather than output SPL, the two curves should exactly coincide rather than be separated.)

Knowledge of the hearing aid and/or measurements at further levels will be required to distinguish between gradual nonlinearities such as wide dynamic range compression (see Chapter 6) and simple output limiting. Input-output functions are particularly useful for sorting out in what ways a hearing aid is nonlinear, and can usually be measured in the ear just as easily as in the coupler (see Section 4.1.5). Preferably though, the clinician will have become thoroughly familiar with the characteristics of the hearing aid (from test box

---

[n]   For hearing aids that are linear over a wide range of input levels, the gain that is measured at any input level within the linear range will also apply at any other input level within the range.

What to do when you need, but cannot use, a broadband test signal

Many older real ear gain analyzers do not have broadband noise test signals. Even when they are available, background noise often limits the use of broadband test signals to higher input levels. Swept warble tones can be used instead if:

- The hearing aid is operating in a linear region at the desired test level, or

- The hearing aid has no filters preceding any of its compressors (see Section 4.1.3). This can be assessed from the hearing aid's block diagram. Note that a directional microphone acts as a filter, unless it contains circuitry to compensate its inherent low-cut characteristics.

If the hearing aid is nonlinear, and has filters preceding its compressor(s), the following alternatives avoid the measurement of real-ear gain at low input levels with a broadband signal:

- Verify the gain-frequency response at high input levels only, and rely on the programmer or a test box to confirm that all compression ratios and compression thresholds are correct;

- Verify the real-ear I-O curves, rather than gain-frequency response, using narrow band signals like warble tones;

- Measure the patient's RECD curve, calculate a corrected coupler-gain target, and do all measurements and adjustments in a test box (see Section 10.6.2);

If you are unable to test with any technique, all you can do is adjust the hearing aid controls carefully to nominally match the prescription and then evaluate the response subjectively using the methods described in Chapter 11. The ideal, however, is to have a real-ear gain analyzer with broadband measurement capability, located in a quiet place such as a test booth.

---

measurement, the specification sheet, or the fitting software) long before its performance is measured on a hearing aid wearer.

4.4.5 Loudspeaker orientation

People listen to sound coming from all directions, but are probably interested in sound coming from approximately frontal directions more often than from any other direction. Why then would we want to measure the real-ear response of a hearing aid from any direction other than from directly in front? (Angle in the horizontal plane measured from the front is called *azimuth*.) The answer is that measurement from another direction is more reliable.[471] The control microphone controls the test level only at the position of the control microphone itself. If the source is positioned straight ahead, and the person being tested turns his or her head so that the test ear is away from the source, complex diffraction patterns occur on the side of the head away from the source. Consequently, the test level at the ear canal entrance and/or the aid microphone may be different from the level at the control microphone.[471] If however, the source is positioned 45° from the front, on the same side as the hearing aid, the subject would have to turn his or her head a long way before the ear being measured was in the acoustic shadow region of the head. Thus, the 45° azimuth will allow greater head movement between aided and unaided measurements than will the frontal direction, without adversely affecting measurement accuracy.

Practical tip: Positioning the aid wearer and the loudspeaker

- Whatever angle of the source relative to the head is chosen, position an interesting object in the direction in which the patient should be facing and have the patient look directly at it during the measurement. If 45° is chosen (see text), two such objects will be needed, one on either side of the source, for testing left and right ears.

- Choose a test position about 0.5 to 0.75 m away from the source. This is a compromise. If the spacing is too close, a small head movement can result in a large change of angle between the source and the patient. If the spacing is too large, room reflections are more likely to cause significant standing waves in the vicinity of the head.

- Avoid large, flat reflecting surfaces near the client.

- The tester should stand well back from the client, and should remain in the same position for aided and unaided testing, so as not to alter the reflections from the room.

For CIC hearing aids, the unaided ear and the hearing aid microphone have the same directionality, because in both cases sound is picked up after it has entered the ear canal. The insertion gain will therefore be the same no matter what azimuth is chosen, assuming no head movements during testing. For other hearing aids, where the microphone is not located within the ear canal, insertion gain will depend on azimuth, but below 5 kHz, and within the range from straight ahead around to 45° on the hearing aid side, azimuth has little effect on insertion gain.

For measurement of REAG, rather than insertion gain, the gain-frequency response obtained will depend on azimuth. For omni-directional hearing aids, head baffle effects will cause high-frequency gain to increase as azimuth increases from 0° to 60° or more (depending on frequency and aid type). For directional hearing aids, the combined effects of head baffle and microphone directionality will also make the gain and response shape depend a little on azimuth, with maximum gain at most frequencies occurring for azimuths between 20° and 50°. It may be most reasonable to test directional aids with an azimuth of about 30°, but any choice from 0° to 45° could not be criticized because the directionality of hearing aids is currently not large enough to have substantial effects on the measured response.

4.4.6 Measurement signal characteristics

There are two aspects to be considered in selecting a signal for measuring real-ear gain. The first of these is choosing a signal that will make nonlinear hearing aids operate in a realistic manner. This issue is no different from measuring hearing aids in a test box and has been covered in Section 4.1.3.

The second aspect is choosing a signal type that assists in control of the signal level. Although the measurement equipment uses a control microphone, this controls the level precisely only at the location of the control microphone. How well the level is controlled at other positions around the pinna depends on the signal bandwidth and the test environment. If reflections (e.g. from room boundaries, nearby objects, the subject's shoulders) cause standing waves to develop in the vicinity of the head, then large variations in SPL will occur within small regions, especially for the higher frequencies. Standing waves have their most pronounced effects for pure tones, because very pronounced minima (nodes) can occur when the reflected wave cancels the direct wave. As stimulus bandwidth is broadened, the acoustic field becomes smoother, because it is impossible for a range of frequencies to all have a node at exactly the same point in space.[238]

Consequently, the control microphone does a better job of keeping SPL constant at points a small distance from it if the signal has the widest possible bandwidth. Bandwidths of about 1/6th octave provide a reasonable compromise between getting a smooth acoustic field but still having a frequency-specific stimulus. These bandwidths are commonly achieved by using warble tones, narrow bands of noise, or a broadband noise. In the latter case, the analyzer creates the necessary bandwidth as it analyzes the output.

An alternative way to average across frequency is to measure with pure tones, at closely spaced frequencies, but average the results across adjoining frequencies prior to displaying the measurement. This is referred to as *post-measurement smoothing*.

4.5   Aided Threshold Testing and Functional Gain

Prior to the introduction of probe-tube equipment, hearing aid real-ear gain was tested by finding the hearing thresholds in a sound field while the person was aided and while he or she was unaided. The difference between these thresholds is known as *functional gain*. Except in certain circumstances, functional gain is identical to insertion gain.[233, 584] If the hearing aid is operating in a nonlinear region for either measurement, then insertion gain and functional gain are equal only if they are measured at the same input level.

The similarity and difference between the two gains can be summarized as follows:

- for insertion gain, the field level is the same for the unaided and aided measurements, and the acoustic effect of inserting the hearing aid on eardrum SPL is measured;
- for functional gain, the eardrum level is the same for the unaided and aided measurements, and the acoustic effect of inserting the hearing aid on field SPL is measured.

In both cases, the difference is the effect of inserting the hearing aid on the transfer function from free field to eardrum. Although insertion gain and functional gain are similar in concept, they have different measurement errors associated with them. Small random measurement errors prevent the measured insertion gain from being *precisely* equal to the measured functional gain.

Insertion gain has a number of advantages over functional gain because insertion gain:

- is the more accurate;
- can be measured in less time;
- gives results at many finely spaced frequencies instead of just the audiometric frequencies;
- can be measured at a range of input levels (see below);
- is not affected by the problem of masked aided thresholds (see below); and
- requires the hearing aid wearer only to sit still.

A severe disadvantage of functional gain testing is that it can conveniently be performed at only one input level for each patient – the level at which threshold is obtained. This is not a problem for linear hearing aids, but for nonlinear hearing aids, gain varies with input level, and we are explicitly interested in the gain at different input levels.

Another disadvantage of aided threshold testing (and therefore of functional gain testing) is that for people with near-normal hearing at any frequency, aided thresholds will often be invalid. A problem occurs when noise in the environment, or noise internal to the hearing aid, masks the test signal.[564] The result is a functional gain that is lower than the insertion gain of the hearing aid. In this case, it is the insertion gain rather than the functional gain that properly portrays the increase in audibility provided by the hearing aid to most signals in the environment.

Because of these advantages, insertion gain (or alternatively, REAG) has largely replaced functional gain in the clinic. In some circumstances, however, it may be useful to measure aided thresholds in a sound field. Aided thresholds may be the only alternative for a child that is too active to allow a probe tube to be inserted (but see Chapter 15 for some suggestions with this).

Aided thresholds also have the advantage of checking out the entire hearing aid and hearing mechanism. Obtaining an aided threshold provides a check that signal at each frequency will at least be audible, and this check may be especially valuable for clients with a profound hearing loss. Insertion gain measurement may correctly indicate that the hearing aid has a gain of 50 dB, but if the hearing aid OSPL90 is less than the person's thresholds nothing will be heard at that frequency.[841] Aided threshold measurement at least alerts us to this extreme problem, but certainly does not assure us that the OSPL90 is optimal. (Although it is not recommended, insertion gain can even be measured on a cadaver, so high levels of gain are no guarantee of audibility!)

An additional advantage of aided threshold measurement is that the measurement process does not induce feedback oscillations. Insertion of the probe tube around the shell can create additional leakage (see Section 4.6.3). This is particularly a problem for wearers of high-gain hearing aids and deeply seated hearing aids. Measuring the real-ear gain of deeply seated CICs (or other deeply seated hearing aids) can be difficult because of the incompressibility of the bony part of the canal. The probe tube reportedly can also become squashed because of the greater incompressibility of the bony canal. Two solutions to this problem are:

- Order the hearing aid with an additional purpose-drilled hole through which a probe tube can be inserted. The hole can be filled after testing. The only limitation is that the

hearing aid has to have enough space available. This is less likely to be available if it also contains an internal vent. Remember that external vents are always an option.

- Another novel suggestion is to measure the functional gain of these aids, but using earphones as the sound source.[49] Functional gain should be independent of the transducer and signal azimuth for CIC hearing aids and this has been experimentally confirmed.[790] The major limitations are those discussed above – masking by ambient noise if aided thresholds are too good, and the measured gain being applicable to only low input levels if the hearing aid is non-linear. If circumaural earphones (ones that seal against the head) were to be used for this testing, this approach would also have the advantage of substantially attenuating background noise. This makes functional gain testing possible in less than perfect situations.

On balance, and considering the usual clinical time pressures, it does not seem time-effective to measure functional gain or aided thresholds *if* real-ear gain can be measured, and if a systematic procedure has been used to select and fine-tune hearing aid OSPL90. Aided threshold and functional gain measurement may at best be justified for some profoundly impaired patients, for some very young children, and for some wearers of CIC hearing aids.

4.6 Feedback in Hearing Aids

4.6.1   The feedback mechanism

Feedback oscillation (when a hearing aid whistles) is a major problem with hearing aids. The term *feedback* literally means that some of the output of the hearing aid manages to get back to the input of the aid (i.e., it is fed back to the input). Of course, when it does get back to the input, it is amplified along with every other signal arriving at the input. Unfortunately, it is not just any other signal.

It has already traveled a complete loop from the microphone, through the amplifier, through the receiver, into the residual ear canal volume, and then back to the microphone via some path, as shown in Figure 4.17. If it has grown stronger while traversing around that loop once, then it will grow stronger still the next time, and the next and the next, and so on. The process will stop only when the signal is so strong that the hearing aid changes its operating characteristics sufficiently because the signal has grown so large. For a linear hearing aid, this will be when the output limits by peak clipping or compression limiting; for a nonlinear hearing aid, it may be when the gain of the hearing aid decreases because of compression. Notice that the signal will grow every time it passes around the loop no matter how small the original signal was. In fact, there does not need to be an original signal. An infinitesimally small random sound can start the process, and such sounds are always present.

Why doesn't this feedback process happen all the time? Sound is, in fact, always feeding back from the output to the input. It is just that the audible oscillations (whistling) can develop only when enough of it feeds back. Unfortunately, we loosely use the term *feedback* to mean the audible oscillation that results from the combination of feeding back

a signal and then amplifying it sufficiently to cause an oscillation.

How much signal has to be fed back to create this unwanted oscillation? A moment's thought will reveal that if oscillations occur only when the signal gets larger every time it goes around the loop, then *oscillations can happen only if the amount of amplification through the hearing aid is greater than the amount of attenuation from the ear canal back to the microphone.* Thus, if the real-ear aided gain of the hearing aid, (from input to the residual ear canal volume) is less than the attenuation (from the residual ear canal volume back to the microphone) then continuous feedback oscillations cannot occur. We can express this in another way by saying that the **loop gain** of the hearing aid (the total gain travelling forward through the hearing aid amplifier and transducers, and then returning through the leakage path) has to be greater than 0 dB.

Suppose, for example, that a test signal emerging from a hearing aid had a level of 90 dB SPL in the residual ear canal, but had a level of 60 dB SPL by the time it leaked back to the microphone inlet via a vent. This hearing aid could not whistle if the REAG was less than 30 dB, but the hearing aid may whistle if the REAG was greater than 30 dB. One might expect that if the REAG were 31 dB, then the signal would get 1 dB stronger every time it went around the loop. However, every new sound out of the hearing aid adds to the sound that was already there. The combined signal leaks back to the microphone, and so the signal can grow stronger only if the sound adds in phase with the other oscillation already present at the hearing aid output.

This phase requirement is the second condition needed for feedback oscillation to occur: the total delay around the entire loop must be an integer number of periods of the feedback signal. Stated differently, *for oscillation to occur, the phase shift around*

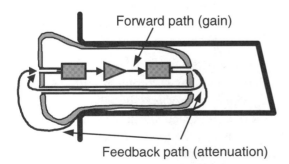

Figure 4.17 The feedback mechanism in hearing aids.

the entire loop must be an integer multiple of 360°, because 360° is the phase shift associated with a complete cycle.[o]

We can turn these two requirements around the other way to determine at what frequency (or occasionally, frequencies) a hearing aid will oscillate: A hearing aid will oscillate at any frequency at which the forward gain is greater than the leakage attenuation, and at which the phase shift around the entire loop is an integer multiple of 360°.

When the sound combines with the sound already in the ear canal in this constructive way, it is called **positive feedback**, irrespective of whether there is enough gain relative to the attenuation of the return path to actually cause oscillations. Positive feedback acts to increase the gain of the hearing aid. Indeed, a whistling hearing aid can be considered to have infinite gain at the frequency of oscillation: it has an output for no input at all. When the complete loop has a phase shift of 180°, 540°, or 900°, and so on in 360° steps, the sound fed back partially cancels any incoming sound. The effective gain of the hearing aid is decreased and we refer to this process as **negative feedback**. Negative feedback can not cause oscillations. As with everyday use of these technical terms, positive feedback causes something to increase, whereas negative feedback causes something to decrease. For hearing aids, the "something" is their gain.

Notice that hearing aid OSPL90 has not been mentioned. For a given amount of attenuation and phase shift, only the gain determines whether feedback oscillations will occur. A high-power hearing aid and a low-power hearing aid, adjusted to have the same gain,

are equally likely to whistle. It is tempting to think that the high-power aid needs a tighter earmold to "hold back the sound." This is simply not correct; it is a high-gain hearing aid that needs a tight mold. The only effect of OSPL90 is that a high-power hearing aid will whistle more intensely than a low-power aid, should they both happen to whistle because of their gain, phase shift, and attenuation of the leakage path.

4.6.2   Effects of feedback on sound quality

Excessive feedback has two adverse effects. The first, audible whistling, is obvious, though sometimes it is obvious to everyone in the room *except* the person wearing the hearing aid. This happens if the aid wearer has so much hearing loss at a frequency that even maximum output from the hearing aid at this frequency is inaudible. This highly embarrassing situation should soon be a thing of the past. A hearing aid can oscillate at a frequency only if there is enough gain at that frequency, and there is no point in providing gain if the aid wearer cannot hear a signal at maximum output SPL at that frequency. As hearing aids become more flexible, it is becoming possible to decrease gain in specific frequency regions to avoid this problem.

The second problem is more subtle. When the hearing aid gain is set a few dB below the point at which the aid continually oscillates, the signal feeding back will still cause the gain to increase at frequencies where the feedback is positive, and to decrease the gain where the feedback is negative. Feedback thus induces extra peakiness in the hearing aid response and these peaks occur at the potential feedback frequencies.[172] Every time

---

[o]   To be precise, this is the phase condition needed for feedback when the loop gain equals 0 dB exactly. The further the loop gain increases above 0 dB, the greater is the range of loop phase responses for which feedback can occur. For a loop gain of 6 dB, for example, oscillation will occur if the phase response of the loop is anywhere within $\pm 60°$ of an integer multiple of 360°. The general condition is that $g \cos\theta > 1$, where g is the multiplicative loop gain, and θ is the phase shift around the loop. The term $g \cos\theta$ can be thought of as the in-phase part of the loop gain.

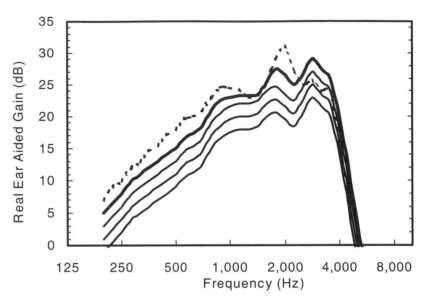

Figure 4.18 Coupler gain of a hearing aid with the volume control adjusted in 2 dB steps. One further increase resulted in oscillation.

a sound with components at these frequencies is put into the hearing aid, the hearing aid *rings* for a little while after the signal has ceased. (The ringing mechanism is in fact very similar to the reason why a bell continues to vibrate and sound after it has been struck: the hearing aid or bell stores energy and gradually releases it at this frequency over the next few hundredths of a second.) Most people have experienced this effect when a public address system is turned up to the point where it is almost continuously oscillating. The sound quality is annoying.

Both the increased peakiness, and the ringing effect rapidly decrease as the gain of the hearing aid is decreased below the point at which feedback oscillation becomes continuous, as shown in Figure 4.18. By 10 dB below the onset of whistling, positive and negative feedback can at most cause the gain to increase by 3 dB and decrease by 2 dB, respectively. It is difficult to say how far below onset the gain must be decreased for the ringing sound to disappear, as it depends on how peaky the hearing aid response is without any feedback being present. However, 5 or 6 dB of gain reduction is likely to be sufficient.

4.6.3 Probe-tube measurements and feedback

A probe tube can *cause* feedback. Inserting the probe between the mold and the canal wall creates small additional leakage paths on either side of the probe, as shown in Figure 4.19. This leakage decreases the attenuation for the return part of the loop. A hearing aid may thus whistle when it is being measured but be totally satisfactory otherwise.

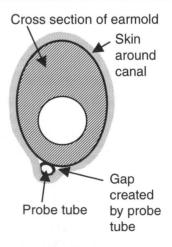

Figure 4.19 Leakage paths created by the insertion of a probe tube between an earmold or shell and the ear canal.

Practical tip: Avoiding probe-induced feedback

- Decrease the gain of the hearing aid by 10 dB (or so) below that which is required and then measure the shape of the gain-frequency response. Mentally add 10 dB to the gain at each frequency when comparing it to the target gain.

- Put some thick lubricating jelly on the mold or shell on the surface where it contacts the probe tube.

Even if there is no leakage around the probe tube, there can be leakage through the wall of the probe. The tip of the probe is in the residual ear canal, so the full output of the hearing aid exists at all points within the probe tube. This high-level acoustical signal vibrates the walls of the probe and hence the air outside the probe near the hearing aid microphone. Both of these leakage paths are significant only for high-gain hearing aids and some CICs. All other hearing aids will have been made with molds or shells sufficiently loose that the extra leakage created by the probe tube is insignificant. Do not attempt to measure the gain of a hearing aid that is oscillating (i.e. whistling). The oscillation can adversely affect the operation of the hearing aid at all frequencies. Agnew (1996) discusses many aspects of feedback in detail in an excellent review.

4.7   Troubleshooting Faulty Hearing Aids

Clinicians do not usually make major repairs to hearing aids. Many repairs, however, are minor and can be done by anyone who can diagnose the problem. Also, when a patient returns a faulty aid, it is usually the clinician that has to decide whether to return the aid to the manufacturer for repair or take some other action. It is inconvenient and unnecessarily expensive for aids to be returned to a manufacturer when a repair could have been done on the spot in a few minutes.

It is useful for the clinician to be able to hear the output of the hearing aid, and there are several ways to achieve this.

- A simple accessory is a *stethoclip*, as shown in Figure 4.20. A stethoclip allows the clinician to hear the output of the hearing aid without having to wear it. For high-powered hearing aids, a damper, or several dampers, can be placed in the stethoclip tubing to decrease the output to comfortable levels for a normal-hearing person.

- There are several electronic devices available in which the hearing aid is connected to a coupler, and the output of the coupler is amplified and presented through headphones. These have the advantage that a comfortable listening level can easily be obtained, even for high-powered hearing aids.

- Most real-ear gain analyzers come with a set of headphones that allow the clinician to hear the sounds present in the client's ear canal. Whenever the probe microphone is inserted, the clinician can listen to the sound while the client identifies precisely what aspect of the sound quality is unacceptable. *This method is invaluable if the clinician is in any doubt about the nature of the noise or distortion that the client is describing.*

Some hearing aid companies offer courses showing how to cut open custom hearing aids and effect straightforward repairs. On the other hand, opening a hearing aid usually (if not always) voids any warranty, and a repair attempted, but badly done, may make it impossible for the manufacturer to then repair the aid.

When diagnosing faults in hearing aids, it is important to be clear about the distinction between noise, distortion, and interference:

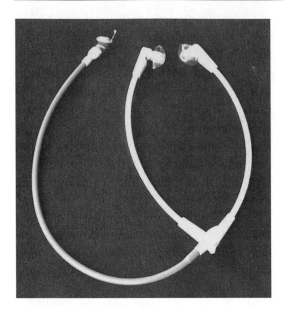

Figure 4.20 A stethoclip attached to a CIC hearing aid.

- *Noise* in a hearing aid output is an unwanted part of the output that is present whether or not a signal is being put into the hearing aid. It may originate totally from within the hearing aid, in which case it is referred to as internal noise, or it may originate in some external non-acoustic source, in which case we will refer to it as interference.

- *Interference* is the creation of a noise in the output of a hearing by a magnetic, electrostatic, or electromagnetic field near the hearing aid.

- *Distortion* is an unwanted part of the output that is present only when a signal is being amplified. It will usually be audible as a signal of poor quality rather than as something that is present in addition to, or in the absence of, the signal.

Interference of hearing aids by other electronic devices is currently receiving a lot of attention at the design stage of hearing aids. This increased interest has occurred because the signal transmitted by digital mobile telephones is particularly effective at stimulating hearing aids. These signals have a frequency high enough for the short wires inside hearing aids to act as receiving aerials. Also, the digitally coded speech sent out by GSM (global system mobile) phones comprises regular bursts of energy that produce a loud buzzing sound if the hearing aid accidentally demodulates the radio frequency signal. Hearing aids are now being **hardened** against this and other forms of interference by a combination of metallic shielding, capacitors to short circuit the radio frequency energy, and shorter wiring routes.[523, 525]

There is very little that can be done to make an existing hearing aid more resistant to interference. The only practical option is to replace an older style microphone with a newer model that has improved performance. Some modern hearing aids that use newer microphones combined with other forms of hardening against interference can be used with a digital phone placed against the ear. The use of a hands-free set (a remote microphone and receiver) for a mobile phone is another way that many hearing aids can be used with digital mobile phones, including those that use the GSM transmission system. The receiver of the hands-free accessory is placed next to the hearing aid microphone or close to the hearing aid telecoil. Alternatively, the telephone can drive a neck loop. Mobile phones using either analog coding or CDMA (code division multiple access) digital coding radiate a less pulsatile signal of lower power than the GSM telephones, and hence produces less audible interference.

The following tables list some possible causes of hearing aid faults, and the remedial action required for each, grouped according to the symptom. The comments apply to all types of hearing aids, except where otherwise indicated. Where the hearing aid operates intermittently from one second to the next, look particularly for problems with the battery contacts (see Table 4.8 and 4.9) or the connections to the transducers. Where the hearing aid output diminishes in strength or quality each day, returning to good performance each morning, look for cerumen build-up in the wax guard, dampers, sound bore or receiver screen. This is referred to as the rainforest effect because each day the high humidity in the ear canal reactivates and expands the dried-out cerumen lodged in the hearing aid (see Table 4.8).

As discussed previously, feedback is always caused by a signal leaking from somewhere back to an earlier point in the chain. Figures 4.21 and 4.22 show the major points in ITE/ITC/CIC hearing aids and BTE hearing aids, respectively, at which sound leaks.

4.8   Concluding Comments

Every clinician has to be competent at measuring hearing aids. The clinician must know the different types of hearing aid gains and be familiar with the various methods of displaying performance. If a clinician can not confidently measure a hearing aid in a test box, the clinician has no way to determine whether a hearing aid is operating to the manufacturer's specifications. If a clinician can not confidently measure a hearing aid in a patient's ear, the clinician has no way to determine whether the hearing aid is adjusted as closely as possible to the prescription target believed to be appropriate for that patient.

As with all measurements, hearing aids can be measured reliably and accurately only if the clinician has an appreciation of what can go wrong with each measurement, techniques for minimizing the chance of an error occurring, and an understanding of what a correct measurement would look like.

Table 4.8 The audio output from the hearing aid is weak.

Possible cause	Diagnosis	Remedy
Weak battery	Test battery or try a new one	Replace battery
Dirty battery contacts	Visual inspection	Clean with eraser
Corroded battery contacts	Visual inspection	Clean with abrasive paper, or return to manufacturer
Clogged sound bore or receiver	Visual inspection	Clean with loop
Clogged wax-guard (ITE/ITC/CIC)	Visual inspection, plus output restored when wax-guard removed	Replace wax guard
Clogged damper (BTE)	Output restored (and hearing aid feeds back) when earhook is removed	Replace damper
Clogged microphone inlet port	Visual inspection, or thump audible when the aid is tapped	Clean inlet port with a fine pick. Replace tubing if it is perished.
Inadvertent re-programming or de-programming	Check program settings (only applicable to programmable aids)	Re-program. Return to manufacturer if fault re-occurs.
Faulty microphone	Aid works on telecoil or audio input (if present), and internal noise audible at high volume control setting	Send to manufacturer
Faulty amplifier or transducer	No other discernable fault	Send to manufacturer

Table 4.9 There is no audible sound from the hearing aid. Consider all of the items in Table 4.8, plus the following.

Possible cause	Diagnosis	Remedy
Dead battery	Test battery or try a new one	Replace battery
Bent battery contacts	Visual inspection, plus jiggling battery compartment causes intermittent operation	Bend contacts carefully (this may provide a temporary cure only), or send to manufacturer for replacement of contacts
Faulty wiring	No other discernable fault	Send to manufacturer

Table 4.10 The output from the hearing aid is distorted.

Possible cause	Diagnosis	Remedy
Weak battery	Test battery or try a new one	Replace battery
OSPL90 excessively decreased (if a peak clipper)	Problem disappears for low input levels or higher OSPL90 settings	Increase OSPL90, or fit a hearing aid with compression limiting and/or wide dynamic range compression
Dirty battery contacts	Noise occurs when battery or battery compartment is moved slightly	Clean contacts with eraser
Faulty transducer or amplifier	No other discernable fault	Send to manufacturer

Table 4.11 The output of the hearing aid is noisy

Possible cause	Diagnosis	Remedy
Faulty volume control or tone control	Noise increases or decreases markedly when the control is moved slightly	Send to manufacturer for replacement of component
Interference from computer, electric motor, transmitter, mobile phone, car ignition, or other electromagnetic source	Interference noise is present at particular times, or in particular places	Avoid the source of interference, or upgrade hearing aid to one with greater immunity to interference
Hearing aid is switched to the T position!	Hum disappears and signal reappears when switched to M position	Re-instruct user about the function and use of the M-T switch, or disable the T position
Dirty battery contacts	Noise changes when battery or battery compartment is moved slightly	Clean contacts with eraser
Faulty transducer, wiring, or amplifier	No other discernable fault	Send to manufacturer
Faulty microphone	Noise like radio static which increases with changes to gain	Send to manufacturer

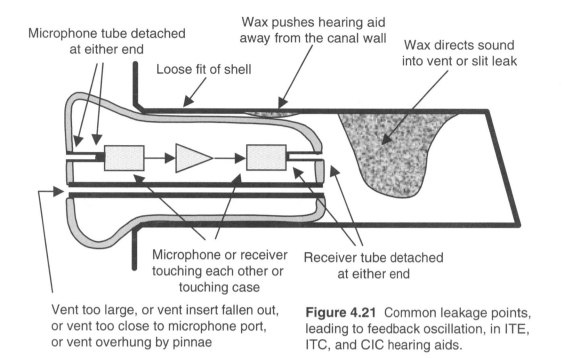

Microphone tube detached at either end

Wax pushes hearing aid away from the canal wall

Loose fit of shell

Wax directs sound into vent or slit leak

Microphone or receiver touching each other or touching case

Receiver tube detached at either end

Vent too large, or vent insert fallen out, or vent too close to microphone port, or vent overhung by pinnae

Figure 4.21 Common leakage points, leading to feedback oscillation, in ITE, ITC, and CIC hearing aids.

Table 4.12 Feedback causes an ITE/ITC/CIC hearing aid to whistle

Possible cause	Diagnosis	Remedy
Shell improperly inserted	Visual inspection	Re-instruct patient on insertion technique
Shell no longer fits ear snugly (especially for unvented aids)	Whistling stops when thick lubricating jelly is smeared over the canal stalk, or when a Comply™ Soft Wrap or E-A-R Ring™ Seal encircles the canal stalk	Add build-up material to shell, or re-make shell
Venting insert or plug has fallen out	Visual inspection, compared to record of fitting on file	Insert (and glue in!) a new venting insert or plug
Microphone or earphone has moved and is touching the case or the other transducer	Whistling continues when the microphone inlet port is blocked with a finger	Return to manufacturer for re-positioning
Microphone tubing detached from microphone or case	Whistling continues when the microphone inlet port is blocked with a finger	Return to manufacturer for re-attachment
Receiver tubing detached from receiver	Whistling continues when the outlet hole is blocked with a finger	Return to manufacturer for re-attachment
Receiver tubing detached from tip of earshell	Visual inspection; whistling continues when the outlet hole is blocked with a finger	Grip carefully with fine tweezers, reposition, and glue (or return to manufacturer)

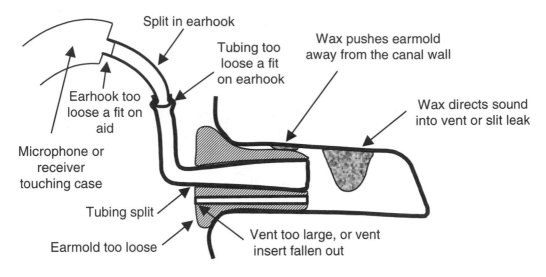

Figure 4.22 Common leakage points, leading to feedback oscillation, in BTE hearing aids.

Table 4.13 Feedback causes a BTE hearing aid to whistle

Possible cause	Diagnosis	Remedy
Mold improperly inserted	Visual inspection	Re-instruct client on insertion technique and/or modify mold shape
Mold no longer fits ear snugly (especially for unvented aids)	Whistling stops when thick lubricating jelly is smeared over the canal stalk, or when an E-A-R Ring™ Seal or Comply™ Soft Wrap encircles the canal stalk	Re-make mold
Microphone tubing detached from microphone or case	Whistling continues when the microphone inlet port is blocked with a finger	Open case and re-attach tubing, or return to manufacturer for re-attachment
Receiver tubing detached from receiver	Whistling continues when the outlet hole of the aid case is blocked with a finger	Open case and re-attach tubing, or return to manufacturer for re-attachment
Receiver tubing detached from case of hearing aid	Visual inspection; whistling continues when the outlet hole of the aid case is blocked with a finger	Grip carefully with fine tweezers, reposition, and glue, or open and re-glue, or return to manufacturer
Split in earhook or leak at junction of earhook and aid (i.e. hook is too loose)	Visual inspection; whistling continues when finger is placed over tip of earhook	Replace earhook
Split in tubing, or tubing a loose fit on the earhook	Visual inspection; whistling continues when finger is placed over tip of earmold	Replace tubing

CHAPTER FIVE

HEARING AID EARMOLDS, EARSHELLS AND COUPLING SYSTEMS

Synopsis

The earmold or earshell (called an otoplastic) is molded to fit an individual's ear and retains the hearing aid on the head. It also provides the sound bore, which is the sound path from the receiver to the ear canal. In many cases the otoplastic provides a second sound path, referred to as a vent, between the air outside the head and the ear canal. Where no vent exists, as in high-gain hearing aids, the mold or shell is said to be occluding.

There are a wide variety of physical styles of both earmolds and earshells. They vary in the extent of the concha and canal that they fill. These variations affect the appearance, acoustic performance, comfort, and security of retention of the hearing aid.

One unwanted consequence of a hearing aid can be an occlusion effect, in which the aid wearer's own voice is excessively amplified by bone-conducted sound. For most hearing aid fittings, vent selection is a careful juggle between choosing a vent that is big enough to avoid an unacceptable occlusion effect, but not so big that it causes feedback oscillations. Vent size also affects the low-frequency gain and maximum output for amplified sounds, but with modern hearing aids, these amplification characteristics are more easily altered by electronic controls.

The shape of the sound bore that connects the receiver to the ear canal affects the high-frequency gain and output of hearing aids. Sound bores that widen as they progress inwards (horns) increase the high-frequency output. Conversely, those that narrow (constrictions) decrease the high-frequency output. Horns have to exceed a certain length if they are to be effective within the frequency range of the hearing aid.

Dampers are used within the sound bore to smooth peaks in the response. Careful choice of the placement and resistance of the damper can also control the mid-frequency slope of the response.

The key to a well-fitting earmold is an accurate impression. This requires an appropriate material (medium viscosity silicone is good for most purposes), a canal block positioned sufficiently deeply in the canal, and a smooth injection of the impression material. Tighter earmolds or shells, that allow less sound to leak from the ear canal, can be achieved by a variety of techniques. These techniques include taking an impression with the patient's jaw open, patting down the impression material before it sets, using viscous impression material, and building up the impression in the patient's ear.

Earmolds are made from a variety of materials. The most important difference between materials is hardness. Soft materials provide a better seal to the ear. On the other hand, they deteriorate more rapidly and are more difficult to modify and repair.

The earmold (for a BTE) and the earshell (for an ITE, ITC, or CIC) perform three essential functions:

- They have a *sound bore* or tube that couples the sound from the receiver to the aid wearer's ear canal, and consequently affects the gain-frequency response of the hearing aid;

• They control the extent to which the inner part of the ear canal is open to air outside the head (**venting**), and consequently affect the gain-frequency response, and electro-acoustic comfort of the hearing aid;

• They retain the hearing aid in the ear in a comfortable way.

There is a bewildering array of earmold and earshell styles and materials, some of them proprietary to particular earmold or hearing aid companies, and some with multiple names. This chapter will help the clinician select an earmold or earshell that achieves a required combination of sound bore acoustic characteristics, venting characteristics, and retention characteristics.

Consider, for instance the two earmolds shown in cross-section in Figure 5.1. These two earmolds look completely different: Earmold *(a)* is a very bulky earmold that completely fills the concha, but it has a vent drilled through the mold. Earmold *(b)* contains very little material in the concha and in the canal, and may be referred to as a **CROS mold** or **Janssen mold**. Provided, however, the cross-sectional area of the drilled vent in earmold *(a)* equals the cross-sectional area of the open space between the sound bore and the canal walls in earmold

(b), and provided the two sound bores have the same length and internal diameter, the two molds will have extremely similar acoustic effects on the gain-frequency response and OSPL90 of the hearing aid. Earmold *(a)* will, of course, be retained much more tightly in the ear than earmold *(b)*.

In this book, *any opening between the inner part of the ear canal and the free air outside the ear will be called a vent*, irrespective of whether it has been formed by drilling a hole (Figure 5.1*a*) or by forming the canal portion of the mold or shell so that it does not completely fill the cross-sectional area of the ear canal (Figure 5.1*b*). These methods can be combined to provide a vent path comprised of a hole drilled through the concha part of the mold or shell leading to an open area within the canal portion. Another way to make a vent is to grind a groove along the outer surface of the mold or shell, all the way from the canal tip to the faceplate. This is called a **trench vent** or an **external vent**.

Earmolds and shells are often described as being **occluding** or **non-occluding**. Occluded molds are those that have no intentional air path between the inner part of the ear canal (the **residual canal volume**) and the outside air. Occluded molds or shells therefore have no vent: The mold or shell completely fills the cross-section of the canal, for at least part

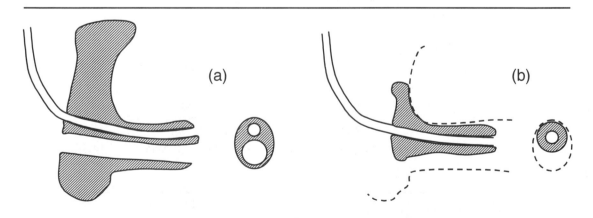

Figure 5.1 Cross sections of (a) a full concha earmold with a wide vent and (b) a Janssen mold that would have extremely similar acoustical properties, but different retention properties. See also Figure 5.3 for perspective views of these molds.

of its length. Occluded molds may, and usually do, have a **leakage path** around them as a consequence of imprecision in either making the impression of the ear or making the mold or shell from the impression, or because of the flexibility of the ear canal. This leakage path has properties similar to those of a vent, and is sometimes referred to as a **slit-leak vent**.

Unfortunately, the term *non-occluding* is used in so many ways it is practically meaningless. By non-occluding, some people mean that there is some vent path, no matter how small. Other people would describe a mold or shell as non-occluding only if most of the canal cross-section were left open. Some people may define *non-occluding* in terms of the hearing aid wearer's subjective impression

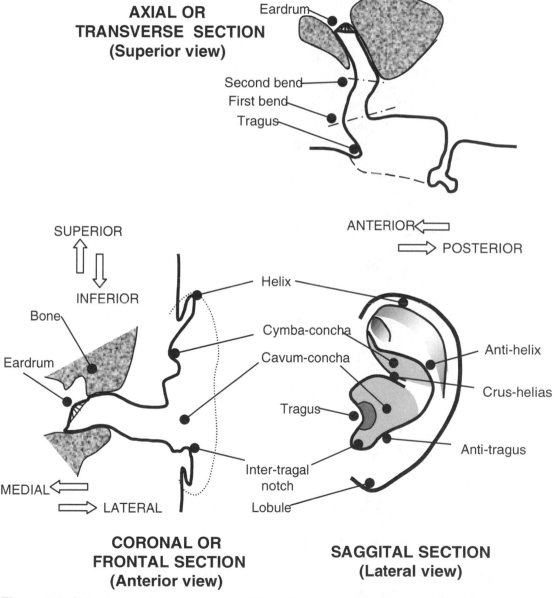

Figure 5.2 Side view and cross section of the external ear, drawn to average full-size dimensions and typical shape (Salvinelli et al., 1991; Staab, 1999), and the names given to various parts of the ear (Shaw, 1975).

of the earmold, as discussed in Section 5.3.2. There is, of course, a continuum of openness from being completely occluded to being completely open. The term non-occluding, if used at all, should be used in a way that makes its intent clear. All "non-occluding" earmolds are, in fact, partly occluding.

5.1 Earmold and Earshell Physical Styles

Earmolds and shells of different styles fill different portions of the concha and the canal. The parts of the molds and shells can be described by the corresponding parts of the ear in which they fit. Let us therefore review some names for parts of the ear, and for an earmold or earshell[18] as shown in Figures 5.2 and 5.3. Some features of the ear have particular significance for hearing aid fitting. The inner half of the ear canal, the *bony canal*, is bounded by smooth skin only 0.2 mm thick overlaying bone[17] and is very sensitive to applied force. In the outer half of the canal, the *cartilaginous canal*, the skin is much thicker, overlays cartilage, and is less sensitive. Cerumen is produced by glands and these are located only in the cartilaginous part of the canal. Earmold manufacturers refer to the section of the canal just inside the ear canal opening as the *aperture*, and the corresponding part on the earmold can be called the *aperturic seal* (because the earmold most readily seals to the ear canal in this region).

The earmold has two easily recognizable bends. The *first bend* (the most lateral bend) although a pronounced feature on a mold or impression, is less evidently a bend when looking at the ear. The posterior surface of the tragus is continuous with the posterior wall of the canal. The first bend is, in fact, coincident with the ear canal entrance or a few mm inside the canal, depending on where one considers the entrance to be. The *second bend* marks the start of the transition from the cartilaginous canal to the bony canal, first on the posterior wall, and further in on the anterior wall. The first and second bends are

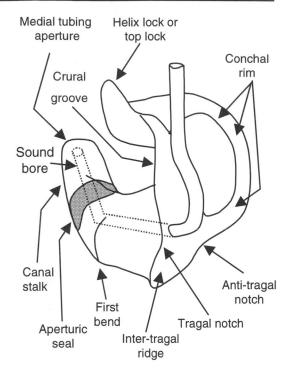

Figure 5.3 Names given to various parts of an earmold or ear shell, based in part on Alvord, Morgan & Cartright (1997).

much more acute for some people than for others. When people have a sharp first bend, however, they also tend to have a sharp second bend, so that the most inner and most outer segments of the canal tend to be parallel to each other.[708]

5.1.1 BTE earmold styles

One of the difficulties in describing different styles of earmolds is the lack of standardization of names. Although the American National Association of Earmold Laboratories (NAEL) agreed on some standard names in 1976,[156] many new styles have been invented and re-invented since then. Some earmolds are usefully given a descriptive name (e.g. *skeleton*), some are named after their inventor (e.g. *Janssen*) and some are confusingly named after the application in which they were originally used (e.g. *CROS*), even though they are subsequently used more frequently in other applications.

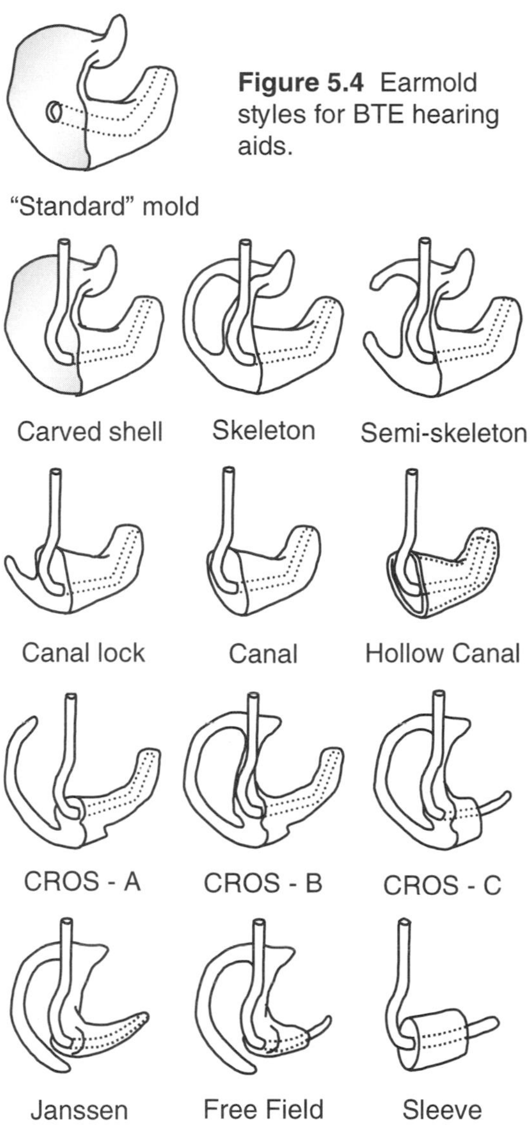

Figure 5.4 Earmold styles for BTE hearing aids.

"Standard" mold

Carved shell   Skeleton   Semi-skeleton

Canal lock   Canal   Hollow Canal

CROS - A   CROS - B   CROS - C

Janssen   Free Field Sleeve

Figure 5.4 shows a number of earmold styles that are available from different earmold manufacturers. The names may vary from manufacturer to manufacturer. The diagram does *not* include styles that differ only in the diameter of the sound bore. Every one of the styles shown could include a sound bore that widens or constricts along its length, so it is unnecessarily confusing to give a new name to an earmold on the basis of its sound bore internal diameter(s). The effects of sound bore variation, and names for several commonly used sound bore shapes, will be covered in Section 5.4.

The **receiver mold** (confusingly called a **standard** or **regular** mold, despite being rarely used these days) is the only one that can be used for a body aid: a button receiver clips firmly into the ring on the surface of the mold. It can also be used for a BTE aid by clipping a plastic angle piece into the ring. A length of tubing connects the angle piece to the hearing aid earhook. For BTE use, however, its disadvantages (leakage of sound, appearance, potentially decreased high-frequency response) outweigh its advantage (easy replacement of tubing).

A better way to enable tubing to be easily replaced is to have an elbow mounted in the earmold, to which the tubing is connected, as shown in Figure 5.5a. The sound bore inside the mold consists of a drilled hole rather than a tube. To avoid decreasing the high-frequency response of the hearing aid, the internal diameter of the elbow should be the same as that of the tubing. One particular brand of elbow that achieves this is known as a **continuous flow adapter (CFA)**™, as shown in Figure 5.5b.

The top seven earmolds shown in Figure 5.4 can be ordered as occluding earmolds, or they can be ordered with vents drilled through them. The remaining five molds can never be completely occluding, because the canal stalk does not fill the entire cross-section of the ear canal at any point along its length. The **sleeve mold**[131] has been designed to be as non-occluding as is possible.

The top four molds in Figure 5.4 are shown with the **helix lock** segment intact. Each of these molds can be ordered with the helix lock removed, or the helix lock can be cut or ground away by the clinician. Retaining the helix lock helps the mold stay in place, and thus maximizes security of the aid, provided the user can fully insert the mold with the helix lock properly tucked in under the helix and anti-helix. By helping retain the earmold in its correct position, the helix lock can also slightly decrease the likelihood of feed-

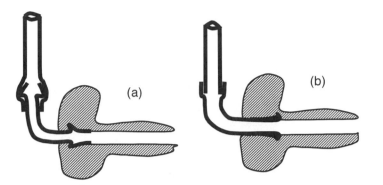

Figure 5.5 Two types of elbows used in BTE earmolds. In (a) the tubing fits around the elbow, which creates some constriction. In (b) the tubing fits inside the elbow.

back.[506, 598] Unfortunately, many people can not tuck in the helix lock properly, in which case its presence pushes the mold *out* of position, thus *increasing* feedback. The helix lock area of the mold can also create pressure discomfort. Consequently, some clinicians order molds without a helix lock for all patients, whereas others start with it attached, and remove it if it creates problems.

There are systematic procedures that can be followed for determining how open (i.e. non-occluding) an earmold should be for a particular aid wearer, as outlined in Sections 5.3 and 5.7. It is not so clear how to systematically choose between molds that differ only in appearance, fragility, and degree of retention properties (e.g. shell versus skeleton versus semi-skeleton, or CROS-A versus CROS-B). There is no difference in the retention properties or occlusion properties of a shell versus a skeleton, because the material removed to turn a shell into a skeleton comes from the center of the concha region. As a general rule, the mold becomes less firmly anchored in the ear as more and more segments are removed from around the rim of the concha, and as the diameter of the canal stalk is decreased below the diameter of the ear canal itself. For people who have pinnae that move excessively during talking, chewing and head turning, however, the mold or shell may be best retained if it makes minimal contact with the concha, in which case a canal-sized mold or shell may be optimal.[429]

5.1.2 ITE, ITC, and CIC earshell styles

Because the electronics of the hearing aid has to be included inside the shell for an ITE, ITC or CIC hearing aid, there are fewer possibilities for alternative shell styles within each of these classes of hearing aids. ITE hearing aids that extend above the crus-helias are classified as *full-concha ITEs*, and those that are fully contained below the crus-helias are referred to as *half-concha ITEs*. If either of these does not extend laterally sufficiently far to fill the concha, they are referred to as *low-profile ITEs*. ITC hearing aids that extend only part of the way along the posterior-medial wall of the tragus are sometimes referred to as *mini-canal* hearing aids. Mini-canal hearing aids can be thought of as low-profile ITCs.

The distinction between ITEs, low-profile ITEs, ITCs, and CICs can best be seen in an axial section through the ear, as shown in Figure 5.6. The faceplate of ITEs (whatever their thickness in profile) is approximately parallel to the plane containing the lateral surfaces of the tragus and helix. The faceplate of ITCs, however, is approximately at right angles to the posterior-medial surface of the tragus. The faceplate of CIC hearing aids may be at the ear canal entrance or medial to the entrance. Any hearing aid that extends to within a few mm of the eardrum is referred to a *peri-tympanic* hearing aid, but it is rare for any hearing aid other than a CIC to extend this far.

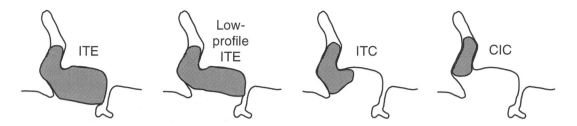

Figure 5.6 Axial view of typical placements for ITE, low-profile ITE, ITC and CIC hearing aids.

Many of the comments made about BTE molds are also true of earshells. In particular, earshells can be occluding or partly occluding, and in general, the hearing aid becomes less securely anchored in the ear as more of the concha material is removed. Despite this generality, ITC and CIC hearing aids, with little or no material in the concha, can usually be retained in the ear provided that an appropriate impression technique is used (see Section 5.8).

When the vent path in an ITE or ITC hearing aid is opened out by removing some of the shell at the medial and lateral ends of the vent, leaving only a short, wide vent path, as shown in Figure 5.25b, the style is called an IROS vent.[a]

5.2   Overview of Earmold and Earshell Acoustics

The earmold or earshell affects the shape of the gain-frequency response of the aid when it is mounted in the ear, the comfort and appearance of the hearing aid, the self-perceived quality of the patient's voice, and the likelihood of feedback oscillation.

The three acoustic aspects of the coupling system are the *sound bore,* the *damping*, and the *venting*. These primarily affect the frequency response in different frequency regions, as shown in Figure 5.7. Sound bore dimensions affect only the high-frequency

response (above 2 kHz for BTE aids and above 5 kHz for ITE/ITC/CIC aids). Damping mainly affects the response shape in the mid-frequency region (from 800 Hz to 2500 Hz for BTE aids, and from 1500 Hz to 3500 Hz for ITE/ITC/CIC aids) although it has some effects outside this range. Venting mainly affects the low-frequency response (from 0 Hz up to approximately 1 kHz, with the frequency range affected depending strongly on the vent size and hearing aid gain).

5.3   Venting

Although this section on venting may seem to be excessively comprehensive, it is the author's experience that the effects of vents and leakage paths lie behind much of the seemingly inexplicable behavior of hearing aids. A good understanding of vents is essential to hearing aid fitting.

The vent size must be selected so that the target gain is achieved, but without the ear

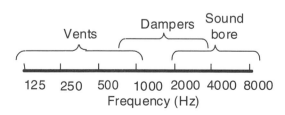

Figure 5.7 Frequency regions affected by each of the components of the hearing aid coupling system.

---

[a]   The term stands for ***Ipsilateral Routing of Signals,*** meaning that sounds reach the ear canal by two paths in the same ear. This is not a particularly helpful term, because all hearing aids result in some mixture of amplified and non-amplified sound in the same aided ear canal.

canal being excessively occluded, and without the hearing aid oscillating. These three issues are covered in Sections 5.3.1 to 5.3.3 respectively. Vents also enable an exchange of air between the air that would otherwise be trapped in the ear canal and the outside air. This air exchange helps avoid excessive moisture build-up. The venting action can enable people with perforated ear-drums to wear hearing aids, provided the perforation is not too large.[19]

Our understanding of the effects of vents will be greatly increased if we first understand the concept of *acoustic mass*. A vent is a column of air surrounded by the walls of a tube. Air, like any other substance, has mass, and there-fore has inertia. For a vent to transmit sound, this inertia has to be overcome (or else the air does not move). Overcoming inertia is much easier at low frequencies than at high frequencies and is much easier for small masses than for large masses. Pick up a small weight, like a pen and shake it sideways in

front of you at a rate of once per second (i.e. 1 Hz). Increase the rate to 3 or 4 Hz. You will notice the increase in force that you have to provide. Now pick up a heavier weight, like a 1-kg (2-pound) bag of sugar or flour and repeat the exercise. The higher frequency will require considerable force, and if you provide only a very small force at the 3 Hz rate, then only a very small motion will result. The analogy is that the column of air in a vent will not move much and so not transmit much sound if the stimulating frequency is high and if the vent has a large acoustic mass. As shown in the panel, vents have a high acoustic mass if they are long and narrow.

Real vents are not always tubes with uniform diameter. The concept of acoustic mass helps us understand how their performance varies from that of a constant diameter tube. For a vent like the one shown in Figure 5.8 the total acoustic mass equals the sum of the acoustic masses of each segment. In this particular case, the acoustic mass of the narrow segment

---

Underlying theory: Calculating the acoustic mass of vents from their diameter and length

Although it is never necessary in clinical practice to calculate acoustic mass, the calculation formula is simple and helps our understanding of how changing the vent dimensions will vary the effects of a vent. Acoustic mass is not the same thing as the physical mass of the air in the vent. The acoustic mass of a column of air (i.e. a tube) of length* L (in meters) and cross sectional area A (in square meters) is equal to (Beranek, 1954):

$$Ma = 1.18 \ (L/A) \quad ..... \ 5.1$$

The units are kg/m^4, but by analogy with electrical inertia, the units can be referred to as Henrys. The quantity 1.18 is the density of air in kg/m^3. Because vents are usually circular in shape we can make the calculation more convenient. If the internal diameter of the vent is d (in mm) and the length is l (in mm), the acoustic mass can be calculated as:

$$Ma = 1500 l/d^2 \quad ..... \ 5.2$$

As an example, a vent 20 mm long with diameter 2 mm would have an acoustic mass of 7500 Henrys. The acoustic mass of a vent increases as the vent gets longer or narrower. *Thus long vents transmit less sound than short vents, and narrow vents transmit less sound than wide vents.*

* To precisely calculate acoustic mass, it is necessary to add a length correction to each end of the vent that opens out into a larger space (such as free air at the lateral end or the residual ear canal at the medial end). This end correction is equal to 0.4 times the diameter of the tube. Thus, the tube in the example above actually acts like a tube that is 21.6 mm long, so that its acoustic mass is really 8100 Henrys. The end correction can be neglected for vents that are much longer than they are wide, but otherwise should be included, and the correction is especially important for short wide vents.

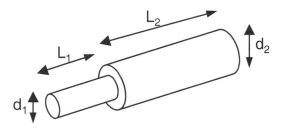

Figure 5.8 A vent made up of two tubes of different lengths and diameters.

will be much greater than the acoustic mass of the wider segment, so the total acoustic mass will be approximately equal to the acoustic mass of the narrow segment. The acoustic mass of vents with more than one diameter has a practical application to vents with adjustable apertures and vents that have been widened at one end.

Because it can be difficult to predict exactly what size a vent should be, the clinician often needs to adjust the vent after a preliminary fitting has been made on the aid wearer. One way to do this is to enlarge the vent diameter by drilling or grinding, or decrease the vent diameter by filling it with wax or plastic materials that cure, and then re-drilling it if necessary. Vents can be modified more quickly and easily if they are ordered with an exchangeable *vent insert plug*. One such system is shown in Figure 5.9. It comprises a vent tube connected to a widened cylindrical

receptacle at the lateral end of the vent. A "tree" of inserts, any one of which seats firmly in the receptacle, completes the system. The inserts all have the same length (2.5 mm) but differ in the diameter of their internal hole. The different inserts thus change the acoustic mass of the vent but only provided:

- The rest of the vent (the vent tube) is not so long or so thin that its acoustic mass dominates the total mass,[165] and,

- The leakage around the mold or shell is not so big that the size of the vent is inconsequential.

It will commonly be the case that the inserts with the few largest holes will have almost identical effects (because the total vent mass is dominated by the vent tube), and the inserts with the smallest few holes will have similar effects to each other (because the natural leakage dominates the venting effect). The insert system is nevertheless worthwhile in that it offers an easy way to obtain two or maybe three effectively different vents. If one does need the maximum flexibility in venting, then:

- For the narrowest inserts to be useful, leakage must be minimized by making the mold a tight fit (which may be uncomfortable and is not very sensible if one ends up using a wide insert).

- For the widest inserts to be useful, the vent tube must be short and wide, which may

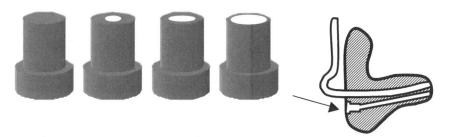

Figure 5.9 The inserts (larger than life-size) from a vent insert system, and the earmold and vent receptacle (approximately life-size) into which they fit. Positive Venting Valve (PVV) and Select-A-Vent (SAV) are two such systems commercially available.

not be possible if the ear canal is narrow, and the canal has to contain other large objects, like a horn for BTEs or a large receiver for ITEs.

It is thus useful to be able to predict approximately how much venting is necessary, and this is taken up in the next three sections.

5.3.1 Effects of vents on hearing aid gain and OSPL90

Vents (including leaks) affect the low-frequency gain and OSPL90 of hearing aids by allowing low-frequency sounds *out* of the ear canal and by allowing low-frequency sounds *in* to reach the residual ear canal volume without passing through the hearing aid amplifier. These are two separate effects of vents, so let us consider them in turn, and then consider their combined effects.

Effects of vents on the amplified sound path
When amplified sounds emerge from the sound bore into the residual ear canal volume, they generate sound pressure in that volume. It is this sound pressure that is sensed by the eardrum. The smaller the residual canal, the greater will be the SPL generated. If there is an escape route, such as a vent, some of the injected sound will leave by that route rather than contribute to the sound pressure within the residual canal. How much sound leaves and how much stays? The proportion leaving depends on the impedance of the escape route relative to the impedance of the residual canal. The vent pathway, being an acoustic mass, has an impedance that rises with frequency. Conversely, the residual ear canal volume, being primarily an acoustic compliance, has an impedance that falls as frequency increases. For both these reasons, the vent becomes more attractive as an escape route as frequency decreases. Consequently, for sounds injected into the ear canal by the amplifier and receiver, the vent provides a low-cut to the frequency response.

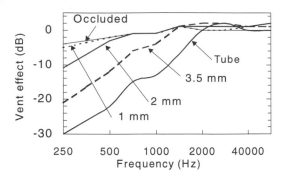

Figure 5.10 Effect of different sized vents on the frequency response of amplified sound, relative to the response with a tightly fitting earmold or earshell (Dillon, 1985).

The extent of the low-frequency cut depends on the size of the vent (because the vent size determines its acoustic mass). Figure 5.10 shows the degree to which vents of different sizes cut the low-frequency response of the amplified sound path relative to a tightly fitted earmold or earshell. Because these data are so useful in selecting a vent, they are presented in tabular form at the audiometric frequencies in Table 5.1. Vents of other sizes, but with the same acoustic mass, would have the same effect on the amplified sound path.[b]

The amount of attenuation that a vent provides to an aid with a canal stalk extending beyond the second bend would be greater than that shown in Table 5.1, though no experimental data exist. The reason for the greater effect is that if the residual ear canal volume is smaller, the acoustic impedance of the residual canal is greater. Consequently, a vent of a given length and diameter provides a more attractive escape route for sound than it would for larger residual canal volumes.

Effects of vents on the vent-transmitted (acoustic) sound path
Vents will transmit low-frequency sound waves no matter which end of the vent they enter. Sound waves reaching the head will

---

[b]   The data in Figure 5.10 were obtained with vents averaging 17 mm in length. Equation 5.2 can be used to generalize the data to vents of different lengths. For example, if the vent length were to be halved, the acoustic mass (and hence the size of the low cut) would remain constant if the vent diameter were to be decreased by $\sqrt{2}$.

Table 5.1 Effect of different sized vents, in dB, relative to a tightly sealed earmold or shell, on the gain of the amplified sound path. Note that the acoustic masses shown do not allow for leakage around the mold, which reduces the total acoustic mass.[220, 898]

Vent size	Vent acoustic mass (Henrys)	Frequency (Hz)								
		250	500	750	1000	1500	2000	3000	4000	6000
Unvented, average fit		-4	-2	-1	-1	1	0	0	0	0
1 mm	26,700	-5	-2	-1	-1	1	0	0	1	1
2 mm	7,000	-11	-3	-1	-1	1	1	1	1	2
IROS (ITE/ITC)	4,700	-16	-11	-4	-3	2	4	2	-1	0
3.5 mm	2,400	-21	-12	-6	-4	1	2	2	1	1
Janssen (ITE)	2,100	-23	-13	-3	-3	1	6	4	-1	1
Tube (BTE)	800	-30	-22	-15	-13	-7	0	2	0	0

thus be transmitted directly *into* the ear canal by a vent. This sound path is totally non-electronic. The range of frequencies over which the vent transmits sounds into the ear canal without attenuation is the same as the range over which it attenuates sound that has been electronically amplified. In particular, sounds are transmitted into the ear canal without significant attenuation up to the vent Helmholtz resonant frequency. Above that frequency, the vent increasingly attenuates sound so the hearing aid, when turned off, begins to act like an earplug.

Figure 5.11 shows the ***real-ear occluded gain (REOG)*** of the ***vent-transmitted sound path*** averaged across ten subjects. That is, it shows what the insertion gain of the complete hearing aid would be if the hearing aid amplifier were to be turned off. Vents of other dimensions, but with the same acoustic mass, would have the same effect. For hearing aids that extend beyond the second bend, vents of a given size will provide 0 dB insertion gain up to a somewhat higher frequency than one would expect on the basis of Figure 5.11.

Effects of vents on the combined amplified and vent-transmitted sound paths

The hearing aid user does not hear either the amplified sound path, or the vent-transmitted

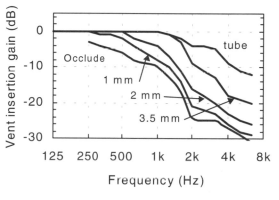

Figure 5.11 Insertion gain of the vent-transmitted sound path for vents of different sizes in an earmold or shell with a mean canal stalk length of 7 mm (Dillon, 1985).

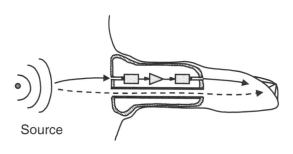

Figure 5.12 Sound travels from a source to the eardrum via the amplified path (solid line) and the vent or leakage path (dashed line). An ITE is shown but the same principle holds for BTE or body aids.

Theoretical diversion: The "*vent-associated resonance*" and its impact on how hearing aids should be measured

Books and articles on earmold acoustics often mention the "*vent-associated resonance*". This is a Helmholtz resonance between the acoustic mass of the vent and the compliance of the residual ear canal volume and eardrum. This type of resonance is analogous to the resonance that occurs when a mass is dangled on the end of a spring. It results in large volumes of air rushing in and out of the vent at the resonant frequency. (This is the frequency at which the impedance of the vent is equal in magnitude, but opposite in phase, to the impedance of the cavity.) When a hearing aid is measured in a HA-1 type 2-cc coupler, adding a vent causes such a vent Helmholtz resonance, and this causes the gain to *increase* at the resonant frequency. Below this resonant frequency the vent causes a low cut and above it the vent has little effect. Long thin vents, with a high acoustic mass, have a low resonant frequency (typically around 500 Hz). Short wide vents, with a low acoustic mass, have a high resonant frequency (typically around 1500 Hz; Tecca, 1992).

When the response of the vented aid is measured in an ear simulator, the magnitude of the resonance decreases. When the hearing aid's response is measured in real ears, the magnitude is smaller still and may be apparently absent (i.e. there may be no bump in the frequency response). The reason for this is that although the resonance is still present, it is damped by any acoustic resistance present. There is more resistance in the ear simulator than in the 2-cc coupler, and there is even more in the real ear, especially if the person has a loosely fitting earmold, because the slit leak around the earmold adds acoustic resistance. The net result is that the vent Helmholtz resonance has little effect in real ears, unless the earmold or shell is very tight. This is hopefully an uncommon situation, as it does not make sense to inflict a tight mold on someone when the mold also has a vent drilled through it! When the resonance is referred to, the term **vent Helmholtz resonance** or **vent-cavity resonance** should be used because vents can also have wavelength resonances in the high-frequency region.

A practical consequence of the resonance causing different effects in couplers than in real ears is that *vents should be blocked whenever hearing aids are measured in a 2-cc coupler*, and the vent effect allowed for separately (e.g. by using Table 5.1).

sound path, in isolation.[458] Rather, as Figure 5.12 shows, sounds arrive at the eardrum via both routes. The sounds arriving via each path combine in the residual ear canal volume.

Figure 5.13 shows an example of how the two paths combine.[221] Notice that whenever the insertion gain of one path exceeds the insertion gain of the other path by 10 dB or more, the insertion gain of the combined paths is almost the same as the insertion gain of the path with the higher gain. This is because the amount of sound arriving via the path with the lower gain is inconsequential

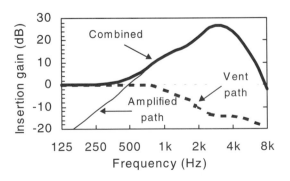

Figure 5.13 Insertion gain of the vent-transmitted path and the amplified path and the way these might combine to form the insertion gain of the complete hearing aid.

compared to the sound arriving via the dominant path. When the insertion gain (or alternatively, the real-ear aided gain) of a hearing aid is measured, the only curve that is apparent is the combined response. It is evident from Figure 5.12, however, that this combined curve arises from two entirely different paths, and it is useful to divide the response into three separate regions: the *vent-transmitted region*, the *amplified region*, and the *mixed region*. In the vent-transmitted region, which can extend up to 1500 Hz in some hearing aids fittings, the microphone, amplifier, and receiver play no part in the sound received. In the amplified region, however, the vent can have an effect if it attenuates part of this region by allowing sound out of the ear canal, as detailed earlier.

In the mixed region, the final result depends on how the vent and amplified paths combine, which in turn depends on the phase difference between the two paths. Figure 5.14 shows three possibilities for how the two paths can combine in the mixed region. A dip or notch occurs in the combined response when the phase difference between the two paths is close to 180 degrees. In practice, the notch is rarely more than 10 dB deep, because deep notches require a phase difference of almost

exactly 180 degrees at the frequency at which the two paths have identical gains. Minor dips probably do not have any adverse perceptual consequences, although peaks in the frequency response can.[232] In fact, the dip, when it does occur, provides a convenient marker to distinguish the vent-transmitted region from the amplified region.

It must be remembered that because vents affect the sound coming out of a hearing aid, they affect the maximum output in much the same way they affect the gain. An OSPL90 control, for example, will have no effect on maximum output in the vent-transmitted region.

There has been some conflicting research, for understandable reasons, on whether people prefer the low-frequency response of hearing aids to be achieved by the use of vents or by the use of electronic tone cuts. Conventional electronic low cuts, when combined with a well fitting earmold will produce negative low-frequency gains (i.e. an attenuation of

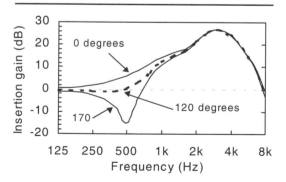

Figure 5.14 Insertion gain of the combined response for phase differences of 0, 120, and 170 degrees between the vent-transmitted and amplified sound paths shown in Figure 5.12. The combined path in Figure 5.12 assumed a phase difference of 90 degrees.

Practical tip: Matching a real-ear gain target

- *Adding or widening a vent moves the insertion gain towards 0 dB* (causing a low-frequency gain reduction in the amplified region, but a low-frequency gain increase if the aid was previously acting like an earplug).

- *Varying an electronic tone control has no effect in the vent-transmitted region*, and therefore may have no effect at all if the tone control only affects the same frequency range as covered by the vent-transmitted region.

- *Varying an electronic tone control can have unpredictable effect in the mixed region*, with the result depending on the phase relationship between the two sound paths.

Achieving high-quality, low-frequency sound

If a patient needs a gain of 0 dB below some frequency, no electronics can compete with the low distortion, flat frequency response that a vent can provide.

For such people an earmold or shell that attenuates sound below this frequency should be used only if:

- The required high-frequency gain cannot be achieved if a vent is used, or
- The hearing aid has a directional microphone and listening in low-frequency noise is important to that patient.

---

sound), whereas vents decrease the low-frequency gain only to 0 dB and then provide 0 dB gain for all lower frequencies, as discussed earlier. Consistent with this, Cox & Alexander (1983) and Kuk (1991) found that vented hearing aids produce superior sound quality. Lundberg et al. (1992), however, used a more complex filter that better simulated the real effect of the vent and consequently found no difference in perceived sound quality. In general, the quality of an amplified sound will also depend on distortion, and this depends on the signal level relative to the level at which the hearing aid saturates. Distortion is never a problem with vent-transmitted sound!

Effects of vents on directivity

Conventional directional microphones produce their greatest directivity at low frequencies. This directivity, however, will be apparent to the user only at those frequencies where the amplified sound path dominates over the vent-transmitted sound path. To maximize the benefits of a directional microphone, the amplified sound path should therefore extend to as low a frequency as possible, which in turn means the vent should be as small as possible.

Effects of vents on internal noise

The level of internal noise, like other amplified sound, will be decreased in the low frequencies by vents. For people with near-normal low-frequency hearing, perception of internal hearing aid noise will therefore be minimized by making the vent as large as possible.

Effects of vents on compressor action

Although a large vent may cause a hearing aid to provide no gain over an extended low-frequency region, the vent does not affect the sound reaching the microphone, and therefore does not affect the sound reaching any compressors within the amplifier. Consequently, low-frequency sounds may still be activating or even dominating the activity of a compressor, even though all the low-frequency sound heard by the patient arrives via the vent. This is an undesirable situation. One solution is to use multiple channels of compression, as will be discussed further in Chapter 6.

5.3.2 Venting and the occlusion effect

When an ear canal is occluded by a mold or a shell, people with low-frequency hearing thresholds less than about 40 dB HL will complain that their own voice sounds hollow, boomy, like they are speaking in a drum or a tunnel, or that it echoes. These are all descriptions of the occlusion effect.

Experience the occlusion effect yourself

1. First say the vowels *ah*, *ee*, and *oo*. Notice that they sound approximately equally loud.
2. Now block both ear canals by squashing the tragus firmly across the ear canal with your fingers.
3. Repeat the same sounds and notice that the *ee* and *oo* sounds have become much louder than the *ah* sound. The *ee* and *oo* sounds are also much boomier than before.

Why the occlusion effect occurs

As can be inferred from Figure 5.2, the residual ear canal is bounded by the eardrum, the medial end of the mold or shell, and the walls of the canal comprising the cartilaginous section and the bony section. If any one of these boundaries vibrates with respect to the others, the volume of the residual canal changes, and an intense sound pressure is generated within the residual ear canal. What can cause such a vibration? When a person speaks, vibrations in the vocal tract are coupled to all the bones of the skull (including the jaw), and to any tissues connected to these bones. Because the bones and other tissues have mass and elasticity, they do not move as a single unit, so there will be phase differences between the movement of one structure and the movement of others (von Bekesy, 1960). Consequently, in the cartilaginous portion of the canal, the inferior and anterior canal walls (which are in close contact with the jaw) will vibrate with respect to the other two walls (which are in close contact with the temporal bone) thus generating a sound within the residual canal volume. When a person is not wearing a hearing aid this does not create a problem, as there is no enclosed cavity within which sound pressure can be generated. The air vibrations created by the vibrating canal wall just leak out into the outside air.

Why is the occlusion effect most noticeable for the *ee* and *oo* vowels? Looked at one way, their first formant is around the frequency of maximum occlusion effect (300 Hz) and so is most reinforced. Looked at differently, these vowels are formed as closed vowels, so there is a higher SPL present in the vocal tract than for open vowels like "ah" (Killion et al., 1988).

Figure 5.15 shows the increase in SPL, relative to the SPL in an unoccluded canal, measured in one person's ear canal, as the person talked. The subject wore an occluding earmold with no sound bore. The length of the canal stalk was progressively shortened. For these measurements, a reference microphone in front of the subject was used to remove the effects of any variation in vocal effort. Data for the octave centered on 315 Hz are shown, because this is the frequency range in which the occlusion effect was largest. As the canal is progressively blocked by an earmold, the SPL rapidly increases, then decreases slightly, and then rapidly decreases. A similar variation of SPL with canal stalk length has been reported by Mueller (1994) and by Pirzanski (1998). These changes are caused by changes in three things as the canal stalk is lengthened:

- The seal to the ear increases, thus trapping more of the bone conducted sound within the residual canal.

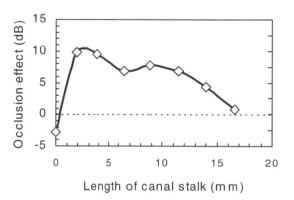

Figure 5.15 Increase in ear canal SPL (relative to no earmold) for the octave centered on 315 Hz when an aid wearer talks. Ear canal length was measured from the ear canal entrance along the center axis of the ear canal. For this person, the transition from cartilaginous to bony canal, as evidenced by the texture of the impression surface, commenced 9 mm into the canal (on the posterior wall, at the second bend) and completed 16 mm into the canal (on the anterior wall).

- The residual volume decreases, which by itself would lead to a higher SPL.
- The area of the vibrating cartilaginous canal wall that causes the occlusion sound decreases. By itself this would lead to a lower SPL. The decrease in SPL from this cause occurs at a rate faster than the decrease in volume, particularly as the end of the canal stalk approaches the end of the cartilaginous canal. Once the canal stalk fills the cartilaginous portion, only the bony portion of the canal remains, and this is not an effective generator of occlusion sound. Because the same (temporal) bone[c] surrounds all sides of the bony canal, phase differences between the top, bottom, front, and back walls are presumably minimal.

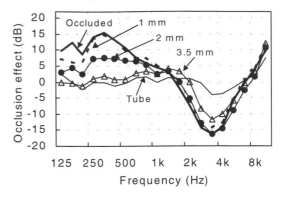

Figure 5.16 The mean increase in SPL (relative to no earmold) in the ear canal for 10 subjects, as they talked while wearing earmolds with vents of different sizes (May & Dillon, 1992).

There are at least two ways to decrease the SPL induced by the occlusion effect. The first is to open out the residual ear canal volume with a vent. Figure 5.16 shows the increase in SPL in the ears of 10 subjects as they talked while they were wearing earmolds with vents of different sizes.[d] Subjects' ratings of the acceptability of their own voices were significantly correlated to the degree of low-frequency SPL increase (r=0.63). It is clear that a 1 mm vent is not large enough to decrease the occlusion effect because a vent this small does not increase the venting significantly beyond that which occurs by leakage around the mold. With the 3.5 mm vent, the opening is sufficiently large that the SPL increase is only a few dB. Not surprisingly, the subjects (who all had normal hearing) rated their own voice as normal with a vent of this size.

For each patient, however, own-voice quality will become more acceptable as the mold or shell is made more open. A 2 mm vent is only partially effective in solving the occlusion problem. It decreases the size of the SPL increase but does not eliminate it. A 2 mm vent can be regarded as a good starting point for fixing the occlusion problem, but in many cases, the vent will have to be widened to 3 mm before the patient is satisfied with the sound of his or her own voice.

The above results for different vents were all obtained with earmolds having a conventional canal stalk length, averaging about 7 mm. As the residual ear canal volume decreases, its impedance rises, and a vent of given size becomes increasingly effective. The key parameter is the acoustic mass, and hence impedance, of the vent relative to the impedance of the residual ear canal volume and eardrum. For more deeply seated hearing aids, smaller vents can thus be used to achieve the same release from occlusion.

The second way to solve the problem of the occlusion effect is not to create one in the first place! As explained earlier, if the mold or shell completely fills the cartilaginous portion of the canal, there will be less occlu-

---

[c]   The **tympanic plate** forms the floor and anterior walls of the bony canal; the **squamous part** forms the roof and posterior walls; but these bones are both parts of one rigid **temporal bone**.

[d]   The vents and subjects are the same as those for which the data in Tables 5.1 and 5.2 were obtained. Data for an occluded skeleton earmold was very similar to that shown for the occluded carved shell mold. A reference microphone in front of the subject was used to remove any effects caused by variations in vocal effort.

sion-generated sound compared to molds or shells that terminate within the cartilaginous portion.[97, 465] While this sounds like an easy solution, there are practical difficulties for some hearing aid wearers. First, extra care must be exercised when taking the impression, as detailed in Section 5.8.2. Second, the resulting earshell (or less commonly, earmold) may be difficult for the aid wearer to insert or remove. Third, the earshell may be uncomfortable when worn for long periods if it extends into the bony portion of the canal. Comfort is improved if the shell is made with a soft tip.[676] If the soft material is made of compressible foam, the disadvantage is that the foam has to be replaced regularly, and if it is made of a soft plastic, the life of the earmold or hearing aid may be decreased.

As well as controlling the length of the canal stalk, it is important that the most medial parts of the earmold or shell be in close contact with the canal walls.[465, 744] Earshells that receive a heavy build-up during manufacture cause less occlusion SPL than those made from open-jaw impressions (which achieve a tight fit in the lateral, flexible parts of the canal).[709] Figure 5.17 show three earmolds of the same length. For earmold A, the tight seal near the ear canal entrance and the loose fit more medially traps the vibration-induced sound within the ear canal and so ensures that a high level reaches the eardrum. For earmold B, by contrast, the path of least resistance is outwards, so little vibration-induced sound will reach the eardrum. Earmold C should produce intermediate effects. Addition of a vent to any of the three will decrease whatever occlusion effect does occur.[e]

For people with more than 40 dB loss at 250 Hz and 500 Hz, the occlusion effect is rarely a problem. These people need significant low-frequency amplification, so it does not matter if there is an increased sound level when they speak. The only complication is that the hearing aid amplified sound will add (constructively or destructively, depending on the phase relationship) to the occlusion-generated sound, and this can affect the shape of the frequency response in the low-frequency region for the person's own voice.

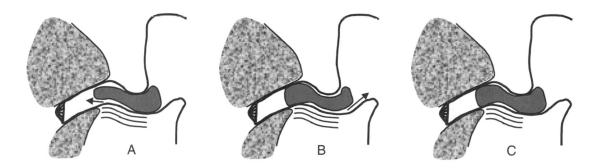

Figure 5.17 Axial view of earmolds or shells that produce a very strong occlusion effect (A), and a very weak occlusion effect (B). The mold or shell shown in (C) will produce a weak occlusion effect and will also have minimal leakage of sound from the hearing aid. In each case, the wavy lines show the vibrating anterior wall and the arrow shows the primary direction in which bone conducted sound will travel once it enters the ear canal. The looseness of fit in each diagram has been exaggerated for clarity.

[e]The level of vibration-induced sound reaching the eardrum may be affected in another way by earmold tightness. It may be that inserting a tight earshell or mold into the canal partly couples the canal walls and so decreases the vibration of the tissues on one side of the canal relative to the tissues on the other side. If so, even the unfilled part of the cartilaginous canal would become a less effective generator of sound. This suggestion is merely an untested supposition.

When the electronically amplified sound is out of phase with the bone conducted sound, increasing the degree of low-frequency amplification can cause a *decrease* in the SPL in the residual canal. This may be the reason behind the anecdotal reports of solving the occlusion effect by *increasing* low-frequency gain.[874]

The clinician can use real-ear gain analyzers to monitor the magnitude of sound when the patient speaks, whether this arises from bone conduction alone or from the combination of bone conduction and amplification.[630, 744] It is unlikely that this measurement is worthwhile doing routinely, as in the end, the amount of occlusion that is acceptable depends on a subjective judgement by the aid wearer rather than on a physical measurement. Measurement of occlusion would, however, be worthwhile when the aid wearer continues to complain about the sound of his or her voice, even after the clinician believes venting or deep seating should have largely eliminated the occlusion sound build-up. For deeply seated molds or shells, measurement will be possible only if the mold or shell contains a hole through which the probe tube can be placed. The skin of the bony canal does not have sufficient flexibility to enable the probe to be placed between the hearing aid and the canal wall without affecting either comfort or leakage.

So far, the "occlusion effect" has been defined as the increase in SPL that occurs in the ear canal when the aid wearer talks. Another consequence of a fully occluded earmold or shell is that the lack of ventilation and increase in moisture may increase the likelihood of external ear disease. Information on the effectiveness of ventilation is scarce. One study showed that even a 2 mm vent did not decrease reports of itchiness and moisture in the ear canal.[557]

5.3.3 Effects of vents and leaks on feedback oscillations

As explained in Section 4.6.1, feedback oscillation occurs when the signal leaking from the ear canal back to the microphone is larger than the forward gain given to the signal by the hearing aid. Measurements of the amount of signal leaking back at each frequency can therefore be used to deduce the maximum possible insertion gain before feedback oscillation occurs.[f] The maximum possible insertion gain without feedback is shown in Tables 5.2, 5.3, and 5.4 for BTE, ITE and ITC hearing aids, respectively. Not surprisingly, the maximum achievable gain decreases as the mold or shell becomes more open. In Table 5.2, data for shell and skeleton styles have been combined because the same maximum insertion gain is possible for both styles. Kuk (1994) also reached the conclusion that concha bulk does not affect leakage. Removing all material from the crus-helias upwards (a canal lock style – Figure 5.4) results in a 5 to 10 dB reduction in useable gain for non-vented molds,[506] presumably because the mold can more easily move within the ear. Unfortunately, comparable data are not yet available for CIC hearing aids.

The information contained in Tables 5.2 to 5.4 can be used to select the maximum possible vent size without feedback. It is simplest to first compare the value in the 3 kHz column to the target insertion gain at

---

f   As explained in Chapter 4, IG equals REAG minus REUG. In turn, REAG equals the microphone location effect from the free field to the microphone plus the hearing aid gain from the microphone to the ear canal. The maximum value of the gain from microphone to ear canal (without oscillation) is approximately equal to the attenuation of the sound leaking back from the ear canal to the microphone. Consequently, the maximum insertion gain equals the leakage attenuation, plus the microphone location effect, minus the REUG. The maximum achievable gain at each frequency can thus be determined. When maximum gain is determined just by turning up the gain of a particular hearing aid until it oscillates (e.g. Gatehouse, 1989; Kuk, 1994), the results are applicable only to the frequency at which oscillation first occurs, which depends on the particular hearing aid used.

Table 5.2 Maximum possible insertion gain (in dB) before feedback oscillation, for BTE hearing aids connected to hard acrylic earmolds with vents of different sizes. The data are average results for ten subjects.[220] Higher insertion gains are possible with tight earmolds and/or soft earmold materials.

Vent size	Vent acoustic mass (Henrys)	Frequency (Hz)							
		500	750	1000	1500	2000	3000	4000	6000
Occluded average fit		65	66	64	60	56	41	45	50
1 mm	26,700	65	64	61	58	52	39	45	47
2 mm	7,000	60	60	57	54	49	36	41	48
3.5 mm	2,400	51	53	52	48	43	31	35	41
Tube	800	41	43	42	40	34	23	26	37

Table 5.3. Maximum possible insertion gain (in dB) before feedback oscillation, for ITE hearing aids containing vents of different sizes.[898] The occluded tight shells had a special build-up during shell construction.

Vent size	Vent acoustic mass (Henrys)	Frequency (Hz)								
		250	500	750	1000	1500	2000	3000	4000	6000
Occluded tight fit		62	56	56	56	47	41	23	24	12
Occluded average fit		62	54	52	49	44	33	24	22	13
1.5 mm	14,200	61	57	54	53	48	37	26	25	15
2 mm	8,000	54	50	46	46	42	33	24	23	13
IROS	4,700	44	42	40	38	38	32	19	16	12
Janssen	2,100	42	41	40	39	36	31	17	16	13

Table 5.4. Maximum possible insertion gain (in dB) before feedback oscillation, for ITC hearing aids containing vents of different sizes.[898] The occluded tight shells had a special build-up during shell construction.

Vent size	Vent acoustic mass (Henrys)	Frequency (Hz)								
		250	500	750	1000	1500	2000	3000	4000	6000
Occluded tight fit		58	52	49	52	45	39	31	33	13
Occluded average fit		52	48	44	45	42	37	23	28	11
1.5 mm	14,700	47	47	44	45	39	34	28	31	12
2 mm	7,800	44	41	38	38	38	32	21	27	17
IROS	4,500	39	34	31	31	29	26	15	23	7

3 kHz, as this frequency usually provides the strictest constraint. This occurs because target REAG curves often have a maximum at 3 kHz, reflecting the maximum at this frequency in the REUG curve. Consequently, hearing aids must provide a REAG at least equal to the REUG before they start to give the aid wearer a greater signal level than is received without a hearing aid. For non-linear hearing aids, the maximum gain is needed at low input levels, so it is this low-level gain that should be compared to the maximum achievable gain.

The maximum vent size should be selected with considerable caution. For a given vent size, there is some variation between people in the maximum gain achievable without feedback. This variation is greatest for unvented styles because leakage around the mold or shell is more variable than leakage from a vent of known dimensions. Also, when the hearing aid gain is set a few dB below the point at which the aid continually oscillates, sound quality is adversely affected, as explained in Section 4.6.3. It may therefore be appropriate to allow a 10 dB safety margin when using these tables to select the maximum safe vent size.

The bottom row in Table 5.2 contains data for a *tube-only* earmold. The particular earmolds tested had a tube extending 7 mm past the ear canal entrance. The amount of gain that can be achieved before feedback varies with insertion depth.[466] To achieve maximum gain for high frequencies, the tube should be inserted only a few mm, whereas to achieve maximum gain at low frequencies (for reverse slope hearing losses) the tube should be inserted as far as possible.[466]

It might be expected that the shape of the vent, rather than just its acoustic mass, would have an effect on the likelihood of feedback oscillation. It is sometimes recommended that vents be widened at the medial end rather than the lateral end, so that the vent has a reverse horn shape for sounds exiting from the ear canal. While a reverse horn does decrease the amount of high-frequency sound leaking back to the microphone (relative to a vent that has been widened at the lateral end), the differences are confined to frequencies above 6 kHz.[217] Consequently, the variation in shape has little effect on feedback oscillation, because oscillation usually occurs at frequencies below 6 kHz. A more effective way to decrease high-frequency leakage while maintaining a low acoustic mass to decrease the occlusion effect is to use a cavity vent.[561] This vent comprises a cavity within the earmold, accessed via two small openings at the medial and lateral ends, which combine to form an acoustic low pass filter. It requires a relatively large earmold to be effective.

5.3.4   Parallel versus Y (or diagonal) vents

Other than their propensity to cause feedback oscillations, one of the biggest difficulties with vents is fitting them in! This is especially a problem at the medial end. Figure 5.18 shows an alternative way to fit in a vent when space is tight. This is called a *Y-vent, diagonal vent*, or *angle vent*, as opposed to the *parallel vent* shown in Figure 5.1, and which has been assumed until now. *The Y-*

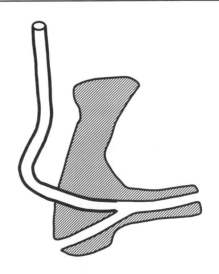

Figure 5.18 Cross section of a Y-vent (or diagonal vent) in a BTE earmold.

vent should be avoided unless there is absolutely no alternative, as it creates two serious problems.[165] High-frequency sounds propagating down the sound bore will be partially reflected at the Y junction where the sound bore meets the vent tube. This reflection decreases high-frequency gain and also makes high-frequency feedback oscillation more likely.

If a Y-vent absolutely has to be used, the sound bore and the vent tube should intersect as close to the medial end of the mold as possible. Furthermore, the diameter of the sound bore medial to the Y-junction should be widened as much as possible. This decreases the impedance of this section of the sound bore and minimizes the loss of high-frequency energy back up the vent. Of course, if there is room for extensive widening, there is probably room to avoid the Y-vent altogether!

5.4   The Sound Bore: Tubing, Horns and Constrictions

The sound bore provides the path between the receiver and the residual ear canal volume. In a BTE hearing aid it comprises:

- 8 to 15 mm of tubing connected to the receiver (usual diameter approximately 1 mm);
- 17 to 25 mm of earhook (usual diameter approximately 1.3 mm); and
- 35 to 45 mm of tubing from the earhook, connected to, and/or through the earmold to its medial end (usual diameter 1.93 mm).

The typical total length of the sound bore is 75 mm, with a range of 60 to 85 mm.[165] The final section of this (from 10 to 20 mm long) is contained within the earmold itself.

The sound bore in ITE, ITC and CIC hearing aids is much shorter, and typically contains a tube 5 to 12 mm long of approximate diameter 1.5 mm.

So far, all the diameters mentioned in this chapter have been internal diameters, because

Table 5.5 Diameters, in mm, of commonly used tubing.[953]

Tubing type	Inner diameter (mm)	Outer diameter (mm)
#12 Standard	2.16	3.18
#13 Medium	1.93	3.10
#13 Thick wall	1.93	3.31
#13 Super thick	1.93	3.61
#15 Standard	1.50	2.95
#16 Standard	1.35	2.95

it is this that affects the passage of sound *along* a tube. The thickness of the tubing wall, and hence the outer diameter, affects the leakage of sound out *through* the walls of tubing. Such leakage can be a problem in high-gain hearing aids, and tubing with extra thick walls is available. Inner and outer diameters of commonly used tubing, along with their NAEL classifications, are shown in Table 5.5. For new tubing, the #13 super thick wall (double wall) tubing provides 2 dB more attenuation of sound leaking through the walls than is obtained with #13 standard tubing (Flack et al., 1995). This difference may seem small but is consistent with the difference in wall thickness. Because a common source of leakage is the junction between the tubing and the earhook, the thicker wall tubing may provide greater advantages over time if it is better able to retain the integrity of this joint.

In areas with high humidity, moisture-resistant tubing should be used. This tubing is made of a different plastic that decreases the likelihood of moisture droplets forming inside. The tubing is stiffer than conventional tubing.

5.4.1   Acoustic horns and constrictions

Varying the internal diameter of the sound bore along its length will modify the high-frequency response of the hearing aid. If the diameter increases (either smoothly or in steps) it is referred to as an ***acoustic horn***,

Theory: How acoustic horns work

Horns help overcome the ***impedance mismatch*** between the acoustic impedance of a receiver and the much lower acoustic impedance of the ear canal. If the receiver and the ear canal are directly connected together, or are connected via a constant diameter tube, much of the power is reflected back from the medial end of the tube rather than being transferred to the ear canal. By gradually changing the diameter of a connecting tube, and hence its impedance, there is a more gradual transition from the high impedance receiver to the low impedance canal, and hence less reflections. This gradual transition is only effective for those high frequencies for which the wavelength is less than, or comparable to, the dimensions of the tube. Because reflections are less marked, so too are standing waves in the tube. Consequently, the response is less peaky, resulting in improved sound quality.

The effects of horns can be quantified. The approximate boost provided to high frequencies can be calculated from:

$$Boost = 20 \cdot \log_{10}\left(\frac{d_o}{d_i}\right) \ \text{dB} \qquad \dots 5.3.$$

That is, horns with the biggest outlet diameters will give the biggest high-frequency boost. However, this boost only occurs for frequencies well above the ***horn cut-off frequency***, f_h. Below the cut-off frequency, no boost occurs. For a continuous horn with an exponentially growing diameter, the cut-off frequency can be shown to be (Beranek, 1954):

$$f_h = \frac{c \cdot \log_e(d_o / d_i)}{2\pi l} \ \text{Hz} \qquad \dots 5.4,$$

where c is the speed of sound, and $\log_e$ is the natural logarithm (shown as *ln* on most calculators). Thus, the shorter the horn, the higher the cut-off frequency of the horn. As an example, for a horn with an inlet diameter of 2 mm, an outlet diameter of 4 mm, and a length of 25 mm, the horn cut-off frequency is 1520 Hz. The boost *commences* at this frequency and does not reach its full extent until an octave higher than this.

If a horn is made in a stepped manner, as in Figure 5.19, the stepped portion has an additional effect: standing waves will occur within the widened section of tube because reflections occur at each change of diameter. The ***quarter-wavelength resonances*** caused by these reflections can be used to shape and extend the frequency range of the hearing aid (Killion, 1981; Dillon, 1983; Killion, 1988).

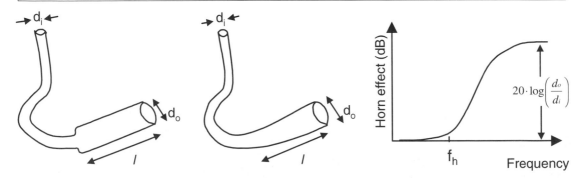

Figure 5.19 Two acoustic horns, one stepped and one continuous, each with inlet diameter di, and outlet diameter do, and the boost (an increase in gain and maximum output) given to the frequency response by the continuous horn.

and if it decreases it is referred to as an *inverse horn, reverse horn,* or *constriction*.

Horns

Acoustic horns increase the efficiency with which high-frequency power is transferred from the receiver to the earmold, and hence increase both the gain and the maximum output in the high-frequency region. This boost is achieved only above a certain frequency, which depends on the inlet and outlet diameters of the horn, and on its length (see panel). The shorter the horn, the higher the range of frequencies affected. Horns attached to a BTE earmold can be much longer than horns contained within ITE hearing aids, and are thus able to boost amplification over more of the frequency range where a boost is often needed. Horns in BTE fittings can typically provide significant boost at 3 Hz and above, while those within ITEs cannot provide any significant boost below 6 kHz.

Horns can be built into BTE earmolds in a number of ways. A simple method is to insert tubing only a few millimeters into the earmold. The outlet diameter of the horn will then be determined by the size of the hole drilled into the medial end of the earmold. Although a horn with one or more steps can be made in this way, the method has two major disadvantages:

- The length of the horn will always be less than the sound bore length of the earmold (typically 15 to 22 mm), so the boost may not extend sufficiently far down in frequency.

- The tubing is poorly retained in the earmold. Furthermore, glue may have to be applied at the lateral end of the mold, and over time this will cause the tubing to stiffen, and crack, just where the tubing is most stressed in daily life.

One alternative is to use an elbow securely mounted in the lateral end of the mold, to which the tubing is attached. This has the advantage that the tubing can be replaced without having to replace the mold, or without doing any gluing. It does not solve the problem of having only a limited length available, but is a good solution unless the biggest possible boost is required over the widest possible frequency range.

An alternative which allows the horn to be longer than the earmold is to use a molded plastic horn, such as a *Libby horn*.[533] It is very common for BTE hearing aids to have insufficient high-frequency gain relative to their mid-frequency gain and relative to the prescribed frequency response. Very commonly then, it is desirable to include the widest horn possible. One limiting factor is simply fitting it in, especially if the mold also has to fit a vent. Figure 5.20 shows two ways in which a Libby 4 mm horn can fit into a mold. In the method on the left, the horn is fully inserted through the mold, for which a hole of approximately 5 mm diameter is required. In the method on the right, however, the final 15 or so mm of the horn is cut off and then the remainder of the horn is glued into the lateral end of the mold. Because the mold itself forms the final section of the horn,

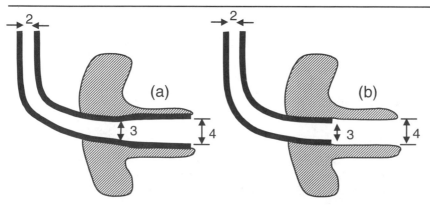

Figure 5.20 A Libby 4 mm horn (a) fully inserted into the earmold, and (b) partially inserted, with the mold forming the final section of the horn. Diameters are in mm.

only a 4 mm hole has to be drilled into the canal portion of the mold. Furthermore, it is the area of the sound bore that matters, not the shape, so an oval-shaped outlet hole can be made if needed.

Using the same method of construction, a 3 mm Libby horn requires only the same space that is needed to fully insert a 2 mm constant diameter tube. The potential disadvantage of this *half-tubing* construction method is that if the horn is glued at the lateral extremity of the mold, the life of the tubing is shortened.

Both the horn effect and the quarter wavelength resonance rely on there being a difference between the inlet and outlet diameters of the horn. Instead of increasing the outlet diameter, the inlet diameter can be decreased relative to a #13 tube. This is the basis of the ***Lybarger high-pass tubing*** configuration: a tubing of internal diameter 0.8 mm connects the earhook to the final 15 mm section of 1.93 mm diameter tubing. The narrow inlet tubing decreases the mid-frequency gain, however. The small size of the outlet diameter makes it particularly suitable for creating a horn in an earmold for an infant.

Note that a fully effective horn can *not* be made just by ***belling*** (i.e. gradually widening), or drilling, the last 5 mm of sound bore at the medial tip of the earmold. Such a practice does make a horn, but because it is very short, its major effects will be above the amplification range of most hearing aids. Belling is likely to increase the frequency of the various tubing resonances, which, in a particular fitting, may be advantageous or disadvantageous. Figure 5.21 shows the effects of drilling a 4 mm diameter hole of different lengths at the medial end of an earmold. Notice that the bore has to be at least 10 mm long before a worthwhile effect is achieved at 4 kHz. An exception to this is when the original, *nominally* constant diameter, tube had been inadvertently constricted at the medial end. A short horn

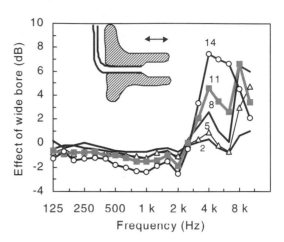

Figure 5.21 The effect of drilling a 4 mm diameter hole at the medial end of an earmold, relative to a constant 2 mm diameter sound bore. The number next to each curve shows the length, in mm, of the widened bore.

can sometimes provide a significant high-frequency boost, not because of a horn effect, but because adding the horn removes the constriction.[457]

Table 5.6 shows the effect on gain and OSPL90 provided by various acoustic horns relative to a constant diameter #13 tube. The overall high-frequency boost provided by a horn of specified dimensions is reliable – it is an acoustic inevitability, and so does not depend on the characteristics of an individual patient's ears or the model of hearing aid.[219] The boost in dB at specific spot frequencies, will, however vary from person to person and from aid to aid. This is because the horn shifts resonant frequencies slightly, as well as providing the overall high-frequency boost. The reason for the small decrease in gain at low frequencies is that horns slightly increase the total volume connected to the hearing aid. The data for the Lybarger high-pass tubing were measured with the one-piece molded plastic version (ER-12 HP).

Table 5.6 includes data for a glued #13 tube, which can produce a high-frequency cut relative to a #13 tube of truly constant

Table 5.6 Effect on gain and OSPL90 (in dB) of various sound bore profiles relative to a #13 (2 mm) tube of truly constant diameter.[217, 219]

Sound bore	Frequency (Hz)								
	250	500	750	1000	1500	2000	3000	4000	6000
Libby 4 mm	-1	-2	-3	-3	-1	-2	6	10	6
Libby 3 mm	-1	-1	-2	-2	1	1	5	5	2
CFA #2 horn	0	0	-1	-1	0	-1	4	6	4
CFA #3 stepped bore	0	0	-1	-1	0	-1	4	6	2
Lybarger high-pass tube	2	4	0	-11	-13	-12	-10	-1	-1
#13 glued-tube	0	0	0	0	0	0	0	-1	-5
6C5	0	1	0	0	0	0	-4	-6	-11
6C10	0	2	0	-2	-1	-5	-10	-12	-17
1.5 LP tube	1	3	0	-9	-10	-9	-10	-10	-12

diameter. These data are indicative only: The magnitude and extent of high-frequency reduction depends strongly on the degree to which the tube is accidentally constricted when it is glued into a more or less tightly fitting hole in the earmold. Horns can also suffer the same fate. If they are squeezed into a hole that is too small for them, Killion (1988) showed that the high-frequency boost obtained will be less than that expected.

Constrictions

Constrictions have the opposite effects of horns: They decrease the efficiency with which high-frequency power is delivered to the ear canal. They are needed far less often than horns, partly because hearing loss usually is greatest at high frequencies, and partly because hearing aid receivers become less effective above their primary resonance

of 2 to 3 kHz. By combining a constriction with a small cavity, achieved by widening the sound bore, an even greater degree of high-frequency cut can be achieved.

Figure 5.22 shows the dimensions of three constricting sound bores. The 6C5 and 6C10 configurations are part of a family of sound bores, and are so named because at *6* kHz, they nominally *C*ut the response by *5* and *10* dB, respectively.[467] The 6C5 configuration can be made by inserting 14 mm of #16 tubing inside an earmold with a 3 mm horn.[458] To make the 6C10 configuration, 13 mm of #19 tubing is inserted inside 13 mm of #13 tubing which is inserted inside a 3 mm horn.[457] This structure makes it possible to vary the high-frequency gain to meet a target or patient preferences if the desired response cannot be obtained by an electronic tone control. The

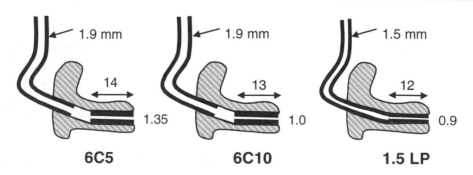

Figure 5.22 The dimensions of the constriction configurations known as 6C5, 6C10, and 1.5 LP (Etymotic Research Catalog; Killion, 1981).

1.5 LP (low-pass) configuration is available as a one-piece molded tube (ER-12LP). The acoustic effects of constrictions are shown in Table 5.6.

5.4.2   Special-purpose earhooks

Several earhooks have been designed to modify the gain-frequency response in ways that particularly suit patients with unusual audiometric configurations.[466] The earhooks described in this section contain acoustic components (small tubes and cavities), and are therefore a little larger than conventional earhooks.[g] The audiometric configurations for which each earhook has been designed are shown in Figure 5.23. These are indicative only; the actual range of hearing loss configurations depends on the coupler response of the BTE hearing aid used. If the hearing aid contains sophisticated tone controls, a much wider range of audiogram configurations is suited to each earhook. Alternatively, with such hearing aids, it may be possible to obtain the response required without using a special earhook.

Low-pass earhook: The ER12-1 earhook directs the sound sequentially through cavities and narrow tubes so that low frequencies are passed without attenuation but high frequencies are markedly attenuated. Relative to a conventional undamped earhook, it provides a 6 dB boost at 500 Hz, 13 dB attenuation at 1 kHz, and in excess of 40 dB attenuation above 2.5 kHz.[217] Even further high-frequency cut is obtained when it is used with the 1.5 LP sound bore configuration. The low-pass earhook is used for patients who have hearing loss at low frequencies but near-normal hearing at high frequencies. It must be used with an open mold (e.g. a tube fitting) so that high-frequency sounds can enter the ear canal via the open acoustic path.

Notch-filter earhook: The ER12-2 earhook attenuates the signal at 2 kHz by approximately 15 dB but has negligible effect below

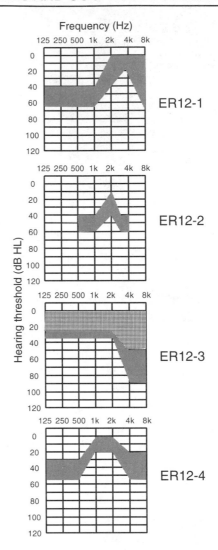

Figure 5.23 Audiometric configurations for which each of the special earhooks has been designed. The hatched area in the ER12-3 audiogram is applicable if a non-occluding earmolds is used and the solid area if an occluding earmold is used.

1 kHz or above 3 kHz.[217] It is based on the principle of adding a side-branch resonator that absorbs energy at its resonant frequency.[559] The earhook is suitable for any patients who have considerably better hearing at 2 kHz than at higher and lower frequencies, and it is used with a conventional earmold.

High-pass earhook: The ER12-3 earhook, in combination with the Lybarger high-pass

---

g   The earhooks described in this section are proprietary to Etymotic Research.

Table 5.7 The typical effect on gain and OSPL90 (in dB) of the dampers placed at the nub or tip end of the earhook of a BTE hearing aid. Values shown are averages across several hearing aids; the attenuation varies slightly from hearing aid to hearing aid. The colors are the coding system used by Knowles Inc. Other values available are 1000 ohms (brown), 3300 ohms (orange), and 4700 ohms (yellow).

Damper impedance (ohms)	Damper position	Frequency (Hz)								
		250	500	750	1000	1500	2000	3000	4000	6000
330 (gray)	Nub	0	0	0	-1	-1	-1	-1	0	0
680 (white)	Nub	0	-1	-1	-3	0	-1	-1	0	0
1500 (green)	Nub	-1	-2	-3	-7	-1	-2	-4	-1	-1
2200 (red)	Nub	-1	-1	-2	-6	0	-3	-3	-4	-1
330 (gray)	Tip	0	0	-1	-3	-1	-1	0	-1	0
680 (white)	Tip	0	0	-2	-6	-1	-1	-1	-1	-1
1500 (green)	Tip	-1	-2	-6	-11	-3	-1	-2	-4	-1
2200 (red)	Tip	-3	-4	-9	-16	-4	-1	-1	-5	-1

tubing, attenuates the signal from 1 kHz to 2 kHz by 20 to 25 dB but has negligible effect below 500 Hz or above 4 kHz.[217, 466] When used with an open mold, it enables an insertion gain of 25 dB to be provided at 4 kHz without any amplification being provided below 1500Hz.[466] It can also be used with a closed mold for patients who have hearing loss at all frequencies, but whose hearing deteriorates steeply above 2 kHz. (But see Section 9.2.4 for discussion on the extent to which such people *should* receive amplified high-frequency sound.)

Cookie-bite earhook: The ER12-4 earhook, in combination with the Lybarger high-pass tubing, attenuates the signal at 2 kHz by approximately 35 dB but has negligible effect below 500 Hz or above 5 kHz.[217] It is thus similar to the ER12-2 notch-filter earhook except that a broader range of frequencies is attenuated and the attenuation at 2 kHz is greater.

5.5   Dampers

Dampers are used to decrease gain and maximum output at frequencies corresponding to resonances in the sound bore (See Sections 2.6.2 and 2.7). Dampers are most effective if they are placed at loca-

tions where the resonance causes the largest flow of air particles. For wavelength resonances, particle velocity is least at the end of the tube that joins to the receiver. In a BTE, the 1, 3, and 5 kHz resonances are therefore damped increasingly effectively as the damper is moved down the sound bore from the receiver towards the lateral tip of the earmold. Conversely, the receiver resonance near 2 kHz is damped increasingly effectively as the damper is moved towards the receiver. Figure 5.24 shows the effect of a 1500-ohm damper placed at the tip (earmold end) and the nub (hearing aid end) of an earhook.

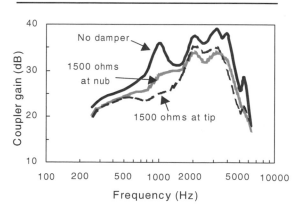

Figure 5.24 Frequency response of a hearing aid with no damper, and with a 1500 ohm damper placed at each end of the earhook.

Practical tip: Shaping a BTE mid-frequency response with dampers

- To maximally damp 1 kHz and minimally damp 2 kHz, place the damper as close to the earmold as possible. The tip of the earhook is the most practical position. Dampers placed at the medial end of the earmold would be more effective, but quickly become clogged with wax and moisture, and should therefore be avoided.

- To maximally damp 2 kHz, and minimally damp 1 kHz, place the damper as close to the receiver as possible. The end of the earhook where it attaches to the hearing aid case is the most practical position, but only some earhooks have been designed to accept fused mesh and sintered steel dampers in this position.

Table 5.7 shows the effect on gain and OSPL90, in dB, of dampers with different impedances when they are placed at each end of the earhook.

In some cases it might be necessary to use dampers at both ends of the earhook to achieve a sufficiently smooth gain and OSPL90 response that is sufficiently close to the target gain.

Dampers can also be placed in the tubing of ITE/ITC/CIC hearing aids, but they are likely to need replacing more frequently because of blockage by wax and moisture. They can also be inserted in microphone tubing to decrease the high-frequency response of a hearing aid (typically to prevent feedback). Dampers are available with diameters of 2.08, 1.78, 1.37 and 1.12 mm to accommodate these various applications.[914] For the three smaller sizes, the damping screens are not encased within a metal ferrule.

5.6 Specific Tubing, Damping and Venting Configurations

Earmold laboratories offer a range of earmolds that have particular combinations of tubing, venting and damping. These earmolds are given particular names or numbers. Instead of thinking of each of these as a unique style with unique acoustic properties, identify the shape and dimensions of the sound bore, the size of the vent path, and the value and location of any dampers. The acoustic performance of the complete earmold will readily be understood on the basis of these three elements.

5.7 Procedure for Selecting Earmold and Earshell Acoustics

The following steps can be used to select suitable earmold acoustics prior to fitting the hearing aid. The procedure assumes that a tentative choice for the rest of the hearing aid has already been made (see Chapter 10). Sometimes, performing these steps will show that the first tentative choice was not a good one, and that a new choice should be made.

1. Find the maximum vent size possible. The target insertion gain is calculated, and the appropriate one of Tables 5.3, 5.4 or 5.5 is used to find the *maximum vent size* that can be used without feedback. For non-linear hearing aids, the target gain for low-level inputs should be used, as gain is greatest for low-level inputs. (Remember to allow a 10 dB safety margin, especially for the smaller vents, unless you are inclined to gambling.) If the target gain prescribed is unrealistically large for the high frequencies (in that it is more than is beneficial for the person), then the maximum vent size allowable will be unrealistically small. Some prescription procedures can lead to unrealistically high gains, so choose your selection procedure carefully! (More on this in Chapter 9.) Similarly, if the high-frequency target gain is greater than can be achieved with any hearing aid, the vent size constraint will also be unrealistic.

2. Estimate the minimum vent size needed. Based on the patient's hearing thresholds at 250 and 500 Hz, estimate the *minimum vent size* needed to overcome the occlusion effect. Good research data on this are not available, but as a guide, low-frequency losses greater than 45 dB do not need a vent, and low-frequency losses less than 30 dB must have at least a 2 mm vent, and preferably will have a larger one. Although a 1 mm vent is usually too small to have any effect on occlusion, the inclusion of such a vent will make it easier for the clinician to drill or grind a wider vent if it proves necessary.

3. Decide on the vent size. Given the constraints determined in steps 1 and 2, this will be an easy choice for many patients, as the maximum and minimum vent sizes will be the same, or the maximum vent size will be slightly larger than the minimum. More difficulty will be found for patients with near normal low-frequency hearing thresholds and 60 to 90 dB loss in the high frequencies. The maximum vent size will turn out to be less than the minimum vent size. These are indeed difficult fittings, and will require careful adjustment of vent size, after fitting, if feedback and occlusion are both to be avoided. Even then, feedback-canceling circuits may provide the only complete solution. It is well worth while ordering adjustable vents for patients with difficult audiograms, and it is probably worth while ordering adjustable vents for anyone where there is not a big range between the minimum vent size and the maximum vent size.

4. Select a sound bore profile. The details outlined in this step are aimed at earmolds for BTE hearing aids, partly because of the limited effectiveness of horns for ITE/ITC/CIC hearing aids, and partly because selection of the sound bore for these hearing aids is carried out by the manufacturer. For

---

> **Practical tip: Will it fit?**
>
> Before finalizing your choice of sound bore and vent, ensure that the larger diameter of the canal stalk on the impression is at least 2 mm bigger than the total of the sound bore diameter and vent diameter.

BTEs, the sound bore has the greatest effect on the response shape in the 2 kHz to 4 kHz octave, so selection can be based primarily on these frequencies. First calculate the slope (in dB/octave) of the coupler gain target (i.e. the 4 kHz target gain minus the 2 kHz target gain). Then calculate the slope of the coupler gain of the chosen hearing aid. If the target slope rises more steeply than the hearing aid slope (as will usually be the case) then a horn of some type is required. If, in rare instances, the target slope of the response from 2 kHz to 4 kHz is *less* than the hearing aid gain slope, then a constriction of some type is required. If the target slope and the hearing aid slope are approximately the same, a #13 tube is appropriate.[h]

The data in Table 5.8 will help you decide which horn or constriction to choose. Simply find the sound bore configuration whose slope in the 2 to 4 kHz octave matches the discrepancy you calculated between the target slope and the slope of the hearing aid you are going to fit. Note that the Lybarger high-pass tube achieves its slope, relative to a #13 tube, by suppressing the mid-frequencies rather than boosting the high frequencies, as shown in Table 5.6. Also note that the 1.5 LP tube achieves its cut from 500 Hz to 2 kHz, and so has little affect on the slope above 2 kHz. If you adopt a simple rule (without doing any calculations) of always choosing the biggest horn that will fit in the ear canal, you will be right most of the time!

---

[h]   The CORFIG figures used in this book for BTE hearing aids are based on the 2 cc coupler response being obtained with a HA2 earmold simulator, but the insertion gain being obtained with a constant diameter (#13) sound bore in an occluded, and non-leaky earmold. Consequently, when there is no discrepancy between the target coupler response and the actual hearing aid response, the appropriate sound bore is a #13 tube.

Table 5.8 Sound bore profile needed to resolve a discrepancy between a target response slope (calculated as 4 kHz gain minus 2 kHz gain) and the response slope available from the hearing aid in a coupler.

Sound bore profile	2 to 4 kHz slope (dB/octave)
Libby 4 mm horn	12
Libby 3 mm horn	4
CFA #2 horn	7
CFA #3 stepped bore	7
Lybarger high-pass tube	11
#13 glued-tube	-1
6C5	-6
6C10	-7
1.5 LP tube	-1

If the selection of a hearing aid and earmold is based on insertion gain instead of coupler gain, Table 5.8 can still be used to select the sound bore. In this case, base the selection on the discrepancy between the target insertion gain slope and the expected insertion gain slope for the chosen hearing aid.

5. Select a damper. Selection of the damper is most efficiently made after the hearing aid has been fitted. The first reason for this is that Table 5.7 does not show what effect the damper has on the frequencies between the audiometric frequencies. Second, the precise effects of dampers at a given frequency will vary depending on whether that frequency coincides with a peak or with a trough. Third, peaks and troughs in the insertion gain response of a hearing aid will depend on the shape of the individual's real-ear unaided response. Fourth, unlike a vent or a sound bore profile, the size of a damper can be changed at a fitting appointment within a few seconds. It therefore seems easiest to make the first measurement of real-ear gain with whatever damper comes as standard with the hearing aid, and then to vary the damper as needed, guided by the data in Table 5.7 and

---

> **Practical tip: Changing dampers quickly**
>
> Dampers can be changed quickly and without damaging the damper to be removed if a small stock of spare earhooks for the hearing aids most commonly used is maintained. These earhooks can be pre-loaded with dampers of different sizes.

the information in the panel *Shaping a BTE mid-frequency response with damping*.

5.8　Ear Impressions

Although this chapter has commenced with the acoustic effects of earmolds and earshells, there can be no earmold or earshell without first taking an impression. This section describes techniques and materials for making an impression

5.8.1　Standard ear impression techniques

Examine the ear canal. Taking an ear impression begins with an otoscopic examination.

- Do not proceed if cerumen is present in amounts large enough to disrupt the accuracy of the ear impression. Opinions vary as to how much this is, but it certainly depends on the accuracy required. More cerumen can be tolerated for a low gain, vented, BTE earmold or full concha ITE hearing aid than for a high gain occluded aid or a CIC.

- Do not proceed if there is any visible sign of outer or middle ear infection or inflammation, a distended eardrum, or a perforated eardrum. Medical clearance should first be obtained in each of these cases.

- Do not make a deep impression if the ear canal widens sufficiently (relative to the outer parts of the canal) that removal of the impression will be difficult. It is common for ear canals to widen slightly in the anterior-posterior dimension just medial to the second bend.[17] Ear impression material is able to compress *slightly* during removal (see Section 5.8.3), but there is a limit. An extreme case of widening is when a mastoidectomy has been performed to remove diseased portions of the mastoid bone. ENT clearance should be sought before taking an impression of such an ear. An additional block is used to pack the surgically created cavity prior to inserting the block that protects the eardrum. Sullivan (1995) recommends the use of cotton blocks rather than foam blocks, and the same web site contains additional instructions and pictures.

- Trim any hair in the concha that is long enough to be cut with scissors, as it will be less likely to distort the impression or to get caught in the impression and make removal difficult.

Insert a canal block.. A ***canal block*** is a small amount of cotton wool or foam that fills the cross-section of the ear canal to prevent impression material flowing further into the canal than is required. Canal blocks are also called ***oto-blocks***, ***impression pads*** and ***ear-dams***. The resistance to flow provided by the block enables the impression material to completely fill the canal cross-section right down to the desired length, rather than gradually tapering off in width. A piece of strong thread is knotted around the block to aid in removal, although the thread is usually needed only if the block has to be removed without an impression being taken. Blocks can be custom-made or, more conveniently, can be purchased in a range of sizes, with pre-tied thread. The correct size must be used: Blocks that are too small may get pushed down the canal by the impression material, or allow the material to flow around the block. Blocks that are too large will not go in far enough, and may be uncomfortable. Blocks with decreased thickness in the medial-lateral

---

> **Caution: unintended consequences**
>
> A canal block of adequate size *must* be used. The pressure that can be exerted during syringing with normal viscosity material is sufficient to rupture the eardrum. This has resulted in impression material being forced into the middle ear cavity (Schimanski, 1992).

dimension are available for taking deep canal impressions. The block is most conveniently inserted by pushing it with an illuminated plastic stick, referred to as an ***ear-light***, ***oto-light***, or ***light-stick***. Your little finger should be braced against the side of the head whenever using the ear-light. If pushing the cotton block deeper suddenly becomes easier, beware – the canal may widen suddenly and removal of the impression will be difficult. The depth of insertion of the canal block is very important. Earmold or aid manufacturers can make the finished device with a canal stalk shorter than the impression, but they cannot make it longer. Err on the long side of what you need. The block should be at or past the second bend, unless you are sure you need a very short canal stalk on the finished device. If you wish the earmold or shell to be shorter than the impression you can mark the desired length on the impression.

Mix the impression material. Use only the recommended proportions of the ingredients. Although changing the mixture may let you decrease the viscosity (i.e. make it runnier for easy syringing) or vary the setting time, the change will probably also adversely affect the finished impression. Excessive liquid in a liquid/powder acrylic, for example, will make the impression more readily melt or change shape in heat[627] and will increase the amount it shrinks.[6] Mixing must be thorough but fast. It should be done with a spatula on a disposable pad or cleanable surface. The reasons for this are:

- To avoid the possibility of health consequences for the clinician arising from repeated absorption of impression chemicals through the skin.

- To avoid contaminating the impression material with sulfur-based substances that can leak from hand lotions and from latex gloves.[953]

- To avoid raising the temperature of the impression material, because setting time decreases as temperature increases.

Similarly, the impression material can be scooped into the syringe with the spatula, or by pushing the inverted syringe at an angle around the mixing pad.

Fill the ear. Partially depress the syringe (or gun) until the material starts to flow out of the tip. Pull the pinna up and back so that the syringe can be inserted as far as possible. Syringe extension tips can be used for long narrow canals. Depress the syringe until the material has covered the syringe tip to a depth of about 6 mm (0.25 inches). Continue to depress the syringe plunger but simultaneously withdraw the syringe tip at the rate required to keep it buried by the same amount. After the canal is filled, and the concha is nearly filled, lower the plunger end of the syringe and push the tip upwards along the back of the concha (close to the anti-tragus and anti-helix) towards the helix. After the cymba-concha is filled, raise the big end of the syringe and push the syringe tip down the front of the cavum-concha (close to the tragus). Finish syringing when the concha is completely filled and is slightly overflowing on all sides. The earmold/earshell laboratory must be able to recognize all the landmarks on the ear, and this is not possible unless the concha is over-filled. The whole operation should be one complete motion with a constant pressure being applied to the syringe. Finishing in such a way as to give an approximately flat external surface will make it easy to glue the impression to a container for shipping should that be necessary.

Wait. After 7 to 10 minutes (depending on the impression material and the temperature), test the impression for hardness by momentarily indenting it with a fingernail or other sharp object. If the indent fully disappears, the impression is sufficiently cured. If the canal is particularly twisty, and/or the canal is particularly long, wait a few minutes longer than usual, so that the impression is less likely to tear as it is extracted.

Remove the impression. Have the patient open and close his or her jaw a few times. Pull down, then back, then up on the pinna. These movements help break the bond between the impression and the ear. Extract the helix part of the impression (the **helix lock**). Grasp the impression and pull it out with whatever twisting motions seem to best suit the individual ear.

Inspect the ear. Make sure that nothing has been left behind!

Inspect the impression. Make sure there are no fold marks, gaps, or bubbles. These blemishes can be tolerated in parts of the impression that will be cut away before the finished product is made, but nowhere else. Good quality in the canal stalk is particularly important. If in doubt, make a second impression. Leave the canal block attached to the impression. Its angle relative to the impression will give the manufacturer some clues about the direction taken by the canal medial to the end of the impression material. *Never* lengthen the impression by adding impression material after the impression has been removed from the ear. It can not be done accurately and is likely to result in discomfort and increased feedback.[708]

Pack the impression. Pack the finished impression in a shipping container in a manner suitable for the impression material (see Section 5.8.3). Any distortion of the impression during shipping will be reproduced in the final product.

Clean up. Appropriate infection control measures are important, as they are for real-ear gain measurement, but it is beyond the scope of this book to cover the degree of risk and type of control measures required. Extremely high care should be taken if any infection is evident in the ear or if any procedure inadvertently causes bleeding in the ear canal.

5.8.2   Ear impression techniques for CICs and high gain hearing aids

CIC hearing aids and high-gain hearing aids may require the earshell or earmold to fit the ear canal more tightly than is necessary for other hearing aids. A tight fit may be needed to avoid feedback oscillation or, in the case of a CIC, to retain the hearing aid in the ear.

CIC hearing aids are retained in the ear by the bends in the ear canal and by the variations in cross-sectional area and shape that occur along the axis of the canal. The widening that usually occurs at the second bend is particularly important.[708] It is essential, therefore, that impressions for CIC hearing aids be sufficiently deep that they clearly contain the second bend, and preferably extend at least 5 mm past the second bend. With the canal block inserted this deeply, the impression material is able to expand the cartilaginous canal along its entire length, and so provide a more secure fit.[707]

Has the impression reached the bony canal?

For hearing aids that are intended to extend into the bony canal, assess the following:

- If the second bend is not clearly visible in the impression, try again – the impression is too short.
- Inspect the impression under a magnifying glass – skin in the bony canal is smoother and less porous than in the cartilaginous canal, and this difference in texture is observable in a good quality impression.

CIC impression technique in brief

- Take an impression to 5 mm past the second bend;
- Use a medium-to-high viscosity silicone impression material (e.g. Otoform A/K, Westone, Silicast, Steramold, Otosil, Dahlberg) (Pirzanski, 1997)
- Use an open-jaw technique

CIC hearing aids, and to a lesser extent, ITC hearing aids may also require a good fit to ensure that the hearing aid does not work its way out of the ear. Movement of the hearing aid can occur because the ear canal changes shape when the patient moves his or her jaw. In particular, the anterior-posterior dimension of the canal between the first and second bend gradually increases as the jaw opens. As the jaw opens, the condyle of the mandible moves forward, and this pulls the anterior wall of the canal forward.[675] Averaged across ears, the canal width increases by 10% for a jaw opening of 25 mm measured between the upper and lower incisors.[674] If the patient's back teeth are missing, the patient has poorly fitting dentures, or the patient has a temporomandibular joint disorder with some other cause, the jaw can over-close, and the variation in canal size with jaw motion will be even greater than normal.[334]

The solution to an overly mobile canal is to take an ear impression with the jaw held open, by having the patient bite on a 25 mm spacer until the material has cured.[706] Although it might be thought that the thicker canal stalk in the mold or earshell would be uncomfortable when the jaw is shut, hearing aids made from open-jaw impressions are equally comfortable to those made from closed-jaw impressions (Fishbein, 1997; Johns, 2000). Pirzanski (1997a) comments that discomfort may result from a *loosely* fitting hearing aid because the patient repeatedly pushes it in deeper than it was intended to go, in an attempt to achieve a more secure fit or to prevent feedback oscillation.

Should open-jaw impressions be made for all CIC hearing aids? Possibly, although it seems likely that the need is greatest for those patients whose canals change shape the most. The clinician can estimate the degree of movement by observing the canal wall movement with an otoscope, or by feeling the degree of motion with an inserted finger.[583]

Greatly excessive movement of the canal wall may preclude the use of a CIC hearing aid.[334] A potential, though untried, solution may be to make the lateral part of the hearing aid a *loose* fit in the canal, but to make the medial part a tight fit within the bony canal (which does not move). A very soft material for at least the medial part of the hearing aid would be essential for comfort.

An alternative way to make a tightly fitting earmold or shell is to progressively build-up the size of the impression in the ear of the patient. The three-stage impression technique (see panel) uses ear impression material with different viscosities to make a tight but very accurate impression of the ear.[282] Each stage expands the walls of canal, with the greatest expansion occurring in those places where the ear has the greatest flexibility.

Both the open-jaw technique and the three-stage technique increase the width of the earmold in the anterior-posterior dimension just inside the ear canal entrance.[560, 707] The relative effectiveness of the two techniques is not known, but the open-jaw technique is considerably faster. A third option is to take a single-stage, closed-jaw impression and have the earmold or hearing aid manufacturer apply special build-up around the aperturic seal region. This is less effective than the three-stage technique because the manufacturer cannot know the flexibility of the patient's ear canal, but even manufacturer's build-up provides enough attenuation for most high gain hearing aids.[560]

The three-stage technique in brief

1. Take an impression using a viscous (i.e. non-runny) impression material, and with an embedded piece of tubing extending to the cotton block. The embedded tubing provides pressure relief as the impression is being removed from the ear, which is particularly valuable for steps 2 and 3. Remove the impression from the ear.

2. Apply medium viscosity impression material over the surface of the canal stalk of the impression. Insert the impression, and apply a gentle pressure to it for a few seconds to assist re-distribution of the uncured material. Remove the impression when dry, ensure that the tube is unobstructed, and then re-insert the impression. Use the air pump of an impedance meter to ensure that a static pressure seal can be achieved. There should be no leakage for 5 seconds after applying a pressure of 200 daPa, while the patient opens and closes his or her jaw. If a leak occurs, repeat this step 2.

3. For this step, the patient's head should be turned to the side and resting on a pillow. Insert a new cotton block, at least as deeply as the first one, fill the ear canal with a low-viscosity material, and quickly re-insert the impression, thus forcing out much of the low-viscosity material. This coating left behind makes a closer match to the fine structure of the ear.

The earmold manufacturer should be instructed not to add any build-up and not to buff the earmold. For further details, see Fifield, Earnshaw & Smither (1980). For a faster, but less accurate procedure, omit step 3.

> ### In summary: Five ways to produce a tightly fitting, but comfortable, earmold or earshell
>
> - Take the impression with the jaw open
> - Take a two- or three-stage impression
> - Request special build-up during earmold construction
> - Use a viscous (non-runny) silicone impression material
> - Pat down the impression material before it hardens
>
> When used in isolation, items near the top of the list are probably more effective than items near the bottom of the list (Macrae, 1990). The use of *all* the techniques simultaneously has not been investigated and is definitely *not* recommended.

5.8.3   Ear impression materials

At least three types of materials are used for taking ear impressions. In each case the impression sets when two materials are mixed and undergo a chemical reaction:

- *Acrylic* material (e.g. ethyl-methacrylate) is mixed by combining a liquid and a powder. Examples are Blend™ and Audalin™.

- *Condensation-cured silicone* material (e.g. dimethyl-siloxane) is mixed by combining two pastes. Examples are Amsil™, Copolsil™, Otoform-K™, Silisoft™, Blue Silicast™, and Microsil™.

- *Addition-cured silicone* material (e.g. polyvinyl-siloxane, vinyl-polysiloxane) is mixed by combining two pastes. Examples are Otoform A/K™, Reprosil™, Pink Silicast™, Silasoft™, Mega-Sil™

Ear impression materials must have a certain combination of properties if they are to lead to a tightly fitting, but comfortable, earmold or earshell.

Viscosity. Low viscosity materials are easy to syringe and are least likely to expand or distort the ear canal.[i] They were previously recommended for making impressions for CIC hearing aids, so as to make the most faithful reproduction of the ear canal. Unfortunately, this recommendation may have overlooked the changes in ear canal size that are caused by jaw motion (Section 5.8.2). Pirzanski (1997) recommends that low viscosity material *not* be used when a tight fit is required, as it does not sufficiently inflate the cartilaginous portion of the canal. One technique that has been recommended for deeply seated CIC hearing aids is to use a low viscosity material for the bony canal, followed one minute later by a higher viscosity material for the remainder of the impression.[830] The intent is that this combination will expand the cartilaginous canal but not the bony canal. The comfort and feedback advantages of the technique have not been quantified.

Dimensional stability. If an ear impression shrinks in the hours or days following its making, the earmold or earshell made from the impression will also be smaller to the same degree unless some compensatory build-up is applied during manufacture of the earmold or shell. Such build-up is applied, but the overall precision of the process from impression to finished earmold or shell is obviously greatest if shrinkage is minimized. In the first 48 hours after the impression is made, the linear dimensions of addition-cured silicone material shrink by 0.1% or less.[662, 663] By contrast, condensation-cured silicones shrink by 0.5%,[662] and acrylic materials shrink by 2 to 5 %.[6, 663]

Stress relaxation. When a force is applied to an impression to remove it, it stretches, compresses, and twists as it is pulled through the bends and tight parts of the ear canal. After removal, it is desirable that the impression spring completely back to the size and shape

---

[i]   Viscosity is measured in units of mPa s. Unfortunately, values are rarely quoted, so we have to describe viscosity by the ambiguous terms of low, medium and high.

of the ear canal. The extent to which this happens is called its stress relaxation. Silicone materials have excellent stress relaxation properties;[j] acrylic materials do not. Forces can also be applied to an impression during shipping, so all impressions should be suitably protected. Crumpled tissues or other lightweight packing material are adequate to protect silicone impressions. Acrylic materials must be more effectively protected against distorting forces, so the concha portion of the impression should be glued to the liner of the shipping container in such a way that nothing can press against the canal stalk.

Tensile strength. Some force has to be applied to the impression to remove it from the ear. It would be a disaster if the impression tore at this stage, so impression materials have to have an adequate tensile strength. Tearing is very rare and is likely to occur only when more medial parts of the canal are considerably wider than more lateral parts.

Release force. Ear impression materials are designed to conform closely to minute variations in the surface of the ear and ear canal. This closeness makes the impression adhere to the skin. To ease removal , a release agent is built into the impression material, which causes the oily feel of an impression.

5.9   Earmolds and Earshells

5.9.1   Earmold and earshell construction

Earmolds and earshells (jointly referred to as ***otoplastics***) are made from the impression, usually by a specialist earmold or hearing aid manufacturer. The impression can be considered to be a negative of the ear. It is placed into liquid silicon or other material that cures around it to make a positive copy of the ear. This positive copy is called the ***investment***, and the finished mold or shell is made from this investment. For ITE/ITC/CIC

hearing aids, the manufacturer trims the shell to the desired size, inserts the electronic and mechanical parts, attaches the faceplate, and sends a complete hearing aid back to the clinician.

Some practices are choosing to maximize their involvement in the supply of hearing aids by doing these tasks themselves. The earshells are constructed of plastic that is cured by exposure to a strong source of ultraviolet (UV) light. The electronic parts are purchased by the practice in bulk and come as a faceplate with pre-wired components. The receiver is on a flexible lead so that it can be suitably positioned before the faceplate is attached.

5.9.2   Materials for earmolds and earshells

Material for earmolds and earshells can be classified at a number of levels. Most simply, there are hard and soft materials. Within each of these categories, there are several base plastics. Within each base plastic there are many variations to the mixture that affect the physical properties. Table 5.9 shows the most common base chemicals used, their range of hardness, and their disadvantages and advantages. The ease with which the materials can be modified refers to the ease experienced by clinicians using the tools commonly found in a clinic. Note that like the other materials, acrylic can be harder or softer. The softer varieties have decreased leakage,[664] but lose some of the durability advantages of the hard acrylic. Otoplastics made from very soft materials may be more comfortable than those made from hard materials, but there is no research on this issue.

It is becoming more common for otoplastics to contain more than one material. Most commonly this comprises a soft material in the canal stalk, or in just the deepest part of the canal stalk, combined with a hard material

---

[j]   Addition-cured silicones appear to have superior stress-relaxation properties to condensation-cured silicones (Nolan & Combe, 1985), but data on this are limited.

The hardness of otoplastics

The material property that most affects the comfort and acoustic performance of an otoplastic is its hardness. Hardness is measured by noting how large an indentation occurs when a standard cone- or ball-shaped object is pushed into the material by a standard force or by a standard displacement. Sharp indentors and large forces are used for hard materials; blunt indentors and small forces for soft materials. The measuring tool is called a *durometer*, and the resulting indentations are expressed as numbers between 0 and 100 on a ***Shore hardness scale***. Larger numbers represent harder materials. Each combination of indentor and force gives rise to a different scale. There are many such scales. Scale A is most suitable for the softer otoplastic materials and scale D is most suitable for the harder materials. For example, a reading of 90 on the A-scale is approximately equivalent to a reading of 39 on the D-scale.

Soft materials are intrinsically more flexible than hard materials. Greater flexibility makes earmolds easier to insert in a tortuous ear canal and may make them more comfortable when the ear canal changes shape. Soft materials also provide a better seal to the ear.

---

in the more lateral parts of the otoplastic. The superior retention, feedback, and perhaps comfort properties of a soft material can thus be combined with the superior durability of the harder material surrounding the lateral parts of the hearing aid. A potential problem is that such mixtures may fracture at the plane where the two materials join.

The advantages of soft materials have to be weighed against the greater deterioration of soft materials with time. Note that a key requirement for comfort is to have some flexibility at the interface between the otoplastic and the ear. If the ear is sufficiently flexible, considering the degree of tightness required, none may be required in the otoplastic. Consequently, the balance of advantages may swing in favor of hard materials for such people. Unfortunately, there is insufficient research for anyone to be dogmatic about the best earmold material in different situations.

A recent innovation for ITE/ITC/CIC instruments is the use of a solid otoplastic instead of a hollow shell.[188] The material is a very soft, very flexible silicone of hardness 10-35 (Shore A scale) into which the hearing aid components are embedded. The soft material is bonded to a conventional hard acrylic faceplate. This approach may make it possible to achieve the advantages of a soft material in an adequately durable package.

The skin of some patients will react to an otoplastic. This may be caused by an ***allergic reaction*** to the specific material, or may be the result of ***prolonged occlusion***, no matter what material is used. A common cause of allergic reactions is that a small proportion of the original monomer did not cure into a polymer when the earmold was constructed.[593] Potential solutions comprise:

- trying an otoplastic that has been heat-cured instead of cold-cured; heat-curing reduces the proportion of uncured monomer;

- trying an otoplastic based on a different, low-allergenic chemical, such as silicone or polyethylene;

- referring the patient for a contact allergy test, so that the presence of a genuine allergic reaction, and the specific allergen, can be detected;[593]

- trying a more open mold, if feasible (as a CROS fitting if necessary – see Section 16.1);

- alternating hearing aid use between ears; and

- when all else fails, using a bone conduction or bone-anchored hearing aid.

Table 5.9 Advantages, disadvantages and hardness of different materials used for earmolds and earshells (Source: Microsonic, Ternens and Westone websites and catalogs)

Type of material	Hardness (Shore durometer scale A)	Advantages	Disadvantages
ACRYLIC **(Poly-methyl-methacrylate)** • Hard acrylic, lucite • Super-alerite, heat-cured acrylic • Soft acrylic – see text	Hard (off scale)	• Little deterioration or shrinkage with time and use • Easy to grind, drill, re-tube, glue and buff • Smooth surface helps insertion and removal • Easy to clean	• Will not compress to insert past narrow areas in the canal • Leaks easily when the ear canal changes shape • Potential for injury when struck, especially if it shatters
ACRYLIC (Hydroxy-ethyl-methacrylate)	Hard (off scale)	Advantages and disadvantages as for poly-methyl-methacrylate, but used for ITE/ITC and CIC shells	
VINYL **(Poly-vinyl-choride)** Rx, Polysheer, Polysheer II, Ultraflex, Superflex, Polyplus, Satin Soft Synth-a-flex II, Formaseal **VINYL (Poly-ethyl-methacrylate)** Vinylflex II, Vinylflex, Marveltex, Marvel Soft, Vinyl Flesh, Formula II, Flexible Plastic	40 - 50	• Comfortable when a tight fit is needed for high-gain hearing aids • Some vinyls (poly-ethyl-methacrylate) soften at body temperatures and harden at room temperatures, helping insertion	• Shrinks, hardens, and discolors with time, necessitating replacement approximately annually • Tubing is difficult to replace: removal is difficult and new tube needs toxic solvent or locking devices to retain it. • Softer vinyls need a toxic solvent to polish them – cannot be worn for 24 hours.
SILICONE (dimethyl-methyly-hydrogen-siloxane) M-2000, W-1, MSL-90, JB-1000, Softech, Soft Silicone, MDX **SILICONE (poly-dimethyl-siloxane)** Medi-Sil II, Mediflex, Emplex, Frosted Flex, Bio-por	20-40 50-70	• Comfortable when a tight and/or long canal fit is needed, especially for the softer grades of silicone • Little shrinkage with time • Low incidence of allergic reactions	• Impossible to grind and buff; difficult to drill • Tubing cannot be glued – a mechanical tubing lock is required
RUBBER ethylene-propylene copolymer) Microlite, Excelite		• Soft, lightweight and floatable • Used for swim-plugs	
POLY-ETHYLENE	Hard (off scale)	• Extremely unlikely to produce an allergic reaction • Easy to grind, drill, glue and buff	• Will not compress to insert past narrow areas in the canal • Leaks easily when the ear canal changes shape • Noticeable plastic appearance

Note that the first three solutions will not help if the cause is occlusion, and the next two solutions will not help if the cause is an allergy. None of the first five solutions will help if the cause is physical pressure as a result of a poorly fitting otoplastic, but a simple physical modification of the otoplastic's shape may solve the problem. Note that impression material can also give rise to an allergic reaction.[797]

5.9.3   Instant earmolds and hearing aids

The earmolds discussed so far are all the results of a two-stage process – an impression is taken and an earmold is made from the impression. An earmold is sometimes needed instantly – for a demonstration, as a temporary solution while waiting for a repair, or because the patient is in a hurry. The following are several ways to achieve an instant otoplastic:

- A temporary earmold can be formed from a foam plug with a tube through it, which can be coupled to an elbow and a tube. These provide a better seal (i.e. less leakage) than a conventional custom earmold,[319] and are more comfortable,[676] but can be more difficult than a custom earmold to insert, and quickly become dirty.

- *Stock molds* are pre-made flexible plastic earmolds and tubing, in a range of sizes. These are suitable only for low-gain hearing aids. One variety of stock molds has compliant plastic flanges to improve the seal in the ear canal.

- A custom earmold can be made in minutes by taking an impression using a two-part silicone material (e.g. *Insta-mold*™). The resulting impression, after some trimming, *is* the final earmold. A variation from the usual impression-taking technique is that the concha should be filled only to the degree required for the final earmold, and the lateral surface should be smoothed to the finished contour before the impression material hardens. Smoothing can be done with a finger or thumb that has been pre-wetted with a special lotion. Twisting and pushing a special punch through the impression can cut holes for tubing and a vent.

- A modular, prefabricated ITE, ITC, or CIC hearing aid of an appropriate size can be chosen. One recent innovation to improve the comfort and fit of these hearing aids

include the use of a shell with an articulated joint, in which the orientation of the canal stalk relative to the concha can be altered, the use of replaceable foam sleeves surrounding the canal stalk, and the incorporation of a controlled venting path inside the sleeve. Another innovation is a disposable soft plastic sheath around a standard module. A third innovation is a hard modular shell combined with a soft, flange-like tip.

If either of the temporary earmold options is used, one must be aware that the acoustic performance, and especially the venting effect, may be very different from that which would normally occur with a custom earmold.

5.9.4   Modifying and repairing earmolds and earshells

The most common reasons for modifying or repairing earmolds and earshells are to:
- Remove helix locks to ease insertion;
- Shorten or taper canal stalks to ease insertion;
- Remove material from the inter-tragal ridge, conchal rim, or the canal stalk to eliminate pressure points;
- Widen or shorten vents to decrease occlusion;
- Constrict vents to decrease feedback;
- Thicken canal stalks to decrease feedback;
- Replace loose or hardened tubing.

Earmolds and earshells can be modified in the clinic with suitable tools and materials. For a BTE earmold, a hand-held motor tool is adequate, but to re-obtain the high luster that is usual on ITE/ITC/CIC hearing aids, buffing and polishing wheels are needed. Two such wheels can be mounted on one side of a ¼ Horsepower dental laboratory motor. Buffing compound, obtained from hearing aid manufacturers, is applied to the buffing wheel, but not to the polishing wheel. Drills and small burrs can be mounted on the other side of the motor, and this leaves both hands free to hold the hearing aids. If such a tool is not available, a relatively high luster can be obtained by applying a hypoallergenic clear lacquer. More detailed instructions on modifying shells can be found in an excellent series of practical articles by Curran (1990a, 1990b, 1991, 1992).

Modifying vents

Earmolds or earshells are made less occluding by enlarging the vent diameter, shortening the vent length, or a combination of both. Vent diameter is easily enlarged by drilling or grinding. Vent length is shortened by grinding away the mold or shell, from either end of the vent. Figure 5.25 shows how the medial end of the vent can be progressively cut away without affecting the sound bore. Prior to modifying any custom earshell, view a strong light *through* it to identify the location of the components and to estimate the thickness of the shell walls. Also check that the shell contains a **poured vent** (also known as a **molded vent**) encased in solid plastic, rather than just a vent made of tubing. The modification shown in Figure 5.25 can be performed only if the aid contains a poured vent. Shortening should be performed progressively, each time removing approximately 30 % of the remaining vent length. If the vent is shortened so much that the hearing aid oscillates, the remaining vent can be partially filled with earshell build-up material. Tables 5.2 to 5.4 will give some guidance as to

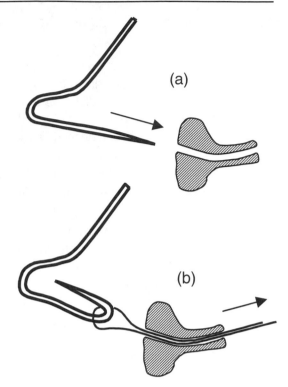

Figure 5.26 Insertion of tubing into an earmold by (a) pushing, or by (b) pulling with a loop of wire.

whether further shortening is likely to induce feedback oscillations. For hearing aids with vents made only from tubing, grinding trench vents in the canal stalk can increase the effective vent size.

Re-tubing earmolds

Replacing the tubing in a BTE earmold is commonly required and easy to perform. If necessary, ream out the existing hole with a drill bit, motorized reamer, and/or a pipe cleaner dipped in solvent to remove any old glue or debris. To facilitate insertion, the end of the new tubing should be cut at an acute angle. Unless the new tubing is an excessively tight fit in the earmold, the new tubing can be pushed into the mold, as shown in Figure 5.26a. If the point does not emerge at the medial end, insert some fine-nosed pliers into the medial end and pull the tubing through. If the tubing fits too tightly to be pushed into the earmold, it can be bent back on itself and pulled through with a loop of fine wire, as

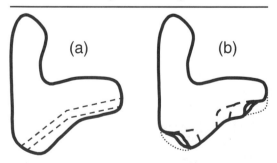

Figure 5.25 An unmodified vent (a) and a shortened vent (b). The dashed lines in (a) indicate the position of the vent. The dashed lines in (b) indicate potential further stages of shortening, and the dotted line indicates the original profile.

shown in Figure 5.26b. Ensure that the lateral end of pre-bent tubing is pointing upwards *in front* of the pinna. If the tubing points too far backwards, it will place excessive pressure on the front of the pinna when the hearing aid is worn.

If the earmold is made from acrylic, the tubing should be glued in. To introduce glue (Cyanoacrylate), bend the protruding tube at the medial end in each direction, and introduce glue into the cracks that open up around the perimeter. Apply glue completely around the perimeter of the tube so that there is no crack for cerumen to penetrate. Finally trim the excess tubing, and optionally withdraw the tubing by 1 or 2 mm. Make sure the glue is thoroughly dry before allowing the patient to handle or insert the earmold. If the tubing is a very loose fit, high viscosity (thick) cement can be used to fill the gap.

If the earmold is made from silicone, the tubing must be held in place mechanically. A collar is slid onto the tubing prior to the tubing being inserted. Some collars are designed to slide in only one direction; these grip the tubing if the tubing is pulled out from the earmold, but these types may constrict the sound bore and decrease the high-frequency response. Other types slide more freely over the tubing and must be glued in place. After fixing the collar onto the tubing at the correct place, the tubing and collar are inserted until the collar is buried a few mm inside the mold material.

Full-length horns (as shown in Figure 5.20a) can be installed in the same manner, except that they are most easily pushed through from the medial end of the earmold. Partly inserted horns (as shown in Figure 5.20b) are preferably installed by pushing the horn in from the lateral end. Glue is applied around the circumference of the medial end of the horn prior to insertion. Provided the horn is inserted very quickly, the glue will act as a lubricant to help insertion.

Building up earshells.
Material has to be added to earshells if a grinding operation breaks through the wall of the shell, thus exposing the inner cavity and the electronic components. Material is added by brushing plastic build-up material on to the earshell. A second reason for adding material to either a shell or a mold is to prevent feedback oscillations. If a hearing aid oscillates, despite the vent being plugged, and provided the feedback is not internal, the otoplastic must be made to fit more tightly within the ear, or else a new otoplastic must be made. (See Table 4.12 and 4.13 for diagnosis of feedback cause.)

Adding build-up material in the region of the aperturic seal most effectively increases tightness. Build-up material should be applied to the canal stalk in the 6 mm medial to the ear canal entrance, and principally in the anterior-posterior dimension. That is, the narrower diameter of the canal stalk should be enlarged slightly. Different types of build-up material are required for hard versus soft earmolds. High-viscosity material is available for those applications where a thick build-up is required.

5.10 Concluding Comments

By keeping in mind the three key functions of earmolds and earshells listed at the start of this chapter, the clinician can easily understand the characteristics of new designs and styles as they are invented (or re-invented!). The three key questions are:

- How does the diameter of the sound bore change along its length from the receiver to the eardrum?

- How large (i.e. long and wide) is the vent path, or if there is no intentional opening, how well sealed is the mold or shell to the canal wall?

- How securely will the mold or shell remain in the ear, and how easily can the aid wearer get it in and out of the ear?

If the answers to each of these questions for any new design are compared to the answers for the most similar structure covered in this chapter, the characteristics of any new designs should be able to be predicted with reasonable accuracy.

The importance of selecting earmold and earshell characteristics to achieve a target real-ear gain is diminishing with time. Hearing aids are incorporating more and more flexible tone controls, which are enabling target gains to be achieved with greater and greater accuracy. Also, it is probable that electroacoustic methods for reducing the occlusion effect will be developed, and electronic methods for increasing the gain that can be achieved without feedback will increasingly be used (see Section 7.3).

Despite these advances, selection of the vent size that minimizes occlusion and feedback problems is likely to be important for many years. Equally, choosing a physical style that provides enough retention, combined with easy insertion and removal, will remain important for as long as hearing aids are taken on and off by the user.

CHAPTER SIX

COMPRESSION SYSTEMS IN HEARING AIDS

Synopsis

Compression's major role is to decrease the range of sound levels in the environment to better match the dynamic range of a hearing-impaired person. The compressor may be most active at low, mid, or high sound levels. Alternatively, it may vary its gain across a wide range of sound levels, in which case it is known as a wide dynamic range compressor. Compressors can react to a change in input levels within a few thousandths of a second, or they can be so sluggish that they take many tens of seconds to fully react. The degree to which a compressor finally reacts as input level changes is best depicted on an input-output diagram or on a gain-input diagram. The compression threshold, which is the input level above which the compressor operates, is clearly visible on such diagrams. The compression ratio, which describes the variation in output level that corresponds to a variation in input level, is related to the slope of the curves on these diagrams. Simple compression systems can be classified as input-controlled, which means that the compressor is controlled by a signal prior to the hearing aid's volume control, or as output-controlled, which means that the compressor is controlled by a signal subsequent to the volume control. This classification is irrelevant for hearing aids with no volume control.

Compression systems have been used to achieve the following specific aims. Different compression parameters are needed for each rationale. Output-controlled compression limiting can prevent the output from ever causing loudness discomfort, or from being peak clipped. Fast-acting compression with a low compression threshold can be used to increase the audibility of the softer syllables of speech, whereas slow-acting compression will leave the relative intensities unchanged, but will alter the overall level of a speech signal. Compression applied with a medium compression threshold will make hearing aids more comfortable to wear in noisy places, without any of the advantages or disadvantages that occur when lower level sounds are compressed. Multichannel compression can be used to enable a hearing-impaired person to hear sounds with the same loudness that would be heard by a normal-hearing person listening to the same sounds. Alternatively, it can be used to maximize intelligibility, while making the overall loudness of sounds normal (rather than normalizing the loudness at each frequency). Compression can be used to decrease the disturbing effects of background noise by reducing gain most in those frequency regions where the SNR is poorest. Gain reduction of this type increases listening comfort and with some unusual noises may also increase intelligibility. Finally, compression can be applied by using the combination of compression parameters that patients are believed to prefer, irrespective of whether there is a theoretical rationale guiding the application. Although these rationales are different, they have various aspects in common. Furthermore, many of them can be combined within a single hearing aid.

Despite the complexity, the benefits of compression can be summarized as follows. Compression can make low-level speech more intelligible, by increasing gain, and hence audibility. Compression can make high-level sounds more comfortable and less distorted. In mid-level environments, compression offers little advantage relative to a well-fitted linear aid. Once the input level varies from this, of course, the advantages of compression become evident. Its major disadvantages are a greater likelihood of feedback oscillation, and excessive amplification of unwanted lower level background noises.

While almost everyone agrees that compression is a good thing, there is much disagreement about the best way to use compression in hearing aids. This chapter describes the different ways that compression can be applied in hearing aids. All of the compression methods have some advantages over linear/peak clipping amplification. All also have some disadvantages.

6.1 Compression's Major Role: Reducing the Signal's Dynamic Range

The major role of compression is to decrease the dynamic range of signals in the environment so that all signals of interest can fit within the restricted dynamic range of a hearing-impaired person (see Section 1.1.2 and Figure 1.2 in particular). This means that intense sounds have to be amplified less than weak sounds. A compressor is an amplifier that automatically turns its gain down as the signal level somewhere within the hearing aid rises (see Section 2.3.5). There are, however, many ways in which the gain can be varied to decrease the dynamic range of a signal.

Figure 6.1 shows three ways in which the amount of gain could change as the input level changes. In the right panel, gain starts reducing as soon as the input level rises above *weak*. By the time a moderate input level has been reached, the gain has been sufficiently decreased, and linear amplification can then be used for all higher input levels. The necessary squashing of the dynamic range of the signal has all been accomplished for low signal levels, so we could refer to this as low-level compression. This can be seen in the upper picture as the lower levels coming closer together after amplification than

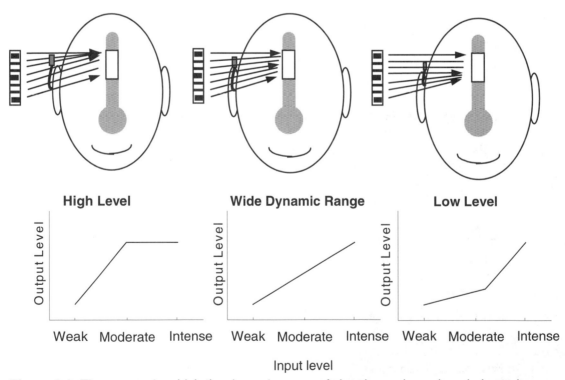

Figure 6.1 Three ways in which the dynamic range of signals can be reduced. In each case, the upper figure shows the spacing of different signal levels before amplification (the left end of the lines) and after amplification (the right end of the lines). The lower figure shows the same data, but as an input-output function.

before, while the spacing of the upper levels is not affected by amplification. In the lower figure, the same squashing (i.e. compression) of levels appears as the decreased slope of the input-output (I-O) function for low-level signals, whereas the linear amplification of higher level signals appears as a 45° slope (see also Section 4.1.5).

In the left panel of Figure 6.1, low-level sounds are amplified linearly, but the inputs from moderate to intense sounds are squashed into a narrower range of outputs. In general, this could be referred to as high-level compression. In the case shown here, all high-level inputs are squashed into an extremely small range of outputs. This extreme case is called *compression limiting*, because the output is not allowed to exceed a set limit.

The center panel represents a third way in which compression could decrease dynamic range. Compression is applied more gradually over a wide range of input levels, and we consequently call this *wide dynamic range compression* (*WDRC*). The overall reduction in dynamic range is the same as for the other two cases. The gradual reduction applies over such a wide range of input levels that there are no input levels for which the corresponding output levels need be squashed closely together. Equivalently, the slope of the I-O curve is never close to horizontal.

It is interesting to note that there are commercially successful hearing aids using each of the three compression strategies, despite the extreme differences between strategies. This is not to say that the differences do not matter, but perhaps the reduction in overall dynamic range of signals that they all achieve is more important than their differences. The relative advantages of different compression systems are discussed later in this chapter, but first we need to define some terms that describe how compressors operate.

6.2   Basic Characteristics of a Compressor

Although a hearing aid employing multiple compressors may operate in a complex manner, the operation of each compressor within the aid can be described with a few simple terms.

6.2.1   Dynamic compression characteristics: attack and release times

A compressor is intrinsically a dynamic device: its job is to change gain depending on changes in the signal level. Figure 6.2 shows an input waveform that rapidly increases, and then decreases in level. When the output level first rises, the detector starts to pass on the increased level to the compressor control circuit. As discussed in Section 2.3.5, the detector first has to convert the waveform to a smooth control signal. This involves *rectification*[a] and then smoothing. A consequence of this smoothing is that following an increase in signal level, the detector output increases gradually to its new value. During the time taken for this to occur, the compressor is not aware of the full extent of the increased signal level, so it does not turn the gain down sufficiently to compensate for the increase. Consequently, the amplifier initially passes the increase without compression, until the compressor reacts to the new input level. The time taken for the compressor to react to an increase in signal level is referred to as the *attack time*.

Because the output gradually approaches its final value, it has to arbitrarily be decided when the final value is reached. Attack time is defined as the time taken for the output to stabilize to within 2 dB (IEC 60118-2) or 3 dB (ANSI S3.22) of its final level after the input to the hearing aid increases from 55 to 80 dB SPL (IEC 60118-2) or from 55 to 90 dB SPL (ANSI S3.22). Eventually, the

---

[a]   In full wave rectification, all negative values are converted to positive values of the same magnitude. In half-wave rectification, the negative values are simply ignored.

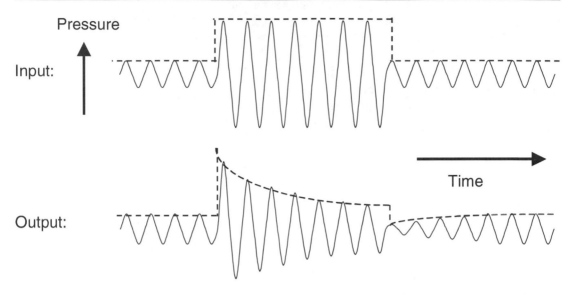

Figure 6.2 Waveforms that are input to a compressor and output from a compressor, showing the attack and release transitions that follow an increase and decrease, respectively, in signal level. The dotted line shows the envelope of the positive half of the signal.

compressor fully reacts to the increased signal level. That is, its gain has been decreased compared to its gain previously.

A similar event happens when the input signal decreases in level. Again, the detector progressively reacts to the new input level, so for a while the compressor amplifies the low-level signal with the gain that was appropriate to the high-level signal preceding it. The control signal decreases gradually, and consequently, the gain and output signal increase gradually. The ***release time*** is the time taken for the compressor to react to a decrease in input level.[b]

Although the attack and release times could be made to have extremely short values (even zero), the consequences are most undesirable. If the release time is too short, the gain will vary during each voice pitch period, so the compressor will distort the waveform.[c] If the attack time is made extremely short, and the

release time long, then distortion will be minimal. However, extremely brief sounds (like clicks) will cause the gain to decrease (because of the short attack time) and the gain will then stay low for a long time afterwards (because of the long release time). It is not necessary for gain to be decreased very much when a very brief click occurs, because very short sounds convey little loudness. It would certainly be undesirable for the gain to remain low long after the brief sound has gone. Attack times in hearing aids are commonly around 5 ms, but can be much longer, as we will see later. Release times are rarely less than 20 ms, and may be much longer.

The attack and release times have a major effect on how compressors affect the levels of the different syllables of speech. First, let us introduce the term ***envelope***, which is an imaginary line drawn through the extremities of a waveform. The envelope gives an

---

[b]   Release time is defined as the time taken for the output signal to increase to within 2 dB (IEC 118-2) or within 4 dB (ANSI S3.22) of its final value following a decrease in input level from 80 to 55 dB SPL (IEC 118-2) or from 90 to 55 dB SPL (ANSI S3.22).

[c]   In the extreme case of zero attack and release times and a high compression ratio, a compressor becomes a peak-clipper.

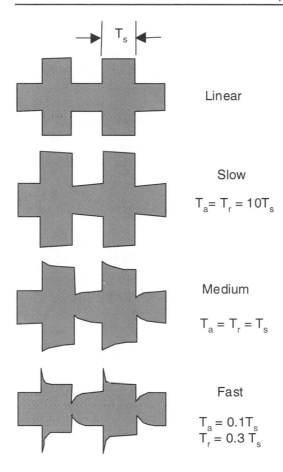

T_s

Linear

Slow

$T_a = T_r = 10T_s$

Medium

$T_a = T_r = T_s$

Fast

$T_a = 0.1T_s$
$T_r = 0.3\,T_s$

Figure 6.3 Envelopes for the output signal coming from a linear amplifier and compression amplifiers with different attack times (T_a), and release times (T_r) compared to the duration of each syllable (T_s) in the signal.

indication of the level of a signal, without showing the fine structure of the waveform. It is useful for showing the effect of compression because compressors intentionally change the envelope while leaving the fine structure almost unchanged. Figure 6.3 shows the envelope of a signal that alternates between two different intensities. An envelope similar to this shape would occur for someone saying the sound *fafaf*.[d] (Notice that there appear to be five "syllables" in the envelope shown.) The first envelope is the output that would occur for linear amplification.

The second envelope shows the output when the attack and release times are both much longer than the duration of a syllable. The compressor starts to turn the gain down or up when each new syllable or phoneme starts, but there is time for only a small gain change to occur before the syllable is finished. The compressor then starts to slowly establish a gain appropriate to the next syllable. Consequently, the gain is almost constant, so the envelope is almost the same as for linear amplification. Is such a compressor therefore doing anything to the signal? As long as the signal level fluctuates around these same values, apparently not. If the input level drops and remains low, however, such as might occur for a distant or softly spoken person, there would be time for the compressor to increase the gain to compensate for the decreased input level.

The third envelope shows the result when the attack and release times are about the same length as the syllables. The level of each syllable is continually changing as the compressor adjusts the gain. The fourth envelope shows the result when the attack and release times are much shorter than the syllables. The full effect of the compressor is applied during nearly all of each syllable, in this case removing most, but not all, of the intensity differences between the syllables. The brief portions of output at the start of each syllable when the compressor is adjusting are known as **overshoot** or **undershoot transients**. In the case shown, the overshoots are shorter than the undershoots, implying that the attack time is less than the release time.

Although it is not shown in Figure 6.3, the shape of the envelope is little affected by compression provided *either* the attack time or the release time is significantly longer than the syllable duration. The sustained syllables of speech are typically 150 to 200 ms long.

---

[d] Note that the complete envelope (comprising positive and negative parts) is shown in Figure 6.3. Because envelopes are usually approximately symmetrical, we often show only the positive part, as in Figure 6.2 and 6.7.

There is no necessity for a compressor to have a single attack and release time. In fact, there are good reasons why the release time, and possibly the attack time, should depend on the signal being amplified. Rapid attack and release is best for protecting the aid wearer against brief intense sounds. Unfortunately, a rapid increase in gain during the pauses in speech will cause greater gain to be applied to background noise than to the speech. As we shall see in Section 6.3.2, the desirability of rapid gain variations during speech itself is hotly debated.

Several hearing aids currently available have an *adaptive release time*. Essentially, the release time is short (e.g. 20 ms) for brief intense sounds, but becomes longer (e.g. 1 s) as the duration of an intense sound increases. When an adaptive release time is combined with a short attack time, a brief intense sound will cause the gain to rapidly decrease and then rapidly increase when the intense sound ceases. This rapid action provides protection against excessive loudness for brief sounds without affecting the audibility of following sounds. Long intense sounds (or a succession of several intense sounds, such as syllables in high-level speech) will, however, cause the release time to automatically lengthen. This slow release means that the gain will not significantly increase during each brief pause between the syllables, or change from syllable to syllable.

Adaptive release times can be achieved by using a single detector with properties that vary with the signal, by controlling a compressor from multiple detectors, or by using multiple compressors in succession. All of these systems are able to provide protection against excessive loudness when brief intense signals occur, without causing rapid fluctuations in gain when high intensity speech occurs. Compressors with variable attack and release times have been used in the broadcast industry for many years,[802] but have been used and evaluated in hearing aids only over the last decade. One compressor

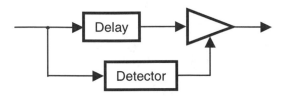

Figure 6.4 A block diagram of a feedforward, look-ahead compression control circuit.

using a combination of fast- and slow-acting detectors, when used at the input of a hearing aid, has been referred to as a *dual front-end compressor*, and has been shown to have the advantages expected of adaptive release time compression.[624]

The advent of digital hearing aids has opened some new possibilities for controlling compressors. Overshoots can be completely avoided if the compressor decreases its gain *before* the signal level increases. Does the compressor have a crystal ball? Effectively, yes! If the signal is delayed for a few milliseconds before it enters the compression amplifier, the detector can fully react to the signal before the signal reaches the compression amplifier.[753, 802, 922] An example of this, which can be called *look-ahead compression*, is shown in Figure 6.4. This figure also shows that a compressor can operate with a *feedforward* control circuit instead of a *feedback* control circuit.

6.2.2　Static compression characteristics

The attack and release times tell us how *quickly* a compressor operates; we need different terms to tell us by how *much* a compressor decreases the gain as level rises. When we measure and specify these gain changes we assume that the compressor has had time to fully react to variations in signal level. Consequently, the *static characteristics* are applicable to signals that are longer than the attack and release times.

The SPL above which the hearing aid begins compressing is referred to as the ***compression threshold***. (For input levels below compression threshold, most hearing aids amplify linearly, but some operate as expanders, as discussed in Section 4.1.5.) Usually, we define the compression threshold as the *input* SPL at which compression commences, but in some circumstances it makes more sense to define it as the *output* SPL at which compression commences (see Section 6.2.3). As can be seen from the I-O diagram in Figure 6.5, the onset of compression can be very gradual. Measurement standards define compression threshold as the point at which the output deviates by 2 dB from the output that would have occurred had linear amplification continued to higher input levels.

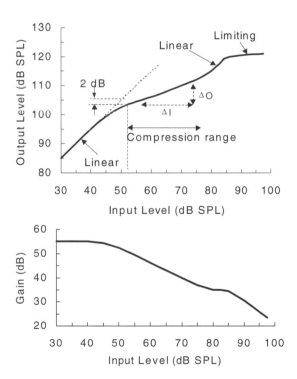

Figure 6.5 Upper: input-output diagram showing the definition of several static compression characteristics. Lower: the graph of gain versus input that corresponds to the I-O curve above it.

Once compression commences, the gain decreases with further increases in input level. The ***compression ratio*** describes, indirectly, how much the gain decreases. Compression ratio is defined as the change in input level needed to produce a 1 dB change in output level. With reference to Figure 6.5, it is equal to the ratio of $\Delta I/\Delta O$, and is therefore the inverse of the slope of the I-O curve.[e] If the slope of the I-O curve varies with input level, so too does the compression ratio. Compression ratios in the range of 1.5:1 to 3:1 are common in hearing aids with wide dynamic range compression.

In the linear part of the curve (below the compression threshold), every 1 dB increase in input level results in a 1 dB increase in output level. Consequently, the compression ratio of a linear amplifier is 1:1. The other extreme is compression limiting, such as that shown at the highest input levels in Figure 6.5. The slope of the I-O function here is close to zero, which means the compression ratio is very large. In practice, any compression ratio greater than about 8:1 would be considered to be compression limiting. Compression ratios can thus have any value greater than 1:1. Compression ratios less than 1:1 are also possible, but these correspond to dynamic range ***expanders*** rather than compressors (see Section 4.1.5).

In the particular I-O function shown in Figure 6.5, there are four distinct regions, two of which correspond to linear amplification. To fully describe this curve, we thus need to specify four compression ratios (two of which are equal to 1:1) and three compression thresholds, with a compression threshold separating each of the regions. Curves like this one might be designed to fulfil a particular purpose (e.g. loudness normalization, as will be described in Section 6.3.5). Such curves might also occur because a compressor is capable of operating only over a restricted range of input levels. A compressor can compress only as long as it can keep

---

[e]   The symbol Δ is pronounced "delta" and in mathematics stands for a small change in any quantity.

on reducing its gain whenever the signal level rises. Once further gain reductions are impossible, compression ceases, and linear amplification resumes. The range of inputs over which compression occurs is called the **compression range**. The I-O function in Figure 6.5 could be generated by a hearing aid with two different compressors: The first has a compression threshold of 52 dB SPL, a compression ratio of 3:1, and a compression range of 30 dB. The second has a compression threshold of 87 dB SPL, a compression ratio of 10:1, and a compression range of at least 15 dB.

An equally useful alternative to the I-O diagram is the input versus gain diagram shown in the lower half of Figure 6.5. Notice how the two curves show the same information:

- in the low-level linear segment, the gain is constant, so the gain-input curve is horizontal;
- in the 3:1 compression segment, the gain drops by 2/3 of a dB for every dB increase in input level;
- in the next linear segment, gain is constant;
- in the high-level compression limiting segment, gain drops by nearly 1 dB for every dB increase in input level;
- for every input level, gain equals output SPL minus input SPL.

Sometimes, I-O curves do not comprise a number of straight lines, but are in fact curved, with the slope (and hence the compression ratio) changing continuously as the input level varies. These are called **curvilinear compressors** - they are no better or worse than compressors with different fixed compression ratios at different input level ranges, just more difficult to describe, except by drawing a picture, as shown in Figure 6.6. In this case, at every input level the curvilinear compressor produces much the same output level as the compressor comprising a fixed 2:1 compression ratio combined with compression limiting of high-level sounds.

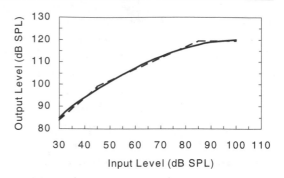

Figure 6.6 Input-output characteristics corresponding to curvilinear compression(solid line) and a fixed compression ratio combined with compression limiting (dashed line).

We must remember that the static characteristics apply only to signals of long duration. As implied in Section 6.2.1, the hearing aid acts in an increasingly linear manner when the intensity fluctuations become increasingly rapid. That is, for rapidly changing signals, the effective compression ratio is less than the static compression ratio. The effective compression ratio is defined as the change in input level divided by the change in output level for a given signal containing high- and low-level components following each other in rapid succession. As can be seen in Figure 6.3, the effective compression ratio depends on the duration of the high- and low-level parts of the signal compared to the longer of the attack and release times.

Phonemes and syllables vary widely in duration, but it is sensible to ask what the effective compression ratio might be for a signal with a typical syllable duration of about 120 ms. Only when the attack and release times are much less than 120 ms will the effective compression ratio equal the static compression ratio. When the attack or release times are much greater than 120 ms, the effective compression ratio will be 1:1. That is, the hearing aid will amplify rapid fluctuations in speech linearly, although its gain will change when the overall level of speech changes. In between these extremes (in which the attack and release times of real hearing aids mostly fall), specification of the effective compression ratio is complex, but it will always be less than the static compression ratio.[853, 923] Both the static and the effective compression ratios are useful: the static ratio tells us how the long-term level of the output changes when the long-term level of the input changes. By contrast, the effective compression ratio tells us how the short-term level of the output changes when the short-term level of the input changes.[f]

6.2.3   Input and output control

As we have seen, compression commences at a certain SPL. How do things change if the user moves the volume control to a dif-

ferent position? The answer depends on the location of the volume control relative to the compressor within the signal chain. Figure 6.7 shows the block diagram of two hearing aids that differ in the relative location of the volume control and the compressor. Consider first the upper diagram, in which the compressor precedes the volume control. What effect does the volume control have on the operation of the compressor? Obviously none, because the compressor acts on the signal prior to the signal reaching the volume control. Consequently, compression commences at the same input SPL for all settings of the volume control. However, once

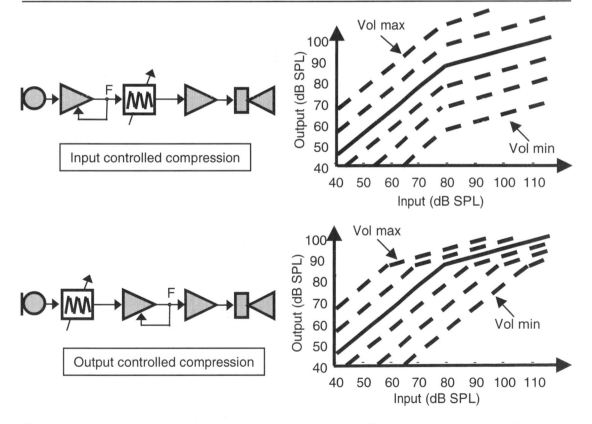

Figure 6.7 Input controlled compression and output controlled compression: their block diagrams and the I-O curves for each as the volume control is varied from maximum to minimum positions.

---

[f]   Note that even the effective compression ratio does not tell the full story for a complex signal like speech. Although the dynamic range of the total signal level is compressed as described by the effective compression ratio, the dynamic range within a narrow frequency range is not compressed to the same degree as is the total broadband level (Verschuure et al., 1996). That is, the width of the speech banana (e.g. Figure 8.2) is not compressed to the extent that one would expect based on the effective compression ratio. This discrepancy occurs whenever the analysis bandwidth is less than the bandwidth of the signal passing through a compressor. The discrepancy is thus greatest for single-channel compressors and least for multichannel compressors with many channels.

Important principle: The effects of user and fitter controls on compressor operation

- Any control that follows the sensing point (i.e. the feedback or feed-forward point) in the signal chain does not affect the amount of compression, but does affect the final level of the compressed signal. Varying these controls causes the I-O curve to shift vertically.
- Any control that precedes the sensing point in the signal chain affects the compression threshold and hence the amount by which a signal is compressed. Varying these controls causes the I-O curve to shift horizontally.

This principle applies to all controls including tone controls.

the compressor has done its job (whether that be linear amplification or compression), the volume control determines the size of the output signal.

The I-O curves corresponding to different volume control settings are thus as shown in the upper I-O diagram in Figure 6.7. Because the compression is controlled from a point (labeled as F) on the input side of the volume control, this arrangement is referred to as **input-controlled compression**. It is also referred to as automatic gain control (input) or **AGC_i**.

Let us now compare AGC_i with an alternative arrangement, called **output-controlled compression (AGC_o)** shown in the lower half of Figure 6.7. In this case, the volume control affects the signal *before* the signal reaches the compressor. Suppose the input level was high enough for the compressor to be just in its compression region. (That is, the input level equals the input compression threshold.) If the volume control were now to be turned down, the amount of signal reaching the compressor would no longer be enough for compression to commence. Consequently, the compression threshold at the input has been increased by the amount of the gain reduction. This variation of compression threshold can be seen in the lower I-O diagram in Figure 6.7. A comparison of the I-O curves for AGC_i and AGC_o shows a basic principle: *For AGC_i hearing aids, I-O curves move up*

and down as the volume control is varied, whereas for AGC_o hearing aids, they move left and right. Equivalently, for AGC_i hearing aids, the compression threshold referred to the input is independent of the volume control, whereas for AGC_o hearing aids, the compression threshold referred to the output is independent of the volume control setting.

Just as the position of the volume control relative to the sensing point determines the effect of the volume control on the compressor, so too the position of any fitter control determines its effect on compression. As discussed in Section 4.1.3, a compressor following a filter or tone control can partially undo the effect of the tone control on narrowband signals. Similarly, a tone control following a compressor can partially undo the effects of the compressor.[g] As the complexity of hearing aids increases, the number of controls and the number of separate compressors within a hearing aid are both increasing. It is thus becoming rather simplistic to describe compression hearing aids as being either AGC_i or AGC_o. For example, compression could be input-controlled with respect to the volume control, but not with respect to the tone controls. It is for this reason that block diagrams are becoming essential if the operation of the hearing aid is to be understood.

With the increased use of compression in hearing aids, it is becoming common for

[g]   If, for instance, a compression limiter removed all intensity differences, a filter or tone control that followed the compressor would create intensity differences that depend on the frequency or spectral shape of the signal.

hearing aids to not have a volume control. For these hearing aids, the main distinction between input and output control disappears.

6.2.4   Multichannel compression

Multichannel hearing aids split the incoming signal into different frequency bands, and each band of signal passes through a different amplification channel (see Section 2.5.1 and Figure 2.2). In a multichannel compression hearing aid, each channel contains its own compressor. There are two basic reasons why we might want to compress different frequency regions by different amounts:

- hearing loss usually varies with frequency;
- signals and noises in the environment have more energy in some frequency regions than in others.

If the amount of compression required at any frequency depends on either the hearing loss at that frequency or the level of the signal in that frequency region, then the degree of compression must also have to vary with frequency. Multichannel compression enables this variation of compression with frequency to be achieved. The degree of compression is greatest for high compression ratios and for low compression thresholds.

Even if neither the hearing loss nor the signal spectrum varies with frequency there is a theoretical argument (i.e. not yet substantiated) why we might want multiple channels of compression. In a single-channel compression hearing aid, when the compressor turns the gain down, signal components at all frequencies are decreased in level. It might not be appropriate to have signal components at one frequency being attenuated just because there is a strong signal, or a limited dynamic range of hearing, at another frequency. Multichannel compression avoids this problem, although it can create other problems, as we will see in Section 6.5.

Although there are many ways in which compression can vary from one channel to the next, the degree of compression often either increases or decreases with frequency. A simple classification scheme describes this overall behavior. When the degree of compression is greater in the high-frequency channel(s) than in the low-frequency channel(s), there will be a greater high-frequency emphasis at low input levels than at high input levels. This characteristic has been labeled as a **treble increase at low levels**, or a **TILL** response.[473] Conversely, when the degree of compression is greater in the low-frequency channel(s) than in the high-frequency channels, there will be less high-frequency emphasis at low input levels than at high input levels. This characteristic has been labeled as a **bass increase at low levels**, or a **BILL** response.[473, h]

6.3   Rationales for Use of Compression

This chapter so far has described how compressors work, but not what we would like them to do. The following sections outline several theoretical reasons why compressors should be included in hearing aids. There is no reason why only a single rationale should be used in any particular hearing aid, but as we will note, some of the reasons are a little contradictory. Section 6.5 will attempt to summarize what we know about the advantages, disadvantages, and effectiveness of these forms of compression.

6.3.1   Avoiding discomfort, distortion and damage

The output of a hearing aid cannot be allowed to keep on getting bigger as the input to the hearing aid increases. There are two reasons why the maximum output must be limited in some way, and one reason why it should be limited using compression rather than peak clipping.

---

h   When the response shape changes in a more complex manner with level or frequency, the characteristic has been labeled as a **programmable increase at low levels**, or a **PILL** response (Killion, Staab & Preves, 1990). This more generic term is less useful than the other two.

Compression to control maximum output

- Output-controlled compression
- Compression ratio >8:1
- Attack time < 5 ms and release time between 20 and 100 ms or adaptive
- Single or multichannel

First, if excessively intense signals are presented to the hearing aid wearer, the resulting loudness will cause discomfort. Thus, the aid wearer's loudness discomfort level provides an upper limit to the hearing aid SSPL.[227] Second, excessively intense signals may cause further damage to the aid wearer's residual hearing ability. As we will consider in more detail in Section 9.7, the SSPL may not be the most important factor to consider in avoiding damage, but it certainly is a factor.

These two reasons explain why the maximum output must be limited (i.e. why the hearing aid SSPL must be set appropriately), but this limiting could be achieved with either peak clipping or compression limiting. The reason for preferring compression limiting over peak clipping in nearly all cases (see Section 9.6.2 for exceptions) is that peak clipping creates distortion, as discussed in Sections 2.3.3 and 4.1.6. So too does compression limiting, but the type of distortion created by peak clipping is far more objectionable than the type created by compression limiting.

When compression limiting is used to control the SSPL of a hearing aid, it must be an output-controlled compressor, or else the SSPL will rise and fall with the position of the volume control. This would be unacceptable, as the user may increase the volume control position (and hence the SSPL) when in a quiet place, only to have an intense unexpected signal occur. A high compression ratio is needed, so that the output SPL does not rise significantly for very intense input levels. The attack time must be short so that the gain decreases rapidly enough to prevent loudness discomfort. This gain reduction must be removed rapidly so that sounds following an intense sound are not too attenuated, hence the release time must be either short or adaptive. As with all compressors, the release time must not be so short that it starts distorting the waveform.

If a hearing aid does not include a compression limiter, peak clipping will occur once the input signal becomes sufficiently intense. If the hearing aid contains wide dynamic range compression, the input level needed to cause peak clipping may be so high that peak clipping seldom occurs. Despite this, all hearing aids will peak-clip once the input signal exceeds some value. For good hearing aids, this value is high enough not to matter; for others it may be so low that patients complain about the quality or intelligibility of amplified sound when they wear their hearing aids in noisy places or listen to nearby talkers.

6.3.2 Reducing inter-syllabic and inter-phonemic intensity differences

The most intense speech sounds (some vowels) are about 30 dB more intense than the weakest sounds (some unvoiced consonants).[i] For people with very reduced dynamic ranges it may be difficult to achieve and maintain a volume control setting that makes the weakest sounds of speech sufficiently audible to be understood without the most intense sounds becoming excessively loud. Even when dynamic range is adequate to hear weak phonemes without intense ones being too loud, there is the potential for the weaker phonemes to be temporally masked by the stronger ones (see Section 1.1.4).

---

[i]   This intensity difference can be judged either from acoustical measurements of intensity, or by assessing how far speech has to be attenuated before different consonants become inaudible (Fletcher, 1929; Kent, Wiley & Strennen, 1979).

A potential solution to both these problems is to include a fast-acting compressor that increases its gain during weak syllables or phonemes and decreases its gain during intense syllables or phonemes. Such compression, not surprisingly, is called *syllabic compression* or *phonemic compression*. Figure 6.8 shows the envelope of the signal for a sentence spoken by a soft talker followed by the same sentence presented at a higher level (representing soft and intense speech). Part (b) of the figure shows the envelope after amplification by such a compressor, and part (c) shows the gain applied by the compressor as it did its job. The dynamic range of the output signal is much less than that of the input signal.

A potential problem is that fast compression alters the intensity relationships between different phonemes and syllables. This might seem like a strange thing to say, because altering the intensity relationships is the aim of the processing. However, if the hearing aid wearer uses the relative intensities of sounds to help identify them, altering relative intensities *may* decrease the intelligibility of some speech sounds, even if it increases their audibility.[720]

Another potential problem is the effect that compression has on brief weak sounds that follow closely after sustained intense sounds. Suppose a sound of higher than average level causes the gain to be lower than would be chosen for a linear amplifier. If the release time is longer than the gap between the intense and the weak sound, then the gain will still be decreased when the brief weak sound arrives. Consequently, such weak sounds will be *less* audible than they would be for linear amplification. Release times of 50 ms or less may be sufficiently short to eliminate this problem.

A more serious problem with fast-acting compression of any sort is that if the gain is fast enough to increase when a soft phoneme occurs, it is also fast enough to increase

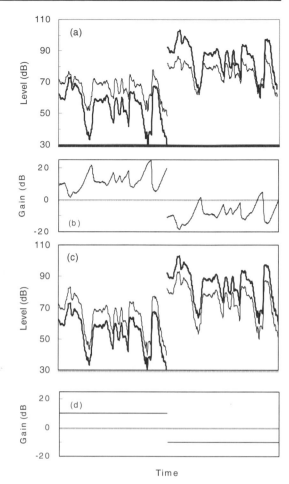

Figure 6.8 (a) Envelope of the signal *The yellow flower has a big bud* put into the hearing aid at two levels. The thick curve shows the envelope for linear amplification and the thin curve shows the envelope for a compressor with a 3:1 compression ratio, attack time of 20 ms, and release time of 200 ms. Part (b) shows the gain applied by the compressor. Part (c) shows the envelope for linear amplification and for compression when the attack and release times of the compressor were increased to 1000 and 2000 ms respectively. The corresponding gain is shown in part (d).

during pauses between words. Does this matter? If there is any background noise, it does. When noise is less intense than the speech, the compressor will increase its gain during the noise, and decrease it during the speech. Amplifying noise by a greater amount than speech is *not* a desirable feature in any

---

Compression to decrease inter-syllabic level differences

- Input-controlled compression
- Compression ratio > 1.5:1, but < 3:1
- Attack time from 1 to 10 ms and release time from 10 to 50 ms
- Compression threshold < 50 dB SPL
- Single or multichannel

---

hearing aid, but this disadvantage has to be weighed against the advantages of fast-acting compression.

For release times between about 100 ms and 3 s, the hearing aid wearer can hear noises grow louder following cessation of a preceding higher level sound. This phenomenon, where the loudness of one sound is clearly affected by the cessation and perhaps commencement of another sound, is referred to as *pumping*. For release times shorter than about 50 ms, compression also amplifies background noise more during pauses than during speech sounds, but the loudness increase may occur too rapidly for the aid wearer to perceive a change in loudness due to compression.[j] Pumping is more evident for single-channel compression than multi-channel compression, and is more evident when speech and background noise come from different directions.[461] Hearing aid wearers are unlikely to actually use the word pumping to describe its effects.

Compressors intended to decrease the intensity differences between syllables must have compression thresholds low enough for the compression to be active across a range of input levels. They must have compression ratios high enough to significantly decrease dynamic range, but low enough to leave some intensity differences intact. Attack and release times have to be short enough that the gain can vary appreciably from one syllable or phoneme to the next, but not so short that

they create significant amounts of distortion to the waveform. Phonemes are shorter than syllables, so phonemic compression requires attack and release times even shorter than syllabic compression. Because phonemic compression will amplify a consonant by a different (usually greater) amount than an adjoining vowel, it changes the consonant-to-vowel level ratio, as discussed in more detail in Section 7.5.

6.3.3   Reducing differences in long-term level

Although the fast-acting compressor discussed in Section 6.3.2 was intended to decrease inter-syllabic level differences, Figure 6.8 makes it clear that it had two effects. As well as changing the inter-syllabic relationships, the mean level difference between the soft and the intense speech has been decreased from 30 dB to 10 dB. An alternative use of compression is to decrease the longer-term dynamic range, without changing the intensity relationships between syllables that follow each other closely in time. This is achieved by using attack and release times much longer than the typical duration of syllables. Parts (d) and (e) of the figure show the envelope of the output signal and the gain applied to the compressor. There are several things to observe. First, notice that the gain now changes much less during each sentence than for the fast-acting compressor. Second, as desired, the intensity relationships between syllables are the same at the output of the compressor as at the input. Third, the desired goal has been achieved: The average level of the first sentence is now only 10 dB lower than that of the second sentence.

This type of compressor is often called an *automatic volume control*. The term is appropriate, because the compressor varies the gain in very much the same way a person would adjust the volume control to partially compensate for differences in the incoming

---

[j]   The loudness of noise during speech sounds is normally less than in the pauses, even without compression, because speech sounds will partially mask the noise.

Compression to decrease long-term level differences

- Input-controlled compression
- Compression ratio > 1.5:1, but < 4:1
- Attack time >100 ms and release time > 400 ms
- Compression threshold < 50 dB SPL
- Single or multichannel

---

levels of sounds. Incoming levels may be high because the talker is close, because the talker has a naturally powerful voice, or because the talker has raised his or her voice above background noise. Incoming sounds of interest may not even be speech. There are no data on what levels of sound people would prefer in different environments, but it seems likely that people would *not* choose to listen to all sounds at the same level. (Life would be less interesting if some gently spoken words and the whistle of a steam train at close quarters were both to be heard at the same intensity and loudness.) Consequently, one would not want the automatic volume control to have an infinite compression ratio. The optimum compression ratio depends on the dynamic range of the hearing aid wearer and the range of sounds to which the aid wearer would like to comfortably listen without having to adjust a manual volume control. The consequence of trying to keep too big a range of sounds within the comfort range of a person is that a high compression ratio is needed. This high compression ratio decreases desirable differences in intensity, perhaps to the point where the differences are no longer perceptible.

The biggest problem with slow-acting compressors is what happens when the input level varies suddenly. Suppose a person has for some time been listening to a softly spoken person in a quiet place. The hearing aid will react by turning up the gain appropriately. If a loud noise then occurs, or a loud talker joins the conversation, the new sound will be amplified with the high gain that was

appropriate to the weaker talker. The output will thus be excessive and must be decreased with an appropriate limiter of some type, preferably a compression limiter. Sudden increases in level are very common: they will probably occur every time the aid wearer talks, because his or her mouth is probably closer to the hearing aid than is anybody else's.

The opposite problem, a sudden decrease in level, also occurs, but is not so easily fixed. If everyone at a gathering suddenly stops talking to hear what one person is saying, the wearer of an automatic volume control hearing aid may miss the important announcement if the hearing aid still has the gain appropriate to the higher input level that was present a moment before. This problem is minimized by having a release time no longer than that necessary to avoid rapid increases in gain during brief pauses in the conversation. Several multichannel hearing aids on the market use separate slow-acting compressors in each channel.

6.3.4   Increasing sound comfort

One might expect that a compression limiter would solve any problems caused by excessive loudness. While it is certainly true that setting the SSPL low enough will prevent loudness discomfort, people may not like the signal being close to discomfort level for a large proportion of the time. It may not be satisfactory to simply further decrease SSPL, as this prevents any sounds from getting close to discomfort, and thus decreases the useable dynamic range by an even greater degree than does the person's hearing loss! One solution to this problem is to use, for higher level inputs, a form of compression that is more gradual than compression limiting.

Figure 6.9 shows the I-O diagram of a compressor that is activated only when the input SPL is at or above typical input levels. There is no agreed name for such compression, but it could be termed either

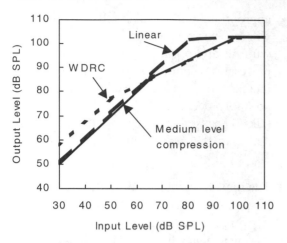

Figure 6.9 Input-output curves for medium level compression, wide dynamic range compression, and linear amplification, all combined with either compression limiting or peak clipping of high level signals.

Compression to increase comfort

- Input-controlled compression
- Compression ratio > 1.5:1, but < 4:1
- Attack time and release time unknown, possibly not important, but release time not too short
- Compression threshold approximately 60 dB SPL
- Single or multichannel

medium-level compression or *comfort-control compression*.[122] Two other I-O diagrams are shown for comparison, all of which have the same output level for an input level of 65 dB SPL. The medium-level compressor provides the same gain for low-level signals as does the linear amplifier, and consequently does not boost soft signals like the wide dynamic range compressor does. Both the WDRC hearing aid and the medium-level compression hearing aid decrease their gain gradually once the input level rises above about 65 dB SPL, and so both increase comfort in noisy places. If, for instance, the SSPL of the hearing aid had been set close to, but below the hearing aid wearer's discomfort level, then for the linear aid, this maximum output level will be achieved whenever the input level is greater than 84 dB SPL. By contrast, the input level has to exceed 99 dB SPL before the output of the medium-level compressor or the wide dynamic range compressor reaches this level.

In summary, a gradual form of compression for medium- to high-level sounds can increase comfort in noise without conveying the advantages and disadvantages of gain increases for weak input sounds. Note that

we do not necessarily expect the compressor to increase intelligibility in noisy places, but we do expect it to increase listening comfort. Of course, a reduction in output level can sometimes result in an increase in intelligibility, for reasons that are not fully understood. The poorer intelligibility at high levels of stimulation may possibly result from the increased spread of excitation (i.e. spread of masking) in the cochlea at high levels.

Before moving on to the next rationale, we should note that the first four rationales have been discussed as though the hearing aid contained only a single compressor covering the entire frequency range. In fact, the comments made about each rationale apply equally well to each channel of a multichannel compression hearing aid. One can thus have:

- multichannel compression limiting - to achieve different SSPLs at different frequencies;
- multichannel inter-syllabic intensity reduction - to decrease the intensity differences between syllables more in one frequency range than in another;[924]
- multichannel automatic volume control - to slowly change the gain and shape of the frequency response as the long-term level and long-term spectral shape of the input signal varies; and
- multichannel comfort control - to decrease gain in noisy places more in some frequency regions than in others.

The justification for all of these is that because hearing characteristics (threshold, comfort level, discomfort level, dynamic range) vary with frequency, so too should a solution that in some way aims to match signals to these hearing characteristics.

6.3.5   Normalizing loudness

Probably the most popular (though not necessarily optimum) rationale for using compression is to normalize the perception of loudness. As mentioned in Section 1.1.2, sensorineural hearing loss greatly affects loudness perception. The principle of loudness normalization is simple: For any input level and frequency, give the hearing aid the gain needed for the wearer to report the loudness to be the same as that which a person with normal hearing would report.

The required amount of gain at each input level can be deduced from a graph showing the loudness of sounds at different levels. Loudness can only be measured subjectively and there are several ways in which it can be measured. Currently, the most popular way is to ask the hearing-impaired person to rate loudness using one of several terms. This procedure is called *categorical scaling of loudness*. The scales commonly have about seven different labels. In variations of the procedure, responses intermediate to the labels are also allowed.

Figure 6.10 shows a graph of loudness category versus SPL (referenced to SPL in a 2-cc coupler) for one hearing-impaired person and for an average normal-hearing person (Cox, private communication). These graphs are often referred to as *loudness growth curves*. Consider first the SPL needed to produce a rating of *very soft*. Whereas the normal-hearing people need only 23 dB SPL, the hearing-impaired person needs 66 dB SPL. The difference between these values, 43 dB, is of course, almost as large as the

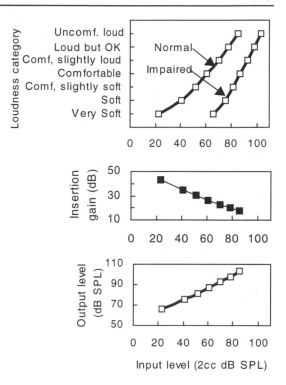

Figure 6.10 (a) Loudness growth curves for normal hearing people and a hearing impaired person with a 50 dB hearing loss. (b) Insertion gain needed for the impaired listener to receive a normal loudness sensation. (c) The corresponding I-O curve.

loss in hearing threshold, which we can think of as the hearing loss for extremely soft sounds. The difference is the insertion gain needed for an input level of 23 dB SPL if the hearing-impaired person is to rate the sound as being *very soft*. This comparison enables us to plot one point on the curve of insertion gain versus input SPL, as shown in part (b). If we know the input level (23 dB SPL) and the gain (43 dB), we can also specify the output level (66 dB SPL), so this also gives us one point on the I-O curve, as shown in part (c).[k] This process can be repeated for all the other loudness categories. For example, the hearing-impaired person needs 98 dB SPL for sounds to be *loud but OK*, which is 20 dB greater than the 78 dB SPL needed for normally hearing people. Consequently, an

---

[k]   Because the gain is an insertion gain, the 2-cc coupler output SPL will equal the input SPL, plus the insertion gain, plus the appropriate CORFIG (see Section 4.3.2). As CORFIG for an ITE at 1 kHz is close to zero, it is ignored in this example.

Compression to normalize loudness

- No volume control
- Compression ratio decreasing as input level increases
- Attack time and release time long or short
- Compression threshold as low as possible
- Different compression ratios needed for different frequencies

---

input level of 78 dB SPL requires an insertion gain of 20 dB and an output SPL of 98 dB SPL.

What can we conclude about the type of compression needed for loudness normalization? The greatest compression ratio is needed for low-level inputs. Consequently, we could refer to this as *low-level compression*. The compression ratio becomes closer to one as the input level increases, but whether amplification actually becomes linear depends on whether the hearing-impaired and normal-hearing loudness functions ever become parallel.

Because the amount of compression needed depends on loudness perception, loudness perception depends on hearing threshold loss, and threshold loss depends on frequency, it will not be surprising that the degree of compression for loudness normalization often varies markedly with frequency. Take for instance a person with near-normal low-frequency hearing and a high-frequency loss. Loudness perception is most different from normal for low-intensity, high-frequency sounds. Consequently, these sounds require the most gain and the greatest compression ratio. Except for people with flat hearing losses, loudness normalization will thus require the shape of the gain-frequency characteristic to vary with input level. High-tone loss is the most usual configuration. For such losses, as input level decreases, loudness normalization results in high-frequency gain

increasing at a faster rate than low-frequency gain. Loudness normalization thus usually requires a TILL response (except of course for flat or reverse-slope losses).

The most common way of achieving loudness normalization is with separate compressors located in each channel of a multichannel hearing aid, such as that shown in Figure 2.2. Alternatively, the hearing aid may contain only two channels, and have a compressor in only the high-frequency channel. It is possible, however, to combine a compressor with a filter that alters its shape with input level, so that even a single channel hearing aid can have a level-dependent frequency response. One well known example of this is the K-Amp™, in which the gain, and the corner frequency of a high pass filter, simultaneously decrease as the input level increases, as shown in Figure 6.11.

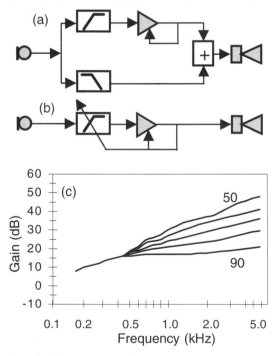

Figure 6.11 Block diagrams of (a) two-channel and (b) single channel processing schemes that can implement approximations of loudness normalisation, and (c) the resulting typical TILL gain-frequency response that increases in slope as the input level decreases from 90 to 50 dB SPL.

Compressors can attempt to normalize loudness for brief sounds by using fast attack and release times, or they can attempt to normalize only the average loudness in each frequency region, by using long attack and release times. Both types of hearing aids are available.

6.3.6   Maximizing intelligibility

Multichannel compression can be used to achieve, in each frequency region, the amount of audibility that maximizes intelligibility, subject to some constraint about the overall loudness. Such an approach will result in loudness *not* being normalized in any frequency region, although the overall loudness of broadband sounds may well be normalized. Further discussion of this rationale requires an understanding of several aspects of hearing aid prescription, and we will return to this topic in Section 9.3.7.

6.3.7   Reducing noise

The interfering effect of background noise is the single biggest problem faced by hearing aid wearers. Not surprisingly, compression is used to decrease the effects of noise. The assumptions behind this approach are as follows:

- Noise usually has a greater low-frequency emphasis than does speech (because of the combined effects of distance, diffraction around obstacles, reverberation, and the nature of many noise sources).

- The low-frequency parts of speech are therefore the most likely to be masked, and hence convey little information.

- The low-frequency parts of noise may cause upward spread of masking and so mask the high-frequency parts of speech.

- The low-frequency parts of noise contribute most to the loudness of the noise.

- Noise is more of a problem in high-level environments than in low-level environments.

Consequently, if the low-frequency parts of the noise cause masking and excessive loudness, and the low-frequency parts of speech do not convey any useful information in noise, then comfort should be increased by decreasing low-frequency gain in high-level environments. Intelligibility may possibly be improved.

Figure 6.12 illustrates this. Part (a) shows the spectrum of a signal and the spectrum of a noise. The remainder of the argument is the same whether these are long-term spectra averaged over a minute or more, or short-term spectra averaged over a few milliseconds. If we assume that information can be extracted from the speech spectrum whenever it exceeds the noise spectrum, then for these particular spectra, only information above 1 kHz is available to the listener. Furthermore, if there was as much upward spread of masking as that indicated by the uppermost dotted line, then nearly the entire spectrum of the speech will be masked by the noise. With or without upward spread of masking, the low-frequency region contributes no useful information in this environment.

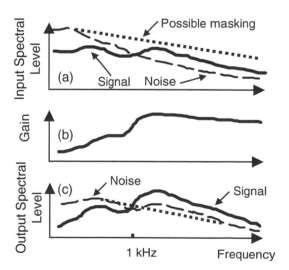

Figure 6.12 (a) Spectrum of the signal and noise input to a noise reduction hearing aid. (b) Gain applied to the signal and noise. (c) Spectrum of the signal and noise at the hearing aid output.

Important principle: the effect of compression on signal-to-noise ratio

- At a given instant in time, everything passing through a compressor (i.e. signal and noise) is amplified by the same amount, thus leaving SNR for simultaneous signal and noise unaffected at every frequency.
- Compressors (and filters) can, however improve the overall SNR, although SNR at every frequency is unchanged (see Figure 6.12 for an example).
- Provided either the signal or noise entering a compressor is above compression threshold, and provided the attack and release times are short enough, signal and noise present at different times will be amplified by different amounts by a compressor. If the (non-simultaneous) SNR is positive, the compressor will decrease SNR.

Despite that, it contributes enormously to loudness. If the level in the environment is much higher than a typical level of approximately 70 dB SPL, the loudness will be greater than is comfortable, and is unlikely to be welcomed by the aid wearer, particularly if it is dominated by unwanted low-frequency noise.

One solution to all of this is to decrease the gain of the troublesome low-frequency region, as shown in Figure 6.12(b). In this particular case, the gain at each frequency is proportional to the signal-to-noise ratio (SNR) at each frequency. (As we shall see in Section 7.2, this particular rule for altering the gain at each frequency is known as *Wiener filtering*.) The corresponding output spectrum is shown in Figure 6.12(c).

Notice that at every frequency, the SNR at the output is identical to that at the input, as it must be, because signal and noise both get amplified by whatever gain is present at that frequency. Consequently, information is still available only above 1 kHz. If the aid wearer can extract information over only the same frequency region, then has this processing helped? Possibly. First, the loudness and annoyance of the noise will have been greatly decreased. Second, there is now no chance that upward masking will further decrease the useful range of frequencies.

In summary, noise reduction should increase comfort (relative to a hearing aid with a fixed gain and frequency response). Noise

reduction should increase intelligibility only when the spectrum of the noise is markedly different from the spectrum of the signal (which is not commonly the case). Both of these expectations have been verified in practice.[231, 275, 510, 678] In those cases where the "noise" is actually one or more people talking nearby, and the signal is also somebody talking, the signal and noise will have similar spectra, and they cannot be separated by filtering (or currently by any electronic means other than directional microphones).

Critics of the noise-reduction rationale have argued that it may be best not to alter the frequency response shape electronically in noisy environments, but rather to present the full spectrum to the aid wearer. This approach relies on the aid wearer's ear and brain being able to separate the signal from the noise.[459]

Hearing aids aimed at noise reduction have often been marketed as *automatic signal processing (ASP)* devices. The term is not very descriptive, as there are many forms of automatic signal processing. Exactly how the signal and noise spectra determine the frequency response depends on the sophistication of the hearing aid. Many hearing aids incorporating the noise-reduction rationale make no attempt to measure the spectrum of either the signal or the noise, but instead simply measure the overall level of the input signal whatever it may be. They then compress the low-frequency components of the signal so that the response becomes more

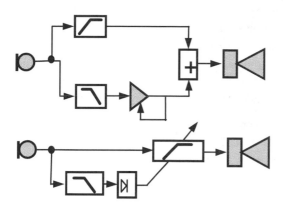

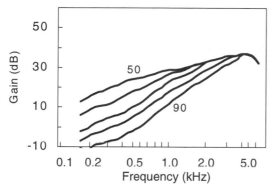

Figure 6.13 Block diagrams of two-channel and single-channel processing schemes that can implement simple noise reduction strategies, and the resulting BILL response that decreases in slope as the input level decreases from 90 to 50 dB SPL.

rising in high-level environments. Most commonly, noise-reduction processing is performed in a two-channel hearing aid, with the compressor located in the low-frequency channel. Alternatively, a high pass filter with a variable corner frequency (controlled by the input level) is used in a single channel hearing aid, as shown in Figure 6.13. The result of either of these arrangements is a gain-frequency response that becomes steeper at high levels; that is, a BILL response.

Noise-reduction processing may have an additional benefit. The aid wearer's own voice has a greater low-frequency emphasis,

> **Compression to decrease noise**
> - Gain reduction where SNR is worst (usually low frequencies)
> - Sometimes approximated by compressing only the low frequencies
> - Attack time and release time long or short
> - Compression threshold medium
> - Usually implemented by multichannel signal processing

and a greater overall level, at the hearing aid microphone than the voice of other people. Consequently, low-frequency compression can help give the aid wearer's own voice a more acceptable tonal quality than would occur for linear amplification.[509]

The noise-reduction rationale can be implemented with slow attack and release times, in which case the frequency response would slowly change, depending on the long-term spectra of the signal and the noise. Alternatively, it can be implemented with fast attack and release times, in which case the frequency response would change rapidly depending on the short-term spectrum of the signal and the noise.

Although the noise reduction discussed so far aims to minimize only low-frequency noise, more advanced multichannel hearing aids on the market can decrease noise (and signal) in any frequency region where SNR is estimated to be particularly poor. Such hearing aids estimate SNR within each channel by taking advantage of the fluctuations in level that are characteristic of speech,[1] in comparison to the more constant level that is characteristic of many background noises. A *speech/non-speech detector* analyzes the envelope in each channel. Higher level parts of the envelope are assumed to represent the peaks of the speech signal. Lower level parts of the envelope are assumed to represent back-

---

[1]   The envelope of a speech signal fluctuates at about 5 Hz, corresponding to the typical syllable rate, but also has some faster and some slower fluctuations covering the range 2 to 50 Hz.

ground noise. The speech/non-speech detector combines these estimates of signal level and noise level to estimate the SNR in each channel. The appropriate gain for each channel can then be calculated. This approach works well when the wanted signal is a single talker and the noise is a continuous babble. By contrast, the hearing aid is likely to make a poor decision about SNR when the wanted signal has little fluctuations (like some music), and the noise has marked fluctuations (like a single nearby talker). In this case, the hearing aid will increase gain at frequencies where it should decrease it and vice versa.

6.3.8 Empirical approaches

The previous seven rationales have all had an underlying theoretical rationale (and perhaps little empirical evidence supporting them). An alternative approach is to experimentally compare different forms of compression and choose the one that is preferred by the aid wearers or that gives the highest speech intelligibility, or hopefully, both. Two hearing aids currently on the market originated from this approach. One of them employs fast-acting, low-level compression of the low frequencies and linear amplification of the high frequencies. The other, a digital hearing aid, employs fast-acting compression for the low frequencies and slow-acting compression for the high frequencies.

The empirical studies behind these hearing aids found that fast-acting compression was more valuable for the low frequencies, although the experimental subjects had their greatest loss and most restricted dynamic range in the high frequencies. Furthermore, subjects who preferred fast-acting compression for the low frequencies were those that had the *widest* dynamic range in the low frequencies.[545] The particular method used to prescribe the compression characteristics may have caused this unexpected result. The prescription resulted in a very high compression ratio for those subjects with the most restricted dynamic ranges. In addition,

even the linear condition contained compression limiting. This compression may have decreased the dynamic range of the signal sufficiently in the high frequencies that there was only minor scope for improvement by adding wide dynamic range compression.

At our current stage of understanding, the empirical and theoretical approaches seem equally reasonable. On the one hand, our theoretical understanding of hearing impairment and the effects of different forms of compression with real world stimuli is incomplete. On the other hand, experiments can answer only the questions their design asks, and under only the conditions their design allows. Neither a theoretical nor an empirical approach to finding the best hearing aid processing should be accepted as being necessarily correct, or dismissed as being the wrong approach. Indeed, we will not be confident that we have the best form of processing for an individual until we have both a theoretical understanding of how the aid is helping *and* empirical evidence that the approach is better than any of several reasonable alternatives.

6.4 Combinations of Compressors in Hearing Aids

There is no reason why a hearing aid should contain a single compressor or be based on a single rationale. Some of the rationales would seem to combine particularly well. As but one of many possible examples, a hearing aid could combine:

- an input compression limiter to prevent very high-level input signals from overloading the circuitry in the rest of the hearing aid (several hearing aids now include these);

- a slow-acting compressor to decrease the dynamic range associated with changes in long-term input level, or alternatively, a multichannel structure, with a slow-acting compressor in each channel;

BILL and TILL: complementary contradictions

For a person with a high-tone loss, the loudness normalization and noise-reduction philosophies lead to contradictory conclusions about what to do. As level decreases, loudness normalization requires a steeper response achieved by high-frequency compression (i.e. TILL; Figure 6.10), while noise reduction usually requires a flatter response achieved by low-frequency compression (i.e. BILL; Figure 6.12). For a person with a high tone loss listening in low-frequency weighted noise, both rationales logically cannot be correct, though both arguments probably have some validity.

If loudness normalization and noise reduction were both implemented with fast-acting compression, the net result would be very similar to single-channel, wide dynamic range compression aimed at reducing the intensity differences between syllables. If both were implemented with slow-acting compression, the net result would be very similar to an automatic volume control.

What the two philosophies have in common is that averaged across frequencies, less gain is needed for high input levels than for low input levels.

- a fast-acting output-controlled compression limiter to prevent the output from exceeding the required maximum output limit, without waveform distortion (many hearing aids have such a limiter).

As we have seen, several rationales require different amounts of compression in different frequency regions. The most straightforward way of achieving this is within a parallel structure, multichannel hearing aid as described in Section 6.2.4. When evaluating how many channels are needed or present in a hearing aid, it is wise not to overlook the effects of venting. As we have seen in Section 5.3.1, any vented or leaky hearing aid has a low-frequency, non-electronic, parallel channel. This will cause apparently single-channel hearing aids to act as though they are two-channel aids. Conversely, hearing aids that are apparently nonlinear in the low-frequency channel may behave as though the low-frequency channel is linear if the vent-transmitted sound dominates the electronically modified sound.

There have been many attempts to classify compression systems into families of similar types. None of the systems does justice to the multitude of ways compression can be used. The most useful system is the TILL-BILL system referred to in Sections 6.2.4. This system is simple but does not distinguish between compression that is most active at higher levels versus compression that is most active at lower levels (see Figure 6.1). Nor does it distinguish between fast-acting, slow-acting, and adaptive attack and release times. A more complex system[223] distinguishes between low- and high-level compression. The only way to unambiguously describe a compression hearing aid is by a block diagram (or its verbal equivalent) and either some I-O curves at different frequencies, or some gain-frequency responses at different input levels, or both.

6.5 Benefits and Disadvantages of Different Compression Systems

In this section we will review the relative advantages and disadvantages of the different compression rationales. This is not a straightforward issue, because the advantage of a compression system or rationale depends on the alternative to which it is being compared, and on how the comparison is carried out. Compression affects the overall level of the output signal, so an important factor in any

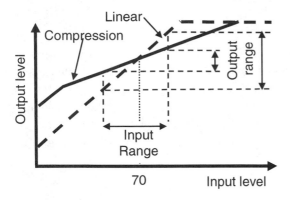

Figure 6.14 Input-output functions for two different hearing aids adjusted to have the same output for a 70 dB SPL input signal.

comparison is how the volume control for each of the systems is adjusted. In this section, we will assume that any amplification systems being compared have been adjusted so that all have the same long-term output level when they are receiving an input signal with an average (70 dB SPL) long-term input level. For example, Figure 6.14 shows the I-O function for two different amplifiers, one linear, and one with a 2:1 compression ratio.

6.5.1 Compression relative to linear amplification

Table 6.1 shows the advantages and disadvantages we *expect* that each type of compression system should have.[223] Unfortunately, there is no experimental evidence to either support or refute some of these expectations. Fortunately, most of the advantages and disadvantages are inevitable consequences of the changes in gain and changes in output level that accompany compression. Suppose, for example, that a compression aid with a low compression threshold and a linear aid have the same gain for a moderate input level. When a low-level sound is input to both aids, the compression aid *will* have more gain, so its output *will* be more audible. On the downside, the compression aid *will* have a greater risk of feedback, which *will* cause a problem if there is enough leakage or a sufficiently large vent. Physical effects such as these are inevitable.

It is much harder to predict the effect of each compression rationale on intelligibility and comfort. Adding just about any sort of compressor will increase the range of input sounds that fall within a person's comfort range without use of the volume control. Unfortunately, there is no theoretical basis for us to predict how much compression is optimal. Hearing aid wearers will need to trade-off the increased loudness comfort and audibility against any extra amplification of background noise occurring in the gaps of speech, and against any adverse change in the quality of speech or other signals. Consequently, we need to look to empirical evidence to assess the advantages of different systems.

A comprehensive review of the relative intelligibility of different compression systems leads to the following conclusions:[223]

1. Limiting. To limit the maximum output of hearing aids, compression limiting should be used rather than peak clipping, except for hearing aids intended for people with the most profound losses. For some people with moderate or severe losses, the compression limiter may offer no advantages over peak clipping, but it will not have any disadvantages. For others, the distortion in the peak clipper will be evident and the compression limiting will be preferred. There is thus no reason not to use compression limiting for everyone except those who will benefit from the additional SPL that can be generated with a peak clipping aid.

2. Typical input levels. If a linear hearing aid is properly prescribed, and the aid wearer adjusts the volume control to get a comfortable loudness, there is no compelling evidence that any form of compression provides superior intelligibility. For speech that is already at an optimal level in the absence of compression, slow-acting compression does not affect the speech. Fast-acting compression will alter the dynamic range of speech (see Figure 6.14), but has

Table 6.1. Summary of compression rationales, methods for implementation, and theoretically expected advantages and disadvantages.

Rationale	Implementation	Expected Advantages (re linear amplification)	Expected Disadvantages (re linear amplification)
Discomfort, distortion and damage avoidance	Fast-acting wideband compression limiting	* No discomfort * Little distortion	* Less SSPL possible than with peak clipping
Reduction of inter-syllabic intensity differences	Fast-acting wideband or multichannel compression with low compression threshold	* Signal kept in audible range without using volume control for a wider range of overall levels and for soft and weak phonemes	* Decreased SNR for noises occurring within the gaps of speech * Increased chance of feedback * Intensity cues may be disrupted
Long-term dynamic range reduction	Slow-acting wideband or multichannel compression with low compression threshold	* Less need to vary volume control * No disruption of intensity cues to different phonemes	* Need further compression to avoid discomfort * Soft and intense phonemes may still fall outside most comfortable range
Comfort increase	Slow- or fast-acting wideband or multichannel compression with a medium compression threshold	* Increased comfort in noisy places without having to decrease the volume control	* Decreased SNR for noises occurring within the gaps of speech
Loudness normalization	Slow- or fast-acting multichannel compression, or adaptive high pass filter (frequency response typically steeper at low input levels)	* Signal kept in audible range without using volume control for a wider range of overall levels (and for soft and weak phonemes if compression is fast acting) * Normal tonal balance at all input levels	* Decreased SNR for noises occurring within the gaps of speech * Increased chance of feedback * Intensity cues may be disrupted (if compression is fast acting)
Noise reduction	Slow- or fast-acting compression in low-frequency band, or adaptive high pass filter (frequency response typically steeper at high input levels)	* Less masking and/or annoyance by low-frequency noise * Signal kept in audible range without using volume control for a wider range of overall levels (and for soft and weak phonemes if compression is fast acting)	* Signal attenuated as well as noise * Abnormal tonal balance * Intensity cues may be disrupted (if compression is fast acting) * Variation of the signal quality as the noise spectrum varies may be objectionable
Empirically determined compression	Fast-acting compression for low levels only in low-frequency band	* Low-frequency components of signal kept in comfort range without using volume control * Signal kept in audible range without using volume control for a wider range of overall levels (and for soft and weak phonemes if compression is fast acting)	* High-frequency components inaudible at low input levels * Intensity cues may be disrupted

Practical advantages of medium or low compression thresholds over linear amplification
• Listening comfort is increased in noisy places.   • Need for a volume control is decreased.

little or no effect on overall intelligibility. The types of confusions may be different for compression than for linear amplification, as one would expect given that compression increases audibility but reduces temporal and/or spectral contrasts.[244] For example, multi-channel compression makes it easier to identify the manner of articulation of consonant (e.g. plosives versus fricatives) but harder to identify the place of articulation.[968] It may be that there is a very slight benefit of fast-acting compression for patients with large dynamic ranges (i.e. mild or moderate losses), and a very slight disadvantage for patients with small dynamic ranges.[921]

3. Low-level inputs. However, as soon as the input sound is decreased (perhaps someone with a softer voice starts talking), any form of compression with a CT less than the original input level can provide intelligibility superior to that of the linear aid (e.g. Humes et al. 1999). This occurs because of the greater gain and hence audibility provided by the compression aid for low-level inputs (see Figure 6.14).

4. High-level inputs. If the input level is then increased above the original level (and above the compression threshold), any form of compression will increase listening comfort. This occurs because of the lower gain (for high-level inputs) provided by the compression aid (see Figure 6.14).

These benefits (items 3 and 4) considerably decrease the need for a manual volume control, although they will not eliminate the need for all patients. Both fast and slow acting

compression provide these benefits. People who have trouble manipulating a volume control will particularly appreciate the benefits. If the compression is fast enough (attack and release times less than about 1 s) the compressor will automatically provide the lower gains that are preferred whenever the aid wearer speaks.[504] Similarly, if the compression is sufficiently fast acting, the hearing aid will be able to decrease the rapid and large variations in level that can occur in some music.[m] With linear amplification, music will often be too soft or too loud.

There is, however, a price to pay for these benefits of compression. Because the hearing aid is often unable to tell the difference between a weak sound that is wanted and a weak sound that is unwanted, it may turn up the gain whenever the sound remains weak long enough for the compressor to react. If this weak sound is actually background noise, the compression aid will sound noisier than the linear aid. (This disadvantage may be avoided if the hearing aid is successfully able to distinguish between wanted and unwanted sounds based on whether these sounds have speech-like characteristics.) In addition, whenever the compressor automatically increases gain, the aid becomes more likely to feed back. The choice of compression threshold is considered further in Section 9.3.9. Lastly, if the compression is fast acting, the compression will lessen some of the natural intensity differences between sounds. If the hearing-impaired person needs these intensity differences to differentiate sounds, the compression may make this task harder.

6.5.2 Benefits of multichannel relative to single-channel compression

Relative to single-channel compression, multichannel compression can increase intelligibility because it increases the audibility of speech. (See the rationales in Section 6.3 for reasons why.) Unfortunately, multichannel

---

m   Classical music usually has a much bigger dynamic range than pop music, so there is a greater need for WDRC when listening to such music.

compression also decreases some of the essential differences between different phonemes. Because compressors give less amplification to intense signals than to weak signals, multichannel compressors tend to decrease the height of spectral peaks and to raise the floor of spectral valleys. That is, they partially flatten spectral shapes. Spectral peaks and valleys give speech sounds much of their identity. Spectral flattening makes it harder for the aid wearer to identify the place of articulation of consonants,[208, 536, 537] and so offsets the positive effect of increased audibility.

Considering these opposing effects of multi-channel compression, it is not surprising that some experiments have shown multichannel compression to be better than single-channel compression[456, 622, 623] and some have failed to show any advantage for multichannel compression.[621, 721, 935] Multichannel compression decreases speech intelligibility for normal-hearing people.[245, 393, 967] If high compression ratios (greater than 3:1) are used in a multichannel compression aid, intelligibility is also decreased for hearing-impaired listeners.[102, 208, 246, 721] In the extreme case of many channels, low compression thresholds, and infinite compression ratios, all sounds would have the same spectrum at the output, no matter how they differed at the input. No one would prescribe such compression, however. Note that for patients with severe losses, and hence greatly reduced dynamic ranges, restoring normal audibility requires large compression ratios. If multichannel compression is applied to these patients in this way, it is detrimental to intelligibility.[246, 537, 967] For smaller compression ratios, the detrimental effects are smaller, so the positive effects (increased audibility) of increasing the number of channels can slightly outweigh the negative effects (spectral flattening).[968]

Whether the positive effects of multiple channels of compression outweigh the negative effects depends on how much audibility is achieved in the reference condition. A net advantage for multichannel compression is thus least likely for sounds that in the single channel condition are comfortably loud and have been amplified by an appropriate gain-frequency response shape. An advantage for multichannel compression over single-channel compression is most likely for very low and very high input levels, but these conditions have not been adequately investigated. (Multichannel compression enables different gain-frequency responses to be achieved at low versus high levels, thus increasing the range of sound levels over which good audibility and comfort can be simultaneously achieved, without using excessively high compression ratios.)

The advantages are, however, unlikely to be large for most patients. One recent extensive laboratory and field study[446] found that, overall, subjects slightly preferred single-channel compression to multichannel compression. For those with steeply sloping loss, two-channel compression was preferred to single-channel compression in real life. For all subject groups, speech scores obtained in the laboratory were insignificantly different for 1-, 2- and 4-channel systems. An overwhelming conclusion was that for most subjects, the choice of number of channels of compression was not an important issue.

There are many reasons other than the use of multichannel compression for choosing a multichannel hearing aid. A multichannel structure enables the gain-frequency response to be most easily and flexibly controlled. Effective strategies for noise suppression rely on being able to control the gain independently in different frequency regions. Some schemes for feedback suppression are based on a multichannel compression structure (see Section 7.3).

Overall, it seems probable that, for most patients, multichannel compression will not have marked advantages or disadvantages compared to single-channel compression. Overall, there are no strong reasons *not* to use multichannel compression provided compression ratios greater than 3:1 are avoided. A significant intelligibility advantage is more likely to be found for patients with a steeply sloping hearing loss. It may turn out that for other patients there will be intelligibility advantages at very low or high input levels, but further research is required before this could be confidently asserted. The full advantages of multichannel compression may not emerge until the aid wearer has had considerable listening experience.[966]

Note that the discussion in this section compares multichannel versus single-channel compression. For low input levels, both multi- and single-channel compression offer intelligibility substantially greater than that available from linear amplification. For high input levels they both result in greater comfort.[537]

6.6   Concluding Comments

It is clear from the preceding section that one cannot yet draw any well founded conclusions about which compression rationale is superior, or even which is superior for hearing-impaired people with particular characteristics (although many people do make assertions along these lines). Why has research not provided answers that are more definite? Part of the problem has been the difficulty, until recently, of comparing different strategies on the same people in their own, realistic listening environments. If the listening environment is highly controlled (or indeed, contrived) almost any compression scheme can be made to look superior to another scheme by a judicious choice of the experimental conditions. The advent of multi-memory programmable hearing aids, and the increased flexibility of digital aids is making realistic research easier. The second part of the problem is that one cannot evaluate a rationale in isolation. Each rationale to be compared has to be implemented for each subject, with appropriate choices made for each compression parameter and for every other amplification characteristic (see Chapter 9). One can never be certain whether a different conclusion would be reached if different choices of amplification characteristics had been made. The result of this is that we will probably have to live with some uncertainty about the best processing scheme (even out of those that are already available) for some time to come. What is clear, however, is that many forms of compression have advantages over linear amplification.

CHAPTER SEVEN

ADVANCED SIGNAL PROCESSING SCHEMES FOR HEARING AIDS

Synopsis

Other than the use of a remote microphone located near the source, multi-microphone directional arrays (including directional microphones) are the most effective way to improve intelligibility in noisy environments. Until recently, directional microphones used in hearing aids have been fixed arrays, meaning that they have the same directional pattern (represented by their polar response) in all situations. These fixed arrays have used subtractive processing in which the signals from two microphones, or the sounds entering the two inlet ports of a single microphone, are subtracted to form a difference signal. A recent development has been the commercial availability of fixed additive arrays, in which the outputs of multiple microphones worn across the upper chest are added together. A more significant development is the introduction of adaptive arrays. These arrays have directional properties that vary dependent on the location, relative to the aid wearer, of background noises.

Adaptive arrays automatically alter the way they combine the signals picked up by two or more microphones so as to have minimum sensitivity for sounds coming from the direction of dominant nearby noise sources. The multiple microphones that provide the input signals can be mounted on one side of the head or on both sides of the head. Like fixed arrays, adaptive arrays work most effectively in situations where there is a low level of reverberant sound.

Single-microphone schemes for noise reduction are much less effective. These schemes, such as Wiener Filtering and Spectral Subtraction, effectively decrease the gain at any frequency at which the signal-to-noise ratio (SNR) is relatively poor. The two schemes have in common the need to make separate estimates of the signal spectrum and the noise spectrum. They differ in how they use these estimates, but some varieties of Wiener Filtering have acoustic effects identical to some varieties of Spectral Subtraction. Although they can improve sound comfort, and the overall SNR, these schemes do not improve the SNR in any narrow frequency band. Consequently, neither do they significantly improve intelligibility, except for unusual background noises.

Feedback oscillation can be made less likely by several electronic means. One simple technique is to decrease the gain only for those frequencies and input levels at which oscillation is likely. A second technique is to modify the phase response of the hearing aid so that the phase shift needed for oscillation does not occur at any frequency for which there is enough gain to cause feedback oscillation. A third technique involves adding a controlled internal feedback path that has the gain and phase response needed to cancel the accidental leakage around the earmold or shell. A final technique involves making the output frequency different from the input frequency. The first and third of these techniques are already available in advanced hearing aids.

For people with severe or profound hearing loss at high frequencies, one way to make the high-frequency components of speech audible is to shift these components to lower frequencies. While such frequency transposition can guarantee audibility, it does not necessarily guarantee better intelligibility, as the speech components shifted down in frequency may interfere with perception of the speech components originally in this lower frequency range. Improvements in intelligibility have, nevertheless, been reported.

The most complex forms of amplification, which are not yet commercially available, involve enhancing speech in ways that vary from one speech sound to the next. These methods include exaggerating the peaks and troughs in the spectrum of a speech sound, lengthening and shortening the duration of particular sounds, and increasing the amount of amplification whenever a consonant occurs. On the evidence available so far, however, none of these techniques will produce a large increase in intelligibility compared to conventional amplification.

This chapter describes several advanced processing schemes for hearing aids. Schemes involving multiple microphones are considered in the greatest detail because they have the most proven benefits, and appear to offer the greatest potential to provide further benefits. These schemes are likely to become increasingly available in commercial hearing aids over the next few years.

7.1 Multi-Microphone and Other Directional Hearing Aids

There are only two proven ways of increasing intelligibility above that obtainable with a well-fitted conventional hearing aid delivering sound at a comfortable level. One way is to move the hearing aid microphone (or some auxiliary microphone) closer to the source. This increases the level of direct sound compared to reverberant sound and background noise, as discussed in Section 3.5. Unfortunately, moving closer to the source, or positioning a remote microphone near the source, is not always practical.

The other proven solution is to use some type of directional microphone. Directional microphones can be constructed from a single microphone with two entry ports or by combining the electrical outputs from two or more microphones, as explained in Section 2.2.4. A microphone or group of microphones with more than one entry port is often referred to as a *microphone array* or as a *beamforming array*. Microphone arrays can be classified into two broad types: those that have directional characteristics that do not

vary from moment to moment (*fixed arrays*), and those that adapt to the environment in such a way as to minimize the pick-up of noise coming from particular directions (*adaptive arrays*). These are covered in the next two sections.

7.1.1 Fixed directional arrays

Fixed arrays, including conventional directional microphones, achieve their directivity by linearly combining the outputs that correspond to the pressure picked up at each port. A linear combination is achieved by filtering each output and adding it to, or subtracting it from, the other outputs. Frontal directivity is achieved if these outputs combine in a more additive manner when the signal is in front of the array than when it is located at most (or hopefully all) other directions. For example, waveforms from two outputs will combine in a more additive manner when the waveforms are in phase than when there is a phase difference between the waveforms. There are two basic types of fixed arrays: additive arrays and subtractive arrays.[a]

The conventional directional microphone, and the two-microphone array that is increasingly being used in BTE and ITE hearing aids, are both examples of *subtractive arrays*. With conventional directional microphones, the subtraction occurs mechanically as sounds from each port press on opposite sides of the diaphragm. When two separate, one-port microphones are used, the electrical outputs of each microphone are subtracted after the output of the rearward microphone has been

---

[a]   More generally, a fixed array can incorporate addition, subtraction, amplification, phase shifts, and time delays.

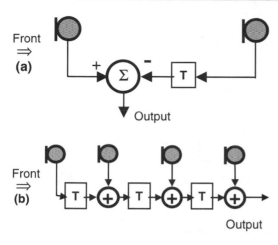

Figure 7.1 (a) Block diagram of a subtractive directional microphone comprised of either a single microphone with two ports, or two separate microphones with one port each. The negative sign next to one of the inputs of the summer indicates that the two signals are subtracted. (b) A delay-and-add directional microphone array with four ports.

electrically delayed, as shown in Figure 7.1(a). The mechanism by which this delay-and-subtract process produces more sensitivity in the forward direction than in any other direction has already been covered in Section 2.2.4.

The subtractive array provides directivity down to an indefinitely low frequency. Unfortunately, the frontal sensitivity also decreases as frequency decreases (i.e. a low cut), and as port spacing decreases, because for low-frequency sounds, the spacing between the ports is much less than the wavelength of the sound. Consequently, the two signals being subtracted become closer in phase, and the difference between them gets smaller. Figure 7.2 shows the calculated frontal sensitivity for two different port-spacings.

A different problem can occur for very high-frequency sounds: the port spacing can approach half a wavelength, and for frontally

incident sounds, the two signals being subtracted will be almost in phase. They will then cancel each other completely. Consequently, the array will be insensitive to sounds coming from the front. As shown in Figure 7.2, however, for small port spacings as used in modern ITE and BTE hearing aids, the frequency at which there is no frontal sensitivity is well above the usual amplification range of hearing aids. If an excessively large port spacing is used, combining the delay with a low-pass filter can solve the problem of decreased frontal sensitivity at high frequencies, just as it is within the conventional directional microphone. This filtering causes the rear port (or microphone) to effectively close at high frequencies. There is then no problem with high-frequency frontal sensitivity, but the microphone is not directional at these frequencies.

Frontal sensitivity decreases as the spacing between the ports decreases (though directivity is maintained). If frontal sensitivity decreases too much, the internal noise of the microphone (see Section 2.2.3) becomes too apparent by comparison with the wanted signal.[b] Consequently, directional microphones can be used only in hearing aids large enough to accept the necessary port spacing.

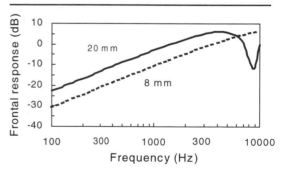

Figure 7.2 Frontal sensitivity of a two-port (or two-microphone) subtractive directional microphone relative to the sensitivity of an equivalent single-port microphone. The parameter shown is the port spacing. The internal delay needed to produce a cardioid polar response has been assumed.

[b]   Subtractive arrays, such as conventional directional microphones, always have greater internal noise at low- and mid-frequencies than omni-directional microphones.

Currently, they are mostly used in BTE and ITE hearing aids. They are never likely to be used in CIC aids, because diffraction by the pinna creates a complex sound field near the faceplate of the hearing aid. Two-port directional microphones have a directivity index up to 5 dB, as shown in Figure 2.9. Every decibel of AI-weighted directivity index (see Section 2.2.4) means a 1 dB improvement in signal-to-noise ratio (SNR), hence an improvement in speech intelligibility of approximately ten percentage points for sentence material.

The *additive array* (also called a *delay-and-add array*) works on a different principle. Instead of trying to produce zero sensitivity for sounds coming from behind, the additive array produces the maximum possible sensitivity for sounds coming from the front, and less sensitivity for all other directions. Figure 7.1(b) shows that the output of each microphone is delayed by an amount T and is then added to the output from the next microphone in line. Consider what happens if the electrical delay T equals the time taken for sound to travel acoustically from one microphone port to the next. Sounds arriving from the front first reach microphone 1, and then continue on to microphone 2. The output from microphone 1, after being electrically delayed, reaches the adder at just the same time as the output from microphone 2 (whose input was acoustically delayed with respect to the first microphone). Consequently, the two signals combine perfectly in phase. The same process happens at the next adder, and then again at the next. The voltage of the final output is thus four times as great (corresponding to a 12 dB increase) as the voltage coming out of any one of the microphones.

But what happens if the sounds arrive from any other direction? When sounds arrive from the side, for example, they reach all four microphones simultaneously. Because of the electrical delays, the two signals going into each adder will no longer be in phase with each other. Consequently, they will not combine as constructively as do sounds from the front. The array must therefore be less sensitive for other directions than it is for sounds from the front.[c] Additive arrays are effective only for high-frequency sounds: i.e., those for which the length of the array is greater than, or comparable to, a quarter-wavelength. For low-frequency sounds, all the microphone signals, and all the adder inputs, will be approximately in phase no matter what direction the sound comes from. They are thus not effective for ITE or BTE aids. Even for a BTE aid with a port spacing of 20 mm, for example, reasonable directivity would be achieved only for frequencies above 4 kHz, so additive arrays require a much bigger style of hearing aid to be worthwhile.

One novel arrangement combined several conventional directional microphones into a delay-and-add array along the side-frames of a pair of spectacles.[826, 827] The directional microphones, with their usual cardioid pattern, contributed directivity at low frequencies and the delay-and-add beamformer contributed directivity at high frequencies. With a total array length of 100 mm the combination had a directivity index, averaged across frequency, of 7.5 dB. At a rate of 10% intelligibility per decibel of SNR improvement, this is sufficient to make the difference between understanding almost nothing and understanding almost everything.

Fixed arrays can also be classified according to the physical arrangement of the microphones. Using terms borrowed from naval warfare, the microphones in an *end-fire array* are in a line pointing towards the source, whereas those in a *broadside array* are in a line perpendicular to the direction from which the wanted sound comes, as shown in Figure 7.3.

---

[c]   The array can be made even more directional by using electronic delays slightly longer than the corresponding acoustical delays between microphones. This is referred to as an *oversteered array* because as the internal delays are increased from zero, the direction of maximum sensitivity is *steered* from a direction perpendicular to the array through to a direction in line with the array (Cox, Zeskind & Kooij, 1986; Kates & Weiss, 1996).

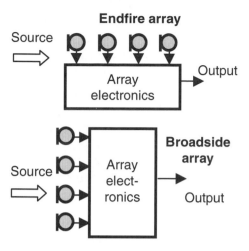

Figure 7.3 End-fire and broadside microphone arrays.

For either type of array, the directivity index generally increases as the number of microphones and the array length increases. For a given number of microphones and array size, however, end-fire arrays are more directional than broadside arrays.[834, d] The reason for this is easy to understand: The end-fire array has its maximum sensitivity in only one direction, whereas there are many directions in three-dimensional space that are at right-angles to a broad-side array (e.g. in front, above, below and behind).

In practice, a broadside array could be mounted across the front of a head on a spectacle frame, on top of the head on a headband, or on the upper chest on a pendant. One commercially available broadside array worn on the upper chest outputs its signal to a neck-loop, which sends a magnetic signal to the hearing aid telecoil. Alternatively, a simple broadside array could be made using one microphone on each side of the head, as in fact happens with a Bi-CROS hearing aid (Section 16.1.2). The signal processing needed for a broadside array is particularly simple: the outputs from each microphone are added. Different directivity patterns are achieved by changing the weights given to each output.[826]

7.1.2   Adaptive arrays

Unlike a fixed array, the directivity pattern of an adaptive array varies depending on where an unwanted noise (referred to as a *jammer,* by analogy with a deliberate interference to radio transmission) is coming from. An adaptive array attempts to make its sensitivity as close as possible to zero for sounds coming from the direction of any dominant noise source or sources, while retaining high sensitivity for frontal sources.

The simple directional microphone shown in Figure 7.1(a) can be turned into an adaptive array by varying the delay time, T, as shown in Figure 7.4. The circuit automatically varies T in whichever direction decreases the total power at the output, after allowing for the effect that variation of T has on the frontal sensitivity of the microphone. Because the power of the output signal equals the signal power plus the noise power, the total power will be minimized when there is no noise in the mixture. If there is a single nearby jammer, T will quickly settle down to the value that minimizes the microphone sensitivity in the direction of this jammer. Figure 2.7 shows several possible responses, but these are just examples from a complete family of responses. The processing scheme shown in Figure 7.4 can position nulls at any angle from 90° through 180° to 270°.

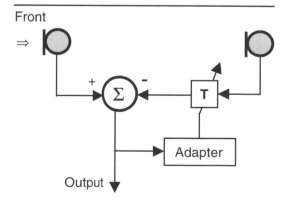

Figure 7.4 A simple adaptive directional microphone with steerable nulls.

d   When arrays are placed on the head and body, their directivity is affected, and it will not necessarily be true that an end-fire array is superior to a broadside array of the same size (Greenberg & Zurek, 1992).

One factor that limits the performance of such a simple adaptive array is that the neat, precisely positioned nulls shown in Figure 2.7 occur only for a directional microphone that is well away from all obstacles, such as a head. The head affects the polar pattern of the microphone (as shown in Figure 2.8b) by different amounts at different frequencies, so the nulls occur at different angles for different frequencies. Consequently, it is not possible to simultaneously remove all frequency components of the jammer. Solutions to this problem involve replacing the simple delay with a more complex circuit that delays different frequencies by different amounts.

The basis of most sophisticated, adaptive, multi-microphone noise-reduction circuits is the **Widrow Least Mean Squares (LMS)** algorithm, with the structure shown in Figure 7.5.[956] The top microphone picks up a mixture of signal plus noise. The bottom microphone is assumed to be positioned such that it picks up only noise. This microphone is referred to as the reference microphone. It is assumed that noise entering the two microphones comes from the same source, but reaches the two microphones by different paths, and thus has a different waveform at each microphone. If the noise at the reference microphone could be filtered to compensate for the difference in acoustic paths taken by the noise to the two microphones, this filtered noise could be subtracted from the mixture of signal and noise picked up by the main microphone. If the filtering and subtraction were perfectly carried out, the result would be speech alone.

The filter approximates the ideal shape by adaptively changing its response in such a way as to minimize the power of the output signal (hence the term LMS, as power is proportional to the square of the signal). Systems typically adapt to this response in less than one second.[e] The Widrow LMS system can increase SNR by 30 dB or more, provided a suitable reference signal is available. For head-worn hearing aids, however, it is not possible to position a single microphone so that it picks up only noise. If the reference microphone contains some signal, the filter will adapt to a shape that partially cancels both the signal and the noise. The situation is not hopeless, however.

Figure 7.6 shows one way in which a noise reference can be obtained in a fully head-worn hearing aid. This array, known as a **Griffiths-Jim beamformer,** is intended to work with one microphone on each side of the head.[336] When the wanted signal is directly in front of the person, there should be little signal coming out of the subtracter in the lower chain, because the outputs from the two microphones should cancel. Consequently, this subtracter output contains mostly noise. The adder in the top chain, however, outputs a mixture of signal and noise. The parts of the Griffiths-Jim beamformer to the right of the dotted line, which are identical to the Widrow adaptive noise-reduction scheme shown in

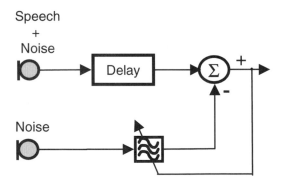

Figure 7.5 The Widrow Least Mean Squares adaptive noise reduction scheme, based on a reference microphone that picks up only the noise. The fixed delay compensates for the delay inherent in the adaptive filter.

---

[e]   The designer can select any adaptation time. If the adaptation is too quick, however, the filter will change excessively when the direction of the noise changes even slightly, and speech quality will deteriorate. If the adaptation is too slow, the filter will not be able to keep up with a changing source position, or movements of the hearing aid wearer's head.

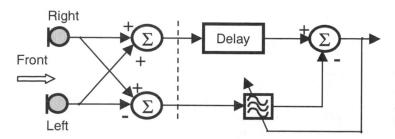

Figure 7.6 A Griffiths-Jim adaptive noise canceller, whereby the two microphone outputs are added in the top chain but subtracted in the bottom chain.

Figure 7.5, then perform the filtering and subtraction necessary to improve the SNR.

Adaptive filtering of the type just described works extremely well under certain circumstances. In particular, where there is only one noise source, no reverberation, and a very poor SNR, the adaptive filter can change its characteristics so that the directivity pattern of the array has an almost perfect null in the direction of the noise. Under these favorable circumstances, the SNR can be improved by as much as 30 dB.[700] There would, however, be few real-life circumstances where improvements this large can be expected. Unfortunately, a beamformer with only two microphones can produce a null in only one direction at a time.[f] Consequently, if there are two noise sources, they both cannot be removed. In general, a beamformer made from n omni-directional microphones can remove only n-1 different noise sources.

Reverberation greatly decreases the effectiveness of adaptive arrays. Unless the wanted talker is very close, reverberation will cause significant speech energy to arrive from all directions. Consequently, the noise reference signal will contain speech as well as noise. This mixture makes it difficult for the filter to adapt, thus reducing the effectiveness of the noise canceling. The subtracter will also remove some of the speech as well as noise, and will thus affect speech quality. The beamformer can be modified in various ways to minimize, but not totally avoid, these difficulties. In one of these modifications, a

speech/non-speech detector, based on the more pulsatile nature and/or overall level of speech signals, is used to stop the adaptive filter from changing its response whenever speech is believed to be present.[332, 357, 908] In another modification, the noise canceler is preceded by another adaptive filter that is used to remove as much speech as possible from the noise.[916] This other adaptive filter adapts only when speech *is* present. By creating such a reference signal that has as *little* speech in it as possible, the main adaptive filter has a much better chance of removing noise.

The presence of reverberation also means that the echoes from a single sound will arrive at the hearing aid for some time after the direct wave arrives. These echoes can be removed only if the adaptive filter is sufficiently complex to store and combine sounds that arrived perhaps many hundreds of milliseconds before.[332] Such complex filters take longer to adapt.

As an example of the substantial benefits obtainable from adaptive filtering, and the limitation that reverberation places on these benefits, Figure 7.7 shows results from Hoffman et al. (1994) for a three- and a seven-microphone array mounted around the forehead.

There are a number of ways in which the two (or more) different combinations of signal and noise (to the left of the dotted line in Figure 7.6) can be obtained. What they have in common is that they must originate from microphones located at two (or more) points in

---

[f]   Actually, nulls can simultaneously occur in other directions, but the beamformer has no control over the directions of those other nulls once it has positioned the first null.

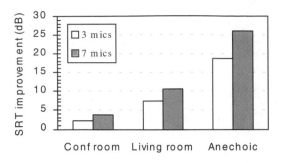

Figure 7.7 Improvement in speech reception threshold for an adaptive array relative to a single microphone. The experiment used frontal speech and a single noise masker at 45 degrees from the front in three simulated environments that differed in the amount of reverberant sound relative to the direct sound. From Hoffman et al (1994).

Noise-suppression systems that combine the outputs from hearing aids on both sides of the head, however, have increased potential to improve sound quality in reverberant situations. One such processing scheme attenuates any narrow frequency band where the signals picked up at each ear do not show the phase difference and coherence appropriate to the direction of the dominant signal.[14, 487] Such processing improves sound quality, but does not improve intelligibility in noise, except to the extent that it also acts as a directional microphone.[71, 487]

The techniques so far described adapt by minimizing the power at some point in the processing scheme. They have the aim of maximizing the ratio of a speech signal arriving from the front to signals arriving from other directions. These schemes must make assumptions about the location of the speech source (e.g. it is directly in front) and/or about the nature of the wanted signal (e.g. it is speech and therefore pulses in amplitude) and/ or about the noise (e.g. it is continuous). A more general technique, referred to as **blind channel separation** or **blind source separation,** is able to separate signals of any type arriving from different directions, as shown in Figure 7.8.[430, 948] The only necessary

space, whether these are on the same, or opposite sides (or front!) of the listener's head. One scheme uses a rearward-facing directional microphone to provide the noise reference and an omni-directional microphone to provide the mixture of speech and noise.[951] Alternatively, the main signal can come from a forward-facing directional microphone. These arrangements have the advantage that all the components can be mounted on one side of the head.

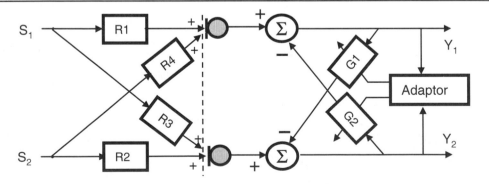

Figure 7.8 Blind source separation of two sources, S_1 and S_2, occurs when the two adaptive filters, G1 and G2, adapt to the response shapes that compensate for the room transmission characteristics, R1, R2, R3 and R4, from each source to each microphone. Note that everything to the right of the dotted line is in the hearing aid, whereas the blocks to the left are the transfer functions of the transmission paths within the room. When properly adapted, the response of G1 = R3/R1 and G2 = R4/R2. The output Y_1 then does not contain any components of S_2. The blocks G1 and G2 can alternatively be feed-forward blocks rather than feed-back blocks.

assumption is that the original sources are statistically independent. This assumption will always be true if the signals originate from different talkers or other sources of noise. The adaptation process varies the filters in the direction needed to maximize the statistical independence of the output signals.

If the input to the Blind Source Separation processing scheme comprises n microphones, each picking up a different mixture of the original sources, the processing scheme can potentially separate up to n sources. Which of the n possible outputs should finally be presented to the hearing aid wearer? To decide this, some assumption must be made, such as selecting the source with the highest level, or the source with the direction closest to the front. Like the other adaptive schemes, this scheme works better in non-reverberant situations than in reverberant situations. In non-reverberant situations, the adaptive filters needed are much simpler, and hence adapt more quickly and accurately.

Where there are many noise sources, adaptive arrays cannot provide better performance than a fixed array, and may provide worse performance. Any adaptive processing scheme that alters its amplification characteristics rapidly while speech is present is likely to introduce unpleasant artifacts to the speech. The hearing aid wearer perceives the rapidly changing response shape as added noises with a musical quality (understandably so, because narrowband components of the signal are suddenly being increased or decreased in level). The artifacts are minimized by slowing the rate at which the processing adapts and/or by not doing any adaptation when speech is estimated to be present, as explained earlier. Adaptive arrays can also inadvertently cancel the speech at some frequencies if the array is not pointed directly at the source. For most implementations, such *misteering* will occur whenever the listener is not looking directly at the source, but its effects can be minimized by statistical techniques.[391]

One advantage of adaptive arrays over fixed arrays concerns the accuracy with which they are constructed. Some fixed arrays (notably subtractive arrays) rely on the separate microphones having characteristics that are well matched to each other. Because adaptive arrays monitor the output signal, the adaptive filter can partially compensate for any mismatch between the microphones.

Although fixed and adaptive directional arrays have been discussed separately in this chapter, they can be combined by using the outputs of two or more fixed arrays as the inputs of an adaptive array.[210, 488, 916] Performance is generally superior to the performance of either array alone for nearby signals and jammers in non-reverberant situations. Adaptive processing is unlikely to provide any additional benefits in reverberant situations in which the signal and/or noise lie beyond the critical distance (the distance at which the direct sound level equals the reverberant sound level).[332] When the SNR is good, adaptive processing can decrease the SNR if adaptation occurs when the speech is present.

7.2   Single-Microphone Noise Reduction

Improving intelligibility when only a single microphone has picked up the signal and noise, is a *much* harder problem. As Levitt (1997) has insightfully said:

> *Our understanding of this problem is so limited that we have not only been unsuccessful in finding a solution, but we do not even know whether it is possible to improve the intelligibility of speech in noise by any significant amount.*

Single-microphone noise reduction has been introduced in Section 6.3.7. In that section, we saw that filtering can be used to decrease the gain in any frequency region where the SNR is poor. It is common for single-input noise-reduction systems to improve SNR when the levels of the signal and noise are measured objectively with a sound level meter. Figure 6.12 provides an example where the SNR at the output will be much greater than that at the input. Except in those cases where the noise is very restricted in bandwidth (compared to the speech), these improved SNRs have not resulted in any increase in intelligibility.[525, 526, 527, 535, 649] The reasons underlying this have already been dealt with in Section 6.3.7. Essentially, if a hearing aid has a single microphone port, then when a noise and signal occur at the same time and at the same frequency there is no known way by which they can be separated.

In principle, improving intelligibility in noise with only a single input relies on the signal and noise having components sufficiently different in frequency or in time to be separable by signal processing, but not by a person with impaired hearing. This *seems* like an achievable goal, especially for people with severe and profound hearing impairment, as these people have the most decreased frequency and temporal discrimination abilities. When noise is restricted to a narrow frequency region, single microphone noise reduction can lead to a substantial increase in intelligibility.[739, 911]

There are several ways to perform single-input noise reduction, but most systems use a variety of either *Wiener filtering* or *spectral subtraction*, and the basics of these are as follows.

A Wiener Filter is a filter whose gain at each frequency depends in a particular way on the SNR at that frequency. Specifically, the gain equals the signal power divided by the sum of the signal power plus noise power. It can be shown mathematically that of all possible filter shapes, the Wiener Filter makes the waveform at the filter output as similar as possible to the signal (without noise) at the input. The problem with making such a filter is evident: how can the filter's gain be calculated when background noise prevents us knowing the power of the signal at any frequency? All we know is the instantaneous

power of the signal plus noise, because that is what our single microphone is picking up.

The answer is that the signal power has to be estimated. When the wanted signal is speech from a single talker, the amplitude of the speech pulses up and down in a distinctive manner. The frequency spectrum also changes in a distinctive manner, and these characteristics can be used to make a *speech/non-speech detector*. If we can estimate the spectral power (averaged over some preceding short or long time) of the noise when there is no speech, and also of the speech plus noise, then we can subtract the first of these from the second to estimate the power of the speech alone. Figure 7.9 shows the block diagram of a Wiener Filter that uses this principle. The filter is being controlled by a signal that reflects the SNR at each frequency.

A Spectral Subtraction system "works" by subtracting the magnitude (i.e. the amplitude) of the noise spectrum from the magnitude of the speech plus noise spectrum. If both magnitudes are known exactly, then the difference will be the magnitude of the speech spectrum alone. The obvious problem with this system is determining the spectrum of the noise, because the microphone picks up the speech and noise combined.

One solution is to estimate the noise spectrum currently present by averaging the noise spectrum that was present during some preceding moments in time, just as for Wiener filtering. Of course, we can measure this preceding spectrum only if we know when the noise was present by itself. Consequently, the Spectral Subtraction system also needs a speech/non-speech detector, as shown in Figure 7.10. Only the magnitudes of the speech plus noise signal are corrected by the processing. There is no known way to estimate what the phase of the speech alone should be, so the final inverse Fourier Transform usually uses the phase of the original speech plus noise. If the spectral

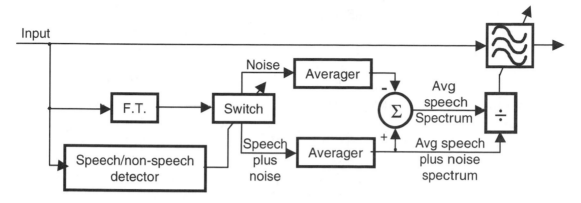

Figure 7.9 A Wiener Filter incorporating a Fourier Transform (F.T) to calculate the spectrum of the combined speech and noise. A speech/non-speech detector classifies the spectrum as noise or speech plus noise, and thus enables the average spectral power of the speech to be estimated.

subtraction process works perfectly, the magnitude of the output spectrum equals the magnitude of the speech spectrum alone, but the phase spectrum remains corrupted by the noise. This adversely affects the quality of the speech, but may be preferable to not removing any of the noise.

A greater problem for Spectral Subtraction (and for Wiener Filtering) is that the noise spectrum is estimated based on the noise characteristics during the preceding seconds (or fractions of a second). Unfortunately, just like speech, background noise can change its character entirely within a short time. In this case, both types of noise reducers are trying to remove a noise that is no longer present!

Furthermore, they know nothing, and can therefore do nothing, about some new noise that has just commenced, or about noise that has just changed its character. Both types of system are most suitable for steady noises (technically called **stationary noises**). These would include some machinery noises, and to a lesser extent, the babble from a large number of other people. Lessening the effects of a single competing talker would be especially difficult with either Wiener Filtering or Spectral Subtraction.

Although Wiener Filtering and Spectral Subtraction may look very different, they have similar effects on a noisy signal. Both decrease the gain most at those frequencies

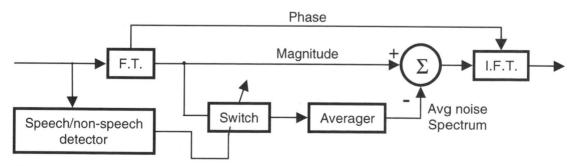

Figure 7.10 A Spectral Subtraction noise reduction system incorporating a Fourier Transform to calculate the power spectrum, a speech/non-speech detector to enable the average spectral power of the noise to be estimated, and an Inverse Fourier Transform to turn the corrected spectrum back into a waveform.

where the SNR is worst, and leave the signal unaltered when there is little noise present. In fact, for some implementations of each, they have mathematically identical effects on the input signal.[535] The precise acoustic effects of each scheme depend on the implementation details.

One important detail is the frequency resolution with which signal and noise power is determined. If a very narrow bandwidth is used, SNR will be greatest at the harmonic frequencies of sustained periodic sounds like vowels. The resulting filter shape will have a high gain at the frequency of each harmonic, and will provide a large attenuation mid-way between harmonics. Because of its alternating, spiky shape, such a filter is referred to as a *comb filter*. Comb filters are very effective at removing noise, but during rapidly changing elements of speech, such as formant transitions, they are also likely to distort the speech signal. Comb filters can be generated by other techniques, such as basing the filter shape on the fundamental frequency of the speech.[540] Unfortunately, the accuracy of fundamental-frequency extraction is adversely affected by noise, and consequently the comb filter passes inappropriate frequencies just when it is most needed.

In conclusion, we must remember that while Wiener Filtering and Spectral Subtraction can definitely increase SNR, and can increase listening comfort, they have not yet delivered improved intelligibility in commonly occurring noises. Still, researchers are hopeless optimists, so despite 30 years of no increase in intelligibility, the search goes on. There are, however, great opportunities for creativity in the combination of Wiener Filters, Spectral Subtraction, and multiple microphones.

7.3 Feedback Reduction

The cause of feedback oscillation has already been discussed in Section 4.6.1. In the following sections we will examine several electronic methods for addressing the problem of feedback. Any of the following methods can help, but none of them can banish feedback oscillations entirely. The need for carefully made impressions and earmolds or shells is unlikely to disappear! More positively, the sometimes impossible task of making a mold or shell open enough to avoid occlusion problems, but closed enough to avoid feedback, is likely to get considerably easier as the following techniques become more widely available.

7.3.1 Feedback reduction by gain-frequency response control

For feedback oscillation of a specific frequency to occur, the gain from microphone inlet to ear canal must be greater than the attenuation from the ear canal back to the microphone at that frequency. Furthermore, at this same frequency, the phase shift around the entire loop must be close to an integral number of periods. Not surprisingly, one way to avoid feedback oscillations is to decrease the gain at all those frequencies where these conditions are met. This can be done in several ways.

The simplest way is to turn the volume control or fitter gain control down below the point required by the patient. This is obviously

---

Reasons for using electronic feedback control

An effective electronic feedback control is useful in the following circumstances:

- When more gain is needed. This is particularly useful for people with severe and profound losses, or people who would like a smaller hearing aid style than could otherwise be provided without feedback.
- When a more open earmold or earshell is needed. This is particularly useful for people with mild loss at low frequencies and severe loss at higher frequencies.

unsatisfactory, as it will give the patient inadequate loudness, audibility, and intelligibility. A better alternative is to decrease the gain at only those frequencies where feedback oscillation is a possibility. This is most likely to be at or near the peaks of the gain-frequency response curve, so anything that decreases the gain at these peaks without reducing the gain elsewhere is likely to be beneficial. Acoustic damping in the sound tube meets this criterion particularly well (see Section 5.5). Unfortunately, it may not always be possible to damp the particular peaks causing the feedback whistling without excessively decreasing the gain in the frequency region around some other resonances.

Instead of decreasing the amplitude of a peak, the frequency of a peak can sometimes be changed. As discussed in Section 2.6.2, variation of the output impedance of the final amplifier can change the center frequency of the receiver resonance, and the phase response around this frequency, which may assist in decreasing feedback. This is not a reliable method, because the feedback oscillation may not originate from frequencies around the receiver mechanical resonance, and because the degree of variation is limited.

Multichannel hearing aids provide a more reliable way to decrease gain in only one frequency region. The degree of control over the gain-frequency response is extremely coarse, however, unless the hearing aid has many parallel channels. If there are only a few channels, gain may be decreased over an unnecessarily wide frequency range, again resulting in inadequate audibility. Figure 7.11 shows the gain-frequency response of a four-channel hearing aid that has had the gain decreased in one band to decrease the incidence of feedback.

Several hearing aids currently available apply this type of feedback control, and apply it in a clever way. Often, feedback occurs only when the volume control is increased above the aid wearer's usual setting, or for wide dynamic range compression hearing aids, at

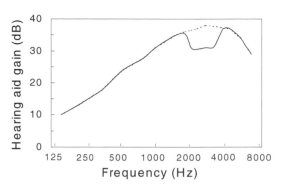

Figure 7.11 The gain-frequency response of a (hypothetical) four-channel hearing aid, where feedback oscillation has been avoided by decreasing the gain of the band from 2 kHz to 4 kHz (solid line) from the original response (dotted line).

low input levels. In such cases it is necessary to decrease the gain in a narrow frequency region only under these specific conditions. Very flexible hearing aids, which tend to be digital hearing aids, limit the maximum gain that can be achieved in each frequency region. (The limit depends on the tightness of fit of the earmold or ear shell.) When feedback is not a problem, the full desired frequency response is provided to the hearing aid wearer. When the overall gain is increased (either manually or automatically) the gain in frequency regions likely to cause oscillations can then be held down to a safe value. The safe value can be determined by:

• the clinician at the time of fitting – this is achieved by the clinician selecting the maximum gain that just avoids oscillation, or by the clinician increasing the compression threshold until oscillation ceases;

• the fitting system at the time of fitting – this is achieved by performing an in-situ feedback test, in which the fitting system automatically raises the gain in each channel until it detects oscillation occurring;

• the hearing aid whenever the hearing aid is worn – this is achieved by the hearing aid reducing the gain in a channel whenever it detects oscillation occurring in that channel.

Digital filters (e.g. Figure 2.17) can provide even finer control of the gain-frequency response shape. Once the frequencies that can cause feedback oscillation are identified, narrow notches can be placed in the gain-frequency response around each of these frequencies. Public address systems have used this technique effectively for many years. It *seems* like this technique should do away with feedback oscillation altogether without excessively reducing audibility.

Unfortunately, the frequencies at which feedback occurs do not remain fixed over time. Remember that oscillations occur at the frequency with the correct phase response. If the earmold were to move a little in the ear, or the person were to move their jaw (and hence their temporo-mandibular joint), wear a hat, or put their hand near their ear, the characteristics of the leakage path can change, so the oscillation frequency can also change. This means that a notch is now needed at some other frequency. Oscillation could be totally prevented only if the notches are wide enough and numerous enough to cover all the possible oscillation frequencies, in which case there may be little gain left at any frequency. The best implementation of such filtering is when the hearing aid continually monitors its own output to detect feedback oscillation, measures the oscillation frequency, and automatically adjusts the gain-frequency response to prevent it from continuing. Such automatic operation is often referred to as *search and destroy* feedback control.

7.3.2   Feedback reduction by phase control

The previous section gave several methods by which the gain of the hearing aid at problem frequencies can be decreased. Some of these methods inadvertently vary the phase response of the amplifier[g]. Depending on luck, this phase variation may help prevent feedback oscillation, or may make it worse! Another method of reducing feedback

oscillation is to intentionally vary the phase response. The aim is to ensure that at any frequency where the gain is large enough to cause oscillations, the phase response around the loop causes the feedback to be negative rather than positive.

Figure 7.12 shows the gain-frequency response and phase-frequency response of the entire *feedback loop* for an ITE hearing aid. This is measured by breaking the connection between the amplifier and the receiver, and then injecting a test signal into the receiver. The test signal travels out of the receiver, back round the leakage path to the microphone, into the amplifier and finally back to the point that normally connects to the receiver. The magnitude and phase of the test signal reaching this point then shows the response of the entire feedback loop. It can be seen that phase is zero at the frequencies of 1200, 3500, and 6000 Hz. Feedback oscillation can therefore occur at any one of these frequencies. Which one depends on the loop gain. For the volume control setting at which the measurement was performed, the loop gain is negative at all frequencies. If the

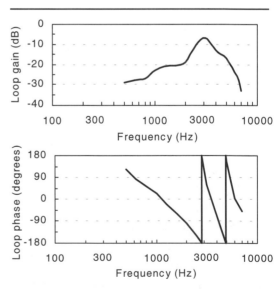

Figure 7.12 Gain-frequency and phase-frequency response of the complete feedback loop for an ITE hearing aid. Redrawn from Hellgren et al., (1999).

---

[g]   Electronic filters affect the phase response of a hearing aid, as well as affecting the gain response.

volume control setting were to be increased, it is evident that of these potential feedback frequencies, the loop gain would first be positive at 3500 Hz. This, therefore, is the most problematic frequency.

If the phase response at 3500 Hz were to be modified so that it was closer to 180° instead of 0°, oscillation would no longer be possible at this frequency. Phase response can be manipulated by adding an ***all-pass filter***: a filter that has the same gain at all frequencies, but which affects the phase at some or all frequencies. Of course, once the first problem frequency has been tamed, (and the gain increased by a few dB) some other frequency will become the problem, and the phase must also be corrected here. Eventually it becomes difficult to simultaneously achieve a satisfactory phase at all frequencies. Like the methods discussed in the preceding sections, this method can thus allow additional gain to be achieved without feedback oscillation but does not remove the problem altogether.

As with the other methods, if the characteristics of the feedback path change, then the required phase manipulations also will change. Devices that continuously (or at least intermittently) monitor the phase shifts needed to avoid feedback are thus more likely to give greater benefit than ones that are adjusted once only at the time of fitting. Hearing aid designers have long used rudimentary control of phase. Reversing the connections to the earphone (when possible) adds 180° to the phase response, which 50% of the time will allow a greater gain to be achieved without oscillation, at least for some settings of the tone controls.

7.3.3   Feedback reduction by feedback path cancellation

The next technique intentionally changes both the gain and phase response of the hearing aid. Rather than manipulating the forward gain of the hearing aid, however, one adds a second, intentional feedback path with just the right gain and phase response to cancel the external leakage path, as shown in Figure 7.13. That is, if at a particular frequency, the two feedback paths leak back the same amount of signal, but these signals have opposite phases, then the two signals fed back will sum to zero, and there is no net feedback. Without any feedback, there can be no oscillation.

This seems like a perfect solution, but like the other solutions, can increase the maximum achievable gain only to a limited extent. To achieve a good cancellation, the gain and phase of the unintentional feedback path must be known with some precision, and changes in these characteristics over time must be allowed for. There are two ways this can be achieved.

In the first method, a test signal is injected, either with or without the amplifier chain being broken.[255] If this is done while the hearing-impaired person is wearing the aid, then whenever the measurement is performed, either the person hears the test signal (and nothing else), or else the test signal appears as a low-level masking noise present along with the amplified sound. The level cannot be too low, or else the measurement cannot be made precisely enough. Amazingly, this seemingly complicated solution has been commercially available in hearing aids for the

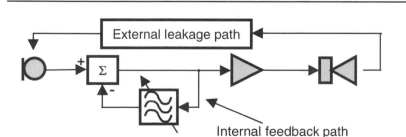

Figure 7.13 Internal feedback path added to cancel the effects of the external, unintentional leakage path.

severely and profoundly impaired for some years. The scheme allows the gain to be increased by approximately 10 dB before feedback commences.[254] The hearing aid uses a continuous noise, approximately 12 dB below the speech level, as a test signal. Its major disadvantage is that if the hearing aid wearer has too large a dynamic range, the test signal is audible or even annoying. This is least likely to be a problem if the aid wearer has a profound sensorineural hearing aid loss, because such people usually have a very restricted dynamic range. They are thus less likely to hear the test signal.

In the second method, the filter shown in Figure 7.13 automatically adapts in such a way as to minimize any signal that continues at a single frequency for more than a certain amount of time, such as feedback oscillation, or the ringing caused by sub-oscillatory feedback.[263] While the filter is adapting (which it should whenever the leakage path, or the hearing aid gain, changes) the filter may also cancel some of the wanted signal. If the wanted signal is speech this may be evident as a reduction in quality during the second or so that it takes the filter to adapt. Another disadvantage of this form of adaptive feedback control is that the feedback canceler will also cancel other sustained periodic signals, such as somebody whistling continuously. The advantages, however, appear to be substantial. A laboratory measure indicated that an additional 20 dB of gain could be achieved without oscillation when the circuit was activated.[263] Commercially available hearing aids using this technique can sustain at least an additional 10 dB of gain.[338]

7.3.4 Feedback reduction by frequency shifting

Feedback oscillation occurs if a sound gets larger every time it goes around the feedback loop. What would happen if a sound came out of the amplifier at a different frequency to that which went in? Because the signal leaking back to the microphone would be at a different frequency from the original input, the two sounds could not remain continuously in phase with each other, and so could not build up in amplitude as effectively. Consequently, the likelihood of feedback would be considerably lessened.

As always, there are disadvantages. To achieve a large increase in gain without oscillation, a large frequency shift is needed.[h] This changes the quality and/or the pitch of the output sound. The method was developed for use in public address systems[779] and has been briefly evaluated in hearing aids.[48] It offers some promise for the future, especially as there are now sophisticated methods for altering the frequencies of speech signals without adversely affecting voice quality.

In conclusion, the advent of digital hearing aids is making it much easier to design complex, continuously adjustable filters. The first three of the above methods for reducing feedback can make good use of such filters. The last method is also most easily achieved by digital manipulation, so there is likely to be an explosion of anti-feedback devices in the near future. Further information about such devices can be found in Agnew (1996).

7.4 Frequency Transposition

Most hearing-impaired people have a greater loss for high-frequency sounds than for low-frequency sounds. For some of these people, their high-frequency loss is so great that they cannot extract any useful information from the high-frequency parts of speech. Because of the distortion associated with hearing loss (see Section 1.1), this unfortunate situation can occur even if the speech is amplified sufficiently to be audible.[147, 392] For most people with sloping losses and high-frequency

---

[h] A frequency shift can be represented as a phase shift that changes with time. A phase-shifted signal can be represented as an in-phase sinusoid plus a second sinusoid phase-shifted by 90°. Thus, even a tone with altered frequency can be thought of as containing a component at the original frequency and phase, and it is this component that will lead to oscillation if the loop gain is high enough.

thresholds of about 70 dB HL or greater, the high-frequency parts of speech apparently contribute no information. Worse still, for some of these people, making the high-frequency parts of speech audible can decrease their ability to recover useful information from the low and mid-frequency parts of the speech signal.[147, 392]

For such people to have any chance of accessing the information that exists only in the high-frequency parts of speech, the information must be moved down to some other frequency region where the person is more able to analyze sounds.[47, 425] This is the basis of *frequency transposition* hearing aids.

The downward shifting can follow a number of rules. A simple technique is to distort sound, such as with pronounced peak clipping. The resulting inter-modulation distortion products occur at frequencies far removed from the frequencies in the input signal, although the spread of frequencies occurs in an uncontrolled manner.[425] In a more sophisticated approach, a certain input range, such as 4 to 8 kHz can be moved down to some lower range, such as 0 to 4 kHz.[918] A modulation process effectively subtracts 4 kHz from each frequency.

The potential problem with this approach is that natural energy from 0 to 4 kHz continues to fall in this range. For sounds with significant energy below and above 4 kHz, such as voiced fricatives, the result may be confusing and ambiguous. For example, does an output component at 1 kHz originate from an input at 1 kHz or from an input at 5 kHz? For an input sound with energy over the whole range, the spectral shape of the output will be a complex mixture of the different input frequency ranges. Important features, like formants, originating in one frequency band may be obscured by speech components originating from the other frequency band. Nonetheless, many people with severe high-frequency hearing loss consider that the scheme improves speech clarity.[918]

Speech cues can also be shifted down in frequency using a *transposing speech vocoder*. In a speech vocoder, speech is filtered into a bank of adjacent narrow bands, and the level within each band is detected. Speech can be re-synthesized by using these levels to modulate the level of narrow bands of noise, or pure tones at the frequency of each original narrow band filter. A *transposing* speech vocoder is constructed by allowing the levels detected from high-frequency bands to modulate low-frequency bands of noise or low-frequency tones.[726]

Not surprisingly, the ability to identify transposed high-frequency consonants improves with training.[726] Even for people who have not received any training, however, transposition of this type allows people to discriminate (i.e. differentiate between) different consonants.[740] Subjects with hearing thresholds greater than 70 dB HL from 4 to 8 kHz benefited from this type of transposition. They could discriminate certain easy contrasts between phonemes but not discriminate certain hard (high-frequency) contrasts.[740]

One way to minimize the problem of transposed sound sharing the same frequency range with unmodified sound is to apply transposition only when the input spectrum is dominated by high-frequency components. Transposed energy will then be available for the sounds for which it is most needed, and will not produce adverse effects when low-frequency sounds are present.[726] Such a scheme increases the intelligibility of stops, fricative and affricates without degrading the intelligibility of nasals and semi-vowels.[726]

Another way to avoid the problem of overlapping spectra is to transpose the entire frequency range by some factor.[895] For example, every input frequency could result in an output frequency that is half the input frequency, such as shown in Figure 7.14. Shifting the entire frequency range avoids the problem of ambiguity, because every input frequency is uniquely associated with only

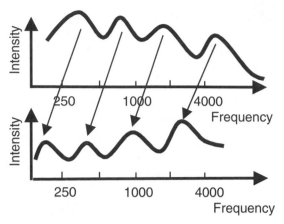

Figure 7.14 Input and output spectra for a frequency transposition scheme in which the output frequency equals half the input frequency. The amplifier also provides some high frequency pre-emphasis. The arrows show the reduction in frequency of each formant.

one output frequency. Furthermore, frequency shifts of this type have the same effect as changing the fundamental frequency and formant frequencies. Such variations occur naturally between talkers.[895] For example, female talkers may sound like male talkers after transposition. Transposition of all frequencies by the same factor is sometimes called *frequency compression*. This term must not be confused with amplitude compression, as discussed throughout Chapter 6.

Unfortunately, lowering the frequencies too far raises another problem. All components will be moved closer together in frequency,[i] and it may therefore be harder for the aid wearer to analyze and identify sounds, even if all components are now audible. This difficulty is all the more likely if the aid wearer has decreased frequency resolution ability in the frequency range to which the signal is transposed. Small improvements in intelligibility have, however, been obtained for some subjects when the frequency was lowered by around 20%.[895]

One commercially available hearing aid transposes different speech sounds downward by different amounts.[204] The *TranSonic* (and its successor the *ImpaCt*) hearing aid transposes high-frequency dominated sounds down by a greater amount than low-frequency dominated sounds. Most commonly, the high-frequency dominated sounds will include all the unvoiced consonants and the low-frequency dominated sounds will include all the vowels. The Transonic hearing aid appears to offer improved speech understanding, relative to a conventional linear hearing aid, for some hearing aid wearers.[204, 689] It is not clear to what extent this improvement is due to transposition, and to what extent it is due to the large low-frequency gain this hearing aid provides, or to the additional boost it provides when it detects a consonant.[588]

An obvious potential difficulty with transposition schemes is that they make speech, and everything else, sound different. It thus takes people some time to become accustomed to, and benefit from, this form of processing.

A side-benefit of frequency transposition is that feedback oscillation is much less likely. Transposition is an extreme version of the frequency-shifting method of feedback reduction discussed in Section 7.3.4.

7.5 Speech Cue Enhancement

For each of the signal processing schemes mentioned so far, including the various compression schemes covered in Chapter 6, the processing applied depends only on the amplitude and spectrum of the input signal. For most of these schemes, a speech signal and a non-speech sound would receive the same amplification if they had the same spectra and variations in intensity. A different class of signal processors is aimed at modifying speech in ways that are believed (or hoped) to make speech sounds easier to

---

[i]   The shifted components are closer together in Hz, although they are same number of octaves apart. Below 1 kHz, it is more relevant to consider the separation in Hz rather than in octaves, because low-frequency critical bands are an approximately equal number of Hz rather than an approximately equal number of octaves.

identify. Any acoustic feature of a speech sound that helps identify that sound, can, in principle, be detected and exaggerated to make recognition of that feature, and hence that sound, easier.

Enhancement of spectral shape

There have been numerous attempts to detect the prominent spectral peaks of speech sounds (usually the formants), and provide them with greater amplification than is provided to the intervening spectral valleys.[11, 31, 32, 98, 234, 809, 852, 912] This is variously called *spectral contrast enhancement* or *spectral sharpening.* The resulting formant structure is sharper, and the locations of formants on a spectrogram become better defined, as shown in Figure 7.15. Unfortunately, improvements in intelligibility have been small or non-existent. It is not as if the detection of spectral peaks is unimportant: When electronic processing is used to smear the shape of the spectrum across frequency, intelligibility in noise is adversely affected.[32, 878, 879] Presumably, the frequency resolution ability of the hearing-impaired test subjects used in some of the spectral enhancement experiments has been so poor that the spectrum of enhanced speech passed on by the cochlea to the rest of the auditory system has been just as smeared and indistinct as it is for unprocessed speech. Indeed, severely hearing-impaired subjects in one study could not detect *any* differences between processed and unprocessed stimuli, even in a paired-comparison listening task, and despite the differences being very evident to normal-hearing subjects.[285] Where differences are discernable, however, there is the potential for benefits to increase with listening experience.[31]

An extreme form of spectral enhancement is *sinusoidal modeling*, in which the few most dominant spectral peaks are replaced by pure tones with the appropriate frequency, amplitude, and perhaps phase (Kates, 1994; Turner, Horwitz & Souza, 1992). The method is very effective at reducing background noise, but has not yet been shown to increase intelligibility. Sinusoidal modeling can also be viewed as a form of speech simplification, as described below.

Enhancement of duration

Another feature that has been modified is the length of vowels. Vowels preceding a voiced consonant tend to be longer than vowels that precede an unvoiced consonant. These differences in the preceding vowel length are one of the cues used by normal hearers to distinguish voiced from unvoiced consonants. Revoile, Holden-Pitt & Pickett (1985) showed that vowel length is a particularly important cue for people with hearing impairment. Exaggeration of the natural differences in length enables hearing-impaired people to better perceive consonant voicing (Revoile et al., 1986). Unfortunately, it is difficult to imagine how this processing could ever be done in real time (i.e. synchronously with the speech signal arriving). The decision to lengthen or shorten the vowel must be made before the vowel ends, and therefore before the final consonant has even reached the hearing aid. Mongomery & Edge (1988) increased consonant duration, though with little success.

In an alternative approach to duration modification, an experimental hearing aid has been developed that lengthens vowels and

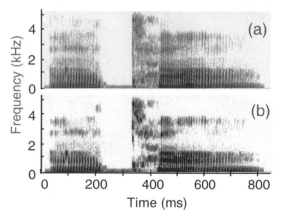

Figure 7.15 Spectrograms of the syllable /ata/ (a) unprocessed and (b) spectrally enhanced, showing more pronounced formants (Fisher, Dillon & Storey, in preparation).

transitions, so that hearing-impaired people have longer to recognize them.[645] Such lengthening alone would make the output of the hearing aid progressively get further and further behind the input. Shortening some of the gaps between speech sounds solves this problem, and so the output "catches up" with the input. This approach increased intelligibility for a small proportion of hearing-impaired people,[645] but decreases intelligibility for normal-hearing people with simulated losses.[646] The negative impact of destroying synchronism between the visual and auditory signals that occurs with this system has not been evaluated to date.

Enhancement of intensity

The ratio of consonant level to vowel level is referred to as the ***consonant-to-vowel ratio***. This ratio is negative in unprocessed speech. The ratio can be increased (i.e. the consonant level made more similar to the vowel level) by increasing the amplification of consonants but not of vowels. Increasing the consonant-to-vowel ratio in this way has little or no effect on the loudness of speech,[612] but increases speech intelligibility.[294, 448, 611, 745, j] When the consonant-to-vowel ratio is increased by decreasing the vowel level, however, speech intelligibility does not generally improve.[769]

It is unquestionable that increasing the level of some consonants makes processed speech more intelligible than unprocessed speech. However, linear high-frequency emphasis and wide dynamic range compression each also increase the level of weak consonants relative to the level of vowels.[383, 731] It has not yet been established that particularly targeting consonants (which requires very complex processing) will give significantly better results than conventional hearing aid amplification comprising compression and high-frequency emphasis. Another consideration is that all of these forms of processing should

be advantageous only in those situations where the audibility of consonants was limited by the aid wearer's thresholds rather than by background noise.

Intensity enhancement has also been linked to the rate of change of intensity. Many consonants with a low level relative to adjoining vowels have rapid intensity changes that must be perceived for the consonants to be correctly identified. There is the potential to increase intelligibility if the rapid variations in intensity can be made more prominent.

Increased prominence can be achieved by a circuit that automatically increases its gain whenever the intensity of the input signal is changing rapidly (such as during a plosive), and decreases its gain whenever the intensity of the input signal is constant (such as during a vowel).[595] The resulting speech is perceived as though all plosives have been articulated with great emphasis. Experiments have so far been unable to verify any improvement in intelligibility, relative to simple, linear high-frequency emphasis[217] or to more conventional compression[486] (both of which also emphasize most of these same consonants). Such a processing scheme can, however, be selected in one hearing aid now available commercially, and has been beneficial in cochlear implants,[321] although here also, the benefit relative to simple compression is unknown.

Speech simplification

If profoundly hearing-impaired people are unable to perceive many of the complex cues in a speech signal, particularly when there is noise present, perhaps they will understand more if less information is presented. Simplification of the speech signal is the concept behind ***speech pattern processing***. At one extreme, the speech signal is replaced by a single pure tone pulsing on and off in

---

j   In the experiments with the most dramatic improvements in intelligibility, masking noise was added after the consonant was amplified (Gordon-Salant, 1986; Gordon-Salant, 1987; Guelke, 1987). Processing thus also improved the SNR for the consonant. This type of processing is not possible in a real hearing aid because the extra amplification added during a consonant would also amplify any noise that was present simultaneously.

time with the speech. The pure tone has a frequency equal to the fundamental frequency of the speech.[758] Other features that have been extracted from the speech and presented in a simple manner include the amplitude of the speech envelope and the presence of voiceless excitation.[276] Speech identification is better with these additional features than with fundamental frequency alone.[277] Presentation of a simplified speech code also helps profoundly impaired people control the fundamental frequency of their own voice.[34] The benefit obtained from speech simplification appears to be restricted to those profoundly impaired people with the least remaining frequency selectivity.[276] People who are likely to be candidates for speech simplification strategies are also likely to be candidates for cochlear implants.

Enhancement by re-synthesis

An extreme example of using the special features of speech would be a hearing aid that recognized speech and then re-synthesized it in a clear, well-articulated, and noise-free way. Of course, there are many problems with this. Just like hearing-impaired people, automatic speech recognizers do not perform well in noisy places, and have trouble with unusual accents. Also, the speech synthesizer would have to transfer many of the features of the real signal if the synthesized voice were to convey emotion, and were to sound like the person really talking. Because hearing-impaired people often use lip-reading cues, the automatic recognizer and synthesizer must output sounds within about 40 ms of the signal arriving.[589, 863] Given the current performance of speech recognizers, except under ideal conditions, a hearing aid of this type still seems far away.

7.6   Concluding Comments

One of the major difficulties in evaluating novel processing schemes is allowing for the effects of familiarity and practice. If sound is markedly altered by the processing, it is likely that experimental subjects will need consid-

erable listening experience, and perhaps even systematic training, before they are able to use the altered or new cues to identify speech sounds. Extensive listening experience is difficult to provide in the laboratory. Increasingly, it is possible to make wearable devices that process sounds in complex ways. Is it reasonable, however, to ask subjects to wear, every day, a hearing aid that produces strange sounds, before there is any evidence that the processing is beneficial? One way to minimize this dilemma is to first test discrimination ability (the ability to differentiate contrasting sounds) after minimal practice. If the processing increases discrimination ability for at least some sounds, then it may be more reasonable to proceed with extensive familiarization, training, and speech intelligibility (i.e. identification) testing.

Most of the processing schemes discussed in this chapter have had sufficiently positive results, either in terms of intelligibility or comfort, to warrant further research or immediate application in commercial hearing aids. Some of the schemes, such as transposition, are applicable only to patients with particular hearing losses, and the signal processing characteristics probably have to be carefully adjusted to best suit each patient. Other schemes, such as directional microphone arrays, would be useful for all patients in some listening situations, and the signal processing characteristics can be identical for all patients.

How does the clinician evaluate the worth of new processing schemes as they become commercially available? Ideally, research will be available to show that with the new processing scheme, experimental subjects obtained higher speech identification scores, and/or preferred the sound quality in their usual listening environments, compared to a reference amplification condition. The reference condition must, as a minimum, have a gain-frequency response appropriate to each subject, and some form of compression. It is essential that the experiment be blinded (so that the subjects do not know which is the new form of processing), and it is desirable that it be double-blinded (so that the experimenter cannot unconsciously influence the subjects).

Before leaving this discussion of signal processing algorithms, it is worth reviewing the effectiveness of signal processing algorithms (i.e. the different forms of compression discussed in Chapter 6, noise reduction, feedback reduction, transposition, and speech feature enhancement) relative to other means for improving intelligibility. By far the best way to improve intelligibility is to remove all noise and reverberation from the signal before presenting it to the hearing-impaired person. The best way to do this is to put the microphone right next to the lips of the person talking and then use enough amplification, frequency shaping and compression to make the speech audible and comfortable at all frequencies. Consequently, FM or other wireless transmission systems, which position the microphone at the talker, still provide the greatest intelligibility improvement.

Another solution, far less effective but still worth having, is the use of directional microphone arrays to decrease (but by no means remove) noise and reverberation. Different solutions are often not mutually exclusive: The more complex forms of signal processing (speech cue enhancement, transposition, adaptive noise reduction) can be combined with either FM systems and/or directional microphones, to obtain greater benefit than any one processing scheme alone can provide.

With the increasing availability of wearable digital technology, we can expect to see a variety of two-microphone, adaptive noise-reduction hearing aids using principles similar to those discussed in this chapter.

CHAPTER EIGHT

ASSESSING CANDIDACY FOR HEARING AIDS

Synopsis

Although the decision to try hearing aids is ultimately made by the patient, many patients will be in doubt as to whether they should acquire hearing aids and so will look to the clinician for a recommendation. This recommendation must take into account many factors other than pure tone thresholds.

Initial motivation to obtain hearing aids has been shown to be a key determinant of whether patients continue to use hearing aids. A patient's motivation reflects the balance of all the advantages a patient expects hearing aids will provide offset by all the expected disadvantages, irrespective of whether all these positive and negative expectations are realistic. The advantages expected by the patient are affected by the degree of disability and handicap they feel they have. Disability describes how much difficulty the person has hearing in various situations, whereas handicap describes the extent to which a person is unable to participate in activities because of the hearing loss. Disadvantages potentially include the impact of wearing hearing aids on a patient's self-image. The expected advantages and disadvantages of hearing aids are affected by what the patient has been told about hearing aids by others. The clinician must attempt to discover a patient's expectations and modify those that are unrealistically low or unrealistically high. Although hearing aids help in quiet and in noise, they help more in quiet, so hearing aids are more likely to be valued and used if the patient needs help hearing in quiet places.

When a clinician encounters a hearing-impaired patient who does not want hearing aids, the clinician should find out whether this is because the patient is not aware of the loss, is aware of difficulty but does not wish to accept the presence of a hearing loss, or acknowledges the loss but does not wish to do anything about it. If the latter is true, the patient's reasons should also be discovered.

Difficulty managing a hearing aid can greatly affect use, so the clinician must consider likely manipulation difficulties when determining candidacy and aid type. People with tinnitus often find that hearing aid use diminishes their problems, so tinnitus positively affects candidacy. The presence of central processing disorders and extreme old age can both affect candidacy, but not in a manner sufficiently predictable to affect the clinician's recommendation.

People with a severe to profound hearing loss are likely to receive more benefit from cochlear implants than from hearing aids. The most useful indicator of which device will be better for them is the speech score they receive for well fitted hearing aids after some years of becoming accustomed to them. For infants, this is not possible so the decision to implant has to be based primarily on aided or unaided hearing thresholds (as well as requiring no medical or psychological contra-indications).

Vibrotactile or electrotactile aids are a worthwhile alternative for those too deaf to receive useful auditory stimulation from hearing aids, but who do not wish to receive a cochlear implant, or for whom a cochlear implant is not suitable on medical or psychological grounds. Training in integrating the tactile information with visual information is essential.

Hearing aids should not be withheld just because speech scores obtained under headphones fall below some arbitrarily determined criterion. There are, however, several audiological/

medical indications that should cause hearing aid fitting to be delayed until the cause of the problems has been resolved.

A clinician therefore has to consider a large number of factors that may affect candidacy for hearing aids, none of which has such a strong effect that the remaining factors can be ignored.

To fit, or not to fit, that is the question. More precisely, when should the clinician encourage an uncertain patient to try hearing aids,[a] and when should the clinician advise the patient that hearing aids will probably not be beneficial, in the patient's current circumstances? The final decision about whether to try hearing aids will be the patient's (or that of an overly dominant close relative). The clinician can greatly influence this decision if the patient is at all uncertain. The hard part for the clinician is knowing which way, and how strongly, to push.

Hearing loss statistics show that many people with hearing loss do not acquire hearing aids. Approximately 10% to 16% of an adult population will report that they have trouble hearing.[483, 961] If we take an audiometric approach to defining hearing problems, 16% of an adult population will have a four-frequency average hearing loss in the better ear of greater than 25 dB HL, and for 7% to 8% it will be greater than 35 dB HL.[202, 961, b] Various studies indicate that of those who consider they have a hearing loss, or who objectively have a hearing loss, only 14 to 24 % own a hearing aid.[30, 200, 483, 724, 848, 900] That is, approximately four out of five people with a hearing loss have not tried hearing aids.

Are these all good candidates for hearing aids, if only they could be convinced to try them, or have they all made a good decision that for them, the practical and psychological disadvantages will outweigh the benefits? Some research suggests that when these people are sought out and given the

opportunity to try hearing aids, many of them find hearing aids to be beneficial and continue to use them.[201, 848] Kochkin (1997) used self-report measures to estimate that the number of people who could benefit from hearing aids is at least double the number who currently own them. Until there is some direct experimental evidence, however, we will not know what proportion of the population will benefit from hearing aids. Epidemiologists are not the only people uncertain about how many people need hearing aids. Every clinician can expect to see many patients who will be uncertain about whether hearing aids will help them.

There are two broad aspects to the question of whether an individual will benefit from hearing aids: is the person deaf enough, and is the person too deaf? As we will see, the first of these questions can *not* be answered from the audiogram. The second question can be rephrased as *will the person benefit more from hearing aids, a cochlear implant, or a tactile aid*? This chapter will identify some factors that should be considered when deciding whether to recommend hearing aids to a patient.

A purely quantitative approach to this decision is not possible at this stage because of the huge number of factors, and because we do not know how best to measure them nor weight them appropriately for each individual. The Feasibility Scale for Predicting Hearing Aid Use (FSPHAU) represents one attempt to quantitatively combine some of the factors that determine whether a person will

---

[a]   From here on, this book will refer to hearing aids in the plural, because more often than not, people will benefit more from two hearing aids than from one. A substantial proportion of the hearing-impaired population will, however, prefer and/or benefit from only one aid. Chapter 14 will cover this issue in more detail.

[b]   Although these self-report and audiologically defined prevalence rates are very similar, the two methods produce considerable differences in *which* individuals are considered to have a hearing loss (Wilson et al., 1989).

find hearing aids to be useful.[766] Unfortunately, the scale (actually a revised version of it) does not appear to be a reliable predictor of benefit.[144] Similarly, although success with hearing aids has been shown to correlate with a combination of factors (handicap, education, number of medications and age), the combination can not predict candidacy with enough accuracy to be useful.[634]

A purely quantitative approach may never be possible, and given the importance of the interaction between patient and clinician, even this quantitatively inclined writer thinks that this may actually be a good thing! Every patient is unique. If you feel uncomfortable with uncertainty and fuzzy human-oriented decisions, you had better find new ways to cope! Other than for patients with moderate or moderately severe losses, there will often be some uncertainty about whether hearing aids will be the best option.

The first section of this chapter is particularly oriented towards adult patients; although most of the factors are also relevant to children, the arguments and evidence are different. The chapter is, of course, directed towards patients who have never previously worn hearing aids, or who have not tried them for several years. For people who have tried and rejected well fitted, modern hearing aids, the candidacy question has probably been answered unless the patient's hearing loss, needs, or attitude changes. It is, nevertheless, worth determining why the person was disappointed, and what it would take for the patient to consider that hearing aids are worthwhile. Options for amplification are expanding rapidly.

8.1   The Lower Limit of Aidable Hearing Loss

There have been many attempts to find the degree of pure tone hearing loss that would distinguish those who benefit from hearing aids from those who will not. All such

attempts have been spectacularly unsuccessful. At first sight this seems surprising. At the extremes, someone with a severe hearing loss will derive enormous benefit from hearing aids, and someone with normal hearing will derive no benefit.[c] Why then is it not possible to find a degree of hearing loss in between that differentiates those who will benefit from those who will not?

The answer is that for these intermediate degrees of loss, other factors influence benefit more than does the audiogram. The strongest of these other factors can be thought of as the motivation of the person to obtain hearing aids. Of course, motivation is really the accumulated result of a variety of other positive and negative factors. These factors include:

- *Acknowledgment of loss*: Does the patient realize (intellectually) and accept (emotionally) that his or her hearing mechanism is not normal? That is, does the patient fully acknowledge the presence of a *hearing impairment*? When patients say that other people mumble, for example, this "cause" of their problem may reflect either a lack of *awareness* of the loss, or a lack of *willingness* to accept that there is a loss.

- *Needs*: How often is the patient in a situation where he or she hears less clearly than is necessary to function effectively? Alternatively, how often is the patient in a situation where so much concentration is needed that fatigue quickly follows? That is, how much *hearing disability* does the patient have? More importantly, how much hearing disability does the patient acknowledge?

- *Consequences*: Does the hearing disability cause the patient to refrain from activities that he or she would otherwise like to do, or does it cause the patient to have negative feelings about life? That is, how much

---

[c]   Because a hearing aid microphone generates internal noise, a hearing aid can only make it *harder* for someone with normal hearing to detect soft sounds in a quiet place, no matter how much gain the hearing aid has (Killion, 1976).

hearing handicap[d] does the patient have? More importantly, how handicapped does the patient feel? Further discussion on the distinctions between impairment, disability, and handicap can be found in Stephens and Hetu (1991).

- *Self-image*: Does the patient consider that wearing hearing aids would make other people view him or her negatively in some way? The presence of hearing aids will lead some people to view the aid wearer as being older[295] or less intelligent,[242] but the important issue is whether, and how strongly, the patient believes this to be the case. Hearing aid wearers actually have a more positive self-image than hearing-impaired people who don't wear hearing aids,[355] though it is unclear whether hearing aids contribute positively to self-image, or whether people with a positive self-image are more likely to acquire hearing aids. Many patients prefer their self-image to be one of social incompetence to one of defective hearing.[380] Their self-image may thus be better preserved by *not* acknowledging their loss.

- *Expected benefit*: How beneficial does the patient believe hearing aids will be, on the basis of what the patient has been told by other aid wearers, by medical practitioners, or by observing other people who wear hearing aids?

- *Influence of others:* Has the patient been encouraged or even coerced into seeking rehabilitation? Nearly half of all hearing aid candidates are positively influenced by their families to obtain hearing aids.[482] On the other hand, many people who have refrained from seeking help have done so on the advice of a health professional.[479]

- *Fear or uncertainty:* Does the patient anticipate having difficulty understanding how to operate hearing aids, or anticipate not having the dexterity to operate them? Does the patient equate a hearing loss with aging, reduced social competence, or even senility, and reject any tangible representation of that loss, such as hearing aids?

- *Costs*: How does the total of all the costs (financial cost, inconvenience, effect on self image) compare to the perceived benefit of wearing hearing aids?[292, 322]

- *Hearing impairment*: Finally, the physiological hearing impairment of the patient influences, but by no means determines, how much impairment, disability and handicap the patient *believes* he or she has. Degradation of frequency selectivity and temporal resolution are only partially correlated with the loss of sensitivity revealed by the audiogram. Despite this, the pure tone audiogram is a very good indicator of the overall degree of physiological impairment, but not of disability, and even less so of handicap.

The patients' acknowledgment of their hearing difficulties, and consequently their degree of motivation to do something about their problem, are strongly related to how much they subsequently wear their hearing aids.[91, 266, 303, 384, 385] Motivation varies on a continuum from being extremely opposed to obtaining hearing aids, to being extremely enthusiastic about obtaining them. Goldstein and Stephens (1981) present four attitude types drawn from this continuum and comment that negative attitudes may be frankly expressed or may require considerable clinical acumen to identify.

If motivation is so important, can it be altered? Even if a patient has unrealistic views about every one of the above factors, his or her overall motivation towards obtaining hearing aids is likely to be a rational consequence of these beliefs.[e] If so, altering motivation would

---

d   The World Health Organization has recently replaced *disability* with *activity limitation* and *handicap* with *participation restriction*. This book will, however, use the earlier terms. The new terms avoid the inherent contradiction in the term *hearing handicap*: a handicap can *affect* many aspects of a person's life, even though it may be *caused* by a single problem such as poor hearing.
e   This conceptualization of the problem is known as the Health Belief Model (DiMatteo & DiNicola, 1982).

be possible only if the underlying beliefs can be altered. Unfortunately, there is little research to indicate whether attitudes can be affected by appropriate counseling prior to aid fitting. Noble (1999) considers that it can lead to people accepting that their hearing loss is the cause of their difficulties, rather than ascribing the cause to the actions of others. Fortunately, we do know that time spent understanding the concerns of patients, and giving information and instructions to them before and after hearing aid fitting, will increase the amount that patients use their hearing aids, regardless of their initial attitude.[91]

Some examples of how unrealistic and unhelpful beliefs of the patient can be challenged will be given in Section 8.1.12. First, we review the evidence for how a number of factors affect the likelihood of a person using, and/or receiving benefit from, hearing aids.

While reading this chapter, you should keep in mind that people with hearing impairments are not indelibly, but invisibly, labeled as *candidates* or *non-candidates* before they walk into your office. It is *not* as if candidacy has been pre-ordained, and it is the clinician's job to wisely discern which camp the individual patient is from. Rather, the patient will be best served if the clinician investigates if there are any factors preventing a person with a hearing loss from receiving benefit from hearing aids, and if so, what can be done to alter these factors.

8.1.1   Pure tone loss and audiogram configuration

The benefit that people will obtain from hearing aids, and the number of hours per day that people use hearing aids, increases with degree of pure tone hearing loss.[273, 326, 901] Unfortunately, if one restricts the analysis to people with only mild and moderate hearing loss, degree of hearing loss is a very poor predictor of use or benefit.[88, 228, 230, 385, 408, 942] One study has shown that people with flat audiograms use their hearing aids more than

those with sloping audiograms,[682] although other studies have shown no such effect.[25, 408] Hearing handicap and disability appear to be more closely related to low-frequency hearing thresholds than to high-frequency thresholds, although both frequency ranges are important to good hearing.[61]

It has long been suggested, nevertheless, that people with three-frequency average losses (average of 500, 1000, 2000 Hz) of less than 25, 30 or 35 dB HL, will not benefit from hearing aids, but that people with greater losses will benefit.[340, 483] There are many problems with such suggestions. There is no data to suggest that pure tone loss is a reliable indicator of who will benefit, and plenty of data to suggest that it is not a reliable indicator. For example, of 98 people with losses less than or equal to 20 dB HL at 500 and 1000 Hz, and less than or equal to 35 dB HL at 2000 Hz, 85% considered that after six months of use, the hearing aids were a worthwhile investment.[46] These people all had three-frequency average losses of 25 dB HL or less.

If pure tone thresholds *are* used as a guide to candidacy, hearing thresholds in the ear with the larger pure tone loss should be used, as they appear to *better* predict hearing aid candidacy than loss in the better ear, at least for people with mild or moderate loss in both ears.[199] Haggard and Gatehouse (1993) point out that hearing in both ears should really be taken into account. For epidemiological purposes, they propose a two-part criterion for hearing aid candidature: four-frequency average loss greater than 35 dB in the better ear, or greater than 45 dB in the worse ear when combined with a difference of 15 to 35 dB between the ears. They caution, however, against using this to decide whether an individual should receive hearing aids.

Another problem with such a criterion for candidacy relates to the match of available technology to the impairment.[343] Suppose a patient has hearing thresholds of 0 dB HL up to and including 2 kHz, and a 25 dB loss at 3

Special issues with a ski-slope hearing loss

- People with good low-frequency hearing are particularly likely to consider (inappropriately) that they do not have hearing problems, and to have been dragged in by relatives. This is especially likely if the hearing loss has been acquired gradually. If so, counseling to assess and modify motivation will be very important (see Section 8.1.12).

- The potential benefit from a hearing aid is least for extremely steep losses and where the high-frequency loss is greatest. The reason for this will be covered in Section 9.2.4, but relates to the diminished ability of an impaired ear to extract useful information from an audible signal when the loss becomes too great. The wider the frequency range where the loss is between 20 and 80 dB HL, the greater will be the benefit of the hearing aid. For all the reasons covered in this chapter, there is unlikely to be a single number (in octaves) that can predict whether hearing aids will be successful.

- The occlusion effect will be a problem that must be dealt with at fitting.

- A hearing aid that provides gain for only high frequencies may improve clarity, but have little or no effect on loudness. This lack of effect on loudness should be explained, and/or the clarity increase demonstrated with a speech test, or the patient may believe that the hearing aid is ineffective.

- Further information about fitting people with ski-slope hearing losses can be found in Harford & Curran (1997), and in Sullivan et al. (1992).

---

and 4 kHz. Few people, including the author, would currently consider that such a person would benefit from hearing aids. But why not? The patient would have a small disability for soft speech or for medium-level speech masked by low-frequency noise. How would the small decrease in disability afforded by the aid, in limited circumstances, compare to the disadvantages of wearing an aid? These disadvantages would potentially include a concern about appearance, a decrease in sound quality for low- and mid-frequency sounds, cost, audibility of internal noise, the possibility of an occlusion effect or feedback oscillation, and the general nuisance value of wearing a prosthetic device.

Suppose the technology available enables hearing aids to provide high quality sound without any occlusion effect or feedback in a cosmetically acceptable package at a cost that is not too great for the patient. If the disadvantages are minor, the patient may consider hearing aids worthwhile even when they provide only a minor benefit. *In general, any audiometric criterion must take account of the technological solutions available.* The flexibility with which hearing aids can match unusual loss configurations is increasing rapidly.

Whether the loss is sensorineural or conductive affects the benefit provided by hearing aids. When listening unaided in low- and medium-level environments, a person with a conductive loss will have poorer speech recognition ability than someone with a sensorineural loss of the same degree.[137] The person with the conductive loss will, however, derive more speech recognition benefit from hearing aids than the person with the sensorineural loss. This greater benefit arises partly because for the person with a conductive loss the unaided score is lower and partly because the aided score is higher. This better aided performance for the person with the conductive loss presumably results from the absence of the distortions that occur within and beyond the cochlea for people with sensorineural hearing loss (see Section 1.1).

Surgical correction of conductive loss should have been considered before providing hearing aids to compensate for the loss.

In short, although pure tone hearing loss has been discussed first, it is unreliable as a sole indicator of who will benefit from hearing aids, except in the cases of normal hearing (no benefit) and severe hearing loss (substantial benefit). For all the people with losses in between, it is best to use hearing thresholds only as a guide for further questioning.

Patients with a moderate hearing loss will not be able to hear parts of the speech signal in most listening situations. If they state that they experience no disability and therefore do not wish to obtain hearing aids, the reason should be investigated. Are they denying a disability they do have? Have they structured their lifestyle and relationships to minimize the impact of the disability? If the latter, then are they happy with the changes to their life they have been forced to make? As a further example, if someone with almost normal hearing was desperately keen to obtain hearing aids, are the problems he or she is trying to solve consistent with the small amount of speech information that someone with such a loss would be missing? Are their expectations of hearing aids realistic? Clearly the person has needs, but are those needs of a type that can be met with an electroacoustic device?

8.1.2   Speech identification ability

It is often suggested that an extremely low speech intelligibility score indicates that a person is *too* deaf to benefit from hearing aids, although this does not seem to be a valid criterion, as discussed in Section 8.2.1. Similarly, high speech scores do not prove that a person does not have enough hearing loss to benefit from hearing aids. Such an approach would not be valid, because speech scores depend strongly on test conditions, such as the speech level, noise level, reverberation, and difficulty of the speech material. Any conclusion that a person had no problems would be applicable only to the conditions under which the speech measurement was performed. Predicting whether a person could increase his or her understanding of speech in the wide range of circumstances that most people encounter would be a very daunting task.

8.1.3   Self reported disability and handicap

Not surprisingly, people who seek hearing aids are more likely to be aware of their hearing disability than people who do not.[79, 512] In addition, people who initially report the most disability or handicap are the most likely to report that they are helped by the hearing aid.[46, 435, 634] A possible approach to determining candidacy would be to administer a questionnaire that assesses disability or handicap while unaided. Unaided scores for the Abbreviated Profile of Hearing Aid Benefit (APHAB),[179] which assesses hearing disability, have been shown to be correlated with eventual reduction in disability following rehabilitation. Further details on the APHAB are given in Section 13.2.2. Similarly, unaided scores for the Hearing Handicap Inventory for the Elderly (HHIE),[919] which assesses hearing handicap, have been shown to be correlated with eventual reduction in handicap. Either could be used to help the patient decide if help is needed (see panel).

A low self-reported disability or handicap may reflect the person's refusal to acknowledge a disability or handicap, rather than an absence of problems. If there is an apparent mismatch between the amount of disability or handicap indicated by the questionnaire, and the degree of pure-tone hearing loss, further questioning of the patient may provide information that helps determine the appropriateness of fitting hearing aids. The situations described in some of the items on the questionnaire may provide a useful starting

---

Assessing the problem to be fixed: Self-report standardized questionnaires

If a patient is in some doubt about whether hearing aids are needed, administering a questionnaire to assess disability (e.g. the unaided part of the APHAB) or to assess handicap (e.g. the HHIE) may be beneficial. Simply doing the questionnaire may help patients reflect on how much their hearing loss is impacting on their life. Scoring the questionnaire can add further information. Cox (1997) has suggested the following:

- Patients with relatively large problems hearing speech unaided and relatively few problems with intense sounds are likely to obtain significant benefit from hearing aids. This translates into unaided scores on the APHAB *Ease of Communication*, *Reverberation*, and *Background Noise* sub-scales of greater than 58, 75, 74 respectively, combined with scores less than 24 on the *Aversiveness* scale.

- Patients with relatively few problems hearing speech unaided, but who find loud noise disconcerting, are unlikely to benefit from a linear hearing aid. A WDRC compression hearing aid may be indicated, but even this may not guarantee success.

---

point for discussion. This may be particularly useful where the patient's response to a particular question was strongly different from that expected based on the measured hearing loss.

Determining motivation to obtain help

In an excellent article on evaluating a person for hearing aid candidacy, Saunders (1997) recommends asking two key questions to quickly determine motivation:

1. *What prompted you to come for a hearing test?* Look for answers that relate to difficulties with hearing on one hand, or prompting from family or friends on the other.

2. *What do you expect to gain from this visit?* The patient may either be hoping for proof that his or her hearing is normal, or may be seeking help with hearing, which may or may not involve hearing aids.

For those who already realize they have a hearing loss and need help, the second question leads naturally to questions about the types of situations in which they need help (see next panel).

8.1.4 Listening environment, needs and expectations

Hearing aids provide much more benefit in some situations (e.g. listening to a softly spoken person in a quiet place) than in others (e.g. listening to a loudly spoken person in a noisy, reverberant place).[178, 225, 586] The reason for this is easy to understand. Figure 8.1(a) shows the long-term speech spectrum at an overall level of 55 dB SPL, in a quiet environment. It also shows the normal threshold of hearing and the thresholds corresponding to a person with a hearing loss that gradually increases from 30 dB HL at 250 Hz to 50 dB HL at 8 kHz. It is clear that much of the speech signal falls below the threshold of the hearing-impaired person. Figure 8.1(b) shows the spectrum of speech at 85 dB SPL in a noisy place where the background level is 80 dB SPL. Much of the speech will again be inaudible, but at most frequencies, audibility is limited by the background noise rather than by the person's hearing loss.

What will a hearing aid do in these two hypothetical, but realistic, situations? In the quiet situation, if the hearing aid has enough gain, the entire 30 dB range of speech could be made audible at every frequency, and intelligibility would increase dramatically. In the noisy situation, the situation is different for all frequencies less than 5 kHz. No amount

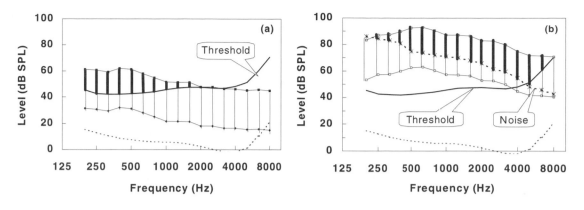

Figure 8.1 The long-term 1/3 octave speech spectrum for a) speech at 55 dB SPL in a quiet place, and b) speech at 85 dB SPL in a noisy place. Each speech spectrum includes the 30 dB dynamic range from the weakest useful elements of speech to the most intense elements (shown as the vertical lines). The portion of the speech range that is audible above noise and hearing thresholds is thickly shaded. The normal threshold of hearing is shown as the lower dotted line.

of gain will make the speech more audible over this frequency range, because the hearing aid will amplify the noise just as much as it does the speech.

How does this affect candidacy for hearing aids? If the patient primarily needs to hear more clearly in places that are quiet, and where speech is at a soft level, hearing aids are likely to be extremely useful. The greater the loss, the greater will be the likely benefit in quiet places.[178] Conversely, if the primary need is to hear better in *very* noisy places, hearing aids may disappoint, irrespective of the degree of the patient's hearing loss. Many real life situations lie between these extremes. Often, background noise will limit audibility for the lower frequencies, and the patient's thresholds will limit audibility for the higher frequencies. In such situations, hearing aids will provide more benefit than they do in very noisy places, but less benefit than they do in very quiet places.

As a rule, people who have not used hearing aids before expect that the aids will be as beneficial in noise as they are in quiet, although they subsequently report this is not the case.[781] On average, patients' expectations about how much hearing aids will improve the clarity of speech in all situations is slightly higher than they subsequently find to be true.[781] Despite this, those patients who arrive with the highest expectations of what hearing aids can do eventually report the greatest use and benefit.[971] It seems important, however, that patients with *grossly* unrealistic expectations (in either direction) be identified prior to their deciding whether to trial hearing aids, so that they can base their decision on the best possible information.

Two provisos should be added to the preceding discussion about different benefits in different environments. Anyone with a hearing loss will undoubtedly have more difficulty hearing in both very quiet and very noisy situations than would someone with normal hearing. Even if a patient initially reports difficulty in only one of these situations, it is worth probing to find out if the other type of situation ever causes problems. If so, the difficulty experienced in the other situation, and the importance of this situation, may have a bearing on the likely overall benefit of hearing aids for this patient.

The second proviso is that if the hearing aids have a directional microphone, or dual microphones that can be selected to function as a directional microphone, considerable benefit from the hearing aids may be experienced

Determining listening needs and expectations: the COSI™

The only way to find out where a patient needs to hear better is to ask! A systematic way to accomplish this is to use the Client Oriented Scale of Improvement (COSI) (Dillon, James & Ginis, 1997). This technique consists essentially of a blank form (see Section 13.3), on which the clinician records the situations that the patient nominates as being difficult. The situations to be recorded often emerge naturally while the patient's case history is taken. If not, the blank form will remind the clinician that something important is missing from the interview.

It is worth continuing to ask the patient for further examples of situations that are difficult as long as he or she is able to keep on nominating them. Five different situations, however, are probably enough to provide a focus for the rehabilitation program. As we will see in Chapter 13, the situations listed at the initial interview can later be used to assess the benefit of rehabilitation. To get full value out of this assessment, the initial needs should be recorded as specifically as possible. For example *hearing my granddaughter when she comes to visit* is more specific than *conversation at home*. Similarly, *understanding Sam and Lou at the club on Saturdays* is more specific than *hearing in noise*.

Determining the situations in which the patient is having problems leads naturally to determining the patient's expectations of hearing aids in each of these situations. Patients will arrive at the initial appointment with expectations that are unrealistically high (especially if the situation is noisy) or unrealistically low (especially if the situation is quiet).[496] In either case, the clinician should modify the patient's expectations so that the patient can make a realistic, personal overall assessment of the benefit of hearing aids.

McKenna (1987) has suggested a very specific way to determine expectations. Patients are asked how well they would need to hear in each situation for them to consider the rehabilitation worthwhile. If the expectation is unrealistic, the clinician and patient jointly negotiate a goal that the patient thinks is worthwhile and that the clinician thinks is achievable. An additional benefit is that both clinician and patient know that the rehabilitation program will be over once these goals have been reached, or when it is apparent that some of the goals can never be reached.

This goal setting approach was implemented in NAL hearing clinics throughout Australia and referred to as **Goal Attainment Scaling (GAS)** (Dillon et al., 1991a; Dillon et al., 1991b). Some clinicians considered that the formal negotiation of realistic goals was useful, whereas other clinicians disliked it. The technique has now been replaced by the COSI technique.

Stephens (1999) recommends mailing information to patients prior to the first interview, and that patients be asked to think about help with hearing. This approach should facilitate COSI, though it is not an essential component of COSI.

in even the noisiest places. When noise is coming from many directions and the wanted signal from only one, hearing aids with directional microphones will allow the patient to communicate in poorer signal-to-noise ratios than would be possible without hearing aids. The directional microphone will decrease the amount of noise being perceived, and except for distant noise sources in reverberant environments, the noise will decrease by an amount approximately equal to the directivity index of the hearing aid, averaged across frequency (see Section 2.2.4). Technology thus directly affects candidacy. The availability of a BTE or ITE with an effective directional microphone can turn a non-candidate for hearing aids into a candidate!

As well as examining the type of situations in which a patient needs help with hearing, it is worth considering how many such situations the person regularly experiences and how often these situations are experienced. The more a person is in contact with other people (or would like to be if poor hearing was not a disincentive) the more likely it is that the advantages of hearing aids will outweigh their disadvantages. A hermit with a loud TV set and radio will not need hearing aids!

At the other extreme, family members can have a powerful effect on people acquiring hearing aids. Approximately 50% of people seeking help with their hearing cite their family members as the primary motivators.[79, 672] It is not so clear how family attitudes affect the extent to which patients actually *use* hearing aids, although it is reasonable to assume that positive reinforcement from family members will encourage ongoing use and that negative reinforcement will have the opposite effect.

Family members certainly influence each other. Prospective patients tend to have the same beliefs about hearing loss and hearing aids that they believe their family members have.[79] In some circumstances, encouragement from others may be very important until the patient has had the opportunity to acquire the skills needed to effectively use hearing aids. On the other hand, patients who have obtained hearing aids *only* to pacify family members may be less likely to use them. Overall, there appears to be no statistical relationship between who motivated the patient to first attend (i.e. self or others) and the resulting use or benefit.[303] There is conflicting evidence about whether satisfaction is affected by who originally motivated attendance.[303, 385]

Patients with long-standing, gradually acquired, high-frequency hearing losses are particularly likely to be brought in by family members. These patients have not had much opportunity to realize the extent of their loss – the gradual acquisition of the loss, the retention of good low-frequency hearing, and in some cases the minimal requirements to communicate with others, can understandably lead these patients to believe that their hearing is normal. Certainly it is true that younger adults feel that their hearing loss causes greater handicap than do the elderly with the same degree of loss.[329, 549]

8.1.5   Cosmetic concerns

Many patients are concerned about the appearance and/or visibility of hearing aids. It is not surprising that some people would rather pay for an ITE hearing aid than have a BTE hearing aid for free.[93] Similarly, when hearing-impaired people who have never worn hearing aids are shown photos of different hearing aid styles, the proportion who say they intend to purchase increases as the size of the hearing aid decreases.[480] Twice as many people say they are likely to purchase a CIC fitted below the ear canal entrance than would purchase a BTE (price considerations excluded). Concern over appearance can apply to patients of any age, but older adult patients are less likely than younger patients to report dissatisfaction with the appearance of hearing aids.[377]

Many adults are concerned that they will be perceived as being older if they wear hearing aids. This is a very understandable concern: hearing aids are worn by a much bigger proportion of the elderly than by younger adults. There have been several studies investigating whether hearing aids make people look older. When judgements are based on photographs, hearing aids do make adults look older, but the age difference is so small (less than one year) that the effect has no practical significance.[632] In addition, the peers of elderly people do not view negatively those who wear hearing aids.[197]

The beliefs of the hearing aid candidate about this issue are, however, more important than the reality. In one study, 26% of hearing aid candidates initially believed that other people would view them as being older if they wore hearing aids.[867] After these people had worn hearing aids for six months, however, only 10% believed this to be the case. It seems reasonable to reassure candidates that they will *not* be viewed negatively if they wear hearing aids. Indeed, hearing aid wearers believe that their hearing loss is *less* likely to be noticed when they wear their hearing aids than when they do not.[867]

Some patients will consider that concern about appearance indicates vanity on their part, and so may not voice any comment about the appearance or visibility of hearing aids, even when asked. The clinician should thus consider that concern over appearance is possible, even where the patient appears to be unconcerned. People who are concerned about the appearance of their hearing aids are less likely to wear their aids unless adequate counseling is provided.[91]

For many patients, choosing a suitably small device can usually overcome cosmetic concerns. (Unfortunately, the emphasis on small size in hearing aid advertising also reinforces the belief that hearing loss should be hidden from others.) Patients who need more gain or power, or who cannot manipulate an aid as small as a CIC or ITC, can be encouraged to reassess the importance of hiding their hearing loss relative to the benefits they could obtain from hearing aids (see Section 8.1.12).

8.1.6   Manipulation and management

Operating hearing aids can be very difficult for many people. Manipulation difficulties may be caused by poor flexibility of joints or by low tactile sensitivity. Low cognitive functioning can also prevent patients from properly operating their hearing aids. The size of hearing aids can make inserting a battery and operating the volume control and on-off

---

> **Checking for ability to manage the hearing aid**
>
> - Before finalizing the aid selection, hand the patient an aid of the style and size you are considering fitting.
> - Assess the patient's reaction to the size of the aid.
>
> Show the patient how to change the battery or turn the aid on and off. Have the patient try it and assess how easily the task is learned. Initial failure does not mean that the task can never be learned, but early success is very reassuring to the patient and the clinician about this aspect of candidacy.

switch difficult. Because the ears are out of sight, insertion of a hearing aid can be a difficult task to learn. If any one of these tasks is too complex, a patient may simply give up trying. Difficulty inserting an earmold appears to be the major reason for ceasing to use hearing aids, at least for BTE hearing aids.[90]

Although management difficulty typically increases with age,[377, 690, 849] there are so many counter examples that age can not be used to reliably predict how much trouble people will have handling their hearing aids. Furthermore, patients may continue to use their hearing aids even if they are having difficulty managing them. A majority of elderly patients, even those over the age of 90, reported using their aids regularly, despite the management difficulties many of them reported.[690, 691]

Ease of management is, however, closely linked to patients' use of their hearing aids[384] so it is a critical issue in aid selection and patient instruction. Section 10.2 contains some recommendations for choosing hearing aids that will help minimize management problems.

8.1.7   Age

Age (either old age or infancy) by itself does not directly affect candidacy for hearing aids.

It can, of course, affect several of the other factors already reviewed (manipulation difficulties, cosmetic preferences, hearing needs, hearing impairment) and so indirectly affect candidacy. Among adults who own hearing aids, daily use is probably less for the old-elderly than for the young-elderly.[828, 866] A number of studies (reviewed in Brooks, 1981), however, have found no relationship between age and use of hearing aids.

Illness often accompanies advancing age. People with a hearing loss may regard other health problems as more pressing than their hearing problem, and may not feel able to deal with more than one problem at a time. This is understandable but unfortunate, as increased ease of communication may make it easier for them to deal with other problems they have.

The younger people are when they first receive their hearing aids (e.g. under 70), the more likely they are to become regular users of their hearing aids.[10, 91, 322] Brooks suggests that advanced age (e.g. over 80) makes it harder to learn the new tasks required to operate hearing aids, whereas these skills are more easily retained into advanced age if they have been learned at an earlier age. It seems feasible for people to be fitted earlier if hearing aids can be given the positive, high technology connotation that they now deserve. Although hearing aid owners are predominantly elderly, there are more hearing-impaired people without hearing aids under the age of 55 than there are over 55.[482]

8.1.8   Personality

A few personality traits have been found to be associated with a greater likelihood of take-up of rehabilitation, and a greater degree of benefit from rehabilitation with hearing aids. Numerous other studies have shown that personality also affects the degree of self-reported disability or handicap.

Locus of control: Patients who feel that they control the things that happen to them (i.e. an internal locus of control) are more likely to use hearing aids than those who feel that things just happen to them (i.e. an external locus of control).[299, 303] An external locus of control has also been referred to as *learned helplessness*.[811] This phrase reflects a belief by some patients that they cannot positively affect their circumstances no matter what they do, so there is no point in doing anything. Counseling for such patients should presumably be aimed at helping them realize they *can* change how well they hear. Those who more strongly believe that their lives are controlled by others are also more adversely affected by loud sounds, but this applies whether they are aided or unaided.[170]

Extroversion: Patients with an extroverted (outward looking) personality report more benefit from amplification than patients with an introverted (inwards looking) personality.[170]

Obsession: Patients who score highly on an obsession scale are likely to report less benefit and satisfaction from their hearing aids.[303]

The association between benefit from rehabilitation and the presence of the above traits is far too weak to establish or preclude candidacy for hearing aids. If a trait is strongly evident, however, this can be one of the many factors taken into account when the clinician arrives at a final recommendation for or against candidacy.

8.1.9   Central auditory processing disorder

As age increases, so too does the likelihood that hearing loss will involve a decrease in central auditory function. The person (or ear) affected will be particularly susceptible to interference from competing signals. Some studies have shown that an auditory processing disorder diminishes the benefit, satisfaction, and use provided by hearing aids.[369, 831] Conversely, one case study showed that a person with central complications but normal pure tone thresholds in both ears benefited from a single hearing aid because it decreased adverse interactions between the ears.[804] Another study showed no relationship at all.[497]

The presence of an auditory processing disorder should therefore *not* prevent the clinician from fitting hearing aids, because the relationship between degree of central deficit and benefit is unclear. The presence of a central processing deficit may, however, help explain why some people report little benefit from hearing aids.

Because central-processing deficits can appear and then increase in magnitude as people age, it is possible for hearing aids to become less effective with time. When this occurs, it is possible that a patient will complain of the hearing aid output becoming distorted, even though the hearing aid electro-acoustic specifications remain unchanged.[833] There are few data on this issue, but the possibility of increasing central deficit, and decreasing hearing aid effectiveness should be borne in mind if a previously satisfied hearing aid wearer indicates a growing dissatisfaction with his or her hearing aids. A more thorough review of the impact of central processing disorder on communication ability, and its implications for hearing aid candidacy, can be found in Stach, Loiselle & Jerger (1991).

Wireless systems provide a potential solution to the problems caused by central processing disorders because of their ability to greatly attenuate unwanted signals and noise. A proportion of people with such deficits will use these systems regularly[832] despite the logistical difficulties associated with their use. A less effective but more convenient solution would be to use a directional microphone, either in the hearing aid or in the form of a highly directional hand-held microphone. If a person (adult or child) has normal pure tone thresholds, good speech discrimination ability in quiet, but unusually poor speech discrimination in noise, for whatever reason, consideration should be given to fitting a wireless system.

8.1.10 Tinnitus

Many people with hearing loss also have tinnitus. The amplification of external sounds can often relieve the adverse effects of tinnitus.[371] The amplified sound can provide partial or even complete masking of the tinnitus, but one cannot assume that either of these will necessarily occur.[596, 865] The presence of tinnitus increases the likelihood that a person will accept hearing aids, and should therefore be considered a positive factor when assessing hearing aid candidacy.[850] The use of hearing aids does not preclude other forms of treatment for tinnitus.

8.1.11 Factors in combination

As we have seen, a difficult audiogram (e.g. a ski-slope loss) does not rule out use of hearing aids. Neither does difficulty manipulating hearing aids, a belief that help is needed only in noisy places, poor speech discrimination, nor a slightly hesitant attitude to trying hearing aids. However, a patient for whom all of these were true is less likely to find hearing aids useful than would a patient for whom there was only one of these difficulties to overcome. The clinician's job is to identify, for each patient, all the potential obstacles to success (see panel), overcome those that can be overcome (with technical solutions or by helping the patient modify his or her beliefs), and weigh up the remaining difficulties against the likely benefits that the patient will receive. A responsible recommendation for or against amplification can then be given.

The clinician's job is also to give the patient all the information that he or she needs to make a well-informed decision about whether to proceed. What impression should the clinician convey if the clinician is uncertain whether the hearing aid will be useful? An obviously negative or uncertain attitude may well be a self-fulfilling prophecy if the patient is not given the confidence to persevere with the hearing aid during any initial difficulties. On the other hand, glowing predictions of wide-ranging substantial benefits without

Summary: Potential obstacles to the acquisition and use of hearing aids

1. Little or no self-perceived disability;
2. little or no self-perceived handicap;
3. stigma, based on an association of hearing loss with old age, low social competence, or even mental disorder;
4. belief that hearing aids provide little help and/or a poor quality of sound;
5. passive acceptance of the inevitability that hearing loss, disability or handicap come with old age (Humphrey, Herbst & Faurqi, 1981);
6. attribution of problems to the actions of others;
7. reinforcement of any of the above beliefs by friends, relatives, or health professionals;
8. difficulty manipulating small objects;
9. low cognitive functioning;
10. other health problems; and
11. financial cost.

Note that for the first six items it is the belief that affects behavior, irrespective of whether the belief is well founded. Experimentally, the first five beliefs have been found to distinguish those who use hearing aids from those who do not attempt to obtain them (Brink et al., 1996).

difficulties will be untrue, and will produce unrealistically high expectations that will make difficulties encountered seem all the greater.

An ethical, but encouraging, summary is that there will definitely be many situations in which the hearing aids will make speech easier to understand, but that there will be some limitations or difficulties to overcome. Furthermore, the patient is the only person who can decide whether the advantages outweigh the disadvantages, and this balance can be judged effectively only when hearing aids are worn.

8.1.12 Counseling the unwilling patient: some examples

Clinicians will frequently encounter patients that have so much pure tone loss that they *must* have trouble hearing clearly in a range of situations, yet the patient seems unwilling to try hearing aids. As an (all too frequent) example, suppose Mr X has been "brought" to the hearing clinic by Mrs X, who is sick of Mr X failing to follow conversations, and is annoyed by the TV volume setting insisted

on by Mr X. (Their neighbors do not like the volume setting either!) Mr X says that he can understand most people most of the time, except for people who do not speak clearly. He can understand the TV just fine, and he came along only because his wife wanted him to. What does the clinician do next (assuming an audiogram has been obtained)?

Any attempt to immediately point out how much benefit hearing aids will give to someone with his degree of loss will probably be meaningless to Mr X, because he has not acknowledged that he has a problem and therefore does not need a solution. Such an attempt may cause Mr X to label the clinician as just another person telling him what to do. Even if he acquiesces to these two insistent people, he has plenty of later opportunities to reassert control over his life by finding the hearing aids to be unhelpful.

Mr X has reasons for his unwillingness and progress is unlikely unless the clinician can first find out those reasons. This knowledge can come only from Mr X. Obstacles can be of three main types.

1. Unwillingness due to lack of awareness:
Mr. X may simply not have noticed that he
has more trouble than others in understanding
speech, or that he needs the TV louder than
anyone else. This is the easiest, but probably
least common reason for the clinician to deal
with. The following are some ways that the
clinician can help Mr. X become more aware
of his loss.

- The clinician can show Mr X his audiogram
  and explain it.

- The clinician can ask Mr X to talk about
  an occasion when he had trouble understanding conversation, and then reflect on
  whether anyone else present seemed to
  have the same trouble.

- The clinician can demonstrate Mr X's
  disability by having him repeat words
  presented in the sound field at a level where
  he cannot hear well, but where Mrs X, or
  any other person with normal hearing, can
  hear well.

2. Unwillingness to accept hearing loss: Mr
X may have noticed that he has difficulty with
conversation, but may not be willing to accept
that his hearing has deteriorated. The course
of action depends on Mr X's reasons for this.

*Mr X may associate hearing loss with aging
and/or senility.* He may have seen hearing loss
in someone significant to him whose health
was deteriorating in some way, and may feel
that hearing loss will be indicative of other
sorts of deterioration in him too. Appropriate
counseling would commence with giving Mr
X basic information about how the hearing
mechanism works, how it deteriorates, and
how the state of the hearing mechanism is
unconnected to mental functioning or other
health issues. Good graphics of the hearing
mechanism can help take Mr X's thoughts
from diffuse concerns about his physical or
mental state to more tangible rudimentary
physiology.

*Mr X may have noticed that he can hear well
in some situations* (e.g. moderate or loud
speech in a quiet setting). He may have

noticed that he can always hear speech, even
if he can not always understand it. He may
also have been told: *He can hear well when
he needs to.* Based on any of these experiences he may conclude that his hearing is
good.

- Appropriate counseling would commence
  with giving Mr X basic information about
  the partial loss of speech cues that accompanies hearing loss and listening in noisy
  places. Again, graphics, such as a trans-
  parent overlay of the speech range to
  superimpose on Mr X's audiogram, can be
  helpful. Figure 8.2 shows one such picture.
  The vertical overlay can be moved upwards
  to simulate softer speech. Mr X may
  develop confidence in the clinician if the
  clinician can nominate situations in which
  Mr X has had difficulty but has not ascribed
  the cause to his hearing mechanism. Such
  situations include listening from another
  room, listening to a softly spoken person
  in quiet, and listening in the presence of
  various background noises.

- The benefit of amplification can be
  demonstrated to Mr X by having him listen
  to a list of words played at a weak to
  moderate level, with and without a demonstration hearing aid. The demonstration
  hearing aid can be a BTE in a temporary
  mold, or an ITE/ITC mounted in a
  stethoclip, although the former may scare
  people if they are fearful of leaving the
  clinic with a large hearing aid.[915] There is
  no need to precisely prescribe the hearing
  aid's response, although its gain, power and
  response shape (including the effects of the
  stethoclip) should not be grossly inappropriate, or the demonstration will have an
  effect opposite to that intended!

*Mr X may associate hearing loss with shame
or guilt.* In the mind of Mr X, accepting that
he has a hearing loss may require him to
accept a sense of shame for being defective,
and/or a sense of guilt for being the cause of
communication problems.[380] Involvement
with other hearing-impaired people can help

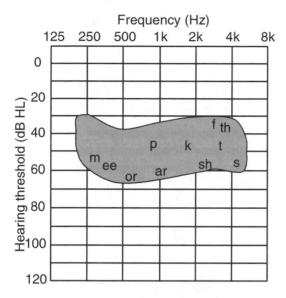

Figure 8.2 The speech spectrum, including a 30 dB dynamic range at each frequency, for speech at a long- term level of 65 dB SPL. The approximate locations of the spectral centre of a few speech sounds are indicated.

Mr X to establish his identity as a whole person with a hearing-impairment. Such involvement can also reinstate his sense of belonging and lead to the realization that difficult communication is the result of hearing loss rather than something for which he should blame himself. [380]

3. Unwillingness to try hearing aids and/or other rehabilitation activity: Mr X may acknowledge that he has a hearing loss, and may acknowledge that he has trouble hearing in some situations, but may still not want to do anything about it. Mr X may believe that the disadvantages of acquiring and wearing hearing aids outweigh the advantages. For Mr X to change his conclusion, he will first have to change his assessment of either the pluses or the minuses of wearing hearing aids. The clinician's emphasis should again be on understanding Mr X's views in an accepting manner. Only when they are understood can the clinician, or perhaps Mrs X, convincingly

give information or suggest actions that may lead him to change his views.

Mr X may consider that hearing aids would not help much, perhaps based on what others have told him, or based on his observations of others.

- After acknowledging that hearing aids do not help some people much, the clinician could comment that often this is for correctable reasons, and that hearing aids have improved a lot in the last few years.

- Mr X could be asked to complete the unaided portion of the Abbreviated Profile of Hearing Aid Benefit (APHAB)[179] or the Hearing Handicap Inventory (HHIE).[919] The poorer the score on either of these, the greater will be the benefit that he is, on average, most likely to experience (see Section 8.1.4), and this can be discussed with Mr X.

- Instead of a discussion about generalized benefit, Mr X could be asked about the difficulties he has in some specific situation that is important to him. He could be asked to imagine what it would be like to be in that situation and not have trouble understanding the conversation around him (provided that is a reasonable expectation in the circumstance).

Mr X may prefer his hearing impairment not to be visible to others, although he accepts that hearing aids may help. This is a difficult issue to deal with, as pressure by the clinician for the patient to reveal his loss to others may simply add one further stress to the life of the patient:

- If Mr X feels that revealing his loss would result in ridicule or embarrassment, he can be encouraged to reveal the loss to just one person and note the reaction (which is most unlikely to be negative).[f] He may then feel able to gradually expand the circle of people to which he is willing to reveal his

---

f   The clinician should not overlook the possibility that in some cases, especially for working-age people, revelation of hearing loss may indeed lead to actual discrimination and disadvantage (Hetu, 1996).

loss. If Mr X is willing, a group of hearing impaired people organized by the clinician or through a self-help group provides a very supportive environment in which to make his loss known (see Section 12.13.4).[388]

- Mr X can be asked if he really is happier with all the consequences of not wearing hearing aids than with the consequences of wearing them. It may be appropriate to ask him whether he thinks other people have already noticed that he misses or misunderstands things.

- The small size of hearing aids now available can be demonstrated.

Mr X may not think his problem is important enough to spend a significant amount of money on solving it. Mr X may have other reasons that he is either unwilling or unable to articulate for not trying hearing aids.

- Mrs X may be able to help Mr X understand all the consequences of his hearing loss. For example, it may be appropriate for Mrs X to say how she feels when Mr X fails to understand the conversation in group situations. Similarly, she could say how she feels about having to act as Mr X's interpreter, or spokesperson, in group situations.

- If there is no significant other person present, the clinician could relate the experiences of other families where one member has a hearing loss and ask if any of these experiences are relevant to Mr X's situation.

- In general, the clinician should make sure that Mr X has the best possible information relevant to his beliefs to help him come to an informed decision. To be balanced, this information may well include the limited help that hearing aids give in very noisy situations.

If at the end of any pre-fitting counseling, the patient still considers that he or she either does not need hearing aids, or does not want hearing aids, the close association between motivation and subsequent benefit suggests

that it would be unwise to in any way coerce the patient to try hearing aids. The negative experience that will probably result may make the patient less likely to return for help when the loss has deteriorated or when the patient otherwise decides that help is needed.

Patients who at least accept that they have a loss may be willing to keep a log, for a specified period, recording any negative impacts that hearing has on quality of life. This may include situations where hearing loss made communication difficult and situations where hearing loss contributed to a patient withdrawing, physically or mentally, from some activity. Some patients may even be willing to attend a *Living with Hearing Loss* program, in which the impact of hearing loss on life is discussed.[492]

The appointment can close with the clinician acknowledging that the patient does not consider that hearing aids are currently necessary, but noting that people can change their assessment of this, either because hearing loss increases, or because their needs change. The patient can be encouraged to seek a reassessment in twelve months.[492]

Some readers may consider that there is an ethical issue in raising patients' awareness of problems. It seems overly timid, however, *not* to probe for problems that are commonly associated with hearing loss, particularly if the clinician is able to assist should any problems be acknowledged by the patient.

8.2   The Upper Limit of Aidable Hearing Loss

Since the advent of cochlear implants and tactile aids, nobody is too deaf to benefit from a prosthetic device. The question is not whether to recommend that the patient receive *any* device, but which *type* of device should be recommended. This section will briefly review the impact of poor speech identification scores on hearing aid candidacy and the relative performance of hearing aids, cochlear implants, and tactile aids. A detailed description of cochlear implant and vibrotactile aid candidacy is beyond the scope of this book. Because cochlear implants provide better speech understanding than tactile aids, the clinician will face decisions in the following order, although not all decisions will be faced for every patient. For example, the first decision may be to recommend hearing aids for both ears.

- Should hearing aids alone be recommended or should the patient also be assessed for cochlear implant candidacy?

- If a cochlear implant is not suitable, should hearing aids be fitted or should the patient trial a tactile device with or without conventional hearing aids?

- If a tactile aid is not suitable, should hearing aids be recommended?

8.2.1   Poor speech identification ability

It is sometimes recommended that word recognition scores, obtained using head-phones, of less than 50% indicate that hearing aid benefit will be limited to help with lip-reading, monitoring one's own voice, and detecting environmental sounds.[390] There are several reasons why speech identification scores obtained using headphones are not a good indicator of whether a person will benefit from hearing aids.[226]

A hearing aid does more than just amplify. It also re-shapes the speech spectrum, which means that for a given loudness, greater speech identification is possible than with the flat frequency response that is available within an audiometer. Christensen, Lee & Humes (1994) showed that for people with steeply sloping hearing losses, speech scores obtained with a high-frequency emphasis filter adjusted to match the NAL-RP prescription for each person were usually greater than those obtained without such a filter. Often, they were much more. Pettersson (1987) reached similar conclusions for a group of 50 children, including those who had flat audiogram configurations.

Even the maximum score possible with a flat frequency response may not be discovered during routine testing. Speech identification scores have an inherent random component. If the true score (i.e. based on an extremely large number of items) was 50%, a score based on 50 items, for example, will be greater than 61% on 5% of occasions and will be less than 39% on 5% of occasions.[341, 881] As the number of test items used decreases, the spread of scores from test to retest widens. Speech scores also depend on the level at which they are presented. The only way to be sure that the test is presented at the level giving the highest possible score is to test at several levels. Time constraints make it impossible to test at many levels with a large number of items per level. Reliability can be improved by testing at several levels, plotting the results, and drawing a smooth line through the resulting psychometric function. Despite this, some uncertainty over the maximum score is likely to remain.

Both of the above problems can potentially be rectified by spending a lot of time testing, and by doing the testing with an amplification system that has a gain-frequency response appropriate to the patient. A more fundamental problem is determining what cut-off score separates hearing aid candidates from non-candidates. It does not seem likely that any particular cut-off could ever be shown to be valid. Some people with a profound loss wear hearing aids because they help with lip-reading, and because they give the aid wearer an awareness of sounds in their environment, which decreases stress, tension and insecurity.[272] These people may not be able to score anything on a speech test unless the material is particularly easy, such as a closed set test where the response choices differ in the number of syllables. In general, any cut-off value chosen would be highly dependent on the type of speech material.

A related problem is that the increase in intelligibility offered by hearing aids is highly dependent on the levels of speech and noise used. There is no logical reason why the intelligibility increase available in any situation should be predicted by the highest score obtained under headphones.

One should thus be very cautious in concluding, based on speech identification scores obtained with a flat frequency response under headphones, that a hearing aid will not help in any situation. Not all authors or clinicians will agree with the preceding statement.

8.2.2 Hearing aids or cochlear implants?

There are many factors that must be considered before a person can be fitted with a cochlear implant (see panel). The requirement that will be considered in more detail here is that there should usually be a reasonable expectation that the cochlear implant will provide speech identification ability superior to that which can be achieved with hearing aids. One exception might be a patient with a progressive hearing loss, where there may be reasons to consider implantation for a patient with a lesser degree of loss than would be considered for a patient with a stable hearing loss.

A difficulty in deciding the likely benefit is that cochlear implants work much better for some people than for others. Some predictions about likely performance can be made based on duration of loss, age at implantation, age at onset of deafness, pre-implant residual hearing, specific pathologies, and motivational factors,[66, 67, 163, 298, 896] but considerable unexplained variability of outcomes remains.

Figure 8.3 shows, for adult implanted patients tested with three speech tests, the probability

of exceeding the speech score indicated on the horizontal axis, based on results reported for the Cochlear Ltd SPEAK processing scheme.[814, g] Even for very low speech scores with hearing aids, the probability of improvement is less than 100% because a small proportion of implanted patients do not achieve any open-set speech discrimination. Zero scores for open-set discrimination, for a proportion of patients, also occur for other types of cochlear implant.[451] On the other hand, many patients achieve very high open-set sentence scores in quiet when implanted.

A commonly applied criterion for implantation is that for adults, open-set speech sentence scores in quiet with hearing aids should be less than 40%. Figure 8.3 shows that there is a 67% chance of obtaining a score higher than this with a cochlear implant. Even if the performance of the implant were to only equal the performance of the hearing aid in the other ear, there would be many real life situations in which the patient received significant benefit from the cochlear implant. (This assumes that both devices are worn after implantation.) The implications of head shadow on bilateral advantage are just as applicable to head-worn cochlear implants as they are to acoustic hearing aids (see Section 14.2.1).

Candidacy for a cochlear implant becomes much more uncertain if the likely change in speech identification performance is predicted based on hearing thresholds alone. The additional uncertainty arises because it is not possible to accurately predict speech identification ability with hearing aids based on hearing thresholds. For adult patients with a long-standing hearing loss this problem should not arise, because there should have been ample opportunity for the patient to have

---

g   Before calculating the probabilities shown in Figure 8.3, the published results were adjusted to allow for the 25% of patients who were not included in the study, and who presumably had low speech scores. They have all been assumed to have a score equal to the mean difference between the score obtained with the SPEAK processor and the score obtained with the Multipeak processor, averaged across the subjects who were measured. As this assumption is undoubtedly not correct, the left-hand half of the curves in Figure 8.3 should be regarded as a very crude approximation of the true situation and no probabilities are shown for scores lower than the assumed score. Disregarding the 25% of patients would however, be an even worse approximation.

Cochlear implant candidacy

The following considerations for cochlear implant candidacy reflect those in common use, and should be considered as an approximate guideline only. Criteria vary somewhat from country to country, from implant center to implant center and from implant company to implant company. Criteria are changing rapidly as implant performance increases and as experience with implanting people with less hearing loss accumulates. As with hearing aid candidacy, many factors affect the likely outcome. The following must be considered in combination, not as separate criteria that individually enable or preclude implantation.

Adults and children

- A hearing loss greater than 90 dB HL at some frequencies and greater than 60 dB HL at all frequencies, in both ears.
- No medical contraindications such as cochlear ossification, an absent cochlea, chronic middle-ear infection, or retrocochlear hearing loss. Etiology of the hearing loss will be a strong consideration in the decision to implant.

Adults

- A postlinguistic hearing loss. That is, a profound hearing loss occurred after the patient had acquired language aurally and was able to speak. Some exceptions are made for those who have been able to make adequate use of their residual hearing.
- A score of 40% or less on open-set sentence recognition when optimally aided.
- Motivated, emotionally stable patient, with realistic expectations, who is willing to attend for the required number of assessment, mapping, and training sessions.

Children

- Over the age of 18 months, although younger children are increasingly being implanted.
- For older children, the vocalization of varied sounds while communicating.
- Expectation of being in an aural and oral education program that includes appropriate rehabilitation.
- Insufficient access to speech cues via hearing aids. For example, aided thresholds above 2 kHz out of the 30 dB dynamic range of speech at 70 dB SPL overall level.
- Cooperative, motivated family (and patient if old enough), with realistic expectations.

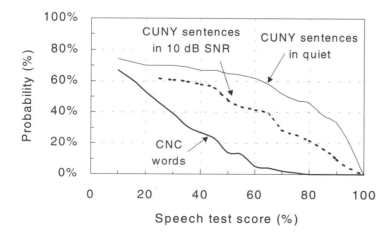

Fig 8.3 Probability of implanted adults exceeding the indicated speech score for CNC (consonant-nucleus-consonant) words, CUNY/SIT sentences (City University of New York speech intelligibility test) in quiet, and CUNY/SIT sentences in noise with a 10 dB SNR.

been fitted with hearing aids, for the hearing aids to be fine-tuned to get the best possible performance, and for speech identification ability to be measured. This rosy situation may not always apply, but even when it does not, a hearing aid trial can be performed prior to implantation.

At what level of hearing loss should a clinician perform a measurement of open-set sentence identification ability for the purpose of determining implant candidacy or the need for referral to an implant clinic? Figure 8.4 shows some data that can help answer this question. By statistically comparing the distribution of scores obtained for adult implanted patients[814] to the distribution of scores for similar[h] speech tests obtained by hearing aid wearers with various degrees of hearing loss,[290] the probability of the anticipated implant score exceeding the anticipated hearing aid score can be calculated. Unfortunately, as can be seen from Figure 8.4, the answer depends somewhat on the type of speech test upon which this calculation is based.

Figure 8.4 also shows the results of the same calculation for children with cochlear implants and hearing aids. This curve is based on data obtained with the IMSPAC (Imitative Speech Pattern Contrast) test.[74, 76] The curve is consistent with Boothroyd's conclusion that

children with an implant, on average, perform about as well as children with pure tone average hearing thresholds in the 90 to 99 dB range when wearing hearing aids.[74] The implanted children whose data were used for the purposes of these calculations used an earlier version of the implant (using the Multipeak processing scheme), which is known to give scores inferior to those possible with the SPEAK processing scheme. Consequently, the somewhat higher curves based on CUNY sentence data for adults may also give realistic expectations of the effects of implantation for children.

The IMSPAC-Multipeak data shown in Figure 8.4 are consistent with the findings from several studies using the Multipeak processing scheme: Children with a pre-implant hearing loss exceeding 100 dB HL can be expected to perform better with cochlear implants (even using the earlier Multipeak scheme) than with hearing aids.[308, 573, 599] They are also consistent with a small study comparing the results of children using hearing aids to children using the Clarion implant with CIS processing.[257] This study showed that across a range of speech tests, aided children with a three-frequency average loss of 71 dB performed better than implanted children. By contrast, aided children with a three-frequency average loss of 88 dB performed a little worse than

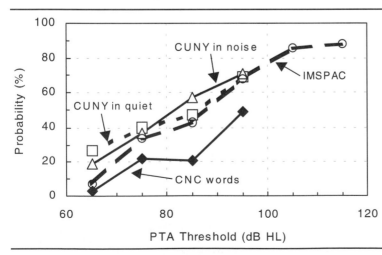

Figure 8.4 Probability of a speech identification score for an implanted adult or child being greater than the anticipated score obtained with hearing aids, as a function of pure tone hearing levels.

---

[h]   The speech tests used for the hearing aid patients were nominally the same as those used for the implant patients, but employed different talkers, so equivalence of the material cannot be guaranteed (Flynn, Dowell & Clark, 1998).

implanted children in an oral communication setting but better than implanted children in a total communication setting.[i]

The probability of improvement is one way to examine the question of whether to refer for an implant assessment. An equally important decision is the degree of improvement expected. Figure 8.5 presents the expected increase (or decrease) in score if the person were to be implanted. These curves are calculated from the same data as used for Figures 8.3 and 8.4.

It is evident from Figures 8.4 and Figure 8.5 that there is a large range of hearing levels for which the relative performance of hearing aids versus cochlear implants is uncertain. This reinforces the importance of obtaining actual speech identification ability with hearing aids before making a recommendation about cochlear implants, whenever possible.

What is a reasonable level of probability to set before recommending, on speech identification grounds, that a cochlear implant be considered? There is no single correct probability. We can note, however, that for a three-frequency average loss of 85 dB there is a 50% chance that the ability to understand sentences will improve after implantation.

This increases to a 70% chance for a loss of 95 dB. Patients (or their families) can be advised about the likelihood of their doing better with a cochlear implant. They can then make up their own mind whether they wish to pursue an implant.

For child patients, uncertainty over the performance possible with hearing aids is a very serious problem. On the one hand, if a child is going to be implanted, it is in the child's interest to receive the implants as early as possible.[143, 243] On the other hand, it may take some time for the full benefits of hearing aids to appear.[308] In one study, out of ten post-meningitic children who initially appeared to receive little or no benefit from hearing aids, three children displayed excellent benefit after 16 to 25 months.[84] For the other seven, delaying implantation for this amount of time could have had very adverse consequences: Delay can decrease the ability to learn to use the information provided by the implant, and ossification may make it impossible to implant the electrodes or may decrease their effectiveness when they are implanted.

One problem with the statistical treatment used in the preceding paragraphs is that it assumes that performance with hearing aids

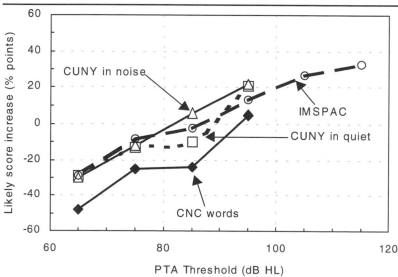

Figure 8.5 Average increase in scores (implant minus hearing aids) as a function of pre-implant hearing threshold.

---

[i]   One cannot infer whether the education setting has determined the effectiveness of the implant or whether the efficacy of the implant has determined the type of education that is possible.

is independent of performance with an implant. This does not appear to be true. Those patients with the best speech recognition ability and/or aided hearing thresholds prior to implantation are likely to end up with the best ability after implantation.[163, 980] This would have the effect of increasing high probabilities, and decreasing low probabilities, relative to the values shown in Figures 8.3 and 8.4.

Another limitation of the preceding discussion is that it totally focuses on speech identification performance. Implantation also improves children's speech production ability, but the effectiveness of implants relative to hearing aids seems to be similar to that observed for speech perception, at least up to five years of age.[604, 886] Furthermore, it is common for pre-lingually deafened adults to get open-set speech scores that are no higher than those they obtained prior to implantation. Despite this, many are successful implant users. They report that:[979]

- they use the device regularly;
- they are satisfied with it;
- it helps them monitor their own voice; and
- it enables them to detect and recognize environmental sounds, which increases their feeling of security.[955]

8.2.3   Hearing aids or tactile aids?

Some patients are so deaf that they receive only vibratory information from hearing aids. They are able to receive time-intensity information, but little or no spectral information. For such people, it is likely that more speech information will be correctly perceived if a purpose-designed vibrotactile or electrotactile aid is used.[716] These aids can encode more speech information into the sense of touch than is accidentally encoded by hearing aids designed to provide an acoustic stimulus. All commercially available tactile aids use vibration as the stimulus. An alternative used in several research studies is electrotactile stimulation, in which small electrical discharges stimulate nerve bundles under the skin. If the characteristics of the electrical discharge are appropriately adjusted, the stimulation will be felt as a tactile sensation.[164]

Although tactile aids can unquestionably provide information that supplements lip-reading, they do not on average provide as much information as a multichannel cochlear implant.[13, 139, 309, 310, 605, 751, 815] This does not mean that every person with an implant will have better speech identification ability than every person with a tactile device.[680]

Vibrotactile aids primarily provide supra-segmental cues, such as intonation and stress.[57] Even simple, single-stimulator vibrotactile aids can indicate whether consonants are voiced, and whether they are stops or continuants.[714] These cues are not available by lip-reading alone.[717] Multi-stimulator tactile aids can also provide more detailed information, such as the format frequencies of vowels.[68, 164] There is some evidence that perception of supra-segmental information may then be more difficult.[140, 710] Such conclusions may, however, be very dependent on the design of the individual device and the extent of training.

Integrating the tactile information with visual cues obtained from lip-reading is not easy. It is not unusual to initially find no improvement when tactile information is added to visual information[69] or even to find a decrease in score relative to visual perception alone.[57, 554] Training has substantial effects on performance, however, and the new skills are maintained after the training is complete.[12, 949] Training is also likely to benefit people with a severe or profound hearing loss who receive a cochlear implant or hearing aids, but the need for training is probably even greater for those who receive a tactile aid.

Although this brief discussion has focussed on the benefits of tactile aids for speech recognition, tactile aids can also help people monitor their speech production, and this helps with speech production training.[297, 681, 713, 950]

In summary, the clinician can be confident that a tactile device will provide information that supplements lip-reading and helps speech production. It is unwise to provide a tactile device without also ensuring that the patient will receive appropriate training for some weeks or months following provision of the device. If training can be provided, tactile devices should be recommended to any patient who receives little or no benefit from hearing aids and who is unwilling to obtain a cochlear implant or for whom a cochlear implant is unsuitable. It seems likely that multi-stimulator tactile devices will provide more information than single-stimulator devices, but may also require more training. More detailed information about tactile devices can be found in Plant & Spens (1995). Training procedures can be found in Plant (1994, 1996).

8.3   Medically Related Contra-indications to Hearing Aid Fitting

Any factor that would cause a clinician to refer the patient for medical assessment will temporarily, or in some cases permanently, halt the process of hearing aid fitting. These factors include:

- a hearing loss of sudden onset;
- a rapidly progressing hearing loss;
- pain in either ear;
- tinnitus of sudden recent onset, or unilateral tinnitus;
- unilateral or markedly asymmetrical hearing loss of unknown origin;
- vertigo (i.e. dizziness);
- headaches;
- conductive hearing loss of any origin;
- otitis externa or otitis media (i.e. infection in the external ear or middle ear and/or drainage);
- cerumen filling more than 25% of the cross-section of the ear canal (unless the clinician has been trained in cerumen removal), or a foreign body in the ear canal; or
- atresia (i.e. missing external ear) or deformity of the external ear.

Whether hearing aids are fitted to the patient after medical intervention will, of course, depend on the medical diagnosis, treatment, and outcome; the doctor's recommendation if appropriate, and the patient's wishes.

8.4   Concluding Comments

This chapter systematically sets out the factors that affect candidacy for hearing aids. In the end, however, the decision about whether to recommend amplification requires a qualitative judgment by the clinician. The decision about whether to accept amplification requires a qualitative judgment by the patient. The clinician's task is to ensure that the patient is well informed about every factor relevant to the individual patient.

Hetu (1996) points out that reluctance to accept rehabilitation or even the existence of a hearing loss is not simply an irrational denial of something that is evident to everyone. To many hearing-impaired people, accepting a hearing loss is equivalent to accepting a spoiled self-identity, and such acceptance may engender feelings of shame for being defective or guilt for being the cause of communication problems with their loved ones and peers. In many instances, it is less painful for a person to endure communication difficulties and social isolation than it is to view oneself as a hearing-impaired person. Helping the patient change these feelings is a more difficult task for the clinician than prescribing and adjusting hearing aids, but until the patient actually wants some form of hearing rehabilitation, there is little point in pursuing a technological solution.

CHAPTER NINE

PRESCRIBING HEARING AID PERFORMANCE

Synopsis

Amplification can be prescribed using a formula that links some characteristics of a person to the target amplification characteristics. This contrasts with an evaluative approach in which the hearing aid characteristics selected are those that are empirically observed to best suit the person. Prescription formulae can be based on hearing thresholds, supra-threshold loudness judgements, and the situations in which the hearing aids are to be worn.

Popular procedures for linear hearing aids include POGO, NAL, and DSL. For all of these, gain can be prescribed based on hearing threshold alone. These formulae all contain variations of the half-gain rule, but the variations are so different that the resulting prescriptions differ greatly, especially for people with a sloping hearing loss.

For nonlinear hearing aids, all available prescription procedures include some aspect of normalizing the loudness of supra-threshold sounds. Several procedures (LGOB, IHAFF, DSL[i/o] curvilinear, and FIG6) adopt loudness normalization as their sole goal, at least for sounds above the compression threshold of the hearing aid. Other procedures vary from loudness normalization in some way. ScalAdapt decreases the loudness of low frequency sounds. DSL[i/o] linear fits a wider than normal dynamic range into the dynamic range of the hearing impaired person. NAL-NL1 normalizes only the overall loudness, whereas the loudness balance across frequencies is based on maximizing calculated speech intelligibility. Several of these nonlinear procedures require the measurement of supra-threshold loudness; the other procedures predict supra-threshold loudness growth based on hearing thresholds. Not surprisingly, the different procedures can produce greatly different prescriptions. Although several of the procedures prescribe compression threshold, none of them have well-developed rationales or evidence for how it should be prescribed. There are no well-developed procedures for prescribing compressor response times.

Maximum output (OSPL90) has to be prescribed so that loudness discomfort is prevented, but so that enough loudness can be obtained without the hearing aid becoming excessively saturated. In many procedures, the target OSPL90 is assumed to just equal LDL, in others it is predicted from threshold, in which case it may fall above or below an individual patient's LDL. For patients with mild to severe hearing loss, an acceptable sound quality is more likely if compression limiting controls maximum output than if peak clipping controls maximum output. Many patients with a profound loss, however, will benefit from the additional SPL that is achievable with a peak clipper.

People with conductive and mixed hearing loss require greater gain and OSPL90 than people with sensorineural loss of the same degree. For a variety of reasons, the gain needed to compensate for a conductive loss seems to be less than the amount of attenuation that the conductive loss causes in the middle ear. The same is consequently true of OSPL90.

Multi-memory hearing aids require a different prescription for each memory. These alternatives can be prescribed as variations from the baseline response prescribed for the first memory. The variations are designed to optimize specific listening criteria in listening environments in which the patient wishes to use the hearing aids. People who wear their hearing aids in many

234

environments, have more than 55 dB high-frequency hearing loss, and require more than 0 dB low-frequency gain, are most likely to benefit from multiple memories.

Neither gain nor OSPL90 should be any higher than is necessary for a patient. Otherwise, a hearing aid may increase hearing loss because of the resulting exposure to noise. The risk of temporary or permanent noise-induced loss is greatest for patients with a profound loss, and can be minimized by using nonlinear amplification.

9.1   General Concepts Behind a Prescriptive Approach and a Brief History

Hearing losses vary widely in their degree, configuration, and type. Consequently, a hearing aid has to be selected, and its amplification characteristics have to be adjusted, to be appropriate for each hearing-impaired person. The only practical way to do this is by using a ***prescription procedure***. A prescriptive approach to hearing aid fitting is one in which some characteristics of the hearing-impaired person are measured, and the required amplification characteristics are calculated from them. Of course, this requires there to be some known (or assumed) relationship between the person's characteristics and the required amplification characteristics.[108] These required amplification characteristics are often referred to as the ***amplification target***.

A prescriptive approach may be contrasted with a hypothetical purely ***evaluative approach***. In such an approach, a number of hearing aids or response shapes would be chosen randomly, and then each tested on the hearing-impaired person to find the best one. Such an approach is totally impractical in its purest form because of the huge number of potential amplification characteristics that could be evaluated. Even in the 1950s and 1960s, when the systematic Carhart evaluation method (or a portion of it) was used to compare the performance of hearing aids on several criteria, the hearing aids to be evaluated were selected using a vaguely defined prescriptive approach.[133] Low gain, low power hearing aids, for example, would

never be evaluated on someone with a profound hearing loss.

In fact, all hearing aid selection and fitting invariably uses some combination of prescription followed by evaluation of the end result. A clinician may carefully prescribe, select, and adjust a hearing aid to meet some target, but it would be rare not to ask *how does that sound*? This question comprises a *very* rudimentary evaluation. If the answer is *terrible,* the clinician is bound to investigate further, and potentially alter the amplification characteristics away from the carefully matched prescription. More sophisticated methods for evaluation and fine-tuning are considered in Chapter 11.

Prescriptive selection procedures have a long history. As early as 1935, Knudsen and Jones proposed that the gain needed at each frequency was equal to the threshold loss at the same frequency minus a constant. This is often referred to as ***mirroring of the audiogram***, because the shape of the gain-frequency response equals the inverse of the shape of the hearing loss. With mirroring procedures, every 1 dB increase in hearing loss requires 1 dB of additional gain to compensate. In sensorineural hearing loss, the gain needed to restore normal loudness perception is equal to the threshold loss only when the person is listening at threshold. For all higher levels, this amount of gain would be excessive, as can be seen in Figure 6.10. Mirroring thus leads to excessive gain, especially for those frequencies with the greatest hearing loss.

The next development was to base the gain needed on the person's most comfortable level (MCL) rather than on their thresholds. Watson and Knudsen (1940) suggested that speech should be amplified sufficiently to make speech energy audible and comfortable. Their specific formula involved MCL, but surprisingly did *not* take into account the variation of speech energy across frequency. Shortly after, Lybarger (1944) made a very important observation: the amount of gain chosen by people was approximately half the amount of threshold loss. This is known as the ***half-gain rule***, which as we shall see, underlies several current prescriptive procedures.

These two ideas (raising speech to MCL and the half-gain rule) are really two sides of the same coin. For mild and moderate sensorineural loss, the threshold of discomfort is little different from normal, as shown in Figure 9.1. MCL is approximately half way between threshold and discomfort, so MCL increases by 0.5 dB for every 1 dB increase in hearing loss. This explains *why* gain is approximately half the hearing loss. Of course, if the aim is to raise *speech* to MCL,

then we cannot predict how much gain is needed at each frequency unless we take into account the speech intensity at each frequency. Because the low-frequency components are more intense than the high-frequency components, the half-gain rule has to be modified. Either a little less low-frequency gain has to be given, or a little more high-frequency gain, or both. We will return to this with some specific examples in Section 9.2.1.

The half-gain rule has to be further modified for severe and profound losses. For hearing thresholds greater than 60 dB HL, discomfort thresholds are significantly above normal. MCL remains approximately midway between threshold and discomfort; this relationship means that MCL is elevated by more than half the hearing threshold loss. The gain, consequently, must be more than half of the hearing loss.

It can be seen that even 50 years ago it was recognized that there were two different auditory attributes that could provide a useful basis for prescription. One approach was to measure some supra-threshold loudness percept (such as MCL). The second was to measure hearing threshold. The link between these is made clear in some procedures: threshold and discomfort are measured, but are used to estimate MCL by assuming that MCL ***bisects*** the person's dynamic range.[937]

As we shall see in Section 9.3, this dichotomy between basing gain prescription on threshold or on loudness perception survives through to the most recent procedures for nonlinear hearing aids. The relative effectiveness of the two types of procedures remains a controversial issue, in part because there has been little comparative evaluation of nonlinear procedures. In the past, the procedures based on hearing threshold have been most popular, probably because threshold is easier and faster to measure and can be measured on infants and on people who have low mental ability. Gain prescription procedures based at least in part on loudness (MCL, discomfort, or entire loudness scales) include:

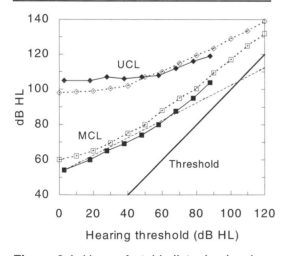

Figure 9.1 Uncomfortable listening level and most comfortable level for people with sensorineural hearing loss, averaged across 500, 1k, 2k, and 4 kHz. Data shown with filled symbols are from Schwartz et al. (1988) and those with open symbols are from Pascoe (1988). The dashed line has a slope of 0.5, illustrating the relationship between MCL and the half-gain rule.

- Shapiro (1976);
- CID (Central Institute for the Deaf; Pascoe, 1978; Skinner et al 1982);
- LGOB (Loudness Growth in half Octave Bands; Allen, Hall and Jeng, 1990; Pluvinage, 1989);
- IHAFF/Contour (Independent Hearing Aid Fitting Forum; Cox, 1995; Valente & Van Vliet, 1997);
- ScalAdapt (Kiessling, Schubert & Archut, 1996); and
- DSL[i/o] (Desired Sensation Level Input-Output, curvilinear compression version; Cornelisse, Seewald & Jamieson, 1995).

Gain prescription procedures based on threshold alone include:

- NAL (National Acoustic Laboratories; Byrne & Tonisson, 1976);
- Berger (Berger, Hagberg & Rane, 1977);
- POGO (Prescription of Gain and Output; McCandless & Lyregaard, 1983);
- NAL-R (NAL-Revised; Byrne & Dillon, 1986);
- POGO II (Schwartz Lyregaard & Lundh, 1988);
- NAL-RP (NAL-Revised, Profound; Byrne, Parkinson & Newall, 1991);
- FIG6 (Killion & Fikret-Pasa, 1993); and
- NAL-NL1 (NAL nonlinear; Dillon, 1999).

Some procedures have given the user the option of basing the gain-frequency response prescription entirely on threshold, or on a combination of threshold and uncomfortable listening levels:

- MSU (Memphis State University; Cox, 1988); and
- DSL[i/o] (linear compression version; Cornelisse, Seewald and Jamieson, 1995).

For linear hearing aids, prescription of gain has received far more attention than the prescription of maximum output (OSPL90), despite the probable high importance of OSPL90 for linear hearing aids. For nonlinear (compression) hearing aids, the level at which

hearing aids limit the maximum output is less important than for linear aids because some of the gain reduction that occurs when a hearing aid limits is provided by the more gradual form of compression that commences at lower input levels. In addition, OSPL90 can be considered to be just one of the many output curves (each for a different input level) that can be specified for a nonlinear hearing aid.

Prescribing the best response for a given patient *seems* like a simple problem, but prescription formulae have changed often during the several decades that this topic has been researched. Finding a simple relationship between hearing loss and gain has not been easy because:

- The optimum gain-frequency response probably depends on the type of input signal, and its level and spectral shape, whereas the hearing aids used for clinical practice and research until the last decade have been linear, and hence have not been able to provide this variation;
- The optimum gain-frequency response *may* depend on things such as supra-threshold loudness perception and frequency resolution ability in a way that can not be predicted from threshold (although no such relationships have as yet been established); and may depend on other unknown factors;
- The optimum gain-frequency response for a person may depend on the nature of the auditory input to which the person has become accustomed during the preceding months or years;
- For a particular person listening to speech at a particular time and input level, there may not even *be* a single optimum response. Rather, the optimum may depend on whether the person wishes to maximize intelligibility, or comfort, or some other perceptual attribute of sound.[443]

More thorough reviews of the development of prescriptive procedures and evaluative procedures can be found in Byrne (1983) and

---

Understanding the nature of prescriptive procedures

The prescription procedures listed in this section vary in many ways other than whether they are based on threshold or loudness data. When confronted with a new procedure, there are three essential questions to ask:

1. On what type of patient data is the procedure based? Most commonly this will either be thresholds or the levels needed to achieve certain ratings of loudness;

2. What type of amplification characteristic is being prescribed? For a linear aid, this will most commonly be gain and/or the maximum output (OSPL90). For a nonlinear aid, it will most commonly be the gain prescribed for several input levels, or some other characteristics derived from these gains, such as compression ratio.

3. What is the aim of the selection procedure, and what relationships have been assumed in the link between the patient data and the amplification characteristics?

---

in Hawkins (1984). Some of the more recent and popular procedures for gain and OSPL90 are described in more detail later in this chapter.

Prescription rules invariably involve some sort of formula. Once a prescription method has been chosen, there are several ways to calculate the results of its formula. Most obviously, one can use an electronic calculator to find the required gain or output level at each frequency. Some procedures are also published in graphical or tabular form, and some are available on a slide rule. Increasingly, these manual calculation or look-up methods are not necessary, because the formulae are being included within computer-based fitting software. With these, the user needs only to input the necessary patient data (such as the audiogram), and the computer performs the calculations. There are three broad types of computerized methods for calculating the target.

First, several computer programs are specifically designed to calculate prescription targets:

- MSU (Memphis State University);
- HASP (Hearing Aid Selection Program, for the NAL-RP procedure);
- DSL3.1 (Desired Sensation Level, for linear aids);

- DSL 4.0 (Desired Sensation Level I/O method);
- VIOLA (Visual Input-Output Locator Algorithm, for the IHAFF/Contour procedure);
- FIG6;
- NAL-NL1 (for the NAL nonlinear procedure); and
- HAS (Hearing Aid Selection, for various procedures).

See de Jonge (1996) for a detailed review of most of these packages.

Second, software programs provided by hearing aid manufacturers for fitting their programmable hearing aids often include formulae for one or more of the better known prescription targets. Usually, the programs also automatically adjust the hearing aid to approximately match the target.

Third, real-ear gain analyzers also include the better-known formulae, so targets can easily be compared to the measured real-ear response.

The emphasis in this chapter will be on real-ear gain, both real-ear aided gain (REAG; see Section 4.2) and real-ear insertion gain (REIG; see Section 4.3). An REAG prescription specifies how much the SPL at the eardrum should exceed the SPL in the incoming field. Insertion gain, by contrast, describes how much more signal should be at the eardrum when the person is aided than when they are unaided. Of course, either type of gain can be converted to the other by adding or subtracting the real-ear unaided gain (REUG) curve (see Section 4.3). No matter how real-ear gain is calculated, it can be converted to a 2 cc coupler gain or ear simulator gain, using the principles described in Sections 4.2.2 and 4.3.2 and the specific procedures described in Section 10.7.

POGO formula

$IG_i = 0.5 * H_i + k_i$

Freq	250	500	1k	2k	4k
k_i (dB)	-10	-5	0	0	0

POGO II formula

$IG_i = 0.5 * H_i + k_i$,   for $H_i < 65$

$IG_i = 0.5 * H_i + k_i + 0.5 * (Hi-65)$,

                           for $H_i > 65$

9.2   Gain and Frequency Response Prescription for Linear Amplification

Linear hearing aids have the same gain-frequency response for all input levels, until the output level is high enough to cause the aid to limit. The following three sections will present the concepts and calculation details, as applied to sensorineural hearing losses, for three procedures that are in common use today. In each of the formulae presented in the panels in this chapter, IG_i will represent the insertion gain at the *i'th* frequency, k_i will represent an additive fitting constant at the same frequency, and H_i will represent the hearing threshold (in dB HL) at the same frequency.

9.2.1   POGO

The original POGO (prescription of gain and output) procedure,[587] is a straightforward application of the half-gain rule, with an additional low cut. The low cut was intended to decrease upward spread of masking from low-frequency ambient noise. The low cut could, of course, also be justified by the greater intensity of speech at low frequencies and by the lesser importance of speech information in the very low-frequency region. The amount of low-frequency cut specified was based on the originators' experience. Insertion gain at each frequency is equal to

half the hearing loss at that frequency, plus a constant, as shown in the accompanying panel. The procedure was intended to be used only for hearing losses up to 80 dB HL.

In 1988, the procedure was extended to provide additional gain for people with severe and profound hearing losses.[782] The revised procedure, known as POGO II, prescribes the same gain as POGO for losses less than 65 dB HL. For greater losses, however, gain increases by 1 dB for every 1 dB increase in hearing loss. The amount of additional gain prescribed in POGO II was based on an experimental observation that people with severe and profound hearing losses prefer to listen to speech at a low sensation level.[a] For sensation level to be held at a small, but constant level as hearing threshold increases, the gain has to increase by the same amount that hearing loss increases (see Figure 9.1).

9.2.2   NAL

The NAL (National Acoustic Laboratories of Australia) prescription formula has also been revised since it was first published in 1976.[132] From the outset, the aim of the NAL procedure has been to maximize speech intelligibility at the listening level preferred by the aid wearer. Intelligibility is assumed to be maximized when all bands of speech are perceived to have the same loudness (i.e. *loudness equalization*). Does it matter if one

---

[a]   On average, the long-term rms 1/3-octave speech levels were only 7 dB above threshold (Walden et al., 1983).

frequency region is much louder than the rest? Yes! If one frequency region dominates the overall loudness, the patient will turn down the volume to make this region comfortable. Varying the volume control will also decrease the loudness of all other frequency regions, which may then be at too low a level to contribute optimally to intelligibility. This logic can best be understood in the context of the Speech Intelligibility Index method of predicting intelligibility (see Figure 8.1).[b]

The 1976 formula was derived as follows. Empirical observations indicated that preferred insertion gain at 1 kHz equaled 0.46 times the 1 kHz threshold (a minor variation of the half-gain rule).[125] It was assumed that at all frequencies an extra dB of loss required an extra 0.46 dB of gain. To deduce how much gain was needed at the other frequencies relative to 1 kHz, two additional data sources were used. Gain at each frequency was adjusted by an amount that mirrors the shape of the long-term average speech spectrum (LTASS), so that less gain was given to those frequencies where the speech is most intense (the low frequencies). Finally, gain was adjusted so that for someone with normal hearing, speech was raised to MCL, which for normal hearers was estimated to be the 60-phon equal loudness contour. Although the 1976 procedure is no longer used, the concepts behind the formula are still relevant. The *shape* of the gain-frequency response is equal to the shape of the normal equal loudness curve, minus the shape of the speech spectrum, plus 0.46 times the shape of the hearing threshold curve. The *gain* at 1 kHz is equal to 0.46 times the loss at 1 kHz. The NAL 1976 formula is very similar to the original POGO formula and to the recently published Cambridge formula for linear hearing aids.[617]

The type of gain prescribed by the NAL response is insertion gain (or equivalently,

in those days, functional gain). The original publication also expressed the formula in terms of the coupler gain likely to be needed to achieve the target insertion gain. These coupler gain targets included a reserve gain of 15 dB so that the hearing aids could be measured in the coupler at their maximum volume control setting, but be worn at a mid volume control setting.

During the early 1980s, Byrne extensively evaluated the original NAL formula.[111, 112] These evaluations showed that the aim of the NAL procedure (equal loudness at all frequencies) was correct. Unfortunately, the formula did not achieve equal loudness, especially for people with steeply sloping losses. The evaluation data (and other published data) were used to relate the gain-frequency response shape needed for equal loudness to the shape of the audiogram. This showed that the *shape* of the gain-frequency response, measured in dB/octave, varied at only 0.31 times the *shape* of the audiogram. The revised formula, which became known as NAL-R, reflects this but retains the well-established half-gain rule (actually 0.46) for the three-frequency *average* gain. The gain-frequency response prescribed for a flat 40 dB hearing loss is shown in Figure 9.2. The same shape applies to any other flat loss.

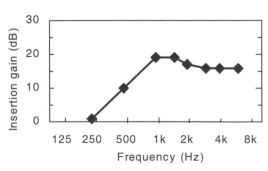

Figure 9.2 The insertion gain response prescribed by the NAL-R formula for a flat 40 dB hearing loss.

NAL formulae

NAL-R formula

$H_{3FA} = (H_{500} + H_{1k} + H_{2k})/3$

$X = 0.15 * H_{3FA}$

$IG_i = X + 0.31 * H_i + k_i$

Freq (Hz)	250	500	1k	2k	3k	4k	6k
k_i (dB)	-17	-8	1	-1	-2	-2	-2

NAL-RP formula

$X = 0.15 * H_{3FA}$ for $H_{3FA} < 60$

$X = 0.15 * H_{3FA} + 0.2 * (H_{3FA} - 60)$ for $H_{3FA} > 60$

$IG_i = X + 0.31 * H_i + k_i + PC$

Values of PC (in dB) to use in the above formula, as a function of frequency and hearing threshold at 2 kHz.

$H_{2\,kHz}$	Frequency (Hz)						
	250	500	1k	2k	3k	4k	6k
≤ 90	0	0	0	0	0	0	0
95	4	3	0	-2	-2	-2	-2
100	6	4	0	-3	-3	-3	-3
105	8	5	0	-5	-5	-5	-5
110	11	7	0	-6	-6	-6	-6
115	13	8	0	-8	-8	-8	-8
120	15	9	0	-9	-9	-9	-9

In turn, the NAL-R formula was evaluated by finding out whether test subjects would prefer to have the response varied from the NAL-R response by an additional high cut, high boost, low cut, or low boost.[117] Few preferred a variation, so the formula was (and still is) considered to be appropriate for people with a mild or moderate hearing loss listening to speech at a comfortable level.

A further series of experiments investigated the preferred gain and frequency response of adults and children with severe and profound hearing loss (Byrne, Parkinson & Newall, 1990, 1991). Compared to the NAL-R prescriptions, these subjects required additional gain, and less high-frequency emphasis. For three-frequency average hearing thresholds above 60 dB HL, the required gain increased at 66% of the increase in hearing loss, rather than the 46% rate that applied to people with less loss.

The additional low-frequency emphasis (or equivalently, the decrease in high-frequency emphasis) needed to maximize speech intelligibility could best be estimated based on the hearing threshold at 2 kHz. The response slope required progressively *less* high-frequency emphasis as the threshold at 2 kHz increased beyond 90 dB HL. (Reasons for this variation from loudness equalization are considered in Section 9.2.4.) Implementing these modifications required the X factor in the formula to be increased for three-frequency average losses greater than 60 dB HL, and addition of a *PC factor* (profound correction) when the 2 kHz threshold is greater than 90 dB HL. The resulting formula is known as the NAL-RP (revised, profound) formula.

The NAL-RP formula, on average, prescribed the gain and frequency response that maximized speech intelligibility for the severely and profoundly impaired test subjects. There was, however, considerable individual scatter around this average (more than for mildly and moderately impaired people). A comprehensive fitting should thus include an evaluation to determine whether the response should be varied from this starting point. Methods for doing this are included in Section 11.2.

9.2.3 DSL

The Desired Sensation Level (DSL) formula aims to provide the aid user with an audible and comfortable signal in each frequency region.[791, 792] It differs from the NAL-RP and POGO procedures in at least three ways.

First, the target it prescribes is a real-ear aided gain rather than a real-ear insertion gain. Second, the DSL procedure has been particularly well integrated with measurement methods that are convenient for use with infants and young children, without the use of average correction factors. The procedure consistently refers all measured quantities to the eardrum so that the aided speech levels and hearing thresholds can be compared as accurately as possible.

Last, the DSL procedure does not attempt to make speech *equally* loud in each frequency region, although it does attempt to make it *comfortably* loud. For any degree of hearing loss, the procedure specifies a target (or desired) sensation level,[c] as shown in Figure 9.3. As hearing thresholds increase, the target sensation level decreases. This is necessary because a person with a profound hearing loss has only a small dynamic range between threshold and discomfort.

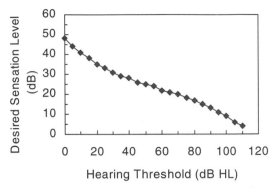

Figure 9.3 Sensation level targets for the Desired Sensation Level method as a function of hearing threshold, at 1 kHz. Values are very similar at other frequencies.

The DSL sensation level targets were derived and revised as follows:[788]

- For profound losses, the desired sensation levels are based on the sensation levels experimentally found to be optimal.[265, 820]

- For mild to severe losses, the sensation level targets for bands of speech are placed one standard deviation below the estimated MCLs for pure tones.[431, 694]

- For normal hearing, the desired sensation levels are those that are experienced by people with normal hearing when listening unaided.

The DSL procedure uses desired sensation levels to calculate its target real-ear aided gain. At each frequency, REAG equals hearing threshold (in dB SPL at the eardrum), plus the desired sensation level, minus the short term maximum speech levels in the field for speech at an overall level of 70 dB SPL. These calculations automated within the DSL 3.1 or DSL 4.0 computer program, or from the implementation of each program within several manufacturers' fitting software. The DSL 4.0 software also performs other calculations related to the implementation and verification of the prescription. These include allowing for the effects of different trans-

---

c   The sensation level of speech is defined as the short-term maximum rms level of a 1/3-octave band of speech minus the person's threshold at the center of the band. This is similar to the definition used in the Speech Intelligibility Index method.

DSL

The target real-ear aided gain values (in dB) used in DSL 4.0 as a function of threshold and frequency. From Seewald (private communication, by permission).

dB HL	Frequency								
	250	500	750	1000	1500	2000	3000	4000	6000
0	0	2	3	3	5	12	16	14	8
5	3	4	5	5	8	15	18	17	11
10	5	6	7	8	10	17	20	19	14
15	7	8	10	10	13	19	23	21	17
20	9	11	12	13	15	22	25	24	20
25	12	13	14	15	18	24	28	27	23
30	14	15	17	18	20	27	30	29	26
35	17	18	19	21	23	30	33	32	29
40	20	20	22	24	26	33	36	35	32
45	22	23	25	27	29	36	39	38	36
50	25	26	28	30	32	39	42	41	39
55	29	29	31	33	35	42	45	45	43
60	32	32	34	36	38	46	48	48	46
65	36	35	37	40	42	49	52	51	50
70	39	38	40	43	45	52	55	55	54
75	43	42	43	46	48	56	59	58	58
80	47	45	47	50	52	59	62	62	61
85	51	48	50	53	55	63	66	65	65
90	55	52	54	57	59	66	69	69	69
95	59	55	57	60	62	70	73	73	
100	62	59	61	64	66	73	76	76	
105		62	64	68	70	77	80	80	
110		66	68	71	73	80	83	84	

ducers used in the assessment of thresholds, allowing for individual RECD values, prescription of OSPL90, and graphical displays of measured and prescribed speech levels relative to threshold and discomfort.

9.2.4 Examples and comparisons: POGO II, NAL-RP and DSL

The three procedures use different formulae, and not surprisingly, lead to markedly different prescriptions for many hearing losses. This section will show the target insertion gains prescribed by each procedure[d] for each of four sample audiograms.

Mild, gently sloping loss. Figure 9.4 shows the audiogram and the insertion gain values prescribed by each of the three procedures. DSL prescribes the most high-frequency gain and NAL-RP prescribes the least. The

difference between DSL and NAL-RP is substantial at the highest frequencies.

Moderate, flat loss. The NAL-RP procedure provides somewhat less gain than the other two procedures for both the low and high frequencies (Figure 9.5).

Moderate, steeply sloping loss. The prescriptions shown in Figure 9.6 are very similar up to 1 kHz, but both DSL and POGO-II prescribe average gains considerably higher than the NAL-RP response, and frequency responses considerably steeper than the NAL-RP response.

Profound, gently sloping loss. The relative average gains and frequency response shapes are again similar for the DSL and POGO-II insertion gain prescriptions, but both prescribe much more high-frequency gain than NAL-RP (Figure 9.7).

[d]   DSL REAG targets have been converted to insertion gain by subtracting the adult average real-ear unaided gain curve (from Table 4.6, for 0° incidence, with no control microphone present).

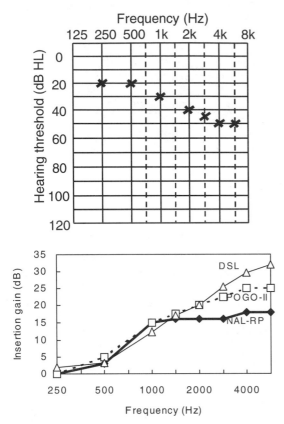

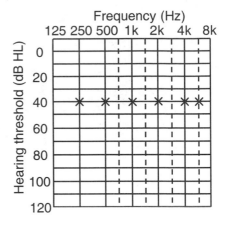

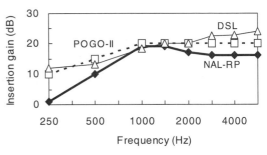

Figure 9.4 Audiogram of a mild, gently sloping sensorineural hearing loss, and insertion gains prescribed by the DSL (triangles), POGO-II (squares) and NAL-RP (diamonds) procedures.

Figure 9.5 Same as Figure 9.4, but for a moderate, flat sensorineural hearing loss.

These differences between the prescriptions can be thought of as a difference in average gain plus a difference in the shape of the frequency response. For adult patients wearing a hearing aid with a volume control, inappropriately prescribed average gain is not a serious problem, because patients will compensate for the clinician's error by adjusting their volume controls. Very young children and adults who cannot vary the volume control (for any reason) do not have this luxury, and the correct prescription of average gain is important. Patients usually can not, however, alter the frequency response shape. It seems likely that, for three or perhaps all four of these sample audiograms, at least one of these procedures is not prescribing an optimal average gain or frequency response.

If the differences between the prescription targets are as great as shown in the preceding examples, why has it not become obvious in clinical practice which, if any, of the three procedures is optimal?

One reason is that with real hearing aids, patients may receive the same frequency response no matter which prescription formula is used. When the NAL-RP method is used, it is common for the measured insertion gain at 3 and 4 kHz to be less than the target gain, because of the restricted range of response slopes that most hearing aids have in the 2 to 4 kHz range. In such cases, substitution of an alternative formula that requires a high-frequency response slope even steeper than the NAL-RP prescription will not result in a fitting with any more slope. Consequently, the large differences that exist between the procedures have rarely emerged in clinical practice *in the past*. Now that hearing aids are becoming more flexible (e.g.

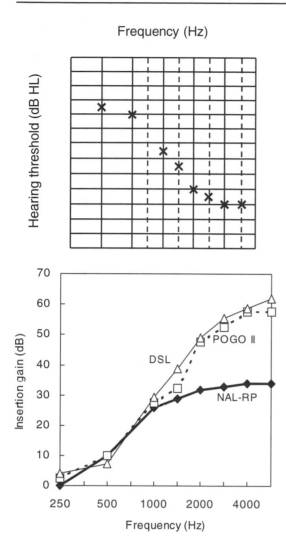

Figure 9.6 Same as Figure 9.4, but for a moderate, steeply sloping sensorineural hearing loss.

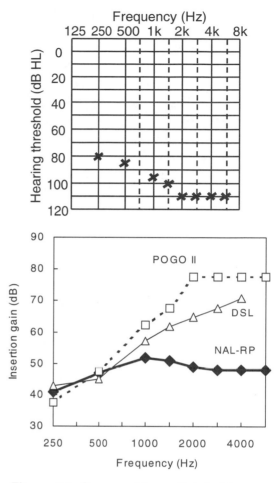

Figure 9.7 Same as Figure 9.4, but for a profound, gently sloping sensorineural hearing loss.

by using digital filters and/or multichannel amplification) they are much more able to match target gains. Consequently, the choice of procedure will have a pronounced effect on the frequency response achieved.

The relatively small high-frequency gain prescribed by the NAL-RP procedure, especially for those with a sloping high-frequency loss, is consistent with experimental data on speech perception. As hearing thresholds increase above about 60 dB HL, the usefulness of high-frequency speech information decreases markedly, even when the high-frequency components of speech are

audible.[129, 147, 253, 392, 738] In many cases, a small sensation level (of 10 to 20 dB) for the high-frequency components of speech is beneficial, but further increases in sensation level provide no additional benefit. For some people, even moderate audibility of high-frequency information decreases intelligibility, possibly because the intense high-frequency components mask the otherwise useful lower frequency components (*downward* spread of masking). That is, increasing audibility can be a bad thing for intelligibility! An excessive sensation level and/or bandwidth of high-frequency components can also lead to poor ratings of speech quality.[636, 859] Note that even for severe hearing loss, a very wide bandwidth can sometimes be beneficial, provided the presentation level of the high-frequency components is not excessively high.[813, 816]

The decreased ability of the impaired ear to extract information from signal even when it is audible has been referred to as *hearing loss desensitization*.[147, 696, 857] If speech intelligibility is estimated using the Speech Intelligibility Index (SII) without allowing for hearing loss desensitization, intelligibility is overpredicted whenever thresholds at any frequency are severe or profound. This overprediction casts considerable doubt on choosing the better response by examining which of two responses makes the greatest proportion of the speech spectrum audible, or by calculating which response gives the larger Speech Intelligibility Index.

Of course, hearing loss desensitization can, in principle, be allowed for when the Speech Intelligibility Index is calculated, but this has rarely been done. It is difficult to combine such an allowance with simplified methods (such as the elegant count-the-dot method) for calculating the Speech Intelligibility Index. Perhaps an extreme example of where hearing loss desensitization must be allowed for is where there is a dead region in the cochlea – a frequency region for which there are no remaining hair cells even though hearing thresholds may give the impression of some remaining hearing acuity.[618]

The impaired cochlea has often been compared to a bottleneck. There may be an abundance of information in the auditory world, and the hearing-impaired person may have a normal auditory system past the cochlea, but if the cochlea can pass only a restricted amount of information, the impaired person can access only a limited amount of information. In such circumstances, it arguably may be better to present less, rather than more, information to the cochlea, and the presentation of speech at a low sensation level is one way this can be done. A more extreme example is the speech simplification scheme discussed in Section 7.5.

The NAL-RP selection procedure is well supported by direct empirical data, and this is not true of any other procedure. The procedure is based on measured speech intelligibility, and subjective preferences for quality and intelligibility, in quiet and in noise, for subjects with losses from mild to profound. Subsequent to formulation of the NAL-R procedure, an experiment using adult subjects revealed that few people significantly preferred any of four alternative frequency response shapes.[117] Averaged across frequency, the prescribed gain agreed closely with the preferred gain. Experiments using older children confirmed that averaged across children with the same audiogram, the NAL-RP procedure neither underestimated nor overestimated the preferred response slope or the preferred average gain.[146, 823] Other studies examining requirements for multi-memory hearing aids also provide support for the NAL-R or NAL-RP response.[442, 447]

Conversely, some studies that have closely examined audibility are sometimes interpreted as showing that other responses will lead to more intelligible speech, or that the response shape does not matter. It is easily possible to provide a prescription that makes speech more audible than the NAL-RP response, and this directly leads to a higher SII value.[403, 738] This is achieved simply by using more gain at some or all frequencies, and hence results in more loudness, which may not be appreciated by the patient. Conditions with a very high SII value (achieved by making speech highly audible at all frequencies) usually do not result in an intelligibility score commensurately higher than that obtained with the NAL-R response, and can sometimes have a lower score.[738]

Kuk & Pape (1992) compared the NAL-R response to a variety of responses individually selected for subjects using a paired-comparison procedure while they listened to several stimuli. For one sub-group of subjects (those with moderate to severe flat loss), the response that maximized clarity in a speech babble was rated more highly in real-life situations than the NAL-R response or any of the alternative responses. Averaged across the subgroup, this response had about 4 dB more gain than the NAL-R response from 250 to 1000 Hz.

Finally, Van Buuren et al. (1995) showed that a wide range of responses produce similar speech reception thresholds in noise. These responses were not compared to those prescribed by any formula. It is noteworthy, however, that the response for which speech was amplified to the middle of the dynamic range at all frequencies received the highest rating for clarity and pleasantness, and was judged to have the ideal loudness and degree of sharpness versus dullness. That is, the results show the desirability of amplifying speech to the middle of the dynamic range, although some variation from the target may have only small adverse consequences. Speech *will* vary from the middle of the dynamic range whenever the input level varies, even for an optimal prescription. If the prescription is sub-optimal, variation from the middle of the dynamic range will be greater than is necessary.

On balance, the experimental evidence indicates that the NAL-RP prescription provides a reasonable starting estimate of the gain-frequency response needed for an individual patient. The best response for an individual may not be identical to the prescription, but this same limitation would seem to apply even more often to any of the alternative formulae based on thresholds alone. The need for individual evaluation and fine-tuning, potentially *away* from the prescribed response, seems greatest for those with severe and profound hearing loss.

There are two notes of caution to this otherwise positive verdict for the NAL-RP response. First, subjects used in all the research studies cited were not used to a high-frequency emphasis greater than that prescribed by the NAL-RP procedure. (Often,

Practical issues associated with the methods

- The NAL-RP formula (as with its NAL predecessors) is based on maximizing speech intelligibility and sound quality in quiet and in noise. A convenient consequence of the procedure, however, is that for people with sloping losses, less high-frequency gain is required than for most other procedures. This makes targets easier to achieve, and makes feedback oscillation less likely.

- The measurement procedures developed as part of the DSL procedure are particularly advantageous with infants, as further discussed in Section 15.2. These excellent measurement methods can be applied to other prescription formula, as outlined in Sections 10.7 and 15.4.3.

not even the NAL-RP gain target at 4 kHz would have been achieved in the subject's usual hearing aid.) It is possible that the subjects may have preferred and/or benefited from a greater high-frequency emphasis if they had enough experience with it prior to participating in the experiments. In the past, limitations with wearable hearing aids prevented the desired responses from being achieved. Multiband hearing aids now make such an experiment possible.

Second, audibility of high-frequency sounds can sometimes be restricted by the high-frequency maximum output of the hearing aid, rather than by the high-frequency gain. It is conceivable that some additional high-frequency gain would be valuable if it could be achieved without saturating the hearing aid. This is very much a supposition, as some of the research showing the decreased value of high-frequency amplification for severe and profound hearing loss has *not* been constrained by high-frequency distortion.

Theoretical conundrum: preserving individual open-ear characteristics. Should we use insertion gain targets or real-ear aided gain targets?

With a REAG target, all people who have the same degree of hearing loss are prescribed the same gain from the free field to their eardrum, irrespective of the gain provided by their unaided ear canal. With an insertion gain target, all people who have the same degree of hearing loss are prescribed the same increase in SPL at their eardrum, relative to the SPL at their eardrum when listening unaided.

One might argue that the IG approach is better, because the job of a hearing aid is to provide more signal than a person gets when unaided, and this is precisely what insertion gain measures.

Alternatively, one might argue that once a person puts on a hearing aid, what they used to receive at their eardrum when they were unaided is inconsequential! Either type of procedure can be converted into the other by adding or subtracting an average REUG (see Section 10.6). For people with a REUG curve that is close to average, the type of target prescribed would then have little effect on the amplification prescribed (though the particular formula chosen may well do so). Consequently, it does not matter which prescription approach is used (Carter, 1993; Palmer 1991). A person whose REUG curve is a little different from average is more likely to prefer an amplification characteristic that incorporates his or her own REUG curve than amplification characteristic that incorporates an average REUG curve (Palmer 1991) - that is, an insertion gain prescription is preferable.

The impact of choosing a REIG versus a REAG target will be greatest for people whose REUG curves are most dissimilar from average. One such group comprises people whose external ears have been altered by surgery, especially mastoidectomy. Their enlarged ear canals cause a Helmholtz resonance in the 1 to 2 kHz range, instead of the expected wavelength resonance around 2.7 kHz. It certainly does not seem appropriate to fit a hearing aid in such a way that this unnatural resonance is maintained (Killion & Monser, 1993). In other words, a REAG target is most appropriate for this group. The same argument applies to a second group of people who have a large perforation of the eardrum, and who hence have a REUG curve with two peaks separated by a valley (Moryl, Danhauer & DiBartolomeo, 1992). Adults with REUG characteristics greatly different from average prefer amplification characteristics based on an average REUG (Palmer, 1991) - that is, a REAG prescription is preferable.

A third group with unusual REUG characteristics is children under about three years of age. At birth, infants have an ear canal wavelength resonance around 6 kHz (Kruger, 1987), decreasing gradually to adult values as their ear canals get longer. It is unclear whether they obtain any advantages from having a high resonant frequency, or whether a high resonant frequency is just the inevitable consequence of a short ear canal, which in turn is the inevitable consequence of a small head. The latter seems more probable, and if so, a REAG target seems more appropriate for this group.

In summary, it seems more appropriate to adopt a REAG target for young children and for people with deformed or surgically altered ear canals, but an insertion gain target for all other patients. This split is convenient, because for young children it is easier to measure REAG (see Section 15.4.3), whereas for adults it is easier to measure insertion gain, because locating the probe microphone for accurate results is easier (see Section 4.3.1). For adults with REUG characteristics that are close to average, it is not critical which type of real-ear gain is chosen as a target.

9.3   Gain, Frequency Response, and Input-Output Functions for Nonlinear Amplification

Nonlinear prescription can be viewed as specifying the gain-frequency response for several input levels. Typically, both the average gain and the shape of the frequency response will vary with input level. Alternatively, the prescription can be viewed as specifying an input-output (I-O) curve for several frequencies. It is necessary to specify the I-O curve for at least as many frequencies as there are channels in a multichannel hearing aid (such as the three-channel aid shown in Figure 2.2).

In principle, if enough frequencies and levels are used, all the information in a set of I-O curves at different frequencies is also contained within a set of gain-frequency responses at different input levels. Both diagrams are useful: The required compression ratios and thresholds are most easily read from a set of I-O curves, and the required filter characteristics are most easily read from a set of gain-frequency responses. Filters are used to form the individual channels in a multichannel aid, and can also be used to shape the frequency response within each of these channels.

If a comprehensive set of gain-frequency curves or I-O curves has been prescribed, compression ratios and compression thresholds at each frequency have effectively also been specified. Such prescriptions do not reveal the compressor response times, however. Currently, no prescription procedures prescribe compressor response times in the sense of matching desired response times to characteristics of the patient. As we saw in Chapter 5, the relative advantages of fast versus slow compression are still being debated. Furthermore, it is not yet clear whether response times have to be individually prescribed, let alone how this should be done.

The reader should absorb the issues discussed regarding linear responses: they all apply to nonlinear amplification, and many further issues arise. Our knowledge about required linear amplification characteristics also provides a useful crosscheck in the still-hazy world of nonlinear requirements. Extensive research into linear amplification tells us about the amplification required for typical mid-level inputs. This knowledge should be equally applicable to nonlinear hearing aids.[114] Additional research is needed to tell us how nonlinear hearing aids should amplify for low and high input levels.

In fact, it has been suggested that the NAL-RP selection procedure can be applied to nonlinear hearing aids for 65 or 70 dB SPL input levels.[904] At higher or lower input levels, the response then varies depending on the compression rationale chosen by the clinician or hearing aid designer. Such rationales might include noise reduction, or loudness normalization, with the typically opposing consequences outlined in Section 6.4.

The first six prescription procedures described in the following sections are based at least partially on normalizing loudness. That is, they aim to give the hearing-impaired person the same loudness that a normal-hearing person listening to the same sound would perceive. They aim to normalize overall loudness as well as normalizing the loudness relationships between different frequency regions. The principles of loudness normalization were introduced in Section 6.3.5. The first four procedures require the loudness scale of each patient to be measured.

9.3.1   LGOB

The idea of using nonlinear amplification to restore normal loudness perception has been around for at least 25 years.[924] The first clinically practical procedure to accomplish loudness normalization, however, was the loudness growth in half-octave bands (LGOB) procedure.[15, 723] In this procedure, the hearing-impaired patient categorizes the loudness of narrow bands of noise using a

LGOB

Triple bursts of half-octave bands of noise are presented at random frequencies and at levels between threshold and discomfort. Testing is performed at the octave frequencies from 250 Hz to 4 kHz. Patients rate their loudness using the following scale:

7.   Too loud
6.   Very loud
5.   Loud
4.   OK
3.   Soft
2.   Very soft
1.   Not audible

The stimuli continue to be presented until the same response is obtained twice for each level.

seven-point loudness scale. The average levels corresponding to each loudness category are then compared to the levels needed to produce the same categories in normal-hearing people. For each input level, the gain needed to normalize loudness is deduced (see Figure 6.10). The procedure is most easily performed using special-purpose software and hardware, such as the ReSound hearing aid programmer or the Madsen Aurical.

If the procedure is applied to any aid with adjustable compression thresholds, then compression thresholds must be prescribed independently of the LGOB results.

9.3.2 IHAFF/Contour

During the mid 1990s, a group of clinicians and researchers noted that there was an urgent need for a practical procedure that could be applied to any hearing aid with adjustable wide dynamic range compression.[176, 906] The group was called the Independent Hearing Aid Fitting Forum (*IHAFF*), and the prescription they devised used loudness scaling to normalize loudness at each frequency. The particular loudness scaling procedure used is called the Contour Test (see panel).

In the IHAFF/Contour protocol, the VIOLA software program presents the results of the loudness normalization as three points on an input-output function at each frequency at which loudness scaling is carried out. These three points show the output levels needed to normalize the loudness of 1/3-octave bands of speech, when the complete speech signal is at the levels needed for normal-hearing people to rate its loudness as *soft*, *average*, and *loud*, respectively.[176, 906] The actual speech levels adopted, and the shape of the speech spectrum assumed in the derivation of the procedure have no effect on the shape of the I-O curve prescribed, but rather determine which three points on the underlying continuous I-O curve are pinpointed as the targets. Figure 9.8 shows an example of an I-O target prescribed by VIOLA. To simplify adjustment of the hearing aid in a coupler, the output scale in this graph is expressed as SPL in a 2-cc coupler.

As with all loudness normalization procedures, it is not possible to read a compression threshold from the I-O target graph, because complete loudness normalization requires that compression be maintained down to input levels corresponding to the threshold of

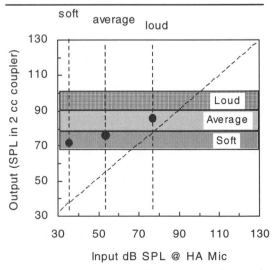

Figure 9.8 An example of the three-point I-O curve, for a frequency of 2 kHz, prescribed by the VIOLA software on the basis of the IHAFF procedure.

IHAFF, Contour, and VIOLA

The Contour test (Cox et al., 1997) is the loudness scaling procedure used with the IHAFF loudness normalization prescription. Pulsed warble tones are presented in an ascending sequence from 5 dB above threshold until the patient indicates that the stimulus is uncomfortably loud. At each level, patients indicate which of the following seven categories best describes the loudness:

7.   Uncomfortably loud
6.   Loud, but O.K.
5.   Comfortable, but slightly loud
4.   Comfortable
3.   Comfortable, but slightly soft
2.   Soft
1.   Very soft

The test is simple enough to perform manually, but software is available to control several audiometers so that the test can be automated. The results of three or four ascending sequences are averaged. It takes approximately 5 minutes per frequency, per ear, for the test to be carried out (Cox, 1995).

A software program called VIOLA (Visual Input/Output Locator Algorithm) simplifies the task of calculating the input-output curve, based on the Contour test results. At each frequency, an input-output curve with two compression thresholds and two compression ratios can be drawn. This is useful when prescribing for hearing aids with compression ratios that either increase (curvilinear compression) or decrease (low-level compression) as input level increases.

---

normal hearing. The IHAFF authors recommend, however, that the compression threshold be chosen in the range 40 to 45 dB SPL.[906] Once power summation across adjacent 1/3-octave bands is taken into account, a compression threshold of 40 dB SPL is low enough that compression is activated at all frequencies for soft speech. Within the high-frequency region, however, only the more intense phonemes within a soft speech signal will activate the compressor.

9.3.3   Madsen Aurical method

At least one audiometer manufacturer has incorporated loudness scaling hardware and software within a combined audiometer and insertion gain analyzer. The loudness scaling method referred to in the Aurical test equipment as the Madsen method is based on the procedure proposed by Kiessling et al., (1995), but with only 7 loudness categories. It has been evaluated for reliability (see

Section 9.3.8). Like the scaling procedures already described, its results are used to normalize loudness for narrow band stimuli.

Madsen Aurical method

Double bursts of narrow bands of noise are presented, and patients rate their loudness using the following scale:

7.   Too loud
6.   Very loud
5.   Loud
4.   Comfortable
3.   Soft
2.   Very soft
1.   Not audible

The stimuli are presented at 10 equally spaced levels, each presented twice, in pseudo-random order (but with a tendency to increase in level) from HTL - 5 dB up to UCL + 5 dB. HTL and UCL are determined prior to loudness scaling.

9.3.4   ScalAdapt

For the loudness normalization procedures discussed in the three preceding sections, hearing aid prescription is a three-step process:

- the loudness scale for the patient is measured;

- at each level, the gain needed to normalize loudness is calculated;

- the hearing aid is adjusted to match the gain target.

ScalAdapt[455] is a clever one-step combination of these three steps. The aid is pre-adjusted using an established threshold-based procedure. Loudness scaling, using an 11-point scale, is then performed while the patient is wearing the hearing aid. Instead of finding the loudness that corresponds to each input level, the clinician adaptively adjusts some characteristic of the hearing aid until the patient gives a desired loudness rating. This desired rating is, of course, the loudness that would be perceived by a normal-hearing person listening unaided.

For instance, if a normal-hearing person would rate a sound of 60 dB SPL at a particular frequency as *comfortable,* then the gain of the hearing aid is adjusted until the hearing-impaired person also rates a 60 dB SPL sound at that frequency as *comfortable.* The hearing aid parameters are adjusted adaptively: If the loudness rating given is different from the target, gain or some compression parameter must be adjusted in the correct direction. The input levels used (and hence the target loudness categories), the order in which they are tested, and the amplification parameters adjusted, have to be appropriate to the filtering and compression characteristics that are adjustable on each aid. Otherwise, the adjustment made in one step may inadvertently undo the normalization for another input level that was achieved in a previous step. Kiessling et al. (1996) show how to apply the procedure to a Danavox

three-channel hearing aid, but it should be possible to apply the concept to any hearing aid.

The procedure seems very efficient and direct: loudness measurements are concentrated around the loudness targets that are used in the prescription, and once the loudness scaling is finished, so is adjustment of the hearing aid. If loudness is then measured using a wideband stimulus and it is found that loudness has not been normalized for this stimulus (because of loudness summation across bands), the hearing aid can be adjusted immediately using the same adaptive procedure. Adjustment of the hearing aid while the patient is wearing it and rating loudness means that there are no calibration difficulties arising from one transducer being used for loudness scaling and another for measurement of the aid response.

The only doubt about the procedure is that which currently exists about every nonlinear procedure: is it based on the correct rationale? The authors comment that in their experience,

---

ScalAdapt

- Double bursts of third-octave noise are presented at the center frequency of each channel of a multichannel hearing aid, while the patient is wearing the aid.

- An appropriate parameter on the aid is adjusted adaptively until the patient gives two consecutive ratings that are within one category of the rating that an average normal-hearing listener would perceive for the same stimulus level.

- The procedure is repeated for some combination of low, mid- and high-level stimuli that is appropriate to the adjustable parameters in the hearing aid being fitted.

- Low frequencies are intentionally made softer than normal.

loudness targets *should* depart from loudness normalization in the low frequencies. They say that complete loudness normalization creates excessive upward spread of masking, so they make low-frequency targets two loudness categories lower than those perceived by normal hearers.

9.3.5   FIG6

The FIG6 procedure specifies how much gain is required to normalize loudness, at least for medium- and high-level input signals. Unlike the previous procedures, however, it is not based on individual measures of loudness. Rather, it uses loudness data averaged across a large number of people with similar degrees of threshold loss. This means that only hearing thresholds are needed to calculate the required gain.

FIG6 gets its name from Figure 6 of the article in which the underlying data were first outlined by Killion & Fikret-Pasa (1993). Gain is directly prescribed for each of the input levels 40, 65 and 95 dB SPL, and is inferred for other levels by interpolation.

For low-level (40 dB SPL) input signals, the gain is prescribed on the basis that people with mild or moderate hearing loss should have aided thresholds 20 dB above normal hearing threshold. In most circumstances, it is not worth providing more gain than this, as background noise will prevent very soft sounds from being perceived, no matter how much gain is prescribed.[462] Except for the first 20 dB of hearing loss, every additional decibel of hearing threshold loss is therefore compensated by an extra decibel of gain. This rule is relaxed to a half-gain rule once the unaided threshold exceeds 60 dB HL because otherwise, the high gains that result are likely to cause feedback oscillation.[468]

For comfortable level (65 dB SPL) input signals, the amount of gain prescribed for any degree of threshold loss is equal to the average elevation of MCL for that threshold loss above MCL for normal hearing, using data published by Pascoe (1988). With this amount of insertion gain, narrow band sounds perceived as comfortable by a normal-hearing person will also be perceived as comfortable by the hearing-impaired aid wearer.

For high-level (95 dB SPL) input signals, the gain is similarly prescribed to be equal to the boost in signal level needed to make sounds as loud for the hearing-impaired aid wearer as they are for the average normal-hearing

---

FIG6 formula

For 40 dB SPL input levels:

$$IG_i = 0 \qquad\qquad \text{for} \qquad H_i < 20 \text{ dB HL}$$
$$IG_i = H_i - 20 \qquad\quad \text{for} \qquad 20 \leq H_i \leq 60 \text{ dB HL}$$
$$IG_i = 0.5\, H_i + 10 \qquad \text{for} \qquad H_i > 60 \text{ dB HL}$$

For 65 dB SPL input levels:

$$IG_i = 0 \qquad\qquad\qquad \text{for} \qquad H_i < 20 \text{ dB HL}$$
$$IG_i = 0.6\, (H_i - 20) \qquad \text{for} \qquad 20 \leq H_i \leq 60 \text{ dB HL}$$
$$IG_i = 0.8\, H_i - 23 \qquad\quad \text{for} \qquad H_i > 60 \text{ dB HL}$$

For 95 dB SPL input levels:

$$IG_i = 0 \qquad\qquad\qquad \text{for} \qquad H_i < 40 \text{ dB HL}$$
$$IG_i = 0.1\, (H_i - 40)^{1.4} \quad \text{for} \qquad H_i \geq 40 \text{ dB HL}$$

Note that the data upon which these formulae were derived extended only to 80 dB HL, so application of the formulae to greater losses should be done with caution.

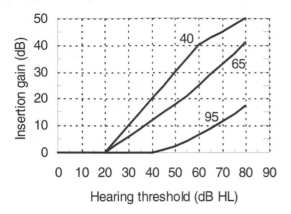

Figure 9.9 Insertion gain prescribed by the FIG6 method at any frequency as a function of hearing threshold, for each of the three input levels 40, 65, and 95 dB SPL.

listener. In this case, the data come from studies by Lippman et al (1981) and Lyregaard (1988).

Killion fitted a multi-line formula to the data referred to in the preceding paragraphs (see panel). Because the gain needed to normalize loudness depends only on hearing threshold and input level, the same formula applies at all frequencies. Software to perform the calculation is available, and this software also prescribes the required coupler response and compression ratios for low and high input levels and low and high frequencies. The FIG6 procedure is easy to use, either with a calculator, or from the special software, or from a graph, as shown in Figure 9.9.

9.3.6 DSL[i/o]

There are two DSL[i/o] procedures, each with its own underlying rationale.[159] The first procedure is called DSL[i/o] linear, where *linear* means that the I-O curve is a straight line over a wide range of input levels. That is, the compression ratio is constant within the wide dynamic range compression region, as shown in Figure 9.10, and should not be confused

with linear amplification. The DSL[i/o] linear procedure uses a compression ratio large enough to fit an extended dynamic range at each frequency into the dynamic range of the hearing-impaired person at the same frequency. This extended dynamic range is equal to the range from a normal-hearing person's threshold up to the hearing-impaired person's uncomfortable level. It thus prescribes a compression ratio greater than that required to normalize loudness.[e] Figure 9.10 shows the basic assumptions behind the DSL[i/o] linear formula. The upper limit of comfort for the hearing-impaired person can either be estimated on the basis of threshold (using the real-ear saturation response recommendations from DSL 3.1 method[791] or can be individually measured for each patient.

The second DSL procedure for nonlinear hearing aids is more conventional in that it *is* aimed at normalizing loudness. This proce-

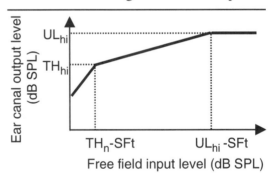

Figure 9.10 The DSL[i/o] method, showing which input levels are mapped to which output levels, using the terminology from Cornelisse et al. (1995). *UL* stands for upper level of comfortable listening, and TH stands for threshold, where both are expressed in dB SPL in the ear canal. The subscripts *n* and *hi* stand for normal and hearing impaired respectively. *SFt* is the sound field transform from free field SPL to ear canal SPL for the unaided ear for the frequency in question, and is synonymous with REUG.

---

e   For people with a mild or moderate loss, average discomfort level is only slightly larger than the normal discomfort level, so the extended dynamic range will only be slightly larger than the normal dynamic range. For people with a severe or profound loss, the difference will be greater (see Figure 9.1 or Figure 9.14). The DSL 4.0 software allows the user to choose whether the prescription is based on mapping a normal or extended dynamic range into the impaired person's range.

dure is called DSL[i/o] curvilinear, because the I-O functions prescribed can be curved lines within the compression region. With this procedure, normal hearing threshold is amplified to the hearing-impaired threshold, and the normal-hearing discomfort level is amplified to the hearing-impaired discomfort level. In between, however, the shape of the I-O curve depends on the rate at which loudness grows for the normal-hearing person relative to the rate at which it grows for the hearing-impaired person. These rates are characterized by the exponent to which stimulus level is raised in the equation that relates loudness category to stimulus level.

The curvilinear procedure is not as fully developed as the DSL[i/o] linear alternative. A potential problem is that loudness category scaling has to be performed in such a way that the exponent that describes loudness growth can be reliably obtained, and any variation of this exponent with level allowed for. As with all nonlinear procedures, the need to precisely normalize loudness at each frequency and level has not yet been established.

9.3.7   NAL-NL1

Unlike the preceding methods, the NAL-NL1 (nonlinear, version 1) formula does not attempt to restore normal loudness at each frequency. The underlying rationale is to maximize speech intelligibility, subject to the overall loudness of speech at any level being no more than that perceived by a normal-hearing person.[224] To derive the gain-frequency response that achieves this at each input level, two theoretical models were used.

The first was a modification of the Speech Intelligibility Index method in which allowance was made for the effects of hearing loss desensitization (see Section 9.2.4), and for the effects of listening at high SPLs. Essentially, hearing loss not only decreases audibility, but also decreases the person's ability to recover useful information, even when the speech is audible, as discussed in Section 9.2.4. Even people with normal hearing are less able to recover information from a signal if they are forced to listen at high levels. People with a severe or profound hearing loss have no choice in this: either they listen at high SPLs or they do not hear anything!

The second model was a method for calculating loudness, again allowing for the effects of sensorineural hearing loss.[620] The only information required by both of these models are hearing thresholds, and the speech spectrum levels input to the ear after amplification.

NAL-NL1

The NAL-NL1 method is based on a complex equation that specifies insertion gain at each standard 1/3-octave frequency from 125 Hz to 8000 Hz. At each frequency, the gain depends on threshold at that frequency, three-frequency average threshold, slope of the audiogram from 500 Hz to 2 kHz, and the overall level of a broad-band signal with a long-term spectrum like that of speech.

Alternatively, the aid can be prescribed in terms of real-ear aided gain. REAG is deduced from insertion gain by adding the adult average REUG to the insertion gain target (see Section 4.3)

The prescription can also be expressed as an I-O curve at any frequency, or as a coupler gain-frequency response. Because these are often measured with pure tones, the NAL nonlinear software allows for the crest factor and bandwidth differences between pure tones and speech signals. The prescription for pure tones, but not the prescription for broadband signals, therefore depends on the number of channels within the hearing aid.

For speech input at any level, gain at each frequency was systematically varied within a high-speed computer until the calculated speech intelligibility was maximized, but without the calculated loudness exceeding that loudness calculated for normal-hearing people listening to speech at the same level. This process was repeated for many representative audiograms, and the optimized gains for each audiogram, for each input level, were found. Because this was a very time consuming process, even for a single audiogram at a single input level, an equation was fitted to the complete set of optimized gains. This equation thus summarizes all the optimizations and can be applied to any audiogram. It is available as part of a computer program called NAL-nonlinear, and is progressively being included in the fitting software provided by the manufacturers of hearing aids and real-ear gain analyzers.

The NAL-nonlinear software program displays the result as either gain curves at different levels, or I-O curves at different frequencies. These curves can be for a 2-cc coupler, an ear simulator, or the real ear. In the case of a real-ear prescription, the gains can be either insertion gain or REAG. For multichannel hearing aids, the software also recommends crossover frequencies, compression thresholds, compression ratios, and gains for 50, 65 and 80 dB SPL input levels.

For a speech input level of 70 dB SPL, the procedure prescribes a gain-frequency response similar to that prescribed by the NAL-RP linear procedure. Also, for most hearing losses, all mid-frequency third-octave bands of speech turn out to have approximately equal loudness. As input level increases, the range of frequencies that are amplified to equal loudness increases. Equal loudness was the critical *assumption* behind the earlier NAL procedures, but in the NAL-NL1 procedure was a *consequence* of maximizing speech intelligibility.

Amplification requirements for people with mixed losses are worked out by applying the procedure to the *sensorineural* part of the loss (i.e. the bone conduction thresholds) and then adding gain equal to 75% of the conductive part of the loss (i.e. the air-bone gap).

9.3.8   Comparison of procedures

This should be a short section! There has been little experimental evaluation of how well any of the nonlinear selection procedures work, which is what we really need to know. Making up a procedure is easier, more fun, and less discouraging than evaluating how well it works! For the most part all we can do at present is compare prescriptions, their theoretical advantages and disadvantages, and the speed and reliability with which they can be administered.

Differences in prescriptions
Differences between the responses prescribed by different methods are evident for many hearing losses. As an example, Figure 9.11 shows the insertion gains that would be prescribed for four nonlinear procedures for one audiogram. Two of the three loudness normalization procedures prescribe more or less flat insertion gains at all levels, corresponding to the flat hearing loss. By contrast, the NAL-NL1 procedure prescribes less gain for low-frequency signals than for mid- and high-frequency signals, particularly at low input levels.

We would not expect the NAL-NL1 prescription to agree with the other prescriptions, because NAL-NL1 is based on different principles. NAL-NL1 attempts to give speech the spectral balance required to maximize calculated intelligibility. Because low-frequency parts of speech are more intense and less important than the high-frequency parts, NAL-NL1 gives the low cut evident in Figure 9.11. The other procedures do not give this cut because they attempt to place speech at each frequency at the level needed to give normal loudness for that frequency. We would expect greater similarity between NAL-NL1 and ScalAdapt, because ScalAdapt aims to make the loudness less than normal at 250 and 500 Hz. Another significant difference becomes evident for sloping losses. The NAL-NL1 procedure never attempts to produce a high sensation level at the frequencies with the greatest loss, because

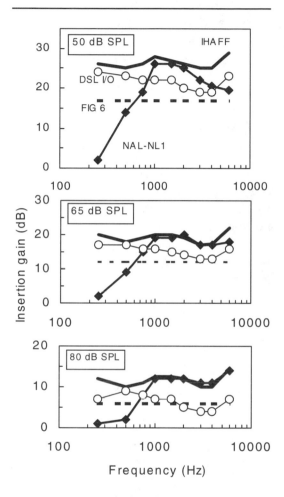

Figure 9.11 Insertion gain at input levels of 50, 65, and 80 dB SPL for each of four selection procedures for a person with a flat 40 dB hearing loss. The IHAFF prescriptions are based on the average loudness growth curves for people with various degrees of hearing loss (Cox, private communication). The DSL [i/o] prescription has been converted from real ear aided gain to insertion gain by subtracting an adult average REUG.

of the decreased ability of the ear to extract information at those frequencies. The gain provided by NAL-NL1 is insufficient to restore normal loudness at these frequencies. The loudness contribution from this region is therefore decreased, and loudness can perhaps be increased more usefully at another frequency.[f] For low input levels, NAL-NL1 may not provide any audibility at the frequencies where loss is greatest and/or where speech is least important for intelligibility.

It is less obvious why the other three procedures produce results different from each other, as their underlying principles all involve the concept of normalizing loudness. There are, however, slight differences in their rationales and in the normative data they use.

As an example of how well the procedures can sometimes agree at isolated frequencies, Figure 9.12 shows the prescription, represented as an input-output diagram for a flat 60 dB hearing loss. The prescriptions are amazingly similar over a wide range of hearing levels.

Experimental comparisons and evaluations

Stelmachowicz et al (1998) compared the gains for 50 and 80 dB SPL input levels prescribed by DSL[i/o], FIG6 and a proprietary algorithm to the gain preferred by subjects wearing the Resound two-channel, fast-acting, wide dynamic range compression hearing aid. DSL[i/o] over-prescribed gain at 500, 2000 and 4000 Hz at both input levels. FIG6 under-prescribed gain for mild and moderate hearing losses, particularly at the 80 dB input level, but over-prescribed gain for severe to profound losses. The proprietary, threshold-based formula more accurately prescribed the gain used. This is not too surprising, as the proprietary formula was a statistical summary of the gains actually used

---

[f]   In hearing aid fitting, we can think of having a loudness budget. If we apply more gain than is needed at a frequency, we spend too much of our loudness budget at that frequency. This leaves less loudness (and hence audibility and intelligibility) available for all the other frequency regions. If we over-spend in total, the patient either turns the volume control down (and destroys what we have carefully provided at *every* frequency) or rejects the hearing aid as too loud if it does not have a volume control.

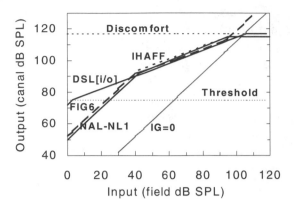

Figure 9.12. Input-output diagrams at 2 kHz, showing the knee-points in the curves, for the FIG6, NAL-NL1, DSL [i/o], and IHAFF procedures, for a person with a flat 60 dB HL hearing loss and a two-channel compression hearing aid. The IHAFF procedure is based on average loudness-growth curves. The DSL[i-o] curve is drawn with the CT used in its derivation. In practice a much higher CT would be used, similar to that of the other procedures.

- The WDRC aid employed compression limiting whereas the linear aid employed peak clipping.
- The linear aid was an old aid, whereas the WDRC aid was a new aid, and was tested second for all subjects.
- The high-frequency gain achieved for a 70 dB SPL input was less than the high-frequency gain prescribed, for both aid types. Because of differences in the two prescriptions and in the two hearing aids, the mean high-frequency gain achieved for the WDRC aid was actually closer to NAL-R than to the DSL[i/o] prescription.

Keidser and Grant (1999) compared two-channel WDRC hearing aids fitted according to NAL-NL1 and according to loudness normalization achieved using the IHAFF protocols (i.e. using individual loudness scaling). Preferences under field conditions and in the laboratory both strongly favored NAL-NL1. Speech identification scores in the laboratory also favored NAL-NL1, particularly in background noise.

Jenstad et al (2000) showed that for both narrow and broad band stimuli, WDRC hearing aids fitted according to DSL[i/o] normalized loudness more closely than could be achieved with linear hearing aids fitted according to a linear DSL prescription. The WDRC aid also produced higher speech identification scores than the linear aid whenever the speech input level was lower or higher than average.[416]

Threshold versus supra-threshold measurements

A controversial issue is whether nonlinear selection procedures should be based on hearing thresholds alone, or on supra-threshold loudness judgments. The FIG6, DSL[i/o] and NAL-NL1 procedures have the advantage of being quicker to use than the others reviewed in this chapter as they require only hearing thresholds as the input data.[g] This difference also makes the other

by wearers of precisely this type of hearing aid. It is possible, however, that the gains used by the subjects were influenced by the gains they were fitted with, which in turn were influenced by the proprietary fitting formula.

Humes et al. (1999) compared a two-channel Wide Dynamic Range Compression (WDRC) prescribed using DSL[i/o] to a linear hearing aid prescribed using NAL-R. The WDRC instrument gave superior speech intelligibility, particularly at lower input levels, and was preferred by 76% of the subjects in a field trial. One possible interpretation is that DSL[i/o] prescribed a more appropriate gain-frequency response for mid-level inputs than did NAL-R. There were, however, several other marked differences in the experimental conditions:

- For low input levels, the WDRC aid provided more gain at all frequencies than the linear aid.

---

g   Discomfort levels are an optional input for the DSL[i/o] procedure.

three loudness-based procedures unsuitable for use with some elderly and very young patients. Plausible arguments for and against using supra-threshold loudness judgments to prescribe nonlinear amplification can be advanced (see panel).

Apart from the issue of practicality, the decision about whether to use individual loudness scaling depends on the importance of individual differences in loudness perception. Although it is true that two people with the same hearing threshold may display different loudness growth curves, it is not apparent what the significance of this is. Two people with normal hearing can also have loudness growth curves that differ from each other. Perhaps if these two normal-hearing people were to obtain identical increases in threshold from identical cochlear damage, they would still perceive loudness differently from each other, just as they did before they had a hearing loss. If so, what would be the most appropriate "normal loudness" target for each of these people?[260] Variations in loudness perception may partly be due to differences in how the instructions or loudness categories are interpreted, or to other random factors, rather than being totally due to fundamental differences in loudness perception. Comparisons of different scaling methods indicate that even for a single person, the slope of the loudness growth curve varies greatly between scaling methods[414, 455]

If loudness scaling is used, it should be as reliable and efficient as possible. Loudness scaling is certainly possible with many elderly patients, though one evaluation showed poorer test-retest reliability for subjects aged 60 to 79 years than for subjects aged 20-29 years.[453] There are at least three procedures that use loudness scaling with a seven-point scale for the purposes of normalizing the loudness of narrow band stimuli (LGOB, IHAFF, Aurical Madsen method).

Choosing a threshold-based or loudness-based procedure?

There are theoretical and/or practical arguments for basing prescription on either threshold or supra-threshold measures.

Arguments for threshold-based

- Fast;
- Usable with all patients;
- Loudness can be partially predicted from thresholds;
- No evidence that loudness (as opposed to audibility) is critically important, especially considering that the world has become louder since industrialization;
- Loudness normalization for narrow band test stimuli in a test booth may not achieve normal loudness for broadband stimuli in the real world;
- "Normal" loudness is ill defined, because it varies considerably across people and across measurement techniques (Elberling, 1999).

Arguments for loudness-based

- Individuals with the same audiogram can perceive different loudness' for the same sound;
- Normal loudness is a worthwhile goal, as well as a means to achieving audibility and intelligibility;
- Accurate loudness prescription is important for automatic volume control aids.

Complexities in truly normalizing the loudness of speech

Because hearing loss varies with frequency, loudness growth characteristics have to be measured with narrowband signals. Differences between these test stimuli and speech can prevent loudness being normalized for speech, although it may be normalized for the test sounds.

- The differences in bandwidth complicate loudness normalization, unless the hearing-impaired person summates loudness across bandwidth in the same manner as does a normal-hearing person.

- Any difference in signal dynamics will create uncertainty in how to normalize. Should bands of speech and the test sounds be compared based on their rms levels, their maximum levels, or something else, and what effect will the compressor attack and release times have on this decision?

The magnitude of these bandwidth and dynamic factors is not well understood. As the need for normal loudness is unknown, the consequence of not achieving it for broadband speech stimuli is also unknown. If a fitting is based on individual loudness scaling, errors arising from differences in loudness between stimulus types can be minimized by a two-step approach, as carried out in the ScalAdapt procedure. After an initial scaling and adjustment using narrowband stimuli, a final scaling and adjustment can be carried out at one or two levels using continuous discourse.

The administration time and internal consistency of the loudness scaling part of these procedures has been quantitatively compared.[454] Whereas the IHAFF procedure required an average of 42 stimulus presentations per frequency, the LGOB required an average of 18, and the Madsen method always required exactly 20. Based on the scatter of individual points around a straight line fitted to the loudness data, the LGOB procedure was less internally consistent than the other two. This decreased consistency is possibly because the LGOB procedure randomizes presentation levels, whereas the IHAFF procedure uses an ascending test sequence and the Madsen procedure uses a partly randomized, partly ascending sequence. The Madsen method thus had the best combination of consistency and efficiency.

9.3.9 Prescribing compression thresholds

Prescribing compression threshold (the lowest input level for which compression occurs) is a problem for all nonlinear procedures. If loudness is to be completely normalized, compression is needed at input levels from the threshold of normal hearing upwards. That is, compression threshold must be around 0 dB SPL! It is easy to see the impracticality of this. The gain for low-level sounds will equal the hearing loss. This requires that the mold/shell be much more tightly sealed than would be necessary for a linear aid with gain equal to only half the hearing loss or less. A likely result would be physical discomfort or adverse effects on the quality of the aid wearer's own voice (i.e., the occlusion effect, see Section 5.3.2). Even if the high gain is achievable without feedback, it may not provide any benefit, and has been referred to as "empty gain".[462]

The high gain will occur only when the input level is around the threshold of normal hearing, and such low input levels occur only rarely in this noisy world. If useful sounds are rarely below, for example, 30 dB SPL, there is no point having a compression threshold below 30 dB SPL, and less gain will be needed.

Going in and out of compression: a non-issue

It is sometimes stated that compression thresholds should be either well below typical speech levels or well above them. Mid-level compression thresholds, it is argued, will adversely affect sound quality as the speech "goes in and out of compression." This argument either comes from a misunderstanding of compression, or reflects side effects that some compressors may once have had.

It is true that compression affects sound quality, but what is heard are the various effects of gain rapidly changing. The size of the quality change depends on how much and how quickly the gain changes. For a fixed compression ratio and attack and release times, the size of the gain change will be *greater* for speech that is totally within the compression region than for speech that is sometimes above compression threshold and sometimes below it.

An additional audible effect as the signal crosses compression threshold can occur only for badly designed compressors that generate a click as the compressor is activated.

Another issue is whether people *like* to have compression extending down to very soft sounds. There have been only two experimental evaluations of this question, both using a fast-acting, single channel compressor with a 2:1 compression ratio.[37, 237] Both studies concluded that most people prefer to have compression thresholds above 60 dB SPL rather than in the 40 to 50 dB range. While it is possible that people need time to become accustomed to hearing the softer sounds of life, there was no tendency for the preferred compression threshold to decrease when the subjects listened to the hearing aids during two successive one-month listening periods in their own environments.[37]

It is possible that different results would be obtained with lower compression ratios, with multiband compression aids, or with slow-acting compressors, but there are no studies upon which to base any conclusion about this.

Wide dynamic range compression for severe and profound hearing loss?

- The major practical problem is that as compression threshold is decreased below about 60 dB SPL, gain for low-level sounds has to be increased. Eventually, further increases in gain will not be possible, either because feedback oscillation occurs or because the maximum gain of the hearing aid is reached. Compared to linear amplification, patients with profound hearing loss certainly prefer such compression as can be achieved.[38]

- People with severe and profound sensorineural losses usually have small dynamic ranges, and many prescription procedures will prescribe big compression ratios. This is especially true of the DSL[i/o] procedure because it maps a wider than normal range into the impaired dynamic range. Authors of DSL and IHAFF express doubt about the wisdom of following the prescription when the result is a compression ratio larger than 4 or so. Nevertheless, something has to be done to decrease a wide range of input levels, wholly or partially, into the narrow dynamic range available to the person. Any combination of slow- or fast-acting wide dynamic range compression, together with fast or adaptive compression limiting will help achieve this aim.

The number of channels and the bandwidths of those channels are likely to affect prescription of compression threshold. Suppose it is considered necessary for speech at, say, 60 dB SPL to be partly in compression. This can be achieved in a single channel hearing aid if the pure tone compression threshold is set a little higher than 60 dB SPL.

For a multichannel hearing aid, lower compression thresholds will be needed if the same aim is to be achieved, because the total speech power is spread across many channels instead of being concentrated in one channel. If one hearing aid channel extended from say 2 kHz to 3 kHz, the speech components within that channel sum to only 41 dB SPL when the overall speech level is 60 dB SPL.[h] The compression threshold for that channel should therefore be much lower than for a single channel aid. The IHAFF and NAL-NL1 procedures both require a lower compression threshold for high frequencies than for low frequencies. In the NAL-NL1 procedure, the thresholds prescribed depend on the number of channels and their bandwidths.

While the advantages and disadvantages of a low compression threshold are easy to state (see panel), it is not yet established how compression thresholds should be prescribed for each hearing-impaired person.

For all nonlinear procedures that include an element of loudness normalization (and that is *all* current procedures), compression threshold is prescribed on the basis of a more or less arbitrary compromise between what the underlying loudness rationale implies, and what seems to be practical, necessary or desirable in real life. Given this lack of certainty about prescription, extra emphasis must be given to evaluating the suitability of compression threshold after the aid wearer has had a chance to try the hearing aid in his or her usual environments (see Chapter 11).

The pros and cons of a low compression threshold

This comparison assumes that the hearing aid is adjusted to amplify typical input levels to the most comfortable level, no matter what compression threshold is adopted.

Advantages of a low threshold

- Soft speech levels and the softer sounds within speech are more likely to be understood.

- The wearer will become aware of soft environmental sounds, like bird calls and clocks ticking.

Disadvantages of a low threshold

- Feedback oscillation is more likely (because of the higher gain for low-level sounds).

- Lower level noise during sufficiently long pauses in speech will be amplified more than the speech.

9.4 Allowing for Conductive and Mixed Hearing Losses

Everything in this chapter so far has been applicable to sensorineural hearing loss. A conductive loss, or a conductive component in a mixed loss, comprises a frequency-dependent attenuation of sound in the middle ear. In pure conductive losses, hearing threshold, MCL, and LDL are all elevated by the same amount and this elevation equals the amount of attenuation occurring in the middle ear.[933] In mixed losses, it seems reasonable to assume that the conductive component also causes all three quantities to increase by approximately the same amount. The size of the conductive component at each frequency is inferred from the size of the air-bone gap on the audiogram.

---

[h] To work out the speech level falling into a channel, add on a power basis all the 1/3 octave bands of speech that fall within that channel.

Given the above information, it might seem that to prescribe for someone with a conductive loss, insertion gain at each frequency should just equal the conductive loss at that frequency. This would seem to result in a normal input to the cochlea, which itself is normal. Similarly, it might seem that a person with a mixed loss should be fitted by prescribing for the sensorineural portion of the loss, and then prescribing additional gain equal to the conductive portion. Although these seem like reasonable deductions, they are probably not true, at least when implemented with current technology. It has long been estimated that when a person with a mixed loss is fitted with a hearing aid, the average gain needed equals half the total loss, plus one quarter of the conductive component.[550] Assuming that the average gain prescribed equals half the total loss, a little arithmetic will show that this is equivalent to providing average gain equal to half the sensorineural loss plus *three quarters* of the conductive component. That is, the empirical observation is that compensation is needed for only 75% rather than 100% of the conductive component. There may be several reasons for this.

First, there is no point in providing additional gain if this gain causes the hearing aid to limit excessively, because limiting causes undesirable auditory effects (see Section 9.6.2).

Thus, the optimum gain will depend on the OSPL90 that can be achieved.[932] If it is not possible to provide a high enough OSPL90 for conductive and mixed losses, then the optimal gain may also be less than theoretically expected. One way to express this is that because of device limitations, the dynamic range available to the listener has been decreased, even for a purely conductive loss.

Second, the acoustic reflex attenuates sound entering the normal-hearing ear at high levels. The acoustic reflex is usually absent in the case of conductive impairment.[669] The hearing loss for high-level sounds is thus a little less than that for low-level sounds. Consequently, for high-level sounds, the gain needed to provide a normal input to the cochlea is less than the elevation in hearing thresholds.

Third, it should not be assumed that normal is best. Normal-hearing people prefer other than a flat frequency response under some adverse listening conditions.[934] Similarly, it is possible that they would prefer to hear many sounds at a lower than normal sensation level. It may be that even if a hearing aid has adequate OSPL90, people would prefer the gain compensating for the conductive component to be less than the attenuation caused by that conductive component, especially in noisy environments.

Otosclerotic hearing losses

Otosclerosis can cause a change in bone conduction thresholds because of stiffening or fixation of the stapes, even in the absence of sensorineural loss.[134, 380] To allow for this change, bone conduction thresholds should be decreased by the amount shown in Table 9.1 before prescribing for either the sensorineural or the conductive parts of the loss.

Table 9.1 Corrections to be subtracted from bone conduction thresholds prior to calculation of the sensorineural and conductive portions of the loss.[134, 380] The values have been derived by averaging across studies, and the 3 kHz figure has been interpolated.

Frequency (Hz)	250	500	1000	2000	3000	4000
Correction (dB)	0	5	10	13	10	6

Although the discussion in this section has referred to the *proportion* of conductive loss that is compensated with gain, the concept of a fixed proportion may not even be correct. It may be that the first 20 dB of loss can be ignored and the remainder fully compensated. Alternatively, it may be appropriate to fully compensate for the conductive loss at low input levels (for which people presumably do not want to hear at a sensation level less than normal), but to decrease the compensation when the input level is high. In short, nonlinear amplification might be appropriate for conductive losses, although the loss itself is essentially linear. If the dynamic range available to the aid wearer is less than normal (because OSPL90 is below discomfort), nonlinear amplification may be just as appropriate for the person as it is for someone whose dynamic range has been decreased by a sensorineural hearing loss.

Given the uncertainty that still exists over how best to prescribe for conductive loss, it is fortunate that conductive components tend to be flat or gently sloping.[931] The appropriate allowance for these losses is thus a gain increase of similar size at all frequencies, though not necessarily the same gain increase at all input levels. If the clinician provides the wrong amount of additional gain to compensate for the loss, the aid wearer can compensate by simply varying the volume control!

Summary: Allowing for a conductive component when prescribing gain:

- First, prescribe gain for the sensorineural part of the loss, using whichever procedure you select.
- Second, prescribe additional gain at each frequency equal to 75% of the conductive loss at that frequency. It is possible that for nonlinear hearing aids, the additional gain prescribed for low-level signals should equal 100% of the conductive loss, but there are no research data on this point.

For the purposes of prescription, people with pure conductive losses can be considered to have mixed losses; the sensorineural part of their loss will just happen to equal zero. Note that, with the POGO, NAL-RP, and NAL-NL1 procedures, the insertion gain provided for a flat loss of say, 10 dB is not a flat insertion gain. This is consistent with the observation that normal-hearing people do not necessarily prefer a gain of 0 dB at all frequencies (Walker 1997).

9.5 Selecting Options for Multi-memory Hearing Aids

Most of this chapter so far is about selecting the gain-frequency response that best suits an individual. For some individuals, there is almost certainly no such single response. That is, in different circumstances, an individual might prefer different gain-frequency responses. Of course, nonlinear hearing aids implicitly provide different gain-frequency responses for different input levels. Even beyond this, however, the aid wearer might prefer different responses depending on the types of signals or noises in their immediate environment. Many hearing aids now on the market have multiple memories or programs (see Section 3.3.2) so that the hearing aid wearer can select the response that best suits each listening situation.

Multi-memory hearing aids can also be used to help find the best single, overall program for a patient, but we will discuss this application of these devices in Section 11.2.6. Multi-memory hearing aids are also particularly valuable for people with a fluctuating hearing loss, such as those with a Stage 2 Ménière's disease. Each of the two or more programs can be adjusted to match different degrees of hearing loss.

Multi-memory hearing aids are sometimes considered as alternatives to hearing aids that automatically adapt to different environments. The two concepts are, however, complementary. An automatic hearing aid that alters the gain-frequency response on the basis of the apparent signal-to-noise ratio at each frequency may adapt inappropriately in some situations (such as when listening to music). If the adaptive processor is enabled in one program, but disabled in another program, the user can obtain all the advantages of the adaptive scheme without having to endure the disadvantages.

The following two sections outline how the gain-frequency response can be altered to suit different listening conditions, and how the clinician can identify which patients are likely to benefit from multi-memory hearing aids.

9.5.1   Response alternatives for different environments and listening criteria

Several research studies have investigated how frequency response or compression characteristics should be varied depending on the acoustic environment and listening criterion. A detailed review of these studies can be found in Keidser, Dillon & Byrne (1996), along with some recommendations for how the aid's response should be altered in different circumstances. Before giving

these response alternatives, it is important to establish the concept of a **baseline response**. The baseline response is individually selected for each hearing-impaired person, and will usually be included as one of the programs in the hearing aid. The alternative responses are then expressed as variations to the baseline response (e.g. a low-tone cut, or additional high-frequency compression). Two people with different hearing loss configurations will thus be prescribed different amplification characteristics, even when they listen in the same acoustic environment, and with the same listening criterion. The combination of an **acoustic environment** with a **listening criterion** will be referred to as a **listening condition**.

The baseline response selected by Keidser et al. was the NAL-RP response. The NAL-RP response was found to be the best response (averaged across subjects) when listening to a talker in quiet or in slight reverberation, or to a talker in a babble noise where the talker and the babble had the same spectral shape. Table 9.2 shows the variations recommended for different listening conditions. For each

Table 9.2 Response alternatives suitable for different listening conditions. The *1, 2* or *3* shown under each response alternative indicates that the alternative is the best, second-best, or third-best alternative, respectively, for that listening condition. (Adapted from Keidser et al., 1996).

Acoustic environment	Listening criterion	Response alternatives					
		NAL-RP	Flatter linear response	Steeper linear response	LF comp	HF comp	Dual band comp.
1. Speech in quiet	Intelligibility	1	2			3	
2. Multi-level speech	Intelligibility		2			1	
3. Speech in LF noise	Intelligibility			1			2
4. Speech in LF noise	Decrease annoyance			3	1		2
5. Speech in HF noise	Intelligibility	1	3			2	
6. Speech in HF noise	Decrease annoyance	2	1				
7. Music	Pleasantness	2	1				

condition, a first, second, and sometimes third choice is shown.

If the clinician establishes the listening situations in which a patient most wants help, Table 9.2 can be used to establish which responses will be most useful. If the first choice response were to be selected for each listening condition, active patients will appear to need more programs than are available on most hearing aids. This is where the second and third choices are useful. It is usually possible to find two, or maybe three, amplification conditions that provide a first, second, or third choice response for every listening condition considered important by the patient. (See Section 8.1.4 for the COSI method of determining where the patient needs hearing aids, in a manner compatible with evaluating the success of rehabilitation.)

The responses in Table 9.2 are based on empirical evidence, but it is easy to see the principles that have led to the data. Where background noise has more of a low-frequency emphasis than speech (e.g. traffic noise, reverberant sounds, machinery noise), the response alternative should de-emphasize low-frequency gain. This can be done with either a filter or a low-frequency compressor. Conversely, where the background noise has more high-frequency emphasis than speech (e.g. impact noise such as printer noise, cutlery and crockery noise), the response should de-emphasize high-frequency gain. Where the wanted signal varies markedly in level, compression is needed to keep the lower level parts of the signal audible. In real life, compression may be needed more often than is implied by Table 9.2, because only listening condition number 2 contained significant variations in stimulus level.

At the time of the Keidser et al. research (and other research drawn on in the compilation of the response alternative table), the NAL-NL1 response was not available and so was not tested. It seems possible that the NAL-NL1 response would be optimal for listening conditions 1 and 2. If subsequent research shows this to be true, then the choice of alternative programs will be simplified.

Although this section has been aimed at prescribing responses for multiple memories, similar considerations apply to prescribing responses for hearing aids with adaptive noise-reduction processing. Such hearing aids can be prescribed and adjusted to optimize intelligibility in quiet with the adaptive noise-suppression disabled. The adaptive noise-reduction circuitry can then be enabled so that it automatically modifies the response depending on the SNR and spectrum of the background noise.

9.5.2 Candidates for multi-memory hearing aids

Multi-memory hearing aids are not for everyone. Estimates of the proportion of patients who will choose to use different programs in different listening conditions vary from 0% to 81%.[445] If a person wears hearing aids in only one situation (e.g. listening to television), it is most unlikely that a multi-memory hearing aid will be beneficial. If a person wears hearing aids in several situations, but the listening conditions are the same in all these situations, it is again unlikely that a multi-memory hearing aid will be beneficial.

There are several other less obvious issues related to candidacy for a multi-memory hearing aid. First, Keidser et al. (1995) found that people with a high-frequency hearing loss (average of 2, 3 and 4 kHz) greater than 55 dB HL were more likely to use multiple programs than those who had less than 55 dB high-frequency loss. The probable reasons for this are the restricted dynamic range and deteriorated frequency resolution of people with severe losses. When dynamic range is large, the sensation level in each frequency region is not critical. When the input spectrum varies in shape and level, the

> ### Recommending a multi-memory hearing aid
>
> Consider recommending a multi-memory hearing aid if all three of the following are true:
>
> 1. The patient plans to wear the hearing aid in at least two situations where the listening conditions differ.
>
> 2. The patient is willing to switch between programs in different environments, and has the physical and mental capability to do this. For most multi-memory hearing aids, this will necessitate the patient being willing to carry and use a remote control.
>
> 3. The patient has a high frequency average loss of greater than 55 dB HL, or, has a baseline insertion gain target at 500 Hz of greater than 0 dB. (Both of these requirements will be met for the strongest candidates.)

consequent variation in the output signal will have little effect on intelligibility or comfort. Conversely, for people with more loss, an inappropriate sensation level in any frequency region is likely to cause poor audibility, masking of one frequency region by another, or excessive loudness. Consequently, whenever the long-term input signal or noise spectrum varies, so too should the amplification characteristics. If an automatic hearing aid cannot adequately do this, there is a strong argument for using a multi-memory aid.

Second, people who have a target gain of close to 0 dB at 500 Hz in their baseline response are not good candidates for a multi-memory aid.[442] The reason for this may lie in the dual transmission paths of hearing aids worn by such people. Recall that a low-frequency gain of 0 dB can most easily be provided to people by simply allowing sound

to enter the ear canal via the vent of the hearing aid (Section 5.3.1). When the vent provides the dominant transmission path, sound at low frequencies will not be affected by which program is selected (or even by whether the hearing aid is on or off). In such cases, the different programs can differ only in the high- and mid-frequency amplification and compression they provide. Altering the hearing aid's volume control thus alters amplification in a similar manner to selecting a new program. This similarity should decrease the advantage of multiple programs, as long as the hearing aid already has a volume control.

Last, it has been suggested that people who encounter a wide variety of listening conditions while wearing their hearing aids are more likely to use a multi-memory hearing aid than those who need help in only a few situations.[508] Although there is no evidence supporting this, it seems highly likely that socially active people are more likely to use a hearing aid in diverse circumstances, and as discussed in the preceding section, the optimal amplification characteristics depend on the listening environment.

9.6   Prescribing OSPL90

As described in Section 4.1.4, the output sound pressure level for a 90 dB input level (OSPL90) is an estimate of the maximum SPL (measured in a coupler or ear simulator) that a hearing aid can put out. The equivalent term when measured in the real ear is the real-ear saturation response (RESR).

OSPL90 may be quoted either at one particular frequency, at every frequency, or at the frequency with the greatest OSPL90, depending on the context. Inappropriately prescribed OSPL90 has the potential to make a hearing aid unusable even more than does inappropriately prescribed gain, as we shall see in the following section. Despite this, there has been little research into the effectiveness of OSPL90 prescription procedures.

9.6.1 General principles: avoiding discomfort, damage and distortion

It is easy to describe a hearing aid with an appropriately prescribed OSPL90 curve.

- The hearing aid will never cause the aid wearer discomfort from excessive loudness. It is desirable for the hearing aid to sometimes make sounds loud, but if it makes sounds uncomfortably loud, the aid wearer will blame the hearing aid, and will be disinclined to wear it. Alternatively, the wearer may turn down the volume control, but this makes the aid less effective once the input sound decreases in level. When a normal-hearing person experiences loudness discomfort, it may be equally uncomfortable, but there is no prosthetic device to blame for the experience.

- The hearing aid will never create sounds intense enough to cause further damage to the residual hearing of the aid wearer. The possibility of damage is affected by more than OSPL90, so this issue is discussed separately in Section 9.7.

- The hearing aid will not distort sounds sufficiently for the aid wearer to perceive the distortion. If OSPL90 is not adequately controlled by a compression limiter (see Section 6.3.1), intense inputs will cause the output to be peak clipped, and the output will contain a lot of distortion.

- If the hearing aid has a larger OSPL90 than is really *needed* by the aid wearer, the hearing aid probably could have been made with a smaller receiver, or battery, or both, without sacrificing battery life. That is, the aid wearer probably could have received a smaller hearing aid without paying any price in performance.

So far, these are all reasons for not making OSPL90 too high. If OSPL90 is too low, there will be several adverse consequences.

- Speech intelligibility may be decreased.

- The aid wearer will not be able to enjoy the full range of loudness sensations that normally hearing people enjoy.

- The aid wearer may compensate for inadequate loudness or clarity by turning up the volume control. Unfortunately, this will further saturate the hearing aid. Consequently, loudness of the primary signal (e.g. speech) will not increase much, although loudness of lower level background noise during the gaps will increase. In the case of peak clipping, there will also be an increase in distortion.

- In extreme cases, the aid wearer will hear nothing within a frequency range if OSPL90 is less than threshold within this range.

In short, the optimum OSPL90 for a person must be low enough to avoid discomfort, damage, distortion, and wasted output, but must be high enough to avoid inadequate loudness and excessive saturation.

9.6.2 Type of limiting: compression or peak clipping

OSPL90 can be controlled by either compression limiting or peak clipping. As mentioned in Sections 2.3.3, and 6.3.1, compression limiting generates less distortion than peak clipping (with distortion defined as the introduction of new, audible frequencies into the waveform). This form of distortion is objectionable to most people with mild and moderate hearing loss, many with severe loss, and some with profound loss.[856]

People with profound losses invariably have decreased frequency selectivity, so they are less able to detect the presence of distortion than are people with mild to severe loss. A peak clipped waveform is at its extreme values for a greater proportion of the time than an unclipped signal as shown in Figure 9.13. Consequently, its average power, and hence its rms SPL will be greater. A peak clipping hearing aid can therefore always

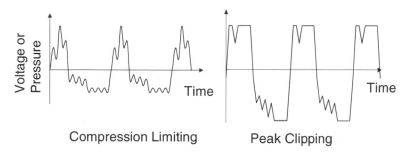

Figure 9.13 A speech waveform after passing through a peak clipper and a compression limiter, where both types of limiter can pass the same peak signal level without clipping.

produce a greater OSPL90 than a compression limiting aid, for the same receiver, amplifier, and battery drain. When measured with pure tones, peak clipping aids can produce about 3 dB more than compression limiting aids. Speech signals, however, have a higher crest factor, and the difference in OSPL90s increases to about 9 dB.[205] For some people with profound hearing loss, this increased OSPL90 more than compensates for the increased distortion in a peak clipper.

It has even been suggested that such distortion can be beneficial, in that intermodulation distortion will create low-frequency distortion products when a high-frequency sound enters the hearing aid. The aid wearer may thus be able to detect the presence of high-frequency sounds because of the low-frequency distortion they generate, much as would happen for a transposition aid (see Section 7.4). Evidence for this argument is scarce and conflicting.

Principles for prescribing compression limiting or peak clipping

- For people with mild or moderate loss do not use peak clipping. For a percentage of these patients it may not matter which you choose, but very, very, few will prefer peak clipping if they have had a chance to try both. Many, however, will prefer compression limiting.

- For people with severe loss, the choice is less critical; an increased proportion will not mind which you use, but again few will prefer peak clipping, so always prescribe compression limiting.

- For people with profound loss, use peak clipping if the patient has a history of preferring maximum volume control settings or complains that the aid does not make sounds loud enough. Otherwise, use compression limiting, though for many people, there may be little difference between the two options.

- For profoundly impaired children too young to indicate whether loudness is satisfactory, the choice is tricky. Such young children will not usually be fitted with the most powerful aids at their maximum OSPL90 setting. When OSPL90 is reduced below maximum, it seems most sensible to reduce it with compression limiting rather than peak clipping, in case the patient has residual hearing sufficiently good to use spectral cues in speech. (Peak clipping will degrade these cues, compression limiting will not.)

- For any degree of loss, if the hearing aid has a form of compression that gradually reduces gain as input level rises above typical input levels, the aid may rarely reach its output limit. If the compression ratio is high enough, the attack time is low enough, and the compression threshold is low enough, the type of limiting will not matter.

9.6.3   OSPL90 prescription

Although many OSPL90 prescription procedures have been devised, only one procedure (NAL-SSPL) has been systematically evaluated. Consequently, that procedure will be described in detail after a brief review of other procedures and some related issues.

Most procedures for prescribing OSPL90 concentrate on avoiding discomfort. There are several procedures based on setting OSPL90 equal to, or just below, the loudness discomfort level (LDL), or uncomfortable level (UCL) of the aid wearer. The rationale behind these procedures is simply that OSPL90 set in this way should not lead to discomfort. Furthermore, setting OSPL90 as high as possible without causing discomfort should minimize the chances of OSPL90 being so low that it causes insufficient loudness or excessive saturation. The POGO procedure,[587] for example, recommends that across frequency, the highest OSPL90 should be made equal to the average of the LDLs at 500, 1000, and 2000 Hz. To allow for the differences in calibration, POGO recommends that 2-cc coupler OSPL90 should be 4 dB below the three-frequency average LDL expressed in dB HL.

One problem with procedures based on individually measured LDL is that LDL can be difficult to measure reliably. The reliability of the values, and the mean values obtained after extensive testing, are both affected by the instructions given to patients and the psychophysical procedure used.[367] Hawkins et al (1987) considered that to get reliable results, patients should understand the purpose of the measurement, and that descriptive labels should be available above and below the target loudness. For some very old and very young patients, it may not be possible to measure LDL, although hearing threshold can be obtained.

An alternative to measuring LDL is to predict it from threshold. Cox (1985) recommends that at each frequency, OSPL90 be set equal to 100 dB SPL plus a quarter of the hearing loss, a relationship also reported by Martin et al. (1976). Again, differences in calibration are allowed for with suitable correction factors. Unfortunately, LDL can not be predicted accurately from threshold. Several experiments have shown that although LDL, on average, increases as threshold increases, measured LDL may be up to 30 dB different from the predicted value.[227, 232, 431, 694, 796] Of course, some of this apparent variability between people will be due to inaccuracies in the measurement of LDL, rather than to a real breakdown in the relationship between LDL and threshold.

A second difficulty with basing OSPL90 on LDL is that OSPL90 is expressed as dB SPL in a 2-cc coupler, whereas LDL is usually measured with headphones calibrated in a 6-cc coupler. While appropriate average correction factors can be used, application of average corrections to individual people causes some error in the inferred value of LDL. There are several ways to obtain LDL without requiring an average correction factor to be used, as shown in the accompanying panel.

A third difficulty with basing OSPL90 on LDL is that OSPL90 has to be low enough to prevent discomfort for all possible sounds. Because loudness generally increases with stimulus bandwidth, broadband sounds may exceed LDL even if narrow band sounds lie below LDL at all frequencies.[51, 936]

Finally, there is no logical reason why OSPL90 has to be as high as LDL. A few authors have suggested that we should think about a range of acceptable OSPL90s.[56, 113] The maximum acceptable OSPL90 is equal to, or just below LDL. The minimum acceptable OSPL90 could be deduced either by assuming that people need access to sounds at least 35 dB above threshold[113] or by assuming that slightly loud speech should not cause the hearing aid to limit.

The NAL-SSPL procedure adopts and quantifies this latter approach.[236] The minimum

Relating OSPL90 to LDL without using average correction factors

If LDL is measured as part of the prescription and fitting process, then there are three accurate ways to directly compare LDL and hearing aid maximum output:

1. Measure LDL with an insert transducer calibrated in a 2-cc coupler.[104, 173, 227, 359]

2. Measure the SPL of the LDL stimulus in the ear canal with a probe-tube while LDL is being obtained.[363, 402, 970]

3. Measure the individual's real ear to coupler difference (RECD) and use it to convert LDL, expressed as 2 cc coupler SPL, into LDL expressed as ear canal SPL.[613]

In the first alternative, ER3A tube-phones can be used if an ITE/ITC/CIC aid is to be fitted. It is important that the tip of the insert phone be inserted to the same point in the ear canal that the tip of the hearing aid will be located. This can be very difficult to judge if the aid is to be deeply seated. Because the SPL generated by the tube-phone will vary by 6 dB for every halving or doubling of effective ear canal volume, the errors with this approach should be acceptable for hearing aids that do not extend beyond about the second bend. For more deeply seated aids, the results should be viewed with caution.

For BTE fittings, the tube-phones can be connected to the tubing of the individual's earmold. This removes the problem of how far to insert the phones, and simultaneously allows for the tubing and venting characteristics of the individual earmold. If the tube-phones are calibrated in dB SPL in a HA2 2-cc coupler (complete with its 25 mm length of tubing), there are virtually no calibration errors involved in setting 2-cc OSPL90 equal to the measured LDL. (Of course, there may be considerable error in the LDL measurement itself.)

In the second alternative, SPL in the ear canal is monitored with a probe-tube microphone either before, during, or after the LDL measurement. Individual calibration errors largely disappear provided the real-ear saturation response (RESR) is also adjusted while ear canal SPL is being monitored.

The third alternative is really a combination of the previous two: LDL is measured with a transducer calibrated in a 2-cc coupler, and so is RECD, but the final result is expressed in ear canal SPL rather than coupler SPL. Procedures for measuring and applying RECD will be given in Section 10.7.

All three approaches are equally accurate and individualized, but may differ in convenience and time efficiency, depending on the overall selection and verification strategy being used. The information in this panel should be taken as suggestions for how LDL *could* be compared to OSPL90, not that LDL *should* be measured.

---

acceptable limit of OSPL90 has been assumed to be that which causes only a small amount of limiting when speech at a long-term rms level of 75 dB SPL is input into the hearing aid. To make this calculation, it was assumed that the hearing-impaired person uses the gain predicted by the NAL-RP gain selection formula. The maximum acceptable OSPL90 was equated to LDL, which was estimated from hearing thresholds. The optimum OSPL90 for a person was assumed to lie midway between the two limits set by discomfort and saturation. In actual use, the midpoint is the only value used, so it is estimated

The NAL-SSPL prescription procedure

For hearing aids in which the shape of the OSPL90 curve cannot be controlled, three-frequency average OSPL90 (average of 500, 1000, and 2000 Hz thresholds) is prescribed on the basis of three-frequency average hearing loss using either Figure 9.14 or Table 9.3.

Table 9.3 The NAL-SSPL selection procedure, for prescription of three-frequency average OSPL90 in 2-cc coupler SPL.

3FA loss (dB HL)	3FA OSPL90	3FA loss (dB HL)	3FA OSPL90	3FA loss (dB HL)	3FA OSPL90	3FA loss (dB HL)	3FA OSPL90
0	89	30	98	60	107	90	123
5	90	35	99	65	109	95	126
10	92	40	101	70	112	100	128
15	93	45	102	75	115	105	131
20	95	50	104	80	118	110	134
25	96	55	105	85	120	115	136

These values can be translated to SPL in the ear canal by adding the RECD, averaged across people and across the three frequencies 500, 1000 and 2000 Hz. This average is 6 dB, so the NAL-SSPL procedure can be used as a real-ear prescription procedure by adopting values 6 dB higher than those shown in Table 9.3 or Figure 9.14. These real-ear values apply no matter what type of hearing aid is used, or whether the person is an adult or an infant. Conversely, the 2-cc coupler SPL values are applicable only to BTE, ITE and ITC aids fitted to an ear of average adult size. A patient with a small residual ear canal volume will need less 2-cc OSPL90 than would an average adult fitted with an average length ITE or BTE aid, if they are both to receive the same real-ear target OSPL90. Methods for accomplishing this are given in Section 10.7.

directly from threshold (see panel). As can be seen in Figure 9.14, there should be a wide range of acceptable OSPL90s for people with mild and moderate hearing loss. For people with severe and especially profound loss, however, the estimated maximum acceptable OSPL90 is less than the estimated minimum. That is, it may not be possible to have an OSPL90 setting that simultaneously avoids discomfort and saturation of the hearing aids, *at least for linear hearing aids*. Because both of the limits are only estimates, the procedure still places the optimum OSPL90 mid-way between the two.

An evaluation of the NAL-SSPL procedure showed that, on average, the procedure neither under-estimated nor over-estimated the OSPL90 found empirically to be best for the experimental subjects.[856] For about 20% of the subjects, however, the OSPL90 prescribed by the procedure was outside the range of OSPL90 values found to be acceptable for each subject. Consequently, the OSPL90 setting prescribed should be evaluated for suitability during the fitting appointment. Methods for evaluating OSPL90 will be covered in Section 10.9.

9.6.4 Prescribing OSPL90 at different frequencies

While it has always been possible to design a hearing aid with an OSPL90-frequency response that could be varied independently of its gain-frequency response, such hearing aids have not been available until the recent advent of multichannel hearing aids.[i]

---

[i]   In a single channel compression limiting hearing aid, control of gain-response and OSPL90-response can be achieved with one filter prior to the sensing point for the compressor, and one filter after the sensing point. Suitable fitting software is needed to make the controls appear independent, because the filter after the sensing point affects both OSPL90 and gain.

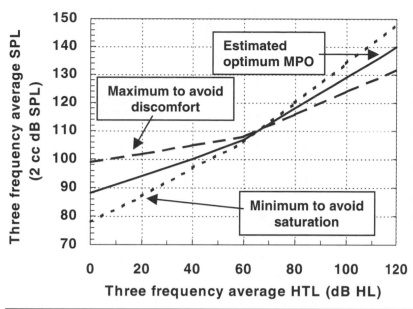

Figure 9.14 The NAL SSPL selection procedure, based on values midway between the OSPL90 needed to avoid discomfort and the OSPL90 needed to avoid excessive saturation.

Before prescribing OSPL90 for those aids where OSPL90 can be varied as a function of frequency, it is essential that the clinician identify whether the OSPL90 is being controlled independently within each channel of a multichannel aid (e.g. Figure 9.15a), or whether the OSPL90 is controlled by a compressor or peak clipper that is operating on the whole bandwidth of the signal (e.g. Figure 9.15b). For hearing aids based on independent control in each of several channels, the effects of power and loudness summation must be allowed for. Suppose, for example, that one channel of an aid was putting out a narrowband sound that by itself just failed to elicit LDL. What would happen if every channel simultaneously put out such a signal? First, the total SPL would be greater than the SPL of any channel by itself. Second, because the combined sound would have a bandwidth wider than any individual channel, the combined sound would be even louder

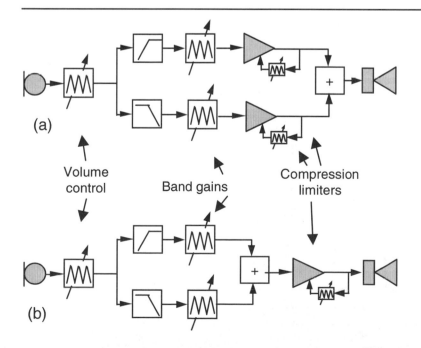

Figure 9.15 A multi-channel hearing aid in which limiting occurs (a) independently in each channel, and, (b) on the wide-band signal after the channels have been recombined.

than would be expected based on the increased SPL. Consequently, the combined sound would easily elicit discomfort.

The more channels there are, the greater the increase in loudness. To compensate for this, the OSPL90 as measured by narrow band signals must be decreased relative to that needed for single channel limiting. Usually multichannel aids will need this reduction in OSPL90 and single channel aids will not, but the hearing aid's block diagram should be examined carefully before deciding whether to make the reduction in OSPL90.

Prescribing frequency-specific maximum output

- At each frequency, read from Table 9.4 the real-ear saturation response appropriate to the sensorineural part of the loss.
- If the hearing aid has independent limiting within each channel, reduce the values by the amounts shown in Table 9.5.
- For conductive or mixed losses, add 87.5% of the conductive part of the loss at each frequency to give the final RESR (see Section 9.6.6).

To express the prescription in terms of 2-cc coupler SPL, subtract individual or average RECD values (Table 4.1) from the RESR values.

Table 9.4 RESR (dB SPL) versus hearing threshold (dB HL). For hearing aids where the maximum output is limited independently in separate channels, the RESR (or OSPL90) should be decreased by the amount shown in Table 9.5.

HTL	Frequency (Hz				
	250	500	1k	2k	4k
0	95	96	95	98	100
5	95	97	96	100	101
10	96	97	98	101	102
15	96	98	99	102	103
20	96	99	101	104	104
25	97	101	102	105	106
30	97	102	104	107	107
35	98	103	105	108	108
40	99	105	107	109	109
45	100	106	108	111	110
50	101	108	110	112	112
55	103	109	111	113	113
60	104	110	113	115	114
65	107	114	115	117	117
70	111	117	118	120	119
75	115	120	121	122	122
80	118	124	123	125	124
85	122	127	126	128	127
90	125	131	128	130	129
95	129	134	131	133	132
100	132	137	134	135	135
105	136	141	136	138	137
110	139	144	139	141	140
115	143	147	142	143	142
120	147	151	144	146	145

Table 9.5 Reduction that should be made to RESR values for multichannel hearing aids with independent limiting in each channel.

Number of channels	Reduction (dB)
1	0
2	5
3	7
4	9
5	10

Theoretical background: Deriving a frequency-specific OSPL90 selection formula

First, discomfort levels were estimated from hearing threshold as shown in Dillon & Storey (1998). Second, the minimum SPL at each frequency that is necessary to avoid saturation was estimated on the same basis as described in Dillon & Storey. The only difference was that gains at each frequency were used rather than three-frequency average gain. Because the gain at each frequency depends on hearing threshold at other frequencies in the NAL-RP procedure, the gain corresponding to each degree of hearing loss was estimated using data from 700 audiograms (Macrae & Dillon, 1996).

These insertion gains were converted to real-ear aided gains, so that the resulting maximum output prescription would be in terms of the real-ear saturation response (RESR). The optimum RESR was then estimated to be the value mid-way between the minimum RESR to avoid saturation and the maximum RESR to avoid discomfort.

For hearing aids where the maximum output is limited independently in a number of channels, the RESR must be reduced, for the reasons outlined in the text. The data of Bentler and Pavlovic (1989a) indicate that to avoid discomfort, the reduction should equal *4 + 13 log(n)*, where *n* is the number of independent channels. Similarly, the maximum output to avoid saturation need not be as great in each channel, because only a portion of the output power falls within each channel. On the assumption that the signal power, after amplification, is equally distributed between channels, the reduction will be approximately *10 log(n)*. The reduction in the optimum RESR, as shown in Table 9.8, is calculated to be midway between the reduction in the maximum and minimum allowable values.

9.6.5 OSPL90 for nonlinear hearing aids

Nonlinear hearing aids are, of course, those in which the gain and/or frequency response shape changes with input level. When gain decreases as input level increases, accurate selection of OSPL90 becomes less critical than for linear aids. If the gain decreases sufficiently at high input levels, the hearing aid may never produce uncomfortable sounds for any input level that the aid wearer is likely to encounter. Killion (1995) argues that for people with mild or moderate hearing losses, limiting is not necessary at all provided the amount of gain is only that required to give normal perception of loudness.

It is, of course, always possible to make the OSPL90 too low, as a hearing aid wearer must be able to receive a certain SPL if the hearing aid is to make sound loud enough. No one has yet devised a simple modification to OSPL90 prescription to allow for the effects

of the nonlinear gain, so a practical solution is to use the same OSPL90 prescription as for linear hearing aids.

9.6.6 OSPL90 for conductive and mixed losses

The general impact of conductive hearing loss on thresholds, discomfort, gain, and amplification requirements was discussed in Section 9.4. Suppose that for someone with a mixed loss, we have already prescribed gain and OSPL90 for the sensorineural part of the loss. The conductive part of the loss will affect the required OSPL90 in two ways. First, we will assume that additional gain, equal to 75% of the conductive loss, has been added at each frequency. This will increase by the same amount the minimum OSPL90 needed to avoid saturation. Second, discomfort level will increase by 100% of the conductive loss.

If we follow the rationale behind the NAL-SSPL selection procedure, the increase in

Prescribing OSPL90 or RESR for conductive and mixed losses

1. If the person has otosclerosis, correct the bone conduction thresholds (see Table 9.1).

2. The sensorineural part of the loss is taken to be the bone conduction thresholds and the conductive loss is taken to be equal to the air-bone gap. It may be reasonable to smooth the air-bone gap across frequency, and it is often necessary to extrapolate the air-bone gap to lower and higher frequencies than can be measured.

3. Prescribe OSPL90 or RESR on the basis of the sensorineural part of the loss alone, using Figure 9.14 or Table 9.3 (three-frequency average OSPL90), or Table 9.4 (frequency dependent RESR).

4. Increase OSPL90 and RESR by adding 0.875 times the conductive portion of the loss. (No, the procedure is not really that precise; adding 90 % of the air bone gap would be just fine.)

optimum OSPL90 will be half way between the increase needed to avoid saturation and the increase needed to avoid discomfort. The required increase in OSPL90 to allow for the conductive loss is therefore equal to 87.5% of the conductive portion of the loss (i.e. the air-bone gap).

9.7 Excessive Amplification and Subsequent Hearing Loss

Hearing aids amplify sound. They therefore have the potential to cause a *noise-induced hearing loss* to someone who already has a hearing loss. Whether a hearing aid causes further loss depends on two factors.

A person's susceptibility to noise-induced loss partly depends on how much loss the person already has. A noise exposure that causes a certain permanent threshold shift to someone with normal hearing will cause much less threshold shift to someone with a severe loss, for example. Essentially, people with hearing loss have already lost the most sensitive detectors within the cochlea, and noise exposure has to be greater to damage the remaining inner and outer hair cells. Methods for calculating the degree of *temporary threshold shift (TTS)* and *permanent threshold shift (PTS)* that noise exposure causes to someone with normal hearing are well understood, at least in a statistical sense. The effect of prior hearing loss on subsequent damage can be calculated theoretically (see panel). For a known input level, the noise-induced loss caused by a hearing aid can be predicted as accurately as it can be measured.[569]

The second factor affecting noise-induced loss is the *daily noise dose* experienced by the aid wearer. This dose depends on the

Theoretical background: predicting noise-induced loss for a hearing-impaired person

Researchers predict noise-induced loss for a hearing-impaired person using a relationship known as the modified power law (Humes and Jesteadt, 1991; Macrae, 1991a):

- The hearing-impaired person's initial loss is transformed to an equivalent internal excitation level;
- The noise-induced loss that a normal-hearing person would undergo is transformed to an internal excitation level;
- These excitation levels are added;
- This total excitation level is transformed back to an external sound level;
- This sound level represents the hearing threshold that the hearing-impaired person is likely to have after exposure to noise.

Practical steps: Avoiding hearing aid induced hearing loss

- Do not prescribe more gain or OSPL90 than is necessary for optimal intelligibility. Choose your prescription procedure carefully! This is particularly important for children too young to operate their volume control, or anyone fitted with a hearing aid that has no volume control.
- Advise the patient to avoid prolonged exposure to high noise levels.
- Prescribe a nonlinear hearing aid in which the average gain decreases as input level rises from typical input levels to high input levels. (Gain may also vary as the input varies from low to typical input levels, but the aid's behavior for low input levels is less likely to affect the likelihood of noise-induced loss.)
- Monitor hearing thresholds over time.
- Wherever doubt exists, check for temporary threshold shift by measuring hearing thresholds after 24 hours without a hearing aid in the test ear and then after 8 hours of hearing aid use. (For school children, measurements first thing on Monday morning and then late on Monday afternoon will be most convenient.) Where it is difficult to achieve enough sensation level without causing temporary threshold shift, consider advising the patient to alternate hearing aid use between the ears to allow the ears greater recovery time.

---

levels at the output of the aid and the amount of time that these levels are maintained. Because the input level fluctuates with time, so too does the output level, and it is not obvious how to describe the output level as a single representative number. The mean value of the short term rms levels (each measured using the *fast* averaging time on a sound level meter) is believed to be the best way to represent a fluctuating level if one wishes to predict how much PTS or TTS will occur.[569]

The output level of a hearing aid at any time depends on three things. First, the greater the gain, the greater will be the output level. Second, the greater the level of sound at the input to the aid, the greater will be the output level. Of course, both of these statements are true only when the output is less than the maximum output limit of the aid. Once the combination of input level and gain is sufficiently great to saturate the hearing aid, the output level is primarily determined by the OSPL90 of the hearing aid (or more precisely, by the RESR). For one group of school children studied by Macrae (1994b), the output of the hearing aid reached its maximum level so infrequently that *the noise dose was almost entirely determined by the combination of input level and gain, rather than by the OSPL90.* This finding is very important as it is often incorrectly assumed that the safety of a hearing aid is determined solely by its OSPL90. There is, however, some evidence that OSPL90 also affects safety, as reviewed in Macrae (1994a). This presumably happens only in those fittings where the maximum output of the aid is reached reasonably often.

PTS will grow towards a final value that is equal to the asymptotic TTS.[499, 569, j] The rate at which PTS grows depends on the amount of noise exposure. First, if TTS exceeds a certain amount, referred to by Macrae (1994a) as the *safety limit*, PTS will begin to accumulate rapidly, reaching its final value in less than 10 years.[9] For normal-hearing people, the safety limit is about 50 dB of TTS.[566, 941] The modified power law can be

---

j   The *asymptotic TTS* is the maximum amount of TTS that occurs when an ear is continuously exposed to noise. The amount of TTS grows exponentially with a time constant of about 2 to 3 hours (Mills, Gilbert & Adkins, 1979; Macrae, 1994a). The TTS is therefore very close to its asymptotic value after about 6 hours of aid use.

used to predict that this safety limit decreases dramatically as hearing loss increases, and is only 2 dB for a hearing threshold of 100 dB HL. Second, if TTS is much smaller than the safety limit, it may take many decades of noise exposure before PTS grows to its final amount.

TTS and PTS are real possibilities with hearing aid use. Using 15 dB more gain than that recommended by the NAL-RP procedure at 1 kHz, for example, is enough to cause TTS of 3 dB (and hence probably the same amount of PTS) for anyone with initial hearing thresholds of 50 dB HL.[568] This example assumes that the mean input level is 61 dB(A) SPL. If the mean input level is significantly higher than this, even a procedure as conservative in gain as the NAL-RP procedure can lead to TTS and PTS. Any TTS should be avoided if possible, even one as small as 3 dB. As well as being a precursor to PTS, TTS has immediate consequences. It will decrease the person's communication ability as soon as it occurs, because they will hear as if their hearing loss has been increased by this 3 dB whenever the TTS is present.[569]

The risk and degree of hearing aid-induced loss increase as hearing loss increases, because people with more loss need more amplification. For hearing losses with a three-frequency average value (500, 1 k, 2 kHz) of less than 60 dB HL, hearing-aid-induced loss should not be a problem if gains similar to those recommended by the NAL-RP procedure are used.[566] By contrast, once thresholds exceed about 100 dB HL, Macrae (1994a) has shown that even the gains recommended by the NAL-RP procedure are likely to be unsafe. The result is a slow downward spiral of hearing, with each increase in hearing loss requiring an increase in gain, and hence causing increased noise exposure, and hence resulting in further hearing loss. The increments of hearing loss are gradual and small and take several years to develop, but for children and younger adults in particular, the concern is obvious. If a hearing aid is to

provide a satisfactory sensation level for people with profound loss, however, it may be necessary to accept that some additional PTS will occur because of the hearing aid.[565] People with this degree of loss are likely to be candidates for a cochlear implant, at least as far as audiometric considerations are concerned (see Section 8.2.2). Finally, the safety calculations have all been performed with linear hearing aids, and the situation *should* be better with nonlinear aids.

Given that one cannot be sure that a hearing aid will not exacerbate a hearing loss, it is important to determine whether such damage is occurring. TTS provides such a check. If hearing thresholds are measurably worse after a day's hearing aid use than after 24 hours without a hearing aid in the ear, TTS is occurring and PTS is very likely to follow unless something is done. Serial audiograms over several months or years can also be used to detect damage. Unfortunately, permanent damage must occur before it can be detected, and it is difficult to differentiate loss induced by the hearing aid from a loss that is progressing for some other reason. It is therefore better to detect excessive amplification by detecting TTS. If it is detected and corrected sufficiently quickly, no permanent damage will have occurred.

9.8 Concluding Comments

The impact of using an appropriate selection procedure should not be underestimated. When the first version of the NAL procedure was introduced to NAL hearing centers around Australia (replacing some vague combination of clinicians' judgment and evaluative procedures), the rate at which batteries were issued nationally increased by 51%.[900, 901] This increase in battery consumption was ascribed mostly to increased usage of hearing aids, because the number and type of hearing aids being issued remained unchanged. Some other changes to service delivery were also made, but these were considered to be less significant.

Some prescriptions in common use have not been mentioned in this chapter. Several manufacturers have a proprietary prescription procedure included in the fitting software for their own products. These procedures have not been reviewed in this chapter because the derivation, formula, and supporting evidence for these procedures are generally not available.

Depending on the prescription formula used, the clinician may need to look carefully at the prescription and compare it to the characteristics of the hearing loss. Most procedures prescribe increasing amounts of gain, without limit, at a particular frequency as hearing loss at that frequency increases. For someone with the audiogram (in both ears) shown by the diamonds in Figure 9.16, there would probably be no point in amplifying above about 2 kHz. For this person, amplified high-frequency sounds may contribute much to the overall loudness, but are unlikely to contribute significantly to speech intelligibility or quality. The large gain needed to achieve audibility of speech above 2 kHz is likely to cause feedback oscillations,

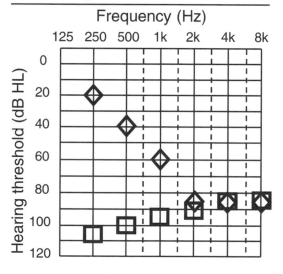

Figure 9.16 Two audiograms with similar losses at 2 and 3 kHz, but different upper frequency limits of aidable hearing.

and so require a tighter earmold than would otherwise be needed. Where the gain prescribed is unlikely to result in any useful contributions to intelligibility at a particular frequency (for speech with typical input levels), the clinician may be well advised to further decrease the gain at those frequencies to minimize the chance of feedback oscillation.

For the person with the audiogram (in both ears) shown by the squares, however, it may be worth extending amplification out to 3 kHz or beyond, even though both people have similar thresholds at 2 and 3 kHz. This person will not be able to extract the full information present in speech in the lower frequency ranges, so the small additional amounts of information at 3 or even 4 kHz may be worth having. The NAL-RP and NAL-NL1 procedures attempt to allow for these factors within their calculation formula, but other procedures do not.[k]

Similarly, some nonlinear formula may prescribe a compression ratio of 4 or much higher, even though in some cases the software implementing the formula gives a warning that such high compression ratios may not be optimal. Empirically, high compression ratios, especially for multichannel compression hearing aids, are associated with poorer speech intelligibility.[208, 626, 721] As mentioned in Chapter 6, fast-acting, multichannel compression with high compression ratios will decrease the availability of spectral cues, and hence decrease intelligibility, even though it increases audibility.

As one reflects on the prescription procedures described in this chapter, it is evident that they have been shaped almost exclusively by speech intelligibility and loudness considerations. There is much more to audition, such as localization, comfort, pleasantness, naturalness, and we can hope that prescriptive procedures of the future give adequate consideration to these issues.[116]

---

k   For the two audiograms in Figure 9.16, NAL-NL1 in fact recommends amplification up to 2 kHz for the diamonds and up to 3 kHz for the squares.

Finally, new technology and fitting procedures should continue to develop in tandem.
Technological advances are of no use unless
the resulting amplification characteristics can
be appropriately matched to the needs of
individual hearing-impaired people.
Conversely, it is not possible to be confident
that a fitting procedure provides the best
results unless the procedure has been
evaluated by comparing it to alternative
prescriptions. For this research to take place,
the technology has to be available in a
convenient, wearable form. Both the
technology and the procedures, in turn,
should be guided by an understanding of what
happens as an impaired cochlea processes
sound. Fortunately, the technology, the
procedures, and our understanding of
impaired hearing are all on an upward spiral
over the last few years. Individual advances
seem small, but their cumulative effect is
likely to be great.

CHAPTER TEN

SELECTING AND ADJUSTING HEARING AIDS

Synopsis

The first decision when a clinician and patient select a hearing aid is whether CIC, ITC, ITE, BTE, spectacle, or body hearing aids would be most suitable. For each style there are advantages relating to ease of insertion, ease of control manipulation, visibility, amount of gain, sensitivity to wind noise, directivity, reliability, telephone compatibility, adjustment flexibility, ease of cleaning, and avoidance of occlusion and feedback. The weight given to each factor will vary greatly from patient to patient. The need for specific features, such as a volume control, a telecoil and switch, a direct audio input, and a directional microphone must be determined on an individual basis. These needs will also influence the style of hearing aid selected.

Next, a signal-processing scheme appropriate to the needs of the patient must be selected. Compression limiting is a more appropriate form of limiting than peak clipping if it can provide a high enough maximum output. In addition to compression limiting, a low compression ratio active over a wide range of input levels is appropriate for most patients. This low-ratio compression will provide advantages whether it is single- or multi-channel, and whether it is fast- or slow-acting. Multichannel compression will provide greater advantages for patients with reasonably sloping hearing loss, and the multichannel structure is consistent with other features such as adaptive noise suppression and feedback suppression. The comfort advantages of adaptive noise suppression are greatest for patients who wear their hearing aids in a range of environments and who also require amplification across a wide range of frequencies. These same considerations apply to multi-memory hearing aids, the only difference being that the patient, rather than the hearing aid, chooses the response variations. Feedback management or reduction schemes are most beneficial for patients with a severe or profound hearing loss, and for patients who have near-normal hearing or a mild hearing loss in the low frequencies combined with a severe loss in the high frequencies. Any signal-processing scheme that requires adjustment for each patient must also be supported by an appropriate prescription method.

The most efficient way to calculate target responses and adjust the hearing aids to meet them depends on the flexibility with which the hearing aid's amplification characteristics can be adjusted. A key goal is to meet a real-ear target response. For hearing aids with inflexible adjustment characteristics, especially when the hearing aids are custom-made, coupler response targets provide an important intermediate goal. Allowing for the acoustic configuration of the earmold or shell when calculating the coupler target will decrease the proportion of times that hearing aids with relatively inflexible adjustment characteristics must be returned to a manufacturer. Coupler targets can be made even more accurate by incorporating the individual patient's real-ear to coupler difference in the prescription. This increased accuracy is probably only worthwhile for hearing aids with very inflexible response characteristics, or for hearing aids intended for infants, where measurement of the final real-ear gain is difficult.

Because it is not possible to prescribe OSPL90 with complete precision, the suitability of maximum output should be subjectively evaluated before the patient leaves the clinic. A variety of intense sounds, including speech and narrowband sounds, should be presented to the patient. The hearing aid should make sounds loud without making them uncomfortably loud.

This chapter uses much of the information in the preceding chapters to give step-by-step guidance on how to choose and adjust a hearing aid. First, we consider how to select a hearing aid style. Second, we consider how to select desired features. Finally, we discuss how to efficiently achieve the prescribed response.

10.1 Selecting Hearing Aid Style: CIC, ITC, ITE, BTE, Spectacle Aid, or Body Aid

There are many factors to take into consideration when selecting hearing aid style. Relative advantages of the different styles are summarized in Table 10.1. Although spectacle and body aids are included, these styles are now rarely used. In those few cases where spectacle aids are used, they are mostly implemented by attaching a spectacle adapter to a BTE hearing aid.

Ease of insertion and removal: ITE, ITC and CIC hearing aids are the easiest to insert and remove because they are easily held, the entire hearing aid is in a single package, and they do not interfere with spectacles.[93, 888, 899] For some patients, ITE hearing aids with a helix-lock may be harder to insert than ITC or CIC hearing aids, or BTE hearing aids with no helix lock on the mold.[597, 849] CICs may be harder for some patients to insert if the patient has difficulty seeing, orienting, or grasping small objects. Removal of CICs is usually easy provided they have removal strings.[631]

Ease of user control manipulation: It is difficult for the aid wearer to manipulate a control on a CIC aid while it is in the ear, especially if the CIC is deeply inserted. Gain adjustment becomes easier if an extended flexible shaft is attached to the volume control, but this detracts from the cosmetic advantages of the CIC. The controls on body aids, spectacle aids, and BTE aids are easier to operate because they are larger and are more easily located by feeling alone. Add-on caps can often be ordered to increase the height and ease of use of a volume control for an ITE or ITC, at some expense to their appearance. Many patients (even new aid users) find rotary volume controls easier to operate than toggle-switch volume controls. Similarly, toggle switches that have two fixed positions cause less confusion than those that

Table 10.1 Relative advantages of different hearing aid styles. Greater advantages relative to the other styles are indicated by a greater number of check marks.

Factor	CIC	ITC	ITE	BTE	Spect-acle	Body
Ease of insertion and removal	✓✓✓	✓✓✓	✓✓✓		✓✓	✓
Ease of manipulating user controls		✓	✓✓	✓✓✓	✓✓✓	✓✓✓
Invisibility	✓✓✓	✓✓	✓	✓		
High gain and maximum output			✓	✓✓	✓✓	✓✓✓
Insensitivity to wind noise	✓✓✓	✓✓	✓✓			
Directivity (for omni-directional mics)	✓✓✓	✓✓	✓	✓	✓	
Directivity (for directional mics)			✓✓✓	✓✓✓		
Reliability				✓✓✓	✓✓✓	✓✓✓
Compatibility with telephones	✓✓✓	✓	✓	✓✓✓	✓✓✓	✓
Flexibility (for non-programmables)			✓	✓✓	✓	✓✓
Flexibility (for programmables)	✓✓✓	✓✓✓	✓✓✓	✓✓✓	✓✓✓	✓✓✓
Ease of cleaning				✓✓✓	✓✓✓	✓
Avoidance of occlusion and feedback		✓	✓✓	✓✓✓	✓✓✓	✓✓✓
Cost		✓	✓	✓	✓	✓

spring back to a centre position. Ease of manipulation of volume controls is not an issue if automatic control of gain via compression is adequate for the patient. For patients whose dexterity causes them to have trouble with any small control, remote controls can be a valuable accessory.

Invisibility: CIC hearing aids are a clear winner on this criterion.

High gain and maximum output: The further the aid microphone is from the receiver, the greater can be the gain without feedback. The larger the receiver and battery, and hence the hearing aid, the greater the OSPL90 can be, particularly for low frequencies.

Insensitivity to wind noise: Most wind noise comes from turbulence created by the head and the pinna.[235] CIC hearing aids pick up less wind noise than the other aid types because the microphone is further from the turbulence-producing parts of the pinna and the head. CIC microphones are also protected from the direct flow of wind. BTE and spectacle hearing aids are strongly affected by turbulence created by the pinna.

Directivity: BTE and ITE hearing aids are the only styles of hearing aids big enough to contain a directional microphone, and are thus best able to suppress sounds coming from the side and rear of the head. Spectacle aids equipped with a multi-microphone array have potentially the best performance, but these microphone arrays have so far been limited to research studies and are not commercially available.[826] If only omni-directional microphones are considered, CIC aids have the best directivity, followed closely by ITC aids, because these aids make the greatest use of the sound collecting and sound attenuating properties of the head, pinna and concha.

Reliability: Hearing aids in which the receiver is located in the ear canal (i.e., CIC, ITC, and ITE) are the least reliable, because cerumen

and moisture limit the life of the receiver. Wax guards are useful for reducing wax ingress.

Telephone compatibility: Hearing aids can pick up either the acoustic or the magnetic signals coming from telephone handsets. For BTE and spectacle aids, telecoil mode is easily selected and used. For body aids, the body-worn unit must be held near the phone handset, and this complicates usage. For ITE and ITC aids, adding a telecoil selector switch makes the faceplate crowded and the controls become increasingly difficult to operate. This difficulty can be overcome if the hearing aid has a remote control, but many patients consider that remote controls are inconvenient. Alternatively, if the hearing aid already has a program selector switch, one of the memories can be assigned as a telecoil program.

For many CIC aids and some ITC aids, the telephone can simply be placed over the ear so that the hearing aid amplifies the acoustic signal. This frees the patient from having to select telecoil mode, but is possible only if the proximity of the telephone does not cause feedback oscillations in the hearing aid. Acoustic damping material placed over the receiver helps avoid this problem. Similarly, a hearing-impaired medical practitioner *may* be able to use a stethoscope while wearing a CIC without causing feedback oscillation, if the CIC does not have too much gain and/or leakage of sound past the shell.[a]

Adjustment flexibility: Any hearing aid that is digitally programmable is likely to have very flexible adjustment of its amplification characteristics. For non-programmable hearing aids, adjustment flexibility decreases with hearing aid size, because there is less room for controls to be mounted on the outside of the aid.

Ease of cleaning: For patients with chronic ear infections, ITE, ITC and CIC styles are unsuitable because the hearing aid cannot adequately be cleaned. BTE or spectacle

---

a   The hard tip on a stethoscope can be replaced with a soft silicone tip available from earmold suppliers.

hearing aids may be suitable, especially if they can be fitted with a large vent (including a completely open style). For these hearing aids, washing of the earmold and/or tubing is possible.

Avoidance of occlusion and feedback: Patients with near-normal low-frequency hearing combined with a severe high-frequency loss are difficult to fit satisfactorily. The low-frequency thresholds require a large vent to minimize occlusion but the gain required at high frequencies will then cause feedback oscillation. These conflicting constraints are more easily met if the distance from the vent outlet to the microphone inlet is increased. The compromise is thus easier in larger hearing aids (e.g. BTEs) than in smaller hearing aids. Although it is often claimed that occlusion is not a problem for CIC aids because the medial end of the aid is in the bony part of the canal, a deeply seated shell or earmold can be used with any hearing aid style, and is thus *not* a special advantage of CIC aids.

Cost: It is common for CIC hearing aids to cost more than the other styles. They are more expensive to manufacture because fitting the components in is more labor intensive, and because they have a higher return rate.

Battery size: A small hearing aid can not be powered by a large battery. As battery size decreases, handling difficulties increase (for some patients) and battery life decreases (assuming no change in gain and maximum output).

Each of the advantages of the different styles has to be weighted according to an individual patient's needs: The ability to provide a high gain, for example, is not an advantage if the patient does not need a high gain. It is therefore illogical to simply add the check marks against each style in Table 10.1. It is worth noting, however, that most hearing-impaired people are elderly, and that many elderly people have trouble manipulating small objects, because of either diminished vision

---

Selecting to minimize management problems

The following choices are appropriate for patients who are expected to have difficulty manipulating hearing aids or their controls.

- Choose a hearing aid with wide dynamic range compression and no volume control.
- Choose the largest hearing aid style and battery size that the patient finds cosmetically acceptable, but choose a half-concha ITE rather than a BTE.
- For patients with good mental capabilities but poor physical manipulation ability, consider an aid with a remote control.
- For patients with poor vision, all controls and the battery compartment opening point have to be easily located tactually.

---

or diminished tactile sensitivity. There is a strong statistical connection between the degree of difficulty patients have in managing different hearing aid styles and the eventual satisfaction they report for each style.[42]

Although not shown in Table 10.1, spectacle aids have a major logistical disadvantage: The eye specialist and ear specialist have to coordinate their activities to ensure that the spectacle adapter on the hearing aid matches the spectacle frame. Also, if either hearing aid or spectacles break down, both devices may be unavailable to the wearer until the repair is completed.

10.2 Selecting Hearing Aid Features

On the basis of electroacoustic parameters such as gain, frequency response, compression ratio, and number of channels, there may be many hearing aids of the desired style that appear to be suitable for the patient.

Identifying additional features that would be useful to the patient is an important step in choosing the best hearing aid.

10.2.1 Volume control

All varieties of compression decrease the need for a volume control, though not necessarily to the same degree. Many patients are very pleased not to have to manipulate a volume control. Fortunately, many patients will not need a manual volume control if the hearing aid has an automatic control. Unfortunately, there are an approximately equal number of patients using automatic hearing aids who say that there are occasions on which they would have liked to turn their hearing aids up or down.[237, 477, 902] Of course, some of these patients would not be able to use a volume control, and some would, on balance, not choose to have one on the hearing aid if the need for one is infrequent. Volume controls can *create* problems for some patients if they are accidentally moved when the aid is being inserted or removed.

There is no effective way to predict which patients are likely to need a control. A safe option is to order (in addition to an automatic control) a manual control that can be electronically locked, unless:

- the patient is expected to have limited ability to manipulate a control;
- the patient has previously used, and been happy with, a fully automatic aid; or
- the hearing aid is so small that inclusion of a volume control is impractical.

Another way to provide some of the benefits of a volume control without actually fitting one is to use a push-button on the hearing aid to select from multiple memories. Each push advances the hearing aid to its next memory, and if these memories differ in gain (possibly along with other response changes) this feature can partly compensate for not having a volume control. If the aid wearer uses a remote control, there is little need for a volume control on the hearing aid.

10.2.2 Telecoil

A telecoil (described in Section 2.8) is essential for anyone with a severe or profound hearing loss. It is also likely to help people with a moderate loss use the telephone. People with mild loss can usually cope reasonably well with the telephone without their hearing aid. People with all degrees of loss will appreciate the reduction in noise and reverberation that telecoils offer when used in conjunction with a room loop. The disadvantages of a telecoil are the increase in size needed to fit in the telecoil and switch, and the increased crowding of ITE and ITC hearing aids when the faceplate contains a telecoil switch in addition to a volume control and on/off switch. This increased crowding can make it hard for the patient to find and operate the correct control. These disadvantages should be weighed against the substantial advantages. Most commonly people with severe and profound losses have telecoils, and people with mild losses do not.

10.2.3 Direct audio input

Direct audio input (as described in Section 2.9) is particularly useful for:

- People who use a wireless transmission system that is electrically coupled to their hearing aids. Adults as well as children can benefit enormously from a wireless system.

- People who use a hand-held directional microphone connected to the hearing aid via a cable. Most commonly it is people with severe or profound hearing loss who choose to use these devices. The increase in signal-to-noise ratio can be substantial. These microphones can provide directivity superior to that of head-worn microphones and often can be held closer to the source.

- People who watch TV in a noisy or reverberant place. A microphone placed near the TV, or a plug coupled to the TV audio output can be connected via a cable to the hearing aid. This can provide a substantial increase in signal-to-noise ratio and a substantial decrease in reverberation.

Eventually, it will be common for hearing aids to contain a wireless receiver, in which case the need for direct audio input connectors will decrease. Currently, some wireless receivers are attached to the hearing aid and connect to it via the direct audio input. Wireless systems are thus currently making the direct audio input more useful than ever.

10.2.4 Directional microphones

Directional microphones can offer a substantial improvement in signal-to-noise ratio, as described in Section 2.2.4. Hearing aids can be ordered with fixed directional microphones, but increasingly, hearing aids enable the user to switch between directional and omni-directional modes. The only reasons for *not* choosing a switchable directional microphone are as follows. Of these, the first is by far the most common reason for denying a patient the advantages of directional microphones.

- The patient wants a low visibility hearing aid (a CIC or an ITC). It is not possible to fit an effective directional microphone in these hearing aids.

- The patient requires amplification over such a restricted frequency range (e.g. above 1500 Hz only) that the benefits of the directional microphone, averaged across frequency, are diminished relative to its cost and size. The hearing aid is directional only over the frequency range where amplified sound dominates over vent-transmitted sound (see Section 5.3.1).

- The patient requires a low- to mid-frequency response *considerably* flatter than can be provided by a hearing aid with a directional microphone. This is rarely a problem in programmable hearing aids, but more low-frequency gain can always be achieved with an omni-directional microphone than with a directional microphone.

- A higher cost than can be afforded, but of all hearing aid features, directional micro-

phones can best be justified on the basis of cost relative to benefit.

Directional microphones have the following disadvantages. It is for these reasons that a switchable directional microphone is better than a permanently directional microphone.

- Directional microphones are even more prone than omni-directional microphones to wind noise. They can therefore disadvantage patients who spend a lot of time outdoors.

- In some circumstances, it is not possible for the patient to always look at the sound source. Examples include someone driving a car and listening to passengers, a pedestrian dodging traffic, and children in a classroom listening to those behind them. In such situations, speech and environmental sounds may be clearer and more audible when an omni-directional microphone is used.

Note that in indoor situations where the talker is some distance away, the hearing-aid wearer will be well outside the direct field of the talker (i.e further than the critical distance) and may remain so even when using a directional microphone. If such situations provide the primary need for hearing aids, directional microphones (whether permanent or switchable) are not likely to offer any advantage.

10.3 Selecting a Signal Processing Scheme and Prescription Method

Signal processing schemes and prescription methods are discussed together in this section because, for nonlinear hearing aids, the two are inextricably linked: Compression and other amplification parameters have to be adjusted in *some* way for each patient. Similarly, there is no point in choosing a prescription procedure that requires a certain parameter to be adjusted to a certain value if the processing scheme chosen does not include this type of adjustment.

10.3.1 Selecting a signal processing scheme

Compression limiting versus peak clipping. Peak clipping should be chosen in preference to compression limiting only for:

- Patients with a profound hearing loss who need the greatest possible OSPL90. If patients prefer the volume control to be turned to its highest setting, it is likely that they would benefit from more gain or more OSPL90 or both. Greater maximum output, especially for speech signals, is possible with peak clipping (see Section 9.6.2).

- Patients who have to be fitted with a larger hearing aid to achieve the required OSPL90 in a compression limiting aid, but who do not want to wear a larger hearing aid. For example, it may be possible to achieve adequate OSPL90 with a peak-clipping ITC or with a compression-limiting BTE. Some patients will prefer the size and appearance of the ITC to the lower distortion of the BTE. For other patients, sound quality will be more important than appearance.

Remember that the choice of peak clipping versus compression limiting is less important for hearing aids that have wide dynamic range compression (see Section 9.6.5). Patients who are used to peak clipping may not initially like a changeover to compression limiting, although most appreciate the change within a few weeks.[205]

Wide dynamic range compression. There is ample evidence that some form of compression with a low compression ratio should be available in all hearing aids (Section 6.5). We will loosely refer to this as wide dynamic range compression (WDRC), whatever the compression threshold may be. While a small proportion of patients may not gain any advantage from WDRC relative to linear amplification, there is as yet no way to *reliably* predict which patients these are.[237] WDRC is, however, most likely to be advantageous for those clients who need their hearing aids in a wide variety of communication situations (Gatehouse, Elberling & Naylor, 2000). It seems safest to initially select some form of WDRC for everyone. For those with a profound hearing loss, relatively high compression thresholds will usually be necessary (see Section 9.3.9).

Multichannel compression. Evidence for additional benefit from more than one channel of compression is less clear (see Section 6.5). It seems *likely*, however, that multichannel compression will provide some additional benefit for patients with a moderately or steeply sloping hearing loss, because a different degree of compression can be used in each channel. A possible criterion would be to use multichannel compression for any patient whose 2 kHz threshold exceeds the 500 Hz threshold by more than about 25 dB. These people are likely to benefit most from a TILL response aid (see Section 6.2.4). Some recent data indicate that patients with a flat loss have a weak preference for single-channel compression, but there is an urgent need for more evaluation of this.[446] On the other hand, the multiple amplification channels needed for multichannel compression are the most common ways by which useful features like adaptive noise suppression and feedback suppression are implemented. Provided compression ratio is less than about 3:1 (or perhaps 2:1), multichannel compression is unlikely to be harmful for anyone.

Fast- or slow-acting compression. Some advanced multichannel hearing aids currently on the market have very fast-acting compression, others have very slow-acting compression, others have combinations of fast and slow, and others have programmable attack and release times. How can the right compressor speed be chosen for an individual patient? As yet there is *no* way of systematically prescribing which type of compressor is best for an individual patient. There are, however, indications that fast acting compression is best for subjects with a high level of cognitive functioning, as measured by their ability to identify target sequences amongst rapidly changing visual patterns (Gatehouse, Elberling & Naylor, 2000).

Fast-acting compression is particularly likely to be beneficial for clients who frequently need to use their hearing aids in communication situations where the sound level varies rapidly by large amounts. Slow-acting compression is more likely to be bencticial for clients who wear their hearing aids in a range of environments that have different mean sound levels (Gatehouse, Elberling & Naylor, 2000). Whichever speed of compression is used, if the patient reports any of the disadvantages of fast or slow compression outlined in Sections 6.3.2 or 6.3.3 respectively, this would be an indication to try the other type.

Adaptive noise suppression. Amplification schemes in which the gain is automatically decreased in those frequency regions that have the poorest signal-to-noise ratio are most likely to be appreciated by patients who wear hearing aids in a wide variety of noisy environments. The benefit of these schemes increases along with the variety of noise spectra that the hearing aid wearer encounters in everyday life. Applying different amounts of compression and/or gain in each frequency region has the potential to improve listening comfort and, more rarely, intelligibility (see Section 6.3.7). Hearing aids that incorporate a sophisticated speech/non-speech detector in each channel are more likely to enhance comfort than are those that react merely to overall input level.

The benefits of adaptive noise suppression will be far greater for patients who need amplification at all frequencies than for those who need amplification of only the high frequencies. If the low-frequency gain of a hearing aid is dominated by vent-transmitted sounds, the effects of adaptive noise reduction are confined to higher frequencies. An adaptive noise-reduction system will then affect sound in much the same way as a far simpler single channel compressor.

Multiple memories. The candidacy issues for multi-memory hearing aids are very similar to those for adaptive noise reduction. Patients are most likely to benefit from multi-memory amplification if they require amplification over a wide frequency range, regularly wear their hearing aids in acoustically diverse listening environments, and have a more severely restricted dynamic range in the high frequencies (see Section 9.5.2). The reason for this similarity is that both multi-memory amplification and adaptive noise suppression aim to vary the amplification characteristics depending on the acoustic environment, and both can achieve useful gain variations only at those frequencies where the gain is greater than 0 dB. In addition, however, multiple memories can be used to access the telecoil or to change the microphone directionality.

Feedback management or reduction schemes. For people with a history of trouble with feedback oscillation, or people whose pure tone thresholds suggcst that feedback will be a problem, some form of feedback management or reduction scheme is worthwhile (see Section 7.3). People with a severe-to-profound hearing loss, and those with good low-frequency hearing combined with poor, but useable high-frequency hearing, will benefit most from feedback management processing.

10.3.2 Choosing a prescription procedure

There is more research evidence supporting the NAL-RP prescription procedure than there is for any other procedure for linear hearing aids (see Section 9.2.4). This procedure can be used with confidence when prescribing for linear hearing aids (whether the aid uses peak clipping or compression limiting to control the maximum output).

There is little research evaluating any nonlinear prescription procedure relative to alternatives (see Section 9.3.8). At this stage, clinicians will have to select the procedure that has the most convincing rationale. The NAL-NL1 procedure is indirectly supported in that it prescribes responses for a 70 dB SPL input level very similar to those prescribed by the NAL-RP procedure. On the other hand, some authors consider that normalizing loudness at each frequency individually is self-evidently worthwhile, so that all of the procedures *except* NAL-NL1 have some validity. Results from an experiment in which the prescriptions from NAL-NL1 and from loudness normalization are compared in the laboratory and in real life strongly favor NAL-NL1, particularly in background noise.[446]

10.4 Overview of Hearing Aid Selection and Adjustment

Let us assume that you have used the prescription procedure in which you have the most confidence to calculate a real-ear electro-acoustic target for a patient. How do you now go about selecting a hearing aid and then adjusting it to match the desired target? The methods described here are most applicable for adult patients and children approximately six years of age and older. Much is also applicable to younger children and infants, but Chapter 15 will recommend some more efficient variations for these younger people.

The prescription formula you use may prescribe in terms of:
- insertion gain (e.g. NAL-RP, or FIG6),
- Real-Ear Aided Gain (REAG) (e.g. DSL for linear aids, or DSL[i/o],
- both insertion gain and REAG (e.g. NAL-NL1).

This book recommends that insertion gain be used for adults and older children, and that REAG be used for children under the age of six (see panel at the end of Section 9.2.4).

Selection of a hearing aid to match a prescription target can be performed systematically only if hearing aid characteristics are expressed in the same way as the required prescription characteristics. For example, if the hearing aid specifications are expressed in terms of the insertion gain that they provide to the average person, these specifications can be directly compared to an insertion gain target for the patient. More commonly, hearing aid specification sheets refer to performance in a 2-cc coupler, so the prescription target also must be expressed as performance in a 2-cc coupler. Unless this is done in a way that takes into account the acoustics of the individual's ear, the 2-cc prescription should always be regarded as a means to an end, not as the final target to be achieved. Ultimately, it is the real-ear performance in which we are interested.

Because hearing aid performance can be expressed as 2-cc gain, ear simulator gain, simulated insertion gain, or simulated REAG, there is no single right method to select and initially adjust a hearing aid. There are, however, some methods that take less time than others.

The most efficient method depends on the degree of flexibility with which the chosen hearing aid can be adjusted, and whether it can be programmed under computer control. Accurate calculation of coupler targets is essential when choosing between hearing aids that have only a limited range of adjustment. At the opposite extreme, an extremely flexible hearing aid is able to meet such a wide range of targets that accurate calculation and matching of the coupler targets is a waste of time, unless it can be done in an automated manner by a computer. Hearing aids can lie anywhere on the continuum between extremely flexible and extremely inflexible. Efficient techniques for choosing and adjusting programmable hearing aids (which invariably have reasonably flexible amplification characteristics) and for choosing and adjusting inflexible hearing aids are shown in the next two sections.

Although non-programmable hearing aids are still in the majority, they are a technology of the past.[b] The steps for non-programmable hearing aids are given in a small font to indicate the diminishing importance that non-programmable hearing aids should have in a modern practice.

10.5 Twelve Steps for Selecting and Adjusting Programmable Hearing Aids

Programmable hearing aids are easier to select and adjust than non-programmable aids, because of the assistance provided to the clinician by the programming computer, and because the response of the hearing aids can easily be changed after their performance has been measured on the individual patient. Figure 10.1 shows an overview of the twelve steps involved in the selection and adjustment process, prior to ascertaining the patient's opinion of sound quality. These steps are described in the following paragraphs. We will assume that the fitting tool is NOAH-based software on a personal computer (see Section 3.3.1). The steps are similar if a dedicated programming device from a single manufacturer is used.

Step 1: Enter Audiometric data. As a minimum, audiometric data will include pure-tone thresholds for each ear to be fitted. Other audiometric data, not necessarily used for the hearing aid fitting, could include patient identifying data, discomfort levels, most comfortable levels, loudness scales, speech identification scores, acoustic reflex data, and tympanometric data. Within NOAH, these data will be entered within the ***Client Module*** and the ***Audiometry Module***. Most procedures will use only the threshold information, but it is a good idea to enter enough

information to unambiguously identify the patient at a later time. Having the audiometric information stored will save time during the fitting appointment. NOAH will store information about the hearing aids selected or

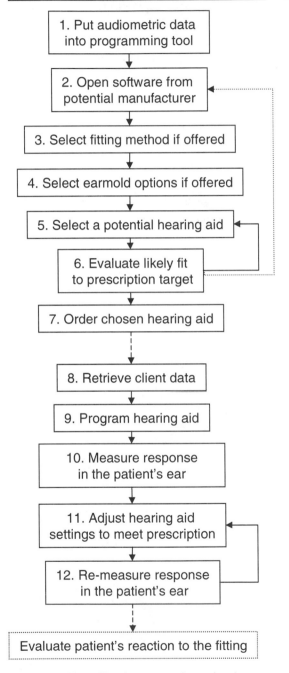

Figure 10.1 Twelve steps for selecting programmable hearing aids.

b   In the public hearing rehabilitation network in Australia, over 90% of patients have received digitally programmable hearing aids for nearly a decade.

adjusted for the patient in each session. This can provide a valuable history of the patient's fittings. Apart from its use in hearing aid fitting, the NOAH database can be used as the sole repository of patient information for the practice.

Step 2: Open manufacturer's software. There is no systematic way to choose a particular brand of hearing aid for a patient. Factors that will affect your decision of which manufacturer to consider first will include:

- The availability of hearing aids with the combination of features required for the particular patient;

- A history of reliable and timely sales and after-sales service in the past;

- Familiarity with the hearing aids and software of a particular manufacturer, especially if that manufacturer has a hearing aid that you have found to give good results for previous patients with similar needs and audiometric profiles;

- Discounts applicable if the requisite number of hearing aids is purchased within a month from the same manufacturer.

Step 3: Select fitting method. Some manufacturers offer you a choice of fitting procedures (NAL, DSL, FIG6, etc). Others offer only a fitting procedure developed by the manufacturer. See Sections 9.2.4 and 9.3.8 for a comparison of different procedures.

Step 4: Select earmold or earshell options. Some manufacturers' software will automatically recommend a vent size (and for BTE hearing aids, a sound bore). Some software instead requires you to specify the earmold or earshell configuration. Other software makes no allowance for the earmold or earshell configuration. If you are able to specify the acoustic configuration, follow the procedure outlined in Section 5.7 to first determine what you should fit. It is important to specify the approximate vent size if a 2-mm or larger vent is used, or else the software

may make large errors in calculating the coupler gain needed to achieve the real-ear gain target. This may result in you choosing an inappropriate hearing aid, and will almost certainly result in the software pre-adjusting the hearing aid to a tone control setting with an inappropriate low-frequency gain.

Step 5: Select a potential hearing aid. With most software, you make an initial specification of the hearing aids you would like to consider. How this is done varies between manufacturers. At one extreme you are required to specify which particular hearing aid style (e.g. ITE) and family of aids, and circuitry (e.g. K-Amp, output compression) you are interested in. At another extreme, you indicate the style and features (e.g. telecoil, directional microphone, and volume control) you require, and the software will list a range of specific hearing aids that meet your requirements to varying degrees. You can then make a selection from this range.

Step 6: Evaluate likely match to the prescription. Once you have chosen a hearing aid, most software programs will indicate graphically how well the hearing aid should meet the prescription targets for your particular patient. For nonlinear hearing aids, the graphical display comprises a gain-frequency response at one or more input levels and/or input-output curves at one or more frequencies. It is often necessary to examine the match to the prescription for several hearing aids before making a final selection. If the match to the prescription is not sufficiently close, or if the hearing aids do not have the features you want, it may also be necessary to return to Step 2 and try the models from an alternative manufacturer.

Step 7: Order chosen hearing aid(s). The software will usually enable you to print out all the information necessary to order the hearing aids you have selected. The information required will vary from manufacturer to manufacturer and from hearing aid to hearing aid, but may include the following if the model number or type does not uniquely specify any of these features.

- Battery orientation (toilet lid or swing-out)
- Battery size
- Telecoil and switch
- Volume control add-on cap
- Removal handle
- Microphone directionality
- Vent diameter and adjustment options
- Sound bore and earmold material (for an earmold)

Step 8: Retrieve patient data. When the hearing aids have arrived and the patient is about to be fitted, you can retrieve the patient data from NOAH.

Step 9: Program the hearing aid. Selecting the ***Fitting Module*** from NOAH. The software will show the hearing aid that you had previously selected for the patient. The desired settings can then be transferred to the hearing aid(s) connected to the HiPro interface.

Step 10: Measure response in the patient's ear. The response of the hearing aid should be measured with a real-ear analyzer employing a probe microphone. The type of measurement to be done will depend on the nature of the prescription target: insertion gain, real-ear aided gain, or real-ear input-output curves. For nonlinear hearing aids, gain-frequency responses should be measured with a broadband stimulus (see Section 4.1.3). For linear hearing aids, broadband stimuli or swept pure tones are acceptable. It is most convenient if the results of the measurement appear on the same screen as the prescription target. This can be a screen within NOAH if the real-ear analyzer is able to send information to NOAH. Otherwise, the audiometric information or the prescription target should be typed into the real-ear analyzer so that the prescription target can be displayed on its

---

Programmable hearing aids are simple – you may have nothing to do!

With programmable hearing aids, the selection and adjustment process to achieve a reasonable match to the target is greatly simplified, provided the hearing aid manufacturer's fitting software includes the prescription procedure you want to use. You must still select the hearing aid (easy, because there will be fewer models to choose from, and each will be highly adjustable) and you must still choose a vent size and sound bore profile, though the fitting software may recommend these to you. Despite this, a programmable aid may take longer to adjust, because the large number of controls tempts the clinician to try numerous combinations to get the best possible match to the prescription and/or to get the best possible subjective reaction from the patient.

If the fitting software is integrated with a real-ear measurement system, it will automatically measure the real-ear response and may adjust the hearing aid for you (Step 11) after the real-ear measurement. Do not worry. Despite all this automation you are still needed because there are many people-oriented aspects of hearing aid fitting (see especially Chapters 8, 12 and 13) for which your human skills will be indispensable!

Irrespective of how easy programmable hearing aids are to program initially, their biggest advantage is found when the patient returns and says something that indicates the electro-acoustic performance should be adjusted. If the hearing aid is an ITC or CIC and is not programmable, it is not likely to have many adjustable controls and may not have any. Even some ITE hearing aids may not have an appropriate adjustment control. Sending a hearing aid back to a manufacturer to have a minor change made to its performance is so much less satisfactory for all involved than instantly adjusting the programming.

Meeting the target: How close is close enough?

- There is no definite rule for how close is close enough. We know that a large majority of people with mild and moderate losses will choose the NAL-RP response over one that deviates from it by 6 dB/octave in either the low frequencies or the high frequencies.[117] We also know that as deviations from the NAL-RP target increase from 0 to 6 dB, self reported benefit from hearing aids diminishes slightly.[42]

- It seems that for mid-level inputs, discrepancies of 3 dB at any frequency can safely be ignored. Discrepancies of 10 dB should certainly not be ignored, but this leaves a large range where you may be uncertain if any further improvement is worthwhile.

- We know even less about the discrepancies that are allowable at low and high input levels.

- The type of discrepancy must be considered. A gain 6 dB above target at one frequency accompanied by a gain 2 dB above target at the remaining octave frequencies is inconsequential if the hearing aid has a volume control, because a reduction in the volume control setting could bring all gains to within 2 dB of target. By contrast, a gain 5 dB above target at one frequency accompanied by a gain 5 dB below target at a frequency one octave away would be worth improving. This represents a discrepancy in the response slope of 10 dB/octave, which should be avoided if possible.

- The speed with which you can make a change to the response and measure its effect, along with the amount of time you have available in the appointment, will often determine whether the response is close enough.

---

screen. It is possible to compare the measurement results on the analyzer with the prescription targets on a different computer, but the comparison is more time consuming.

Step 11: Adjust hearing aid settings to match prescription. If Step 10 reveals a discrepancy between the target and actual response, the hearing aid settings should be modified to minimize the discrepancy.

Step 12: Re-measure the response in the patient's ear. Following each adjustment of the hearing aid, the response should be re-measured. Eventually, you will decide that the measured response is close enough to the target, as discussed in the panel *How close is close enough?* After the prescription targets have been achieved with sufficient accuracy, the patient's reactions to all aspects of the sound quality have to be determined, but this is covered in Section 10.10 (for maximum output) and in Chapter 11 for all other aspects.

10.6 Eleven Steps for Selecting and Adjusting Non-programmable Hearing Aids

Hearing aids with amplification characteristics that cannot easily be adjusted after the aid has been ordered should be selected more accurately than is necessary for programmable hearing aids or non-programmable aids with several controls. Extremely accurate selection (covered in Section 10.7) takes more time, however, and in many cases the additional time may be better spent listening to, informing, instructing, or encouraging the patient.

Figure 10.2 shows an overview of the process of selecting and fitting a relatively inflexible hearing aid (i.e. an aid with one or no fitter controls). The process starts from the audiogram and ends with a real-ear performance that matches the prescription target. Ideally the prescription should be calculated with computer assistance. This might comprise:

- a special purpose program (such as the NAL-NL1 or DSL 4.1 stand-alone software[c]),

---

[c]   NAL-NL1 software is available from NAL, fax: +61 2 9411 8273; www.hearing.com.au; email: Research@NAL.GOV.AU. DSL 4.1 software is available from HHCRU, fax +1519 661 3805; www.uwo.ca/hhcru; email: dsl@audio.hhcru.uwo.ca.

- a real-ear gain analyzer, or

- hearing aid manufacturers' fitting software.

Step 1. Select the prescription procedure in which you have the most confidence. Ideally, linear hearing aids should be prescribed using a linear selection procedure, and nonlinear aids should be prescribed using a nonlinear procedure. Nonlinear procedures should prescribe gain-frequency responses, OSPL90 responses, and input-output curves. If necessary, a nonlinear procedure can be used for linear aids, provided only the prescription for mid-level input sounds and the prescription for OSPL90 are used. Similarly, a

linear procedure can be used to prescribe mid-level responses for nonlinear aids.

Step 2. Calculate the real-ear prescription target. Ideally, the software you are using will specify the prescription target in the form that you want it. If, however, the prescription procedure you select gives only a REAG target, and you need an insertion gain target, you can convert REAG to an insertion gain target by subtracting an adult average real-ear unaided gain (REUG) from the REAG target. Suitable REUG values are given in Table 4.6. Similarly, if the prescription procedure you select gives only an insertion gain target and you wish to use a REAG target, you can convert by adding an adult average REUG. Choose the set of REUG values that correspond to the way you normally measure REAG (e.g. 45° with a control microphone activated). If you are sure what earmold or earshell options you are going to use, all of Step 2 can more efficiently be deferred until the patient returns for the fitting appointment and the calculation can be inserted immediately before or after Step 8.

Step 3. Choose the earmold or earshell options needed for the patient. Choose the vent size of the earmold or earshell, and, for a BTE aid, guess the sound bore profile you will need. (Choose a 3-mm horn if you are unsure at this stage.) Section 5.7, Steps 1 to 4, shows how to make these choices. In a subsequent step you will find out whether you need to revise your estimate of the sound bore profile.

Step 4. Calculate the coupler prescription needed to achieve your real-ear targets. Hopefully, the software you are using will calculate the coupler prescription for you, but if not, the equations in the panel *Calculating coupler targets from real-ear targets* can be used. These equations are based on the equations in Chapter 4, but if you have to use them, or any of the other equations written in small print in this chapter, you should acquire better software! Note that the coupler targets calculated by the equations in this section do not include any allowance for reserve gain. That is, they calculate the gain needed at the used volume control setting. To calculate the full-on gain of the hearing aid, a reserve gain of 5 to 15 dB should be added.

If the insertion gain target equals 0 dB, and if the vent will allow sound into the ear canal without attenuation (see Figure 5.11), the coupler gain

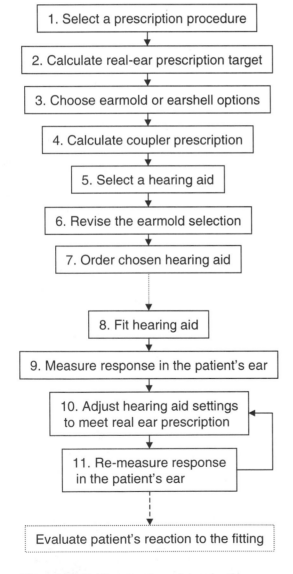

Figure 10.2 Eleven steps for selecting non-programmable hearing aids.

Calculating coupler targets from real-ear targets

When starting from an insertion gain prescription:

Coupler gain = insertion gain + CORFIG – sound bore effects – vent effects   ...10.1.

When starting from a REAG prescription:

Coupler gain = REAG – RECD – MLE – sound bore effects – vent effects   ...10.2.

When starting from a Real Ear Saturation Response (RESR):

Coupler OSPL90 = RESR – RECD – sound bore effects – vent effects   ...10.3.

When starting from a standard OSPL90 target that does not take individual sound bore or vent effects into account (e.g. Table 9.6):

Coupler OSPL90 = Standard OSPL90 target – sound bore effects – vent effects   ...10.4.

Average data for CORFIG, RECD, microphone location effects (MLE), sound bore effects, and vent effects are shown in Tables 4.7, 4.1, 4.5, 5.6, and 5.1 respectively. Note that the vent effects are subtracted, and the vent effects themselves are negative. Consequently, the net effect of the vent is to make the coupler gain larger as the vent gets larger. RECD data for infants are given in Table 15.2. If individual RECD values, measured with the patient's own earmold relative to a HA2 2-cc coupler, are used rather than average values, the sound bore and vent effects will already be included in the RECD measurement and can be deleted from the above equations.

---

target calculated using equation 10.1 or 10.2, should be regarded as the upper acceptable coupler gain, not an actual target. That is, the necessary sound will come in through the vent, and all the hearing aid has to do is not disrupt this natural sound. Excessive hearing aid gain will add to this acoustically transmitted sound in an unpredictable manner. Ideally, the aid coupler gain should be 5 dB or more below the upper acceptable coupler gain prescription to prevent the two paths from interacting (see Section 5.3.1).

Converting a target from real-ear to coupler terms will have no effect on compression ratio, and will have only a minor effect on compression threshold.

Given our uncertainty over how compression threshold should be prescribed, this small effect can be overlooked. Consequently, treat any real-ear compression ratio and threshold targets as though they are coupler targets.[d]

Step 5. Select a hearing aid that matches the coupler response and coupler OSPL90 targets calculated in Step 4. If the hearing aid has some flexibility (e.g. a low-tone cut control) ensure that the response slope needed falls within the range of slopes that can be achieved with the hearing aid. Trying to find a hearing aid whose response matches an entire response curve, or worse, a family of response curves at different levels, can

---

Calculating ear simulator targets from real-ear targets

If the test box you use contains an ear simulator (ES) instead of a 2-cc coupler, all the concepts in the preceding panel still apply. Equations 10.1 to 10.3, however, should be replaced with the following.

When starting from an insertion gain prescription:

ES gain = insertion gain + REUG – MLE – sound bore effects – vent effects   ...10.5.

When starting from a REAG prescription:

ES gain = REAG – MLE – sound bore effects – vent effects   ...10.6.

When starting from a Real-Ear Saturation Response (RESR):

ES OSPL90 = RESR – sound bore effects – vent effects   ...10.7.

---

[d]   To be precise, compression thresholds in the real ear will be smaller than in the coupler by an amount equal to the microphone location effect (see Table 4.5).

be a daunting task. It is usually necessary to simplify the prescription. Some convenient parameters to use when searching for a hearing aid that matches your prescription include:

- **Peak gain.** If you are going to fit an inflexible BTE hearing aid, the peak gain is likely to be at 1 or 2 kHz, depending on the damping you use (see Section 5.5). For an inflexible ITE hearing aid, the peak gain is likely to be close to 2 kHz. For an inflexible ITC or CIC hearing aid, the peak gain is likely to be close to 3 kHz. You therefore need to have a coupler gain target at only one or two of these frequencies in order to select a hearing aid with an appropriate over-all gain.

- **Peak OSPL90.** OSPL90 usually has its peak value at the same frequency at which gain has its peak value.

- **Gain slope.** The difference between the peak gain and the gain at 500 Hz is often referred to as the gain slope. (This is an imprecise, but common, definition; gain slope should really be expressed in dB/octave, rather than as the difference in dB.) The gain slope is often shown on hearing aid specification sheets.

- **Compression ratio.** If you are intending to use a single channel hearing aid, with the exception of a K-Amp, you will need a compression ratio at only a single frequency. For a dual channel hearing aid, it will probably be convenient to use frequencies of 500 Hz and 3 kHz, because these frequencies are likely to fall within the two different channels for any reasonable choice of crossover frequency.

When performing Step 4, be aware of which information you are likely to use in Step 5: do not calculate, look up, or write down the response at any more frequencies or input levels than you are going to use.

Step 6. Revise the sound bore profile (for a BTE). Now that you have selected a hearing aid, you know the coupler performance, so you can compare it to the required coupler performance. If the sound bore profile you assumed in Step 2 results in the coupler gain prescribed at 4 kHz being higher than the hearing aid can deliver, a larger horn should be used if it will fit in the earmold. When making this decision, it is important to look at the slope of the prescription and the slope of the actual coupler gain in the 2 to

4 kHz octave, rather than just the 4 kHz gain in isolation. It is not acceptable to achieve the target gain at 4 kHz if the gain is 10 dB too high at all other frequencies! Much less commonly, the chosen hearing aid will have too much gain at 4 kHz relative to 2 kHz. If so, choose a constant diameter sound bore, or even a constricting sound bore. Step 4 of Section 5.7 has more details.

Step 7. Order the hearing aid(s). Clearly describe the hearing aid and earmold or earshell to the manufacturer, as described in Step 7 of Section 10.5. Additionally, the following features may have to be specified.

- Peak gain
- Gain slope
- Peak OSPL90
- Number and type of fitter controls
- Compression circuit options
- Output amplifier type

For a BTE hearing aid, it is necessary to specify the model number you have selected. This is usually enough to unambiguously describe the features that should come with the aid.

Step 8. Fit the hearing aid. Fitting the hearing aid means making sure that the hearing aid fits comfortably in the ear. It may be necessary to make minor adjustments to the earmold or earshell to ensure that it can be easily inserted and is comfortable. All types of hearing aids can be altered, but earmolds for BTE hearing aids can be more easily and drastically altered than earshells for ITE/ITC/CIC hearing aids. The thinness of the walls in custom shells limits the amount of material that can be ground or sanded away without having to repair the shell.

Step 9. Measure the real-ear response. The type of real-ear gain you measure will be the same as the type of real-ear prescription target you adopted in Step 2. Procedures for measuring REAG and insertion gain have been described in Section 4.2 and 4.3 respectively. The maximum output of the hearing aid can also be checked at this stage, as discussed in Section 10.10.

Step 10. Adjust hearing aid to meet prescription. If the hearing aid you selected has *no* adjustable controls, there is very little you can do in this step. The only option may be to increase or decrease the vent size. More often than not, however, the vent size is dictated by the need to avoid feedback or the occlusion effect, rather than matching the gain-frequency response prescription. For BTE hearing aids you can use different earhooks or dampers to achieve the desired response at mid frequencies (see Section 5.5).

Step 11. Re-measure real-ear response. If the hearing aid does have some fitter controls, these should be adjusted while the probe tube and the hearing aid are still in the ear canal. If the measured response is further from the target than you consider can be achieved with a custom aid, and is sufficiently far to disadvantage the patient, your only option is to send the hearing aid back for re-making. This is a difficult decision (see panel *How close is close enough?*). Sending the aid back is inconvenient, expensive for all parties, and will not necessarily be effective. For this reason it is a good idea to use digitally programmable hearing aids whenever possible.

10.7 Allowing for Individual Ear Size and Shape in the Coupler Prescription

Once the prescribed real-ear gain has been obtained, there is no need to consider the effects of variations in the size and acoustic properties of the patient's external ear. These effects are built into the real-ear gain that has been obtained. The coupler (or ear-simulator) response that is needed to achieve the prescribed real-ear gain, however, depends on the acoustics of the individual patient's ear. If our goal is to achieve a certain insertion gain, the individual patient's real-ear to coupler difference (RECD) and REUG will affect the coupler gain required (see equation 4.10 or 4.12). If our goal is to achieve a certain real-ear aided gain, only RECD affects the coupler gain required (see equation 4.4).

Consequently, a hearing aid that has been pre-adjusted in a coupler or ear simulator to match the prescription will most precisely match the real-ear target if these individual ear effects are known and incorporated into the coupler or ear simulator prescription. Some fitting software (DSL4.1, NAL-NL1) allows this to be done. To make this correction, measure the appropriate individual ear effect, and enter the data into the program at the appropriate

---

> **Practical tip: Is pre-adjustment of response in the coupler worthwhile?**
>
> Pre-adjust the hearing aid in a 2-cc coupler (or ear simulator) when:
>
> - The patient is unwilling or unable to sit still for long enough, with the hearing aid on and a probe tube inserted, for the hearing aid to be adjusted (especially applicable to young children);
> - Real-ear measurements can not be performed for any other reason; or
> - The clinician is not familiar with the effects of all the aid fitting controls, and needs time to learn their effects.
>
> Otherwise, save the time and adjust the hearing aid only while it is in the patient's ear.

---

place. If one wishes to allow for these effects and does not have access to these programs, any coupler prescription can be customized using equations 10.8 to 10.10. To apply these equations to an ear simulator, simply replace *coupler* with *ear simulator* in each equation.

Measurement of the individual's RECD and REUG is worthwhile only in the following cases:

- When fitting a hearing aid with few controls, especially if the average gain of the hearing aid being considered only marginally matches the prescribed average gain.
- For infants (RECD only), as further discussed in Chapter 15.

Other than in these circumstances, measurement of RECD or REUG is not worthwhile, because the hearing aid can quickly be adjusted to match the target insertion gain or REAG while the real-ear response is being measured with a probe microphone, whatever the individual's RECD and REAG are. Individual RECD responses tend to be parallel to the average RECD,[437] and so in most cases, nothing more than a gain change is needed to compensate for the individual response.

Customizing the coupler prescription

If your prescription software prescribes coupler response, and you wish to modify this prescription to allow for the measured characteristics of an individual patient's ears, any of the following corrections can be used.

To accurately meet an REAG target:

Custom coupler gain prescription = standard coupler gain prescription + $\text{RECD}_{\text{average}}$ - $\text{RECD}_{\text{individual}}$

$$...10.8$$

To accurately meet an insertion gain target:

Custom coupler gain prescription = standard coupler gain prescription + $\text{RECD}_{\text{average}}$ - $\text{RECD}_{\text{individual}}$ + $\text{REUG}_{\text{individual}}$ – $\text{REUG}_{\text{average}}$

$$...10.9$$

To accurately meet a real-ear saturation response target:

Custom coupler OSPL90 prescription = standard coupler OSPL90 prescription + $\text{RECD}_{\text{average}}$ - $\text{RECD}_{\text{individual}}$

$$...10.10$$

Average values for RECD (based on HA1 and HA2 couplers) and REUG can be found in Tables 4.1, 15.2, and 4.6 respectively.

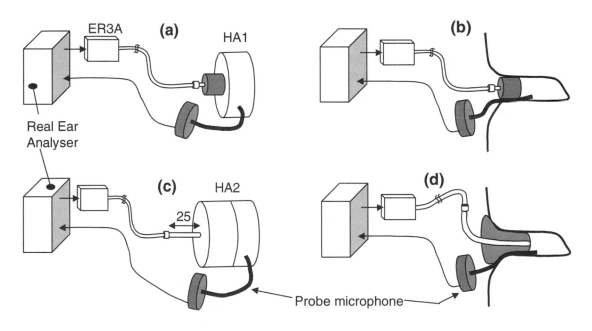

Figure 10.3 Measurement of RECD using a real ear analyser, insert phones, and a probe microphone. For ITEs, the insert phone is connected via foam plugs to (a) a HA1 coupler, and (b) the patient's ear. For BTEs, the insert phone is connected to (c) a HA2 coupler by 25 mm of tubing, and (d) the patient's ear by the individual earmold and tubing. For both measurement types, a hearing aid receiver in a BTE hearing aid case can be used instead of the ER3A earphone if desired.

Measuring Real-Ear to Coupler Difference (RECD)

To measure an individual's RECD response, an insertion gain analyzer is used. Recall that insertion gain is the *difference* between aided and unaided ear canal SPL. We take advantage of the analyzer's ability to measure a difference, but in this case we make it the difference between SPL in the individual ear canal, and SPL in a coupler (or ear-simulator). The steps are as follows and as shown in Figure 10.3 (Moodie, Seewald & Sinclair, 1994). Note that some insertion gain analyzers include RECD measurement as a standard procedure. These analyzers use the standard coupler microphone for the coupler measurement, so it is not necessary to insert the probe microphone into the coupler. For such analyzers, follow the procedure outlined in the analyzer's instruction manual.

1. Connect an ER 3A earphone terminating in a foam sleeve to the insertion gain analyzer loudspeaker output socket. (You may need a suitable adapter.)

2. Insert the probe microphone into a HA1 2-cc coupler. Some couplers have a special hole drilled in the side (initially filled with putty) to accommodate the probe. For these couplers the regular coupler microphone should be in place to seal the cavity, but will not be used. Other 2-cc couplers have a probe adapter that allows the probe to be inserted into the coupler through an adapter that replaces the usual coupler microphone. Alternatively, probe tubes can be inserted through the foam sleeve by first pushing through a crochet needle, and then pulling through the probe tube (Killion, personal communication).

3. Connect the ER 3A earphone outlet to the HA1 2-cc coupler. You can insert the earphone's foam sleeve 1 or 2 mm into the 2-cc coupler, or mount the end flush with the coupler using putty, whichever is more convenient for the coupler you use.

4. Run a baseline response on the insertion gain analyzer. Control the analyzer in exactly the same way you would if you were measuring an unaided response in a person's ear.

5. Insert the probe tube and the ER 3A earphone into the person's ear, with the medial end of the earphone sleeve the same distance down the canal that the medial end of the hearing aid will be.

6. Run a response on the insertion gain analyzer. Control the analyzer in exactly the same way that you would if you were measuring an aided response in a person's ear. The "insertion gain" displayed by the analyzer will in fact be the RECD for the person.

For patients who are going to be fitted with a BTE, the above procedure can also be used. A more accurate assessment of RECD can be made if the patient's own earmold is used for the real-ear measurement instead of a foam sleeve, and a HA2 earmold is used for the coupler measurement. In this case, the "RECD" measurement also allows for the individual's earmold sound bore. It also allows for the *vent out* effects, but not the *vent in* effects (Section 5.3.1). If the patient's own mold/HA2 combination is to be used, Steps 1, 4, and 6 are the same, but Steps 2, 3 and 5 should be replaced with the following:

2a. Insert the probe microphone into a HA2 coupler.

3a. Connect the ER 3A earphone to the HA2 coupler via 25 mm of tubing.

5a. Insert the probe tube and the person's earmold into the ear.

The only slightly tricky part of either RECD procedure is knowing what probe depth to use when measuring the real-ear response. The issues and procedures are identical to those discussed for REAG measurement (Section 4.2.1).

10.8 Allowing for Surgically Altered Ear Canals

As discussed in the panel within Section 9.2.4, it does not seem reasonable to preserve a person's REUG in a hearing aid fitting if that REUG is atypical as a result of surgery. This, however, is what happens if one adopts and achieves an insertion response target for that person. The solution is to use a REAG target rather than an insertion gain target. If the prescription method you use does not specifically give an REAG target (only DSL and NAL-NL1 do), you must add REUG to the insertion gain target to convert it to an REAG target. Suitable values for REUG can be found in Table 4.6.

10.9 Verifying and Achieving the Prescribed Real-ear Response

It is important to verify that the prescribed real-ear response has indeed been obtained. Measurement of real-ear gain is just as worthwhile for nonlinear hearing aids as it is for linear aids. For nonlinear hearing aids, performance can not be summarized by a single gain-frequency response and a single saturation response, as it can for linear aids. This problem can be solved in two ways. Real-ear gain can be measured at three input levels, such as 50, 65 and 80 dB SPL, and compared to the target responses at those levels. If a reasonable match is obtained, it is extremely unlikely that there will be marked discrepancies at intermediate levels. Alternatively, the compression characteristics can be established with the aid of input-output curves. One curve should be used for each channel of a multichannel hearing aid. If these are correct, only a single gain-frequency response curve will then be needed. This should be done at a mid-level input, such as 65 dB SPL.

Nonlinear hearing aids should be measured with a broadband stimulus (see Section 4.1.3). A problem can arise with some hearing aids that view a steady broadband test signal as a noise that should be attenuated! This problem can be overcome by using a more complex test signal (e.g. one that pulses) so that the hearing aid treats it as a wanted signal. Hearing aids manufacturers are aware of this problem and now provide test modes in which these noise-reduction schemes are disabled.

Finally, is there still a role for aided threshold testing to verify hearing aid performance? Possibly, but as the major application is in infant testing, we will address this question in Chapter 15.

10.10 Verifying and Fine-tuning OSPL90

Hearing aid maximum output should be subjectively evaluated for all patients who are capable of indicating excessive or insufficient loudness. Because an excessive OSPL90 can cause an extremely negative first experience with hearing aids, evaluation of maximum output should be performed at the fitting appointment, rather than at the first follow-up. The appropriateness of maximum output should be further evaluated at the first follow-up. Maximum output is evaluated by asking patients about the loudness of intense sounds presented in the clinic, and by asking patients about their reactions to intense sounds after they have had a chance to use their hearing aids in their home environments (see panel). Remember that any variations

> **Caution: Real- ear measurements at 80 or 90 dB SPL**
>
> If OSPL90 is too high, presentation of an 80 or 90 dB SPL input level could be an unpleasant initial hearing aid experience for the patient. Minimize this chance by:
> - first running sweeps at 70 dB SPL;
> - explaining that the sound should be loud, but should never cause discomfort; and
> - reassuring the patient that you will stop the sweep immediately the patient so indicates.

> ### Evaluating hearing aid maximum output
>
> First, ensure that sounds do not cause discomfort.
>
> 1. Present several intense sounds to the patient. Include a pure tone or warble tone sweep at 80 or 90 dB SPL, supplemented by a few complex sounds with low- and high- frequency dominated spectra. These can be generated by the clinician; their exact level does not matter provided they are intense enough to saturate the hearing aids. Suitably high-level sounds can easily be made by hitting a cup with a spoon, clapping hands, and by speaking loudly close to the person (or by using recorded speech). In each case explain to the patient that you are about to make sounds that *should be loud*, but not uncomfortable, and that you need to determine their loudness so that that you can properly adjust the hearing aids.
>
> 2. After you have explained what you are about to do, position yourself such that the patient can see you making the loud sound, so that it does not take him or her by surprise. Ask the patient to rate the loudness, using any of the loudness scales given in Section 9.3. Also carefully watch the patient's expression while the sound occurs. Follow up, with further questioning or instruction, any apparent contradiction between the rating given and the accompanying expression (e.g. a rating of only loud accompanied by a visible flinching or eye-blink, or a rating of uncomfortably loud said without any apparent concern). It should be possible for all the sounds (sweep, impulse sound, hand clapping, and speech) to produce a rating of loud but OK or very loud without any of them being rated as uncomfortably loud.
>
> 3. For bilateral fittings, these sounds should be made with both hearing aids turned on, and it may be necessary to also test each aid separately.
>
> 4. If the patient has already been wearing the hearing aids, ask if any sounds have been so loud that they were uncomfortable, have jarred the patient, have made the patient want to remove the hearing aids, or have given the patient a headache.
>
> Second, ensure that maximum output is large enough.
>
> 1. Play speech (preferably continuous discourse) at approximately 80 dB SPL and ensure that speech is at least *loud* (this is actually done at the same time as step 1 above).
>
> 2. If the patient has already been wearing the hearing aids, ask if there have been any situations in which the level of background noise seems to increase markedly whenever someone stops talking, or in which things that should differ in loudness seem to be equally loud. (But beware, these are also symptoms of an excessively high compression ratio in a wide dynamic range compression system.)

made to the acoustic coupling (vents, dampers, and sound-bore profile) during the fitting will have the same effect on maximum output that they have on gain.

10.11 Concluding Comments

The second half of this chapter describes procedures that enable the real-ear gain of a hearing aid to match a target. It will be apparent that there is no single right way to do this. Some procedures, however, take more time than do others. It is worth reviewing

one's procedures to ensure that the no unnecessary or inefficient steps are being performed.

Finally, it is important to remember that matching a prescription target is only an intermediate goal within the whole rehabilitation process. The ultimate aim is for the hearing aid to provide the clearest possible speech combined with good sound quality. Fine-tuning and troubleshooting methods to achieve this are covered in the next chapter.

CHAPTER ELEVEN

PROBLEM SOLVING AND FINE-TUNING OF HEARING AIDS

Synopsis

Many hearing aid fittings need to be fine-tuned, either electronically or physically, after the patient has had a week or two to try the hearing aids. When a patient has trouble managing hearing aids (inserting, removing, using the controls, changing the battery), re-instructing the patient may solve the problem. If not, the hearing aid should be physically modified. Physical modification will also be necessary when a patient is suffering discomfort from the earmold or shell, or when the hearing aid works its way out of the ear.

Feedback oscillation has several potential solutions: gain reduction at selected frequencies, reducing the vent size, making a tighter earmold or shell, or changing the hearing aid to one that has feedback management or canceling circuitry.

Complaints about the patient's own-voice quality are particularly common. The most common cause is the physical blocking of the ear canal, so the best cure is to add a vent, or increase the size of an existing vent. Where feedback oscillation precludes that, the earmold or shell can be remade with the canal stalk extended down to the bony canal, preferably using a soft material. Own-voice problems are sometimes caused, and cured, by electronic variation of the gain-frequency response for high-level sounds.

Complaints about the tonal quality of speech are fixed by changing the balance of low-, mid-, and high-frequency gain. The hard part is knowing when to ask the patient to persevere with a response in the expectation that it will eventually become the preferred response, and confer maximum benefit to the patient.

When a patient complains about the clarity or loudness of speech, or the loudness of background noise, the patient must be questioned particularly carefully so that the acoustic characteristics of the sounds causing the problems can be identified. The clinician's first aim is to identify whether it is the gain for low or high frequencies, and the gain for low, mid, or high levels, that should be adjusted. Only then can the appropriate hearing aid controls be adjusted.

In those cases where it is not clear which control should be adjusted, or by how much it should be adjusted, a systematic fine-tuning can be performed using one of two general methods. The first of these is paired comparisons, in which the patient is asked to choose between two amplification characteristics presented in quick succession. Multiple characteristics can be compared by arranging them in pairs. Paired comparisons can be used to adaptively fine-tune a hearing aid control if the settings compared in each trial are based on the patient's preference in the preceding trial.

The second general method for fine-tuning relies on the patient making an absolute rating of sound quality. The best amplification characteristic (out of those compared) is simply the characteristic that is given the highest rating by the patient. The absolute rating method can also be used to adaptively alter a chosen hearing aid control. This is achieved by deciding on a target rating (e.g. just right) and adjusting a control in the direction indicated by the patient's rating (e.g. too shrill, or too dull).

The paired comparisons and absolute rating methods are best carried out while the patient listens to continuous discourse speech material. Depending on the complaint being investigated, this can be supplemented with recordings of commonly encountered background noises.

This chapter describes techniques that help the clinician adjust hearing aids on the basis of the patient's comments and preferences. Such adjustment will sometimes involve moving the amplification characteristics *away* from the prescribed response that has so carefully been achieved. Some of the methods described in this chapter can be used when hearing aids are first provided, but more often they will be used after patients have worn their hearing aids for a week or two.

Although the chapter is focussed on fine-tuning the amplification characteristics of hearing aids, the clinician should realize that sometimes listening and talking are all that is required, and/or all that can be done. People with a complaint want to be listened to, and sometimes active listening, plus the provision of additional information (see Chapter 8 and Chapter 12) can change a patient's expectations such that what was perceived as a major problem is now perceived as normal. That is, the clinician has to be able to fine-tune patients' expectations as well as hearing aids.

11.1 Solving Common Problems

After the hearing aid is fitted and the prescription target has been met as well as it can be, the time of problem solving begins. For some patients there will be many problems to overcome before they can gain significant benefit from their hearing aids, for others there may be none. This section describes several common problems and some potential solutions.

11.1.1 Management difficulties

Clients may have difficulty with inserting the aid, removing it, switching it on and off, varying the volume control, or changing the battery. For any of these problems, the first thing to try is further training. The ultimate solution, in some cases, is to train a frequent caregiver to do the task instead of the patient. Training support staff in an aged-care facility, although necessary, may have only short-term effects unless there is some mechanism by

which new staff members are trained as they take up duty.

Some more specific solutions are as follows. In every case, the first step is to closely observe the patient trying to perform the task, so that the clinician can identify precisely which part(s) of which operation(s) the patient is unable to perform.

Difficulty inserting an earmold or ear shell. Options include:

- If the patient picks up the hearing aid differently each time, or in an inappropriate manner, the patient has to be taught landmarks on the aid or earmold, and a specific grip.

- If the patient is unable to insert the helix-lock of the earmold or ITE fully into the cymba portion of the concha, it may be necessary to remove the helix lock entirely (easy for a BTE earmold, but a re-make may be necessary for an ITE).

- Similarly, if the patient is unable to get a BTE earmold under the anti-helix, part of the earmold's conchal prominence (see Figure 5.3) may have to be removed, turning a skeleton into a semi-skeleton, for instance.

- If the earmold or shell is a tight or tortuous fit, a lubricant (water-based for safety) may have to be applied every time the aid is inserted until the patient is more practiced and/or the ear shape adapts to the aid. Alternatively, the earmold or shell can be trimmed (but not the aperturic seal) if feedback oscillation is not likely to result.

- The patient may have to pull the pinna upwards and outwards with the opposite hand, while inserting the hearing aid or earmold with the ipsilateral hand.

Difficulty locating or using a control. If re-training is not successful, the hearing aid may have to be modified or replaced:

- Volume controls on ITE and ITC hearing aids can be made more prominent with add-on caps.

- If the patient is confusing one hearing aid tactile feature (e.g. an MT switch) with another feature (e.g. a volume control), one of the controls may have to be removed so that the more important control (whichever it may be for that patient) can be operated. Some controls can be removed cleanly with electrical wire cutters.

- A hearing aid with an automatic volume control, or with a greater compression ratio, can be fitted instead.

- A hearing aid with a remote control can be fitted instead.

Difficulty removing a hearing aid. Options include:

- If the patient cannot grasp the hearing aid or earmold, a removal handle should be added, or a different hearing aid style used.

- If the patient can grasp the hearing aid but not remove it, and cannot be trained to use an appropriate twisting motion, parts of the earmold or shell will have to be removed.

Difficulty changing the battery. Options include:

- Coloring one side of the battery slot to lessen problems with battery reversal.

- Using a tool to open the battery compartment.

- Using a magnetic tool to hold the battery.

- Re-fitting with a hearing aid that has a bigger battery or a battery compartment that is easier to open or visualize.

- Teaching the patient to distinguish the positive side of the battery tactually rather than visually, or vice versa. The removable tab can help with either of these approaches.

11.1.2 Earmold or earshell discomfort

Earmolds, earshells, and BTE hearing aids can all cause physical discomfort to the external ear if they apply excessive pressure at any point. The problem is diagnosed by asking the patient where it hurts, and by otoscopic or other visual examination of the affected area to look for inflammation. This diagnosis is easier if the patient wears the hearing aid for as long as he or she can reasonably stand the day before, or immediately before, the follow-up appointment. The usual solution to the problem is to grind away, and then polish, the area of the earmold or shell that causes the problem.

For CIC hearing aids, discomfort can also be caused by a hearing aid that is too loose. Discomfort can occur if the patient frequently pushes the hearing aid in further than it was intended to go, in an effort to retain it in the ear or to prevent feedback.[583] Martin & Pirzanski (1998) make the useful analogy with shoes: they cause sore feet whether they are too large or too small. If this is the cause of discomfort, the problems should be viewed as one of poor retention (see next section).

For BTE hearing aids, an incorrectly cut tubing length can create excessive pressure, as shown in Figure 11.1. Pressure spots can arise if the patient has been wearing an earmold only partially inserted. Most

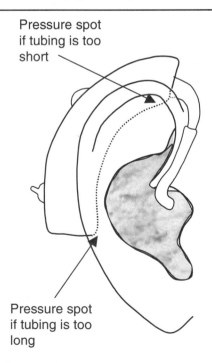

Pressure spot if tubing is too short

Pressure spot if tubing is too long

Figure 11.1 Excessive pressure caused by earmold tubing being cut too short or too long.

commonly, this is because the helix lock has not been properly tucked in.

More generalized inflammation can be caused by an allergic reaction (Section 5.9.2), but this is rarer. The solution is to re-make the earmold or earshell with a different material, or to coat the earmold or earshell with material that the patient is hopefully not allergic to, such as nail polish varnish. Another problem, also rare, is that of the patient trying to use a hearing aid that has been made for his or her other ear, or that has been made for another person's ear! Such a mix-up can happen while the hearing aids or earmolds are being manufactured, or at any time subsequent to the fitting.

11.1.3 Poor earmold or earshell retention

Hearing aids, particularly CIC and ITC styles, can sometimes fall out of the ear. Movement of the patient's jaw when the patient is talking, yawning or chewing can move the ear canal walls sufficiently to *push* the hearing aid out of the ear. Solutions include:

- Remaking the hearing aid in a style that has better retention properties. For example, an ITC could be used instead of a CIC, or a low profile ITE could be used instead of an ITC.

- Remaking the earmold or shell with a longer canal portion.

- Remaking the earmold or shell, and taking the impression with medium viscosity material while the patient's jaw is open, so that the canal width is greater in the flexible part of the canal (see Section 5.8.2). The impression should extend beyond the second bend, even if the hearing aid will not be inserted this deeply.[708]

11.1.4 Own voice quality and occlusion

Any of the following descriptions by a hearing aid wearer about his or her own voice indicate that the spectrum of his or her own voice in the ear canal is inappropriate: *hollow, boomy, echoes, like speaking in a barrel, like having a cold, or feeling plugged.* Because most people are not able to clearly describe different types of spectral emphasis (e.g. insufficient or excessive low-, mid- or high-frequency emphasis), all we can conclude from an adverse description of a patient's own voice is that there is something the patient does not like about the way it is being amplified. If the patient reports that other people's voices also do not sound good, that problem should be fixed first, as it may also solve the own-voice problem (see Sections 11.1.6 and 11.2).

Assuming that other people's voices sound fine, the patient's own voice may sound unpleasant to the patient because of any of the following reasons, the first of which is the most likely.

The earmold or earshell is excessively blocking the ear canal. As discussed in Section 5.3.2, blocking the canal within the cartilaginous section will allow the walls of the canal to vibrate with respect to each other, and hence generate a high sound level in the residual part of the canal that they enclose. For low-frequency sounds, this causes the SPL at the eardrum to increase by up to 30 dB relative to that which would occur for an open ear canal. The problems can be diagnosed and solved, by:

- Increasing the area, and/or decreasing the length, of the vent (but review Section 5.3 to ensure that the way you change a vent significantly affects its acoustic properties).

- Making an earmold or earshell with a canal stalk long enough to extend into the bony part of the canal (see Section 5.1). Possible difficulties with this solution include increased difficulty with insertion and removal, and decreased comfort. These can be helped by constructing the tip (at least) of the earmold or shell out of soft material. The problem with this is that the life of the earmold of shell is likely to be decreased, because soft materials deteriorate in appearance and cleanliness more quickly than hard materials. Invention of a very soft but non-porous material would be welcome! There is no point in extending the earmold or shell into the bony portion of the canal unless the extended section material makes good contact with the walls of the canal. In fact, failure to make good contact can increase the level of occlusion sound generated because it decreases the residual volume without suppressing the source of the vibration.

- In the future, effective electronic means for canceling the occlusion-generated sounds should become available.

The hearing aid is distorting when the patient speaks. The proximity of the mouth to the ear causes the input level to the aid to be higher when the patient speaks than when other people speak, especially if the patient has a loud voice. The possibility of distortion being a cause of the problem can be tested by letting the patient hear, and rate the quality of, another person's loud speech, using either the clinician's live voice or recorded speech as the signal. A presentation level of 80 to 85 dB SPL at the person's ear would be representative of own-voice levels. If distortion is a problem, the solution is to use a hearing aid that does not distort at high input levels, either because it has suitable compression limiting, and/or because wide dynamic range compression (WDRC) causes the gain to be low for low-level inputs. Although an aid wearer is likely to prefer less gain while listening to his or her own voice than when listening to other people,[504] there should not be any special need to adjust the amplification characteristics to suit the aid wearer's own voice. Any aid with compression that gradually decreases gain as the input level rises from 65 dB SPL to 85 dB SPL will provide lower gain for the aid wearer's voice, just as it does for any other intense sound.

The hearing aid amplifier is excessively amplifying low-frequency sounds. The mouth radiates high-frequency sounds forward more than to the side. Also, low-frequency sounds travel around a barrier (the head) more readily than do high-frequency sounds. As a result, the spectrum of the aid wearer's voice near his or her own ear will be more heavily weighted to low frequencies than will anybody else's voice.[158] This bass boost occurs for everybody, but if the hearing aid is also excessively amplifying low frequencies, the combined effect can be a poor own-voice quality, even though the quality of other people's voices is not too bad.[509] The problem is diagnosed by decreasing the low-frequency gain of the hearing aid and seeing if the problem disappears. For nonlinear hearing aids, it should be necessary to decrease only the low-frequency gain for low-level inputs (i.e., a BILL characteristic) but this may conflict with the processing that is best for amplifying other sounds. For hearing aids that do not have a tone control, the problem is more difficult to diagnose, which is one of many good reasons to use flexible hearing aids whenever possible!

The patient has forgotten what his or her own voice should sound like. Because a frequency-dependent hearing loss affects the tonal quality of everything perceived by an unaided person, the new hearing aid wearer may have forgotten what his or her voice should sound like. This is a justification for the oft-repeated instruction *you will get used to the sound of your own voice*. In the author's opinion, this is an unlikely reason for own voice complaints,[a] but there are no data on this question.

---

a   People who most complain about own-voice quality have good low-frequency hearing and poor high-frequency hearing. Such people would be used to hearing a treble-deficient voice when listening unaided, and yet the problem is usually solved by venting, which cuts the bass of the spectrum at their eardrum.

11.1.5 Feedback oscillation

Feedback oscillation may cause patients to report any of the following:

- The volume control cannot be increased to the desired level without whistling occurring.

- Whistling occurs whenever they chew, talk, wear a hat, or put their hand near their ear.

- The hearing aid makes a brief ringing noise whenever certain sounds occur. This is the effect of sub-oscillatory feedback (see Section 4.6.2).

- The hearing aid whistles when they are in a quiet place but stops when a noise occurs. This happens with nonlinear hearing aids, because their gain increases in quiet places.

- The hearing aid appears to stop working or becomes weak or distorted. This observation would come from a person with severe or profound hearing loss at high frequencies who is unable to hear the feedback oscillation itself, but can hear the gain reduction that the oscillation causes.

As explained in Section 4.6, all of these problems indicate that too much sound is leaking from the ear canal to the microphone via some path. Tables 4.10 and 4.11 show how to diagnose the source of the leakage. Assuming that the hearing aid is not faulty, one of the following solutions should be tried. All have potential disadvantages, and all except the first three involve additional appointments and expense.

- Ensure that there are no excessive peaks in the real-ear aided gain (REAG) curve. If so, damp them, which is easiest but also most necessary for a BTE.
  Disadvantage: the peak in the REAG curve may be necessary to achieve the desired insertion gain curve.

- If the hearing aid is vented, decrease the size of the vent with or a vent insert or sealing material.
  Disadvantage: may cause or exacerbate the occlusion effect.

- Decrease the high-frequency gain of the hearing aid, or for a multichannel nonlinear aid, decrease the high-frequency compression ratio or increase the high-frequency compression threshold (Section 7.3.1).
  Disadvantages: may   decrease intelligibility or sound quality.

- Remake or re-coat the earmold or shell so that there is less leakage between the mold/shell and the walls of the canal. Use an open-jaw impression technique if a re-make is necessary.
  Disadvantages: additional time and expense, potential occlusion effect, potential earmold/shell discomfort, and uncertainty of outcome.

- Fit a nonlinear hearing aid with a feedback management system so that the gain increase in low noise environments is limited to that which can be achieved without feedback oscillation (Section 7.3.1).
  Disadvantages: additional time and expense, and may decrease intelligibility at low input levels.

- Fit a hearing aid that has advanced feedback-canceling capability (Section 7.3.2 to 7.3.4).
  Disadvantage: additional time and expense.

Achieving enough high-frequency gain to meet the prescription target and hence obtain good speech intelligibility, while having the vent large enough to avoid occlusion, but simultaneously   avoiding   feedback oscillation, is technically the most difficult part of hearing aid fitting. For people with normal low-frequency hearing and a substantial, but aidable high-frequency loss, it is impossible to achieve all of these with venting alone. Either the patient has to endure sub-optimal intelligibility, or endure poor own-voice quality, or else an alternative method of occlusion or feedback control has to be used. To summarize, these comprise an earmold extending into the bony canal and advanced feedback-canceling circuits.

11.1.6 Tonal quality

Patients may describe the quality of speech and other wanted sounds in a wide range of ways. (Reaction to noise and unwanted sounds will be considered in the next section.) Excessive high-frequency amplification or insufficient low-frequency amplification (compared to their preferred response) may be described as being *shrill, harsh, hissy, sharp, metallic*, or *tinny*. Excessive low-frequency amplification or insufficient high-frequency amplification may be described as *muffled, unclear, boomy or dull*. Patients are more likely to notice or adversely comment about excessive high-frequency emphasis than about insufficient high-frequency emphasis,[117] probably because most patients are used to having deficient high-frequency audibility when they are unaided. Solving these complaints by changing the balance of high- to low-frequency gain is complicated by two factors.

One complication is that an excessively peaky gain curve can produce similar comments, even if the overall balance of low- to high-frequency gain is optimal. The solution to this problem is not to let it develop in the first place. Hearing aid fitting and verification should have included measurement of real-ear gain, and this will have revealed a peaky response if it existed. A peaky response should be dealt with immediately through a suitable combination of filtering and damping. Changing the damping for BTE fittings is easy because the dampers can be added to the sound tubing and can be placed in most earhooks (Section 5.5). ITE, ITC and CIC receivers can also be damped, but this is most conveniently done at the time the hearing aid is manufactured. Microphone inlet ports can also be damped with foam if the problem is in the 3 to 4 kHz range (Section 2.2.2 and 2.7).

The second complication is much harder to deal with. Suppose a patient complains about the high-frequency emphasis of a hearing aid that is providing the prescribed frequency response in a smooth manner. Is it because the patient knows better than the prescription procedure what is best, or is it because he or she has not yet become used to the high-frequency information that he or she has been deprived of for many years? Either of these could be true. People can take months to learn to fully use high-frequency information that they previously have not had.[302] This is known as the ***acclimatization effect*** (see Section 13.5). Initially, patients may choose an amplification characteristic that gives the greatest gain for the frequencies at which they have the least loss, presumably because they are most used to hearing sounds at these frequencies.[944] Patients with a high-frequency loss are a little more likely to prefer high-frequency emphasis four weeks after fitting than at the initial fitting.[755]

A compromise is to provide patients with a response that is mid way between the response they prefer, and the response that is believed to be best for them. The aim is to enable patients to gradually get used to a new response without subjecting them to a sound quality with which they are unwilling to persevere. There is no research addressing whether this is the best management option, but it seems like a very reasonable approach. If patients wear their hearing aids every day, and have not changed their minds about what they prefer within a month, it seems reasonable to give them the response they prefer. The considerations are similar for patients who are used to a peak clipping hearing aid, and are changed over to compression limiting, or for patients who are used to linear amplification and are changed over to WDRC. There are numerous examples of people preferring a compression limiting hearing aid to a peak clipping aid after one to two weeks of use, even though they disliked the compression limiting aid at first.[205]

11.1.7 Noise, clarity, and loudness

Many, many adverse comments by patients will mention noise and/or excessive or insufficient loudness. These can have a multitude of causes, and each cause has a different solution. Careful questioning of the patient is essential to make sure that patient and clinician are discussing the same problem before taking corrective action. Although excessive amplification of noise, inadequate speech clarity, and inappropriate loudness of wanted signals are different phenomena, they are combined in this section because solutions to one problem will affect the others. The total picture should be considered before taking any action. In the following, we will assume that the hearing aid has been adjusted so that typical, mid-level speech is at a comfortable level for the patient.

The hearing aid is noisy in quiet places. This complaint may be an indication that internal hearing aid noise is being amplified sufficiently to be audible in quiet places. It may also indicate that noises in the environment are being amplified and the patient has not realized that these are noises that are present and can be heard by people with normal hearing. Ask if the noise is audible in the clinic. If it is, ask if it is audible while you block the microphone port with your finger or some putty. This should diagnose the noise source as being either internal or external to the hearing aid.

- If the problem is external noise, identify the noise source to the patient and explain that normal-hearing people can also hear these sounds and that they are part of the richness of life. Also explain that the sounds may become less noticeable as the patient becomes used to the sounds being there. Let the person know that the loudness of these sounds can be decreased if the patient really wants it, but that many people come to value being able to hear these sounds when they need to. If complaints persist after further use, it will be necessary to decrease the gain the hearing aid provides for low-level sounds (assuming it is a nonlinear device) by raising the compression threshold or by decreasing the compression ratio.

- If the problem is internal noise, ensure that the aid is within specification by measuring its noise in a test box. If the aid is within specifications, decrease the low-level gain by increasing the compression threshold or by introducing low-level squelch or expansion if they are available. The disadvantages are that the patient will not be able to hear wanted low-level sounds, like soft speech, as well as he or she now does, and that a more expensive hearing aid that has these features may be needed. Internal noise is most likely to be heard at the frequencies where a patient has hearing thresholds that are close to normal. Hearing aids with sophisticated tone controls enable the required gain to be provided at those frequencies where it is needed and not at nearby frequencies where hearing thresholds are close to normal.

Soft speech in quiet places cannot be understood. The solution to this problem is to provide more gain for low-level sounds. Potential difficulties include an increased likelihood of feedback and an increased likelihood that the hearing aid will amplify sounds that the person may rather not hear. In multichannel hearing aids it may be necessary to increase the gain in all channels, or it may be enough to increase the gain in only the low- or high-frequency channels. The frequency range requiring extra gain can be tested by having the patient comment on the audibility of speech sounds that rely on low-frequency cues (e.g., *moon*, *boom*) or that rely on high-frequency cues (e.g. /sh/, /s/). A low overall speech level of around 45 dB SPL should be used.

The hearing aid is sometimes too loud when noises occur. Comments similar to this require especially careful questioning.

- If the noises ever get so uncomfortable that the patient *has* to immediately turn the volume control down or the hearing aid off, the OSPL90 of the hearing aid must be decreased. This can be done by

Which hearing aid control will solve the problem? - The troubleshooting two-step

With nonlinear hearing aids, choosing the correct hearing aid controls and adjusting them in the correct direction, to solve a problem reported by the patient, is potentially very difficult. Use the following approach to break the problem down to two more easily handled tasks.

1. Express the desired change simply. Question the patient until you understand the problem well enough to make a statement like: *I want to decrease the gain applied to low-frequency, high-level sounds.* In any particular case, the words *low-frequency* might be *high-frequency*, or may be absent altogether. That is, you may want to change the gain for high-level sounds at all frequencies. Similarly, the words *high-level* might be *mid-level*, or *low-level* or might be absent. Mentally picture the following table. Your sole aim is to determine which of the gains you need to adjust, and in which direction. This implies that you are also determining which gains are correct and should *not* be altered. If the patient cannot describe the problem and the types of sounds causing the problem well enough for you to know which gains you are targeting, you will have to present sounds in the clinic to gather further information. These sounds might be speech presented at a low-, medium-, or high-intensity, or background noises. Suitable noises can be found on various compact disks. *Notice that this first step is the same no matter what hearing aid the patient is wearing, and no matter what controls or number of channels the hearing aid has.*

Low-frequency, high-level gain	High-frequency, high-level gain
Low-frequency, mid-level gain	High-frequency, mid-level gain
Low-frequency, low-level gain	High-frequency, low-level gain

2. Identify the controls and the direction of change needed. In this step you can forget the patient's complaint and concentrate on the complexities of the particular hearing aid. Unless the hearing aid controls are labeled *low-frequency, high-level gain* (etc.), you will need to understand how each control (e.g. compression ratio, compression threshold, gain, UCL offset) affects each of the gains in the table above. Unfortunately, this varies from hearing aid to hearing aid, so you will need to acquire this knowledge for each type of hearing aid that you use. The knowledge can be obtained from specification sheets, or by measuring a hearing aid in a test box, and altering each control in turn. It may be helpful to sketch some I-O curves showing how the curves alter as each control is varied. Figure 11.2, for example, shows two ways in which an I-O curve might alter as a compression ratio control is varied. In one aid the low-level gain remains constant, but in the other the high-level gain remains constant.

Example. Suppose that a patient complains that crockery noise is too loud, but that most other sounds are fine. In step 1 we deduce that we wish to decrease the high-frequency, high-level gain, but leave the mid-level gain the same at all frequencies (because conversational speech was comfortably loud with a tone quality that was neither hissy nor boomy). Suppose that the patient is wearing a three-channel hearing aid, and that each channel has a selectable compression ratio, which applies to all levels above a fixed compression threshold of, say, 40 dB SPL. To alter the high-level gain while leaving the mid-level gain the same, we need to adjust compression ratio in the high-frequency channel. Depending on whether the I-O curve pivots around low-, mid- or high-level inputs as this control is adjusted, we may also need to adjust the overall gain for high-frequency sounds. Some compromises may be necessary. When we have achieved our aim of reducing the high-level gain but leaving the mid-level gain unchanged, we will find that we have inadvertently increased the low-level gain. Hopefully, this increased low-level gain will be acceptable to the patient. If not, some acceptable compromise between the low-, mid- and high- level gain applied to high frequencies will have to be found.

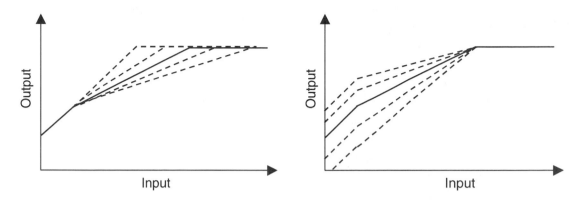

Figure 11.2 Variation of the I-O curve as the compression ratio control is varied for two different hearing aids.

electronic variation or by increasing the damping (in the case of a BTE), but this will also decrease the gain. The loudness may become uncomfortable only for sounds with significant high-frequency energy (like crockery noise, paper rustling, brake squeals, or water flushing); it may occur only for low-frequency sounds (like traffic noise or a door slam); or it may occur for sounds with a wide range of spectral shapes. If the problems seem to stem from only one frequency region, it is necessary to decrease OSPL90 only in that region, assuming the hearing aid has that degree of flexibility. Exposing the patient to a pure tone sweep at 90 dB SPL, from a real-ear gain analyzer provides a rapid cross-check as to which frequency region is responsible for excessive loudness. It may also be desirable to make the changes specified in the following point, if the hearing aid allows it.

- If the patient *can* tolerate the noise, but would rather it was not so loud so often, a change to the input-output characteristics can improve the situation markedly. The compression ratio for input levels above about 65 dB SPL should be increased. This may require that the compression ratio also be increased for lower-level sounds. Ensure, however, that the output level remains comfortable for speech signals of around 65 dB SPL. In a multichannel

hearing aid, the amount of compression could be increased in all channels. If you started from some reasonable prescription where different channels were prescribed different compression ratios, it is probably reasonable to increase all the compression ratios by the same percentage. For example, increase all compression ratios by 50%. If all the noises that are too loud are strongly high-frequency dominated, or strongly low-frequency dominated, it seems more reasonable to increase the compression ratio in only those channels causing the problem.

Background noise makes it hard to understand speech. If the primary complaint is not the *loudness* of the noise, but rather the effect the noise has on intelligibility, the solution is different.

- If the offending noise has a spectrum that is markedly different from that of speech, some small increase in intelligibility may be achieved by applying different amounts of compression in different frequency regions. If the offending noise is low-frequency weighted (traffic noise, some machinery noise), increasing the amount of low-frequency compression, or adding a simple low-frequency cut, will be helpful. If the noise is high-frequency weighted compared to speech (mostly impact sounds), increasing the amount of

---

Handling more than two channels

The procedures in this chapter concentrate on low versus high frequency, simply because it is relatively easy to identify low- versus high-frequency sounds. Many advanced hearing aids have three or more channels. Any mid-frequency channels can be adjusted by amounts intermediate to the adjustments made to the extreme low- and high-frequency channels.

---

high-frequency compression to achieve a TILL response, or a simple high-frequency cut will be helpful.

- If the noise has a spectrum similar to that of speech, which unfortunately is usually the case, and the speech has a satisfactory loudness and tone quality, then intelligibility can be improved only by using an effective directional microphone, or by using a remote microphone with a wireless transmission system.

People in the distance are easier to understand than people nearby. The higher level from people nearby may be causing excess compression or even distortion. A potential solution is to increase the maximum output and/or change from peak clipping to compression limiting.

11.2 Systematic Fine-tuning Procedures

The previous section described *which* hearing aid characteristics should be altered in response to specific adverse comments made by patients, but did not indicate by *how much* they should be varied. This section describes some systematic methods to improve on the initial prescription. Systematic fine-tuning procedures can be used for all patients, or can be used only to help solve problems as they arise. One advantage of routinely fine-tuning hearing aids is that no prescriptive procedure is perfect, and some patients are reticent to complain about sound quality no matter how bad it is. Furthermore, unless

patients previously had hearing aids that provided better sound quality than their new hearing aids, they will not know that better sound is possible, and so will not know to complain. Even when the sound quality of a new hearing aid is very good, it is possible that some variation to the hearing aid characteristics could make it excellent.

We will first review the basic methodology involved in performing paired comparisons, and absolute ratings of quality, and will then consider how these tools can be used to improve hearing aid fittings. They can be used to choose between responses that differ in any manner (Section 11.2.3) or to choose the best setting for any particular amplification control (Section 11.2.4).

11.2.1 Paired comparisons

Different response characteristics with similar perceptual effects can best be selected by allowing patients to choose between two alternative responses heard in quick succession. This process is called *paired comparisons*, and patients can simply be asked which of the two conditions they prefer. The *response criterion* can be made more explicit: patients can be asked which response they prefer on the basis of *intelligibility*, *comfort*, *naturalness*, *pleasantness*, minimizing *annoyance* of any noise present, or just about any other attribute of sound. In many cases, different response characteristics will be best for different response criteria.

Given the time pressures usually present in clinical settings, few clinicians will have time to use more than one criterion. If paired comparisons are being used to help address a specific problem, the criterion should be chosen to match that problem. For example, if the patient is complaining about the comfort of sound in noisy places, the criterion should be listening comfort. If the patient is complaining about the intelligibility of soft speech, the criterion should be intelligibility or clarity (to choose a more easily understood word). If in doubt as to the problem, or if the patient has several problems, the patient can simply be asked to choose the preferred response, with no specific criterion being mentioned.

Another key decision is what *stimulus* should be played to patients while they are choosing their preferred response characteristics. As with the response criterion, the stimulus chosen should be appropriate to the problem being addressed. If the patient is complaining about the effects of a certain type of background noise, there is little point in doing paired comparisons using speech material in quiet. Recordings of various noises are available on several compact discs. If the problem relates to the clarity or tonal quality of speech, a speech stimulus has to be used. To administer the comparisons in the minimum time, speech should be continuously present. There thus seems little reason not to use *continuous discourse* as the primary stimulus. In many cases, patients will be complaining about the disturbing nature of noise when it occurs simultaneously with speech. It is then useful to be able to play continuous discourse combined with selected noises.

If you do not have access to recordings of a wide range of noises, the following set of five stimuli would allow you to assess hearing aid performance in such a way as to address many problems reported by patients.
- continuous discourse in quiet, with the ability to play it at 50, 65, and 80 dB SPL;
- continuous discourse in quiet between three quickly alternating talkers, speaking at levels of 55, 65 and 75 dB SPL respectively;
- continuous discourse at 80 dB SPL with a background noise containing high-frequency impact sounds (e.g. crockery noise) of 80 dB SPL;
- continuous discourse at 80 dB SPL with a background speech babble of 70 dB SPL; and
- continuous discourse at 80 dB SPL with a background traffic noise of 80 dB SPL.

The stimuli are most useful if the speech and noise are recorded on separate channels, so that SNRs larger or smaller than those listed above can be selected when required.

The paired-comparison technique has become practical in a clinical setting since the advent of programmable hearing aids. In one approach, the two amplification characteristics to be compared are programmed into different memories of the aid. The patient can then switch between memories as often as desired until he or she can say which (if either) is preferred. Patients usually take 10 to 30 seconds to make a judgement, though some will take a minute or two. The comparison is easiest (and quickest) for patients if the characteristics of any background noise do not change markedly from any five-second period to the next one.

The second approach also relies on having a programmable hearing aid. In this technique, only one memory is needed, and the clinician changes the value of the parameter being investigated from time to time. The clinician indicates which response is currently selected by pointing to the letter *A* or *B* on a piece of card. The clinician can control the timing of each switch between programs, or the patient can indicate when a switch should occur.

Finally, it is worth contrasting the paired-comparison technique to traditional measures of speech recognition in which the patient has to repeat or choose the syllable, word, or sentence that he or she perceived. When there are only small differences between speech identification performance with different hearing aids, paired comparisons provide a quicker and more reliable way to choose the best option out of several alternatives.[858] Furthermore, paired comparisons can assess aspects of the sound other than intelligibility. The disadvantage of paired comparisons is that it is not possible to discern what types of sounds the patient misperceives, but this is more of a limitation for research than for clinical practice.

11.2.2 Absolute rating of sound quality

One disadvantage of the paired-comparisons procedure is the procedure can never reveal how bad or good the sound quality is – just which of the amplification schemes compared is preferred, and potentially how much better it is than another scheme. Another disadvantage is that if there are many schemes to be compared, and some of these are expected to be much better or worse than the others, many comparisons of different pairs will be needed to deduce which is the best response.

Both of these disadvantages can be overcome by obtaining *absolute ratings of sound quality*. Patients can be presented with a simple chart like either of those shown in Figure 11.3. The labels marked on each scale are explained to the patient. Some patients will find the scale with numbers easier to use; others will like the one with words. Sounds are then presented, while the patient wears the hearing aid. The patient is asked to mark, or state the position, on the scale that corresponds to the sound quality just perceived. It is advisable to let the patient hear a selection, and preferably the extremes, of the amplification conditions to be rated prior to obtaining the judgement for each condition. This makes it less likely that the patient will change his or her internal perceptual scale during the series of judgements.

For increased accuracy, each of the amplification conditions to be tested can be presented on multiple occasions, randomized with the other conditions being tested. Unfortunately, the time to do this is more likely to be found in a research setting than in a clinical setting. Presenting each condition several times is practical if there are less than ten conditions to be tested.

Absolute rating of sound quality is most useful when there are more than five or six conditions to be compared, or when it is expected that some of the conditions will be be much more acceptable to the patient than to others. Absolute ratings can then be used to weed out the amplification conditions that are rated poorly. If four or less of the conditions receive similar ratings, paired comparisons can then be used to select the most preferred condition.

11.2.3 Systematic selection by paired comparisons

If there are just two different responses that one wishes to compare, the procedure described in Section 11.2.1 can be used to make that comparison. What if there are more, and we wish to find the best response? The best way to accomplish this depends on how many different responses we wish to compare, and whether we believe before we commence testing that one of the responses (e.g. the one prescribed by a reliable prescription procedure) is more likely to be preferred than the alternatives. In the following discussion we will assume that we have a

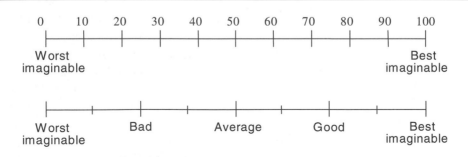

Figure 11.3 Two response scales used for obtaining absolute ratings of sound quality.

baseline response, which is the response that best matches some prescription. If we were not going to perform paired comparisons, this would be the procedure that we would fit to the patient because we believe it is *most likely* to be the best. There are at least three ways that we can organize the various comparisons to find the best response. Let us suppose that there are *n* responses to be compared.

Comparison to the baseline. Each response is paired, in turn, with the baseline response. Because we cannot have a great deal of confidence in the results of any individual trial, it will be necessary to compare each of the *n-1* alternatives to the baseline response several times. Ideally, ten repetitions would be used, but more realistically, time might permit only four repetitions. This requires a total of *4(n-1)* comparisons. For a baseline plus four alternative responses, this means 16 comparisons, which will take about eight minutes on average. If we have any *a priori* belief that the baseline response is right on average, we would not want to select one of the alternative responses unless it is chosen four times out of four in preference to the baseline.[b] If more than one of the responses is consistently preferred to the baseline, further comparisons will be needed to choose among them. The chance of this happening increases with the number of alternatives. Because of this, and because of the total time needed, the comparison-to-the-baseline procedure is probably feasible only for five or less responses.

Round Robin. Each response is compared to each other, and the response that is preferred the most number of times is declared the winner and is permanently programmed into the patient's hearing aid. For reliable results, each response should be involved in about ten preference trials. If the procedure is to be carried out in 10 minutes, this limits the number of responses that can be used to about

four. The Round Robin is particularly suitable for a small number of responses, especially where none of the responses being compared is the baseline response. This can happen when we have already decided to put the baseline response into one hearing aid memory, and are using paired comparisons to decide what should go in the other memory or memories.

Tournament. The responses are organized in pairs, and each pair is compared, say three times. The winners are the ones that are preferred two or more times out of three. These winners advance to the next round, where they are again arranged into pairs. This continues, with half the contestants dropping out each round, until a single winner emerges (see Figure 11.4). The procedure requires between *2(n-1)* and *3(n-1)* comparisons (depending on the consistency of the answers). To be carried out in 10 minutes, the number of responses should be eight or less. It is also particularly well suited to situations in which there is no clear baseline response. You will have to be well organized to keep track of which responses win and progress to each following round.

Irrespective of which of these three arrangements of pairs we use, how do we decide what the alternative responses should be? There is no set of rules for which parameters to vary, just a few guiding principles.

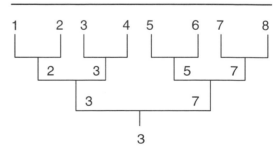

Figure 11.4 A tournament strategy for eight responses, with response number 3 being the eventual winner.

---

[b]   The consistency required before selecting an alternative to the baseline is a complicated balance involving the number of repetitions, the level of *a priori* confidence we have in the baseline, and the number of alternatives we are comparing to the baseline. Use the above recommendation unless you are confident about varying from it.

- The alternative responses should be potential winners. Do not waste time on a response that you strongly expect will be worse than the baseline response.

- Form alternative responses by varying the parameter that you are least confident about prescribing accurately.

- Choose parameter values that are different enough to have clearly audible effects, with the stimulus you are using, but not so extreme that one or the other is very likely to be unsuitable.

- Alternative responses can vary from each other by only one variable (e.g. different values of compression ratio) or they can differ substantially by having different values for many amplification variables.

- The alternatives should all be realistic amplification characteristics. If changing one variable (such as compression threshold) causes the gain applied for typical input levels to vary, it will be necessary to also change some other variable (such as overall gain) to compensate. There is no point in finding a winner under the conditions used for the paired-comparison trial if the patient would not be willing to use the program under typical conditions. (An exception would be if you were attempting to select a program for a second memory, to be used in specific circumstances, such as in very quiet or very noisy places.)

There is a potential logistical difficulty with paired comparisons using multiple responses. The patient cannot make each comparison until the clinician has appropriately set all the controls for the two programs that the patient is about to compare. It is too time-consuming to change multiple control settings prior to each pair being compared. Thus, if it is necessary to alter more than one control to change from one response to the next, all the responses will have to be set up once at the start of the procedure, and stored somewhere. This can be inside the hearing aid (if it has enough memories) or inside the fitting software if it is configured to enable such comparisons. There is no reason why the number of memories in the fitting software has to be limited to the number in the hearing aid. The clinician should not attempt to compare more responses than the number of memories available, with the exception of the special case considered in the following section.

11.2.4 Adaptive parameter adjustment by paired comparisons

A special application of paired comparisons is determining how much a single amplification parameter should be varied. We may strongly suspect, for instance, that we should increase the compression ratio, but by how much should it be increased? The hearing aid may enable a choice of many values above the one that appears to be unsuitable. Which should we choose? With such problems, we start by assuming that some unknown setting of a control is best, and that some aspect of sound quality will deteriorate as the control is increased or decreased from this value.

The paired-comparison method is used *adaptively* to find the best setting of the control. We start by comparing two settings of the control. After each trial, the control setting that was not preferred is replaced with another value. The control is moved in the direction indicated by the winner of the most recent trial. Suppose a patient's difficulty in understanding soft speech led us to believe that a lower compression threshold in a single channel hearing aid would be better and suppose that the hearing aid enables compression threshold to be set anywhere in the range from 30 to 70 dB SPL. Just as when we are finding an audiometric threshold, we must decide what the step size will be. Unlike threshold determination, there is no need to have different step sizes for ascending versus descending runs. In this example, we will assume that we use a step size of 10 dB.

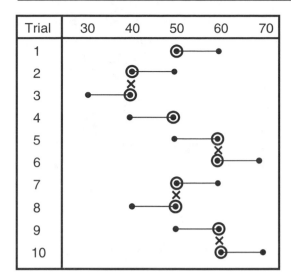

Trial	30	40	50	60	70
1					
2					
3					
4					
5					
6					
7					
8					
9					
10					

Figure 11.5 Worksheet for adaptive paired comparisons of different compression thresholds. Circles show the winner of each trial, and crosses mark the reversals.

Figure 11.5 shows the sequence of trials that might occur. Suppose the current compression threshold is 60 dB SPL and that the first comparison is with a lower compression threshold. The 50 dB threshold is preferred (as indicated by the circle), so in the next trial, this is compared to an even lower threshold. You will notice that the winners of trials 3, 6, 8 and 10 are marked with a cross. These are the values of the winners when a *reversal* occurred. The comparisons are continued until four reversals have occurred. The values at these reversals are then averaged to give the final setting, in this case, 52.5 dB SPL. The more reversals that are used, the greater will be the precision of the procedure, but the longer it will take.[c]

The key to using this method is to choose the step size wisely. The step size must be large enough to make a perceptible difference to the sound quality. If the step size is too small, reversals will occur randomly, and the final answer will also be a random number unless a huge number of reversals is used. It is better to err on the side of making the step size too big. If it is too big, four reversals will be obtained with very few trials, and if it was considered worthwhile, further trials could be done with a smaller step size starting from the result found in the first series of trials.

Patients will often comment that they cannot choose one sound over the other, or even that they cannot hear any difference between two sounds. At first they should be encouraged to make a choice, even if they have to guess. People underestimate their own ability to detect small differences and to reliably choose between two similar sounds. If their pattern of responses and ongoing verbal comments indicate that they really can *not* tell any difference between the pairs, this indicates that something is wrong. Either:

- the step size is too small – increase it;
- the stimulus level or type is inappropriate to the task – change it; or
- the setting of the control is unimportant – cease the adjustment process and use the time for something more worthwhile.

As was discussed in the final dot point in Section 11.2.3, one has to be aware of exactly how the hearing aid response is changing when any control is varied. If changing the compression threshold also changes the gain for mid-level sounds, each change of compression threshold has to be accompanied by an appropriate change in overall gain or compression ratio, such that the gain for mid-level sounds remains the same. This greatly increases the complexity of the adaptive paired-comparison task for the clinician, to the point where it is probably not worth the time required to do it. Fortunately, there are many occasions where a control can be varied without having to compensate for an unwanted effect by varying another control. The adaptive paired-comparison task is then a very efficient way to adjust a control on a hearing aid.

[c]   If the reversal values are averaged as suggested, an even number of reversals should be used. An odd number of reversals *can* be used, but the midpoints between the reversals must be averaged, rather than the reversal values themselves.

Although there are procedures, such as the Simplex procedure,[648] for efficiently adjusting two parameters adaptively, these are too complex and time consuming for clinical use.

11.2.5 Adaptive fine-tuning by absolute rating of quality

Just as we can adaptively vary the hearing aid's response depending on which of two responses is preferred, we can adaptively vary the response depending on an absolute rating of loudness or sound quality. Moore, Alcantara & Glasberg (1998) have described a useful procedure for adjusting the gain-frequency response and compression characteristics of multichannel hearing aids. The goals of this procedure are that:

1. Speech at 85 dB SPL should be judged as *loud;*
2. Speech at 60 dB SPL should be judged as *quiet*;
3. The tonal quality of speech at 85 dB SPL should be neither *tinny* nor *boomy*;
4. The tonal quality of speech at 60 dB SPL should be neither *shrill* nor *muffled*.[d]

To facilitate the adjustment, a patient is shown the appropriate chart, as shown in the first column of Tables 11.1, 11.2 and 11.3. In response to the patient's rating, the hearing aid is adjusted as shown in the remaining columns. The procedure is complete when all four goals are achieved. If the procedure is to be carried out in the minimum possible time, it is important that adjustment of controls at one step does not undo the goals achieved at a previous step.

For one particular two-channel hearing aid, Moore, Alcantara & Glasberg suggest that the adjustment to achieve each goal be carried out in the following order: 1, 2, 1, 3, 2, 4. Note that adjustments for goals 1 and 2 are repeated because of the likelihood of interactions between the different adjustments. It is necessary to repeat all or some of the sequence if any hearing aid control is adjusted to different settings in successive steps. To minimize the number of times the sequence has to be repeated, it may be necessary to adjust more than one control at a time. Simultaneous adjustment of multiple controls is also necessary if the hearing aid has more than two channels of compression. The procedure can be carried out manually, but it is most easily carried out if manufacturers include appropriate software to perform the adjustments within the fitting software provided for each specific hearing aid.

Although this procedure has been presented as a procedure for fine-tuning hearing aids, it can also be used to *prescribe* hearing aids. The procedure takes the least amount of time (5 to 10 minutes per ear), however, if the hearing aid settings are as close to optimal as possible at the start of the procedure. Consequently, it seems most efficient to precede the procedure with a prescriptive procedure. It does not seem sensible to spend time carefully measuring loudness growth curves for the initial prescription, only to depart from the prescription during the adaptive procedure. A combination of a prescriptive procedure based on thresholds followed by the adaptive adjustment described in this section appears to be a reasonable way to adjust multichannel compression hearing aids.

As a group, patients prefer hearing aids adjusted using the adaptive procedure described here to a loudness normalization procedure, whether that procedure is based on individual loudness scaling or on thresholds alone.[616] There has not as yet been any evaluation of the procedure relative to a threshold-based loudness equalization procedure, such as NAL-NL1 or DSL[i/o].

---

[d]   The different adjectives for tonal quality used at the two levels are based on the words that test subjects most commonly use at each level when the low- to high-frequency balance is inappropriate (Moore, Alcantara & Glasberg, 1998).

Rating scales and step sizes for compression fine-tuning

Table 11.1 Gain adjustment for speech at 85 or 60 dB SPL, in response to the loudness ratings shown.

Loudness rating	Gain change at all frequencies for 85 dB SPL	Gain change at all frequencies for 60 dB SPL
7. Uncomfortably loud	-4 dB	-4 dB
6. Very loud	-2 dB	-4 dB
5. Loud	0 dB	-4 dB
4. Comfortable	2 dB	-2 dB
3. Quiet	4 dB	0 dB
2. Very quiet	4 dB	2 dB
1. Can't hear	4 dB	4 dB

Table 11.2 Frequency response adjustments for low-level inputs, in response to tone quality ratings when speech is presented at 85 dB SPL.

Tone quality	LF gain change	HF gain change
7. Uncomfortably tinny	2 dB	-4 dB
6. Very tinny	2 dB	-2 dB
5. Tinny	0 dB	-2 dB
4. Neither tinny nor boomy	0 dB	0 dB
3. Boomy	-2 dB	0 dB
2. Very boomy	-2 dB	2 dB
1. Uncomfortably boomy	-4 dB	2 dB

Table 11.3 Frequency response adjustments for low-level inputs, in response to tone quality ratings when speech is presented at 60 dB SPL.

Tone quality	LF gain change	HF gain change
7. Uncomfortably shrill	2 dB	-4 dB
6. Very shrill	2 dB	-2 dB
5. Shrill	0 dB	-2 dB
4. Neither shrill nor muffled	0 dB	0 dB
3. Muffled	-2 dB	0 dB
2. Very muffled	-2 dB	2 dB
1. Uncomfortably muffled	-4 dB	2 dB

11.2.6 Fine-tuning at home with multi-memory hearing aids

There are two limitations to fine-tuning the hearing aid in the hearing clinic. One, of course, is time. The second is validity. It is possible to reliably choose, from a number of responses, the response that the patient prefers on some criterion while listening to some stimulus. The extent to which this indicates the best response in the real world depends on how good a job we have done of choosing the stimulus and asking the right question. Multi-memory hearing aids make it possible to move the fine-tuning session out of the clinic into the patient's own environment, thus overcoming the second problem and partially overcoming the first.

Suppose a patient has been fitted with a three-memory hearing aid, and the first memory has been programmed with amplification characteristics prescribed by some procedure. Because of the current state of knowledge, we may be unsure whether a lower or a higher compression threshold would be more beneficial. At the end of the appointment we program a lower compression threshold into one memory, and a higher compression threshold into another. The patient is instructed to try the alternatives, and return in a few weeks to tell us which memory (or memories) he or she prefers. At that stage, the unwanted program(s) are removed, and something more generally useful (like a low cut for listening in traffic noise) is put in their place.

This could be the end of the fine-tuning, or it *could* go on for as long as the patient and the clinician have the interest and the time. In some cases, the patients will indicate that they like one program in one environment and another program in other environments. In these cases, both programs can be retained, and the trial will have confirmed the useful-ness of multiple memories for that patient, and given some information on how they should be programmed.

The limitations of continuing the fine-tuning at home are evident: only a few different responses can be compared, and each new set of comparisons takes a new appointment to establish. This is really only practical if a further appointment is already needed for other purposes or if the clinician is easily able to schedule one or more additional short appointments.

As hearing aids continue their rapid advance into the digital age, it is likely that there will always be amplification characteristics that we are not sure how to prescribe, and which we are not able to adjust empirically in the clinic in a reliable or valid way. A role for fine-tuning at home is therefore likely to continue, perhaps combined with remote adjustment of the hearing aid over a telephone line or via the Internet (*tele-medicine*).

11.3 Concluding Comments: Fine-tuning in Perspective

Every clinician will have to fine-tune hearing aids in response to problems reported by patients. Doing this in the most efficient manner will minimize expense and frustration for clinician and patient. The two key skills are asking the questions that will help the clinician understand the problem as precisely as possible, and being able to identify which hearing aid controls should be altered to achieve the desired aim.

The extent to which systematic fine-tuning procedures should be used is a more difficult question. Some clinicians will consider that they do not have time to carry out the systematic procedures described in Section 11.2. It is possible that these procedures will not be used often in busy clinics, but five or ten minutes spent systematically fine-tuning a complex hearing aid may save considerable time in the long run. Fine-tuning may prevent several returns appointments from a client who is dissatisfied with the sound quality provided by expensive and very flexible hearing aids.

Until we know what proportion of patients will benefit from fine-tuning procedures after their hearing aid has been adjusted on the basis of a reliable prescription procedure, we will not know whether it is sensible to include a systematic fine-tuning component in every hearing aid fitting, or just to reserve this process for patients who report problems. Whether or not systematic procedures are used, hearing aids cannot be optimally adjusted unless time is allocated to listen to, and understand, patients' comments about amplified sound.

CHAPTER TWELVE

COUNSELING THE NEW HEARING AID WEARER

Synopsis

People with a hearing impairment benefit from counseling. This counseling may be aimed at giving patients information about their hearing loss, developing skills needed to operate and care for their new hearing aids, or changing patients' beliefs and behavior relating to communication. Providing appropriate counseling increases the likelihood that hearing aids will be fully used.

It is becoming harder to help patients understand the variety of hearing aid styles and performance feature variations that may be suitable for them. The benefits and cost implications of each (including ongoing service costs, warranty, and trial periods) have to be presented in a suitably simple manner. New hearing aid users experience a new world of amplified sound, and may benefit from guidance about how to gradually increase listening experience. The aim is to provide them with the best experiences first, and to avoid them becoming overwhelmed with all the sounds they have not heard for some time.

A major part of counseling the new hearing aid user has nothing to do with hearing aids! A wide range of hearing tactics and strategies can help the hearing-impaired person understand more in difficult listening situations. The first group of hearing strategies requires the listener to look carefully at the talker and the surroundings. The second group requires the listener to alter the communication pattern in some way. The final group requires the listener to manipulate the environment to remove or minimize sources of difficulty. The patients will benefit if their family and/or friends can participate in counseling on these topics. Communication training comprises training in the use of these hearing strategies, plus practice at listening to speech or to the basic sounds from which speech is built.

Patients should be advised about protecting their remaining hearing, and be made aware of where they can obtain support (from peer groups or other professionals) beyond that which the clinician is able to provide. Clinicians should be aware that different people learn in different ways, and that the same material should be taught in different ways to different patients.

Clinicians must be flexible regarding how and when they present information and carry out other procedures. It is, nonetheless, useful to have in mind a standard program from which variations can be made as required. This chapter concludes with a list of activities that can be performed at each of the assessment, fitting, and follow-up appointments. The use of group follow-up appointments, in addition to an individual appointment, is strongly recommended.

A dictionary definition of counseling is: "Giving advice, opinion or instruction to direct the judgment or conduct of another."

At one extreme counseling can be aimed at changing how patients feel about their hearing loss and its consequences, and this may not involve the clinician *telling* the patient anything. At the other extreme,

counseling may comprise giving detailed *instructions* to the client about how to operate a hearing aid. Counseling can be divided into several types, based on its aims or content:

- Making sure the patient **understands** the nature of his or her hearing loss, its consequences, and treatment options (including both devices and procedures).

- Helping the patient *acknowledge* that he or she has a hearing loss, and working through any consequential negative emotions that restrict enjoyment of life.

- Helping the patient *overcome obstacles* that discourage him or her from engaging in any form of rehabilitation.

- Instructing and encouraging the patient in the *use of hearing aids*, or other assistive listening devices.

- Helping the patient acquire additional *communication skills* in the form of hearing strategies. Some of these require some forms of personal adjustment by the patient, such as increased assertiveness.

- Providing *perceptual training* in understanding speech. This training can comprise analytic and synthetic speech training, in either auditory, visual, or auditory-visual presentation modes.

The second and third of these points were covered in Chapter 8. In this chapter, we will assume that the clinician is faced with a patient who desires to improve his or her ability to hear. What information should the clinician give, what should the clinician ask the patient to do, and when is the most appropriate time to do each activity?

The following sections will describe the type of information that patients need to acquire. The chapter will conclude by outlining how this information can be structured into a series of appointments. Or rather, how it might be structured for some patients. If a patient does not absorb critical information, or learn critical skills the first time they are taught, the process must be repeated or varied later. The actual content of appointments must thus remain flexible.

Another reason for flexibility is that some patients will want to know as much as possible about everything. Others will just prefer to be told what to do, accompanied by the minimum possible explanations being given. Those who want to know more than

you are saying will generally let you know by asking questions. Patients who understand less than you are saying may not tell you so. It is a good communication strategy on your part to intersperse your information-giving with questions that test whether the patient understands what you are saying.

Surprisingly, communication with patients is usually not complicated by their hearing loss! Face-to-face communication with a clearly spoken clinician on a known topic, in a quiet, low reverberation environment, does not usually pose much of a problem for people with a mild or even moderate loss. People with a severe or profound hearing loss usually already have hearing aids, and should of course, be encouraged to wear them during all counseling performed prior to re-fitting. When a person with severe or profound loss does not have hearing aids and needs temporary help, options include the talk-over facility of the audiometer, or a body aid fitted with supra-aural or circum-aural headphones.

12.1 Understanding Hearing Loss

Patients understandably want to know about their hearing capabilities and hearing loss. To give a balanced account of their hearing, the concepts of *capability* (i.e. the remaining hearing) and *loss* should both appear in your description. It will help patients to understand their loss, and be able to relate it to significant other people, if they are given a broad understanding of four different aspects of their hearing:

- The *location* of their loss (the middle ear, the inner ear, or the brain), with reference to a suitable wall chart.

- The *degree* of loss (mild, moderate, severe, profound), and *configuration* of loss (flat, sloping etc), with reference to their audiogram, and the prognosis as to how it is likely to change.

- The *disability* that is to be expected (inability to understand speech in noisy places, or quiet speech) even when they

Evidence for the benefit of counseling

Counseling affects the degree to which patients use their hearing aids. In one study using BTE hearing aids, a combination of pre- and post-fitting counseling increased usage from an average of 3.8 hours per day without significant counseling to 5.3 hours per day with counseling (Brooks, 1981). Another study showed that counseling two weeks after fitting increased usage from 3.9 hours per day to 6.3 hours per day (Ward, 1981). Patients are much more likely not to use their hearing aids at all if they do not receive adequate counseling. One major reason is that if patients are not sufficiently taught to insert an earmold or earshell, they will not be *able* to use their hearing aids (Brooks, 1985). Instruction in hearing aid use by volunteer helpers at the patient's home also increases aid use (Kapteyn, Wijkel & Hackenitz, 1997).

Counseling unrelated to the use of hearing aids is also helpful. Patients who are given information about hearing loss, hearing strategies, and communication skills, in addition to being fitted with hearing aids, report less hearing disability and/or handicap than those who are given only hearing aids (Abrams et al., 1992; Andersson et al., 1994; Smaldino & Smaldino, 1988). Similarly, perceptual training can enable people to better understand speech (Walden, Demorest & Hepler, 1981). The increase seems, however, to come more from an increased use of context than from an increased ability to identify individual phonemes (Rubinstein & Boothroyd, 1987; Gagne, Dinon & Parsons, 1991).

There are studies reaching apparently conflicting conclusions about the value of counseling *prior* to aid fitting, although there is possibly no real contradiction. Brooks (1979) showed that a combination of pre-fitting counseling and post-fitting counseling, both carried out at home, will significantly increase daily usage and competence in manipulating hearing aids, and will significantly decrease hearing handicap. In this study, subjects in the control group were seen only twice. In the first visit, the audiogram was measured, and an ear impression taken. The remaining visit was for fitting the hearing aid. Given this minimal contact with the patient, it is not surprising that additional pre- and post-fitting counseling was effective. The pre-fitting counseling appeared to be comprehensive (Brooks & Johnson, 1981). It covered assessment of communication difficulties, modification of attitude and expectations, discussion aimed at reversing many patients' tendencies to withdraw from social activities, provision of information about hearing loss and hearing strategies, and assessment of the need for post-fitting counseling.

By contrast, Norman, George & McCarthy (1994) found that pre-fitting counseling, with these same objectives, does not alone significantly increase satisfaction, usage, or benefit from the hearing aid. What is not clear is whether members of the control group were as bereft of any other counseling as were those in the other control group in the earlier study. Most of the things that should be discussed can probably be done just as effectively before or after fitting. Issues related to attitude, motivation, and the choice of hearing aid must, however, be resolved prior to fitting.

consider that they can easily hear that speech is present. This can be made specific by referring to the situations in which they consider they have trouble hearing, to errors that they have actually made on speech discrimination tests, or to speech sounds for which they are likely to have particular difficulty (see Figure 8.1). Information about their hearing loss configuration and the influence that this has on speech discrimination may be instrumental in people accepting that indeed they do have a hearing loss.

- The ***handicap*** that often results (withdrawal from activities, common emotional reactions, effects on other family members).

All of this has to be strongly tempered by the apparent interest and understanding that the patient is showing. Some patients will be stressed by having their hearing tested and their loss confirmed by a clinician. For this and other reasons, some patients will not absorb much information; giving them too much information will be unproductive and may increase any stress they are undergoing. Close monitoring of the patient's reactions, verbal and non-verbal, is essential.

12.2 Acquiring a Hearing Aid

Discussion about the patient's hearing loss and its consequences leads naturally to a discussion about treatment options, which in most cases will include acquiring one or two hearing aids. After discussing whether or not the patient is likely to benefit from hearing aids (see Chapter 8), and assuming the patient wishes to acquire hearing aids, there are several issues to be discussed.

Hearing aid style

It seems wisest to outline the advantages of each style (See Section 10.1) that apply to that patient before asking the patient which style is preferred. Otherwise, the clinician may have to present information in the context of trying to change the patient's

decision, rather than informing the patient to help him or her arrive at a decision. (Of course, it is possible that the patient will have already decided on a style before the appointment commenced.) The patient should be allowed to physically handle each style. The patient should also be shown pictures of them when worn, or alternatively be shown what they look like when modeled in, or behind, the ear of the clinician.

Hearing aid technology and cost

The clinician has to be highly aware of the advantages and disadvantages of different technologies, and this requires knowledge of complex technology plus the ability to assess the value of each performance feature to each patient. Even more difficult is the task of presenting this to the patient in a way the patient can understand. The patient must have this knowledge, however, to be able to make an informed decision about how sophisticated (and expensive) the hearing aids should be. Table 12.1 gives an extremely simplified list of advantages for each of several technology and pricing levels.[a] The reader should

---

Handling preferences for an inappropriate style

What should you do when the patient wants a hearing aid style that you think is unlikely to be effective (for reasons of inadequate gain, power, or ease of manipulation)? Opinions vary, but here is one opinion:

- If you are reasonably sure that the hearing aid will be ineffective, politely tell the patient that you could not in good conscience fit him or her with a hearing aid that in your judgment will not be suitable, even if some other providers of hearing aids may be willing to do so.

- If you *think* that the hearing aid style is unsuitable, but have some doubt about your conclusion, and the patient is highly motivated to have that style, be specific about the reasons for your doubts. If the patient persists in his or her choice, fit hearing aids of the type the patient prefers. It may be worth gaining the patient's written acknowledgment that the type of hearing aids prescribed are not the ones that you most highly recommend (Sweetow, 1999b).

The rationale behind the first suggestion is that your principled refusal to sell an ineffective hearing aid may cause the patient to change his or her preference. Even if it does not: you have saved the patient money, you have avoided the time wasted on fitting and returning an aid for credit, and you have avoided having an ex-patient walking around telling friends that the hearing aids you supplied were no good. The rationale for acceding to the patient's preference if you have some doubt is that motivation is a very powerful contributor to success with hearing aids.

Table 12.1 Simplified advantages of different technology choices. An additional advantage, *improved intelligibility in background noise,* can be added to the final column for each technology category for which directional microphones are available.

Name	Technology features (typical)	Advantages additional to the preceding technology
Basic analog	Linear / peak-clipping, non-programmable	The baseline, but at least it amplifies sound, even if it distorts it whenever things get loud.
Medium analog	Linear / compression limiting, non-programmable	Cleaner sound because there is less distortion
Premium analog	WDRC (usually single channel), non-programmable	Partially automatic, so less need to manipulate volume control to maintain intelligibility and comfort.
Digitally-programmable analog, or basic digital	Multichannel WDRC, flexible tone controls, feedback management	More accurate match to hearing means better automatic operation, better balance of low-tone, mid-tone and high-tone sounds, and more comfort. Slightly more amplification without feedback.
Advanced digital	Feedback suppression, very flexible tone controls, multichannel noise reduction, adaptive dual-microphone noise reduction	Even more amplification without feedback. Hearing aid more intelligently decreases amplification at specific times and frequencies, so noise is less apparent and disturbing, and overall level is more comfortable.

interpret this in the light of the more detailed discussion in Sections 10.1 and 10.2. Dual microphone technology, though valuable, is not shown in the table because it is available in many of the technology categories.

Depending on the features available in hearing aids at any time, and on the models and brands dispensed in any clinic, it would be possible and desirable to customize and simplify Table 12.1 to suit the clinic. This would comprise the first and third columns (modified as necessary) plus a new column showing the name and price of particular hearing aids in each category. As hearing aids progress it will probably become necessary to subdivide the "Advanced digital" category.

The features listed in the middle column of Table 12.1 are primarily for the benefit of the clinician and would probably be mentioned only to more interested patients. Information about style and technology can be combined in the form of a matrix with the different styles as rows and the different technologies as columns.[189] It is probably simpler, however, to separately consider style and technology wherever possible.

Most patients will be balancing cost against the advantages of the more complex technologies. To help them arrive at a decision you should ascertain whether any concern about cost is driven by a desire to limit the total cost, or by a desire to get the best value for money, irrespective of cost.[63] If the clinician knows of any forms of financial assistance that might be available to the patient, this is an appropriate time to provide this knowledge.

It may help patients place the cost in perspective if they are told the likely life of

a   Although in principle digital is not better than analog, complex processing schemes are more feasible in digital instruments, so digital is becoming synonymous with higher performance, as in Table 12.1.

the hearing aids (perhaps three to six years). It has even been suggested that the total cost of the hearing aids, including batteries and average maintenance costs, be expressed as the average cost per day over the life of the hearing aids.[873]

Responsibilities and rights

Patients have a right to know how much the hearing aid(s) and associated service will cost, what warranty period covers the hearing aids, what service plans are available (and their costs) and what ongoing costs they will have for batteries. They also should be told when payment is due, the period during which they can return their hearing aids, and the extent of refund available during this period.

Government legislation may guarantee patients a right to effective communication in public places. The details vary from country to country, but clinicians should provide patients with written material covering any rights they have in this regard, and details on how they should go about making the most of these rights (e.g. asking at a theatre ticket office for an assistive listening device).

12.3 Using Hearing Aids

Teaching patients how to insert a hearing aid, switch the aid on and off, operate the volume control, manipulate any other controls present, remove a hearing aid, and change the battery are essential parts of counseling. Unless these skills are mastered (by the aid wearer or by a helper if necessary) hearing aid use is not possible. Techniques for teaching these skills vary with the type of the hearing aid. The techniques are similar to those used for re-teaching people who have not mastered these skills by the first follow-up appointment. Some suggestions have already been covered in Section 11.1.1.

Patients will also need to know approximately how long batteries will last. Some patients will appreciate having their own battery tester. If patients are highly reliant on their hearing aids, they will need to carry spare batteries, especially when the battery life is close to an end. A simple way for experienced hearing aid wearers to keep track of when this is likely to occur is to place the battery tag on a calendar on the day that new batteries are used.[946]

The safety concerns related to battery ingestion should also be covered (see Section 15.10).

12.4 Adjusting to New Experiences with Sound and Hearing Aids

When people put on their hearing aids they receive an avalanche of sounds, usually in the high-frequency region, that they are not used to hearing. Many patients will make the transition to hearing aid use more easily if they build up their listening experience gradually,[b] commencing with quiet situations and wearing their hearing aids for only a short time each day.

There are several reasons why a gradual build-up can be useful. It is encouraging for patients to have the most positive experiences first. They can then build confidence in their hearing aids while they are becoming accustomed to hearing more sound and to hearing sound with a new tonal quality. Patients will not instinctively know the situations in which hearing aids are most effective, and so should be guided by the clinician. The following pages show the *Situations To Experience and Practice (STEP)* form that clinicians can hand to patients to guide them through the first weeks of hearing aid use.[c]

---

[b]   The need for gradual exposure is greatest for linear/peak-clipping hearing aids, because they often produce loud distorted sound. With modern hearing aids incorporating both WDRC and compression limiting, sounds need never be uncomfortable or distorted, and should only occasionally be very loud. The need for a graduated exposure may be less marked, but the benefit provided by hearing aids still varies across listening situations.

[c]   The STEP form may be copied and used. An enlarged version will be useful for patients with poor eyesight.

One step at a time

Situations To Experience and Practice

Welcome to some new experiences with sound. You will get the most out of your new hearing aids if you practice using them in certain situations around the home before you progress to situations that are more difficult. Also, do not wear your hearing aids for more than two hours per day for the first week unless you are finding them really comfortable in all respects. Make sure you use them for at least half an hour each day, however.

Try to wear your hearing aids in the following situations in roughly the order shown. Progress through the list as quickly or slowly as you are comfortable with. After you have tried your hearing aids in each situation, write down how helpful they were, and any problems that you encountered. Over the next few weeks, wear your hearing aids while you are:

1. Listening to one other person at home while you can see his or her face.

   Comment: _____

   _____

2. Listening to a TV or radio at home.

   Comment: _____

   _____

3. Walking around inside your home, trying to recognize any sounds you can hear.

   Comment: _____

   _____

4. Listening to one other person at home while you are not looking at their face.

   Comment: _____

   _____

5. Listening to music.

   Comment: _____

   _____

STEP (continued)

6. Listening to your own voice while you read aloud from a newspaper or book.

   Comment:

   _____

   _____

7. Conversing with two or three people in a quiet place.

   Comment: _____

   _____

8. Walking around outside, trying to recognize any sounds you can hear.

   Comment: _____

   _____

9. Shopping or talking to another person in a noisy place.

   Comment: _____

   _____

10. Conversing with two or three people in a noisy place.

    Comment: _____

    _____

11. Conversing in a large gathering or at a noisy restaurant.

    Comment: _____

    _____

12. Special situation: ....

    Comment: _____

    _____

13. Special situation: ....

    Comment: _____

    _____

Source: Dillon - Hearing Aids

Using the STEP form

- Explain to your patient the general principle of gradually stepping up daily listening experience, both in regards to hours per day and the noisiness of the situations encountered.
- Explain that the patient will have to re-learn how to recognize all the sounds that he or she will be hearing.
- Emphasize that like any other learning, this task will require some commitment and application by the patient.
- Tell patients that you are interested in their reaction to each situation, and that you would like them to record how helpful the hearing aid was, and any problems they experienced.
- Make sure that any situations in which the patient particularly needs to hear better are somewhere on the list. These will be evident if you have already carried out the initial phase of the COSI evaluation (Section 8.1.4). Specific situations either can be written in as examples of the standard situations, or can be specifically recorded in the final three blank spaces. In the case of the latter, you will need to indicate which of the standard situations should first be attempted.

The second reason for a gradual build-up of listening experience is that a patient's attitude to hearing aid use may be positively affected if he or she commits to following a specified listening program. It is a well-accepted psychological principal that behavior can affect beliefs.[259, 280] In particular, if patients realize that success with a hearing aid is conditional on them using it in a certain way, they are likely to do so. In turn, the act of using their hearing aids may make them rationalize that the hearing aids are worth-while. This belief then encourages further use. This is not a trick to convince patients to accept a worthless piece of apparatus; it is a technique to help patients overcome what can be a difficult time of adjustment so that they get the most from their hearing aids.

The third reason for a gradual adjustment is that it reinforces to the patient that listening situations *are* different. If hearing aids are found to be of no use in one situation, the patient may be less likely to generalize this conclusion to all situations: *These hearing aids are no use at all.*

There is a fourth reason that has nothing to do with sound. Earmolds and shells can cause discomfort and irritation when they are first worn, even if they fit well (just like new shoes). A gradual increase in daily usage allows the ear to become accustomed to them without pronounced irritation developing. This may be particularly important with any hearing aids that extend into the bony part of the canal.

The benefits of a step-by-step exposure can best be captured if a patient can discuss his or her experiences with the clinician. The clinician may use this information to demonstrate the need for hearing strategies (Section 12.6) or may adjust the hearing aids to provide increased benefits or decreased disadvantages. The STEP form includes space for patients to record their experiences with sound in each situation. These written comments provide an easy discussion prompter for patients who otherwise choose not to talk much about what they have experienced.[271]

The *Active Fitting* program available in Sweden comprises a combination of gradual exposure to sound with several opportunities for patients to discuss their experiences with the clinician. It consists of five appointments interspersed with three periods of home use during which the patient completes a diary called *Try Your Hearing Aid*, and has been shown to increase hearing aid use and satisfaction with hearing aids.[271] The authors comment that the attitude of the clinician is critical: *patients will not regard the listening program as important unless the clinician appears to believe it is important.*

As always, expectations are important. Before new hearing aid wearers start wearing hearing aids, they need to know that they will be hearing background sounds that they have not heard for some years. People with normal hearing hear these sounds, or rather, they *can* hear these sounds, but learn to ignore them when they carry no meaning. The sound of a fan is meaningless except when we believe that we have turned off all the appliances in the house because we are leaving on holidays. Then the sound has great meaning. The clinician should explain to patients that it might take them some time to become so accustomed to hearing these background sounds that they can unconsciously recognize them and ignore them. This advice is particularly important for patients who will be wearing WDRC hearing aids with a low compression threshold, and consequently, a lot of gain for low-level sounds.

Of course, telling patients that they will take time to get used to these sounds is not the same as guaranteeing that they *will* get used to them. When a patient complains about such sounds at a follow-up appointment, the clinician will have to choose between re- instructing about the normality of hearing these sounds, and adjusting the hearing aid so that the patient hears less of them (see Section 11.1.7).

Whether or not patients are gradually exposed to sound, and whether or not they are using WDRC hearing aids, they should be advised that it might take them some months to become used to the sounds provided by their hearing aids, and to receive maximum benefit from them. It is possible that new neural path- ways have to form to allow this to happen, and this process has been referred to as *brain rewiring* and as *acclimatization*.[307] If patients are advised in advance that such a process can occur, they may be less discour- aged by any initial experiences where their hearing aids are not helpful. Section 13.5 con- tains further information about acclimatization.

12.5 Care of Hearing Aids

Patients must be told how to care for their hearing aids. The accompanying panel shows a list of things to do and things to avoid. Although it contains some seemingly obvious statements, they will not be obvious to all

Treating hearing aids kindly	
Don't	**Do**
X Don't wash them.	✓ Do wipe them regularly with a tissue and occasionally with a slightly damp sponge.
X Don't wear them in the shower, the bath, or the swimming pool, but if this happens by accident, don't dry the hearing aids in an oven or a microwave.	✓ Do disconnect a BTE mold from the aid occasionally, and wash the mold in warm soapy water. The tubing may take a day or so to dry out unless you have a hand-pumped air blower to dry it.
X Don't insert anything more than 3 mm up the hole in the end of the aid.	✓ Do clean wax out of the tip, whenever it is present, with a brush, a loop, a pick, or by operating or changing an in-built wax guard.
X Don't spray them with hair spray.	✓ Do store them overnight in their box or some other container.
X Don't leave them in the car in the sun.	✓ Do remove the battery if you are going to store the hearing aid for more than one day.

patients and should therefore be stated. The list can be copied and provided to patients. For individual patients, it may be necessary to vary the 3-mm dimension mentioned in the third point. The appropriate distance can be ascertained by looking at the hearing aid with a bright light behind it.

Patients who frequently need to return their custom hearing aids for maintenance because of moisture build-up or cerumen build-up may benefit from storing their hearing aids overnight in a de-humidifying environment. Storage devices are available that contain various combinations of heat, airflow, desiccant, deodorant, and germicidal electromagnetic radiation. The combined effects of heat and low humidity dry out any cerumen present, which can then more easily be removed with the usual cleaning methods. The battery should be removed prior to placing the hearing aid in the de-humidifier (to avoid drying the chemicals in the battery) and the battery compartment should be left open.

12.6 Hearing Strategies

Hearing strategies (also known as hearing tactics) are methods that people can use to increase their understanding of speech.[926, 927] Patients can use hearing strategies separately from, or in conjunction with, hearing aids or assistive devices. Even people with normal hearing can use hearing strategies in difficult situations. Because hearing-impaired people have decreased ability to discriminate between sounds, they will certainly need to use hearing strategies if they are to function effectively in as many environments as possible.

All hearing-impaired persons should therefore be taught hearing strategies, and should receive some take-home material to remind them of the important points. Patients are likely to already know a few strategies, but there will be many more strategies of which they will not be aware.[281] People who have

received even a brief instruction in hearing strategies report less disability and handicap than those who have not.[939]

Hearing strategies can be grouped into three categories: those that involve *observation*, those that involve *manipulating social interactions*, and those that involve *manipulating the physical environment*.[281] It is as well that multiple strategies are available, because in any given situation, some of the strategies will not be feasible for physical or social reasons.

12.6.1 Observing the talker and surroundings

Lip-reading

Considerable information can be gained from watching people's lips.[65] Most people, including those with normal hearing, probably watch lips naturally, or even unconsciously, in adverse listening situations. Some people, however, may not, and many may not make as much use of *lip-reading* as they could do if they were made aware of its potential. It is therefore important to instruct patients about its value as part of any rehabilitation program. If time permits, the clinician can demonstrate its considerable value. A videotape of a "talking head" such as a newsreader can be played and the patient asked to follow by hearing alone, and then by hearing combined with vision. The difficulty of the task can be varied by adjusting the volume control on the TV monitor, such that the hearing-alone condition is not too easy.

To lip-read, the patient *has* to be able to see the talker's lips. This may involve moving, or asking the talker to remove his or hands from in front of the face. If a patient considers that this would seem rude, some coaching will be necessary. The positive statement *I can understand you much better when I can see your lips clearly* may appear friendlier to both the patient and the talker than *would you move your hands from in front of your face please*,

---

Theoretical background: Why lip-reading is so valuable

The type of information obtained from lip-reading is especially useful to hearing-impaired people. The information most visible is the place of articulation, or constriction, of consonants (lips, teeth against lips, teeth, tongue against teeth, and several places further back inside the mouth). Place cues to speech are, however, the hardest cues for hearing-impaired people to perceive correctly via hearing alone. Lip-reading thus greatly complements audition.

For example, hearing may tell the person that the sound is a /p/, /t/, or /k/ (these are easily confused). Vision may tell the person that the sound is a /p/, /b/, or /m/, as these sounds look identical. The only possible conclusion when hearing and vision are combined is that the sound is a /p/. For either modality alone, there was only a 1 in 3 chance of correct perception (in the absence of contextual cues), but when the patient combines the two forms of perception the correct answer is assured. In this example, no error occurs, but in general, errors will be greatly decreased compared to hearing alone, even if some errors remain.

---

or *would you look at me when you talk please*. These more direct alternatives might sometimes be necessary, however.

Patients who normally place value on eye contact during conversation may be reassured to know that the person talking will not notice whether the listener is watching the talker's eyes or lips.

Non-verbal signals

It is not only a talker's lips that convey information. Facial gestures (e.g. smiling, frowning, surprise, quizzical looks, disgust) all convey the essence of the message that the talker is saying. If the patient understands the essential message, the words can more easily be filled in, or in some cases ignored. Bodily gestures or positions often also reinforce the message. The clinician should advise the patient about the richness of information available from the face and body of the talker. The combination of lip-reading, face-reading, and body-reading is often referred to as *speech-reading*. All the *reading* terms are useful. It is important to point out to patients the various individual sources of information, as well as reinforcing that all of the information combined will contribute greatly to understanding speech.

Filling in gaps

Missing words can often be guessed based on the topic, the talker, facial expressions, or the physical surroundings. Some people are reluctant to guess, so it is appropriate to let the patient know that it is OK to miss words and to guess at meaning based on all the evidence available. When a patient becomes too uncertain as to the accuracy of his or her guesses, the patient can check with the talker about the interpretations that he or she is making by using the techniques described below. Some patients will need to be encouraged to guess more often; others will need to be encouraged to check more often.

12.6.2 Manipulating social interactions

All of the following strategies require hearing-impaired people to modify the way they interact with others. We learn the normal rules of communication from an early age. To the extent that hearing strategies require some variation from these rules, patients require practice and reassurance if they are going to be able to use them comfortably and naturally.

One hearing strategy used (consciously or unconsciously) by some hearing-impaired people is to talk all the time so that they rarely have to listen. If the clinician suspects that a particular patient has adopted this strategy, some tactful reminders about the adverse social consequences of this strategy, and the availability of alternative strategies that induce a more positive reaction from communication partners, would be appropriate.

Clear speaking

Some people are easy to understand, and anyone can more easily be understood when they talk clearly.[703] Consequently, clear speech is more resistant to noise and reverberation than is normal speech.[697] Clear speech differs from conversational speech in several ways. Speaking rate is lower, because speech sounds become longer when they are fully enunciated, and because people speaking clearly insert or lengthen the pauses between words. In clear speech, vowels are fully formed, and stop bursts in word-final consonants are released. The relative intensity of stop consonants is greater.[704] Fortunately, people do not need a course in phonetics to become clear speakers. They just have to be asked to speak clearly, as if communicating in a difficult environment, and to concentrate on producing each speech sound distinctly.

To achieve clear speech amongst family members the clinician can explain the principles to the patient, so that the client can ask communication partners, in a non-threatening way, to speak more clearly. The patient can advise communication partners of his or her need for extra-clear speech, to avoid suggesting to the communication partners that their speech is sub-standard in some way.

There is a range of speaking styles from very indistinct to very clear, and the clearest styles are presumably more likely to be elicited if the clinician directly instructs family members and provides them with feedback about their speaking technique. Schum (1997) says that people take 10 to 15 minutes

of practice to become proficient and that once learned, the effect is maintained for weeks or months without further reinforcement. The effectiveness of clear speech can not be doubted; the only uncertainty is the extent to which family members will continue to speak this way in normal life.

Where there is background noise, increased speech intensity will also improve intelligibility, because it improves SNR. Most guides on hearing strategies advise that shouting is counter-productive, but in noisy circumstances, it may be the only way to achieve adequate intelligibility, just as it is sometimes necessary for normal-hearing people to shout to each other. There is no point in a talker shouting when the SNR is good – if the listener needs more intensity, the hearing aid's volume control (if present) can be increased. Shouting may be less of a problem for modern hearing aids with WDRC and/or compression limiting than it was for linear/peak-clipping hearing aids, but should only be used as a last resort.

Gaining the listener's attention

Because of the importance of speech-reading, a hearing-impaired person can hear best if he or she has the opportunity to speech-read right from the start of an utterance. This is possible only if the listener is looking at the talker right from the first word. Regular conversation partners can be asked (and trained) to gain the attention of the listener before talking. In adverse listening conditions this can be done by a touch, but in most circumstances, it can be achieved just by saying the listener's name, then pausing, then talking. In structured groups, such as at a committee meeting, patients may find it hard to quickly identify who is talking, especially if their localization ability is impaired. The assistance of the chair can be sought to ensure that only one person talks at once, and that people talk only after the chair nominates them. The hearing-impaired person will then find it easier to follow people, aurally and visually, right from the start of their declarations (and everyone else may appreciate the orderly meeting that will result).

Knowing the topic

Knowledge of the topic makes it much easier for a person to correctly guess the words that are not heard or only partially heard. When a hearing-impaired person commences a conversation with others, particularly when joining into an existing conversation, his or her first task should be to find out the topic. Shy or unassuming patients will need considerable encouragement if they are to break into the conversations of others to ask what the topic is. An easier alternative is to take one friend aside and have that person tell them what the topic is. It may seem obvious, but patients should be told the importance of knowing the topic, and reminded that sometimes the only way they will gain this knowledge is to explicitly ask someone.

Repair strategies

When a listener has missed a key word or phrase, the listener can gain the missing information in a way that involves the minimum disruption to the ongoing conversation. The clinician should advise the patient about repair strategies such as:

- Repeating back the words preceding the words not heard, with a questioning intonation, accompanied by a questioning facial expression.

- Asking a specific question that indicates what was heard and what was not, e.g. *What sort of mood did you say he was in?*

- Repeating back or re-phrasing what the listener thought he or she heard to confirm its correctness.

- Asking the talker to say the last sentence or two in a different way.

- When all else fails, spelling out a key word.

All of these techniques reassure the talker that he or she is mostly being understood, and minimize the time needed to gather the missing information.

> **Hearing strategies in summary**
>
> - Watch the talker – lips, face, body
> - Find out the topic
> - Ask the talker to speak clearly
> - Ask the talker to gain your attention
> - Give frequent feedback
> - Ask specific questions
> - Guess meaning and repeat to confirm
> - Get close to talker
> - Get rid of noise
> - Discuss clear speech with significant others

Giving feedback

If the patient is constantly giving feedback to the talker (especially in one-to-one conversations), the talker will quickly learn to talk in a way that best gets a message through without needing further intervention by the listener. Feedback comprises smiles, nods, mmm's, yes's, aha's, frowns, and puzzled looks. Talkers will adapt by varying their talking speed, clarity, voice level, and complexity of expression. People *like* to be understood.

Disclosing the hearing loss

Finally, if the patient is willing to disclose that he or she has a hearing loss, talkers will make some adjustment, as described in the previous paragraph.

12.6.3 Manipulating the environment

Lighting

Because observing the talker is essential for good intelligibility, good lighting is crucial in situations with adverse acoustics. The patient should be advised that it will sometimes be necessary to move or ask the talker to move. Situations that commonly cause problems are when the talker sits with his or her back to a window or lamp. The listener has the double disadvantage of looking into a bright light while trying to see the talker's face and lips which are dimly lit.

Positioning

The key to easy listening is position, position, and position! There are several reasons for this. Close to the talker, signal levels are higher so the SNR is better. Similarly, the ratio of signal to reverberation is better. Both of these ratios are crucial to intelligibility,[542] and both of these ratios deteriorate greatly when the talker and listener are in different rooms.

It is difficult for patients and their communication partners to overcome long-held habits of trying to communicate from another room. The extreme difficulties that such communication creates, even for normal-hearing people, should therefore be strongly pointed out to patients. Getting close to the talker applies whether the talker and listener are the only two people in a room, or whether there are a hundred other people. (It is tricky if they all want to be close to the talker.)

Another aspect of position is relevant to people who have a better side and a poorer side for listening.[d] The head is an effective obstacle for sound waves above about 1.5 kHz. This means that at the better ear, high-frequency sounds arriving from the same side are boosted, but high-frequency sounds arriving from the other side are attenuated (see Section 14.2.1). Consequently, the SNR at high frequencies is much better on the side of the head closer to the talker.

For maximum intelligibility, patients should therefore orient themselves so that the talker is on the good side. If there is a dominant noise source, patients will obtain the highest intelligibility if they point their worse ear towards the noise. That is, the patient should be between the talker and the noise, at enough of an angle to benefit from these head baffle effects, but not so much that speech-reading is impossible.

Minimizing noise

Noise has such a disturbing effect that any reduction in noise level will enable easier understanding. Solutions include:

- Turning the TV or radio off or down,
- Closing a door,
- Moving to a quieter place to talk.

Minimizing reverberation

In the home situation, adding soft furnishings (thick curtains, well-padded lounge chairs, thick pile carpet) to a room will decrease reverberation and hence increase intelligibility. In other situations, patients should choose places with such furnishings for conversations whenever possible. The more absorbent the furnishings, and the bigger the room, the further apart the listener and talker can be and still avoid the adverse effects of reverberation.[e]

Adjusting the source

When the source is an electronic appliance (a TV, a radio, a CD, a public address system) adjusting the tone control of the device may improve intelligibility and naturalness. If the listener is optimally aided, this may not help, but if the listener is not using hearing aids, or if the hearing aids are deficient in high-frequency gain, a treble boost in the electronic appliance should help intelligibility. For good music perception when listening through hearing aids, a bass boost (and possibly a treble boost) may be helpful. There is very little research on this point from which to take guidance.

While all these modifications to the environment (lighting, position, noise, reverberation, and tonal quality) are easy to list, some may be difficult to achieve. Even when there is no physical constraint, the patient may feel that modifying the environment will result in some inconvenience to communication partners. A thorough discussion of these

---

d   Better and poorer sides arise when people with symmetrical hearing loss wear only one hearing aid, or when people have asymmetrical speech identification ability.

e   Close to the talker, the direct sound from the talker over-rides the fuzzy reverberant sounds, even if there is a lot of reverberant sound spread throughout the room.

strategies will elicit how the patient regards this issue, and will enable patients to reflect on how their right to communicate can be balanced against the rights of others. As a generality, the benefit to the patient of a modification far outweighs the disadvantage (if any exists) to communication partners.

12.6.4 Teaching hearing strategies

Hearing strategies can be taught in an abstract manner (rather like the preceding three sections) or can be taught to each patient in an individual, problem-solving way.[494, 940] A method that is bound to capture the attention of patients is to identify a few problem situations that are important to the patient and devise a list of hearing strategies that are appropriate to each situation. For instance, a couple who have trouble hearing each other when they are watching the TV might decide that the following strategies are feasible: They will sit closer together, rearrange the lighting so that they can see each other's face, add some more soft furnishings to the room, and if necessary, acquire hearing aids with directional microphones. If all else fails they will buy a TV with a remote control and turn the sound down before speaking. The situations listed on the patient's COSI form (see Sections 8.1.4 and 13.3) can provide a ready-made starting point.

Teaching hearing strategies using individual problems commences with the patient describing a situation to the clinician in as much detail as possible. The clinician then either suggests strategies, or if time permits, asks leading questions that help the patient work out strategies for him or her self. The latter approach is more likely to result in the patient understanding, retaining, and being committed to the solution.

Hearing strategies are an ideal topic for group discussions (Section 12.13.4) because they enable a good venue for discussion of the social and relationship implications of the strategies. Where hearing strategies involve gaining the cooperation of others, the group provides the opportunity for patients to practice asking for this cooperation.

12.7 Involving Families and Friends.

Although the discussion so far has concentrated on working with patients, both patients and their families can benefit if the families also participate in counseling. There are advantages to having a significant other person (SOP), such as a spouse, parent, child, or friend, participate in all stages of counseling.

Candidacy. If, at the first appointment, the patient understates the difficulties he or she has with hearing, the SOP can add an extra perspective, to the benefit of both clinician and patient. The patient's understatement may be matched by the SOP's exaggeration.

Understanding the consequences of hearing loss. The SOP may be dismissive of the patient's difficulties (*He can hear when he wants to*). If so, the patient will appreciate the clinician explaining and demonstrating to the SOP how a high-frequency loss can make understanding difficult even though the presence of speech may be easily detected. A hearing loss simulation on tape or CD will be helpful to show the difficulties to a caring but non-understanding SOP.[615] It is emotionally beneficial for patients to know that those close to them understand the difficulties they are going through, even with their hearing aids. Patients commonly report (if asked) that *no one really understands*.[511] Furthermore, the patient is not the only one in the family suffering from the problems caused by his or her hearing loss. The SOP therefore also has needs and may benefit from being involved in the rehabilitation process.[381]

Hearing strategies. Most of the hearing strategies covered in Section 12.6 require the cooperation of another person. If the other person has heard first-hand from the clinician what is required, the patient may find it much easier to gain appropriate cooperation, and new behavior patterns are more likely to be maintained.[320]

Learning to use hearing aids. The SOP will witness the clinician instructing the patient to insert, remove, and operate the hearing aid. Unlike the patient, the SOP can *see* the patient's ears, and can considerably assist the patient to learn these skills when they return home. For patients with very poor memory or dexterity, the clinician may elect to teach the SOP, rather than the patient, how to use the hearing aids.

Follow-up questioning. The presence of a SOP can keep the patient honest when he or she is asked about how much the hearing aids have been used and whether there have been any difficulties.

Overall encouragement. A SOP can provide many forms of encouragement as the patient learns to use his or her hearing aids. A clinician will always tell a patient that the hearing aids can be adjusted if the sound quality initially provided is not acceptable. A SOP who knows this can encourage the patient to return for adjustment rather than use inadequate sound quality as an excuse to give up.

After the appointment is over, the SOP can remind the patient about the things that the clinician said. It is very difficult for people to absorb a lot of information when they are in a stressful situation, which hearing-test appointments (and even follow-up appointments) can be.

Although there are many advantages to having a SOP present at all stages of counseling, some patients will prefer to be seen on their own and this choice is theirs to make. Preliminary contact with the patient (telephone or mail) should simply make it clear that that the patient is encouraged to bring along a family member or friend to each appointment.

12.8 Communication Training

People, especially those with a severe or profound hearing loss, may have gradually restricted their activities and communication experiences over several years because of the difficulties imposed by their hearing loss. Many people need to acquire new skills and gain confidence if they are to fully rejoin society. This is the role of ***communication training***. Communication training is also advantageous for people adjusting to a sensory device that processes speech differently than they are used to. This includes cochlear implants and tactile aids, but may also include conventional hearing

---

Confidence building: success breeds success

Probably the major goal of communication training is to build confidence in those being trained. The key to achieving this is to ensure that the hearing-impaired people being trained achieve success in any tasks they are set. The aim is to show people what they *can* do, not reinforce what they *can't* do. Training should commence with tasks that the patient can definitely do, and rapidly increase in difficulty until the tasks are presenting a significant challenge, but are still able to be completed. There are many ways in which the material can be altered to control its difficulties (Garstecki, 1982):

- Syntactic and semantic context, and hence easiness will decrease as the material progresses from familiar stories, through unfamiliar stories, paragraphs, sentences, phrases, words, to individual syllables.
- Background noise can be absent, infrequent environmental sounds, white noise, multi-talker, or a single competing talker. The signal-to-noise ratio can also be varied.
- Situational context can be withheld or described, and the talker's face can be revealed or concealed.

aids. Communication training can be categorized into two general types.

Analytic speech perception training is conducted by presenting speech to the patient, requiring the patient to identify the sounds, or to indicate whether two sounds are the same or different, and then providing feedback as to the correct answer. Analytic training concentrates on developing the patient's ability to differentiate between syllable patterns and between phonemes in syllables or words. The aim is to help patients learn to use speech cues that should be audible to them, but which for some reason they are not using. A possible reason for lack of use is that the patient has only recently begun wearing amplification, and has lost the ability to use the newly audible cues. For analytic speech training, speech material is usually presented one syllable or word at a time, so that the patient can focus on the characteristics of the sound being practiced. The material can however, be presented in whole sentences. Analytic speech perception training is also called *perceptual speech training*, and it is routinely used to help children develop speech perception and production skills.

Synthetic communication training is conducted by presenting speech to patients in a natural manner, such as by conversing with them, or by having them listen to a story. In synthetic training, the emphasis is on the patient understanding the message, even if the patient does not correctly perceive every sound. The origin of *synthetic* in the name is that the listener has to synthesize (i.e. combine) any available pieces of information to correctly interpret the message. As the major part of the training, patients are taught to use any or all of the hearing strategies discussed in Section 12.6. In addition, patients are given practice at understanding speech in a context where they are given feedback about what they perceive and misperceive. Synthetic communication training is also called *active listening training*.[493]

This phrase implies that the listener frequently lets the talker know that the listener has understood the message (also called *reflective listening*), but implies the use of other hearing strategies as well.

It should be apparent that there is considerable overlap between synthetic communication training and hearing strategies. There is also some overlap between synthetic and analytic training, as for example when sentence length material is used for training. Analytic and synthetic training can both be done using hearing alone or can be supplemented with visual cues. If visual cues are excluded, however, so too are many of hearing strategies that could otherwise be taught as part of the synthetic communication training.

Analytic and synthetic training differ in their aims. Analytic training is aimed at increasing patients' correct perception of the individual sounds of speech. Evidence as to whether this aim is achieved is contradictory.[495, 930] Synthetic training, by contrast, aims to alter patients' behavior when communicating and to increase their confidence in engaging in communication. It is unequivocally successful in achieving these aims.[495] Both forms of training are time consuming. Analytic training has the potential to be automated (i.e., computer-based training) so that clinician time is minimized. Because synthetic training usually involves modifying human interaction, the potential for automation is much less. Some parts of synthetic training however, can be carried out in small groups, which decreases the cost of providing the training. Extensive materials for analytic and synthetic training can be found in Plant (1994) and Plant (1996) respectively.

12.9 Avoiding Hearing Aid-Induced Hearing Loss

Patients must be told (but not unduly alarmed) that wearing a hearing aid increases their risk of acquiring further hearing loss because of additional noise exposure. Provided gain and

OSPL90 are responsibly prescribed, and provided the patient does not have a profound hearing loss, the risk is very minor, especially if the hearing aid includes a gradual form of compression for at least mid to high input levels (see Section 9.7). The patient, nevertheless, should be advised to avoid prolonged exposure to loud noise, and to wear hearing protection in very noisy places when intelligibility is not an issue. Interestingly, hearing aids will act as a form of hearing protection whenever the noise level is greater than the SSPL of the hearing aids.[f]

12.10 Assistive Listening Devices

At the assessment appointment, the clinician should briefly consider whether one or more assistive listening devices (see Section 3.11), rather than hearing aids, would meet the needs expressed by the patient. In the vast majority of cases, there will be at least one need that can be met only by hearing aids.[229] Often, however, it will be unclear at this early stage whether hearing aids will fully meet all the needs.

Consequently, it will often be the case that hearing aids are recommended, and a decision about other devices withheld, until the patient can evaluate how well the hearing aids meet all his or her needs. The need for assistive listening devices should therefore be reviewed at a follow-up appointment after aid fitting.

12.11 Ongoing Support

For some patients, needs will become evident that are beyond the ability of the clinician to deal with, or which cannot be dealt with in the time that can be made available to the patient. In these circumstances, the clinician can best serve the patient by referring the patient to an appropriately skilled person or organization. The clinician should therefore have available contact details for:

- peer support groups;
- telephone relay services;
- education services; and
- family counselors.

12.12 Counseling Styles

Everything in this chapter so far has dealt with the content of counseling, not the manner in which counseling is delivered. A clinician will tend to use styles of teaching and questioning with which he or she is most comfortable. Sweetow (1999a) gives a more thorough review of counseling styles and strategies. To be most effective, information has to be delivered in the way that each *patient* can most easily absorb, and in the way that is most likely to change the patient's attitude or behavior, if that is the clinician's intent.

An important distinction to be aware of is that some people learn most easily if they can *see* what is being taught, others most appreciate *hearing* a clear explanation, whereas others most easily absorb things by *doing* them. A problem arises if the clinician is able to teach things only one way, and the patient is able to learn them only in a different way. Flexibility of approach by the clinician is essential if knowledge and skills are to be imparted accurately and in the minimum possible time.

People differ in how they see the world, and there are many ways to express these differences. One psychological profiling method that has become popular in the last decade is the *Myers-Briggs Type Indicator (MBTI)*.[639] The MBTI measures where people fall along each of four dimensions:

- **I**ntroversion-**E**xtraversion,
- **S**ensing-i**N**tuition,
- **T**hinking-**F**eeling, and
- **J**udging-**P**erceiving.

---

[f] This statement is approximately true. The mean aided level at the eardrum relative to the mean unaided level at the eardrum will depend on the individual RECD, the individual REUR, the spectrum of the ambient noise, the dynamics of the ambient noise, and the shape of the hearing aid input-output curve.

Depending on the dominant end of each of these dimensions, people are classified into one of 16 types, such as *ISTJ* or *ESFJ*, etc. The personality of each of the 16 types has been summarized, and linked to things such as the type of occupation likely to be chosen and enjoyed. Traynor and Buckles (1997) summarize these personality types, and suggest that knowing a patient's personality type may help clinicians adapt their counseling appropriately. Such knowledge could help a clinician know a patient's preferred way of operating right from the first appointment, rather than gradually getting to know as the series of appointments progress.[891]

For example, people with an *S* characteristic will respond to facts, whereas people with an *N* characteristic will like reasons and logical arguments for doing things. People with a personality type that includes an *EJ* combination are likely to blurt out any difficulties they face without first thinking them through, and will want to decide how to deal with them immediately. By contrast, those with an *IP* combination will need more encouragement to talk about difficulties if they do not consider they have had enough time to reflect on them and make sense of the difficulties themselves. Patients with an *EFJ* combination are particularly likely to need, and respond well to, encouragement and praise as they learn to use their hearing aids.

Should clinicians spend their time, and their patient's time, gathering data on personality (and presenting these results to the patient) before providing appropriate rehabilitation? In the future – possibly; right now – certainly not. The basic research to link personality type to attitude, motivation, handicap, and effective means of communicating information about rehabilitation has not been done.

Clinicians should definitely be aware, however, that different patients respond best to different approaches and should seek to

---

Handling talkative patients

A dilemma confronting most clinicians is how much to let talkative patients talk. On the one hand, it is essential to find out what concerns patients in relation to their hearing. On the other hand, some patients talk incessantly about seemingly irrelevant things, and the clinician is acutely aware of how many essential things still have to be done or discussed in a limited time. It is useful to be direct with the patient in a positive way. Let them know for example, that you are extremely interested in how well they could hear at the party, rather than telling them (with verbal or non-verbal signals) that you are not interested in hearing what their grand-daughter wore to the party. The difficulty with steering conversation is that people will sometimes not tell you what is most on their mind until you have demonstrated that you will be interested in, and accepting of, the things they fear you may not like hearing.

The major tools available to the clinician are a compassionate nature and ***active listening*** skills. Active listening involves reflecting back to the patient the essence of their message, using either the same words used by the patient or different words that convey the same central message. If the essence of what the patient is trying to convey is a feeling, then so too must be the message reflected back. If a patient continues to produce irrelevant small talk despite you continually bringing them back to your preferred topic, the patient may not be finding acceptance in the reactions you are giving to his or her small talk. In such circumstances, patients often do not feel safe to say the thing that is troubling them most until they are half-way out of the door at the end of the appointment (Luterman, 1997). Interestingly, active listening is also an excellent way to encourage non-talkers to open up.

discover how each patient best operates. Every question a patient asks provides an insight into what type of information he or she prefers. If patients ask for *evidence* of the effectiveness of a high-priced hearing aid, do not give them an *explanation* of how it works, and vice versa. If patients say that something you are asking them to do does not *feel* right, find out why rather than give them a logical, *thinking* argument about why the action you are proposing is the best for them. Similarly, people with a visual orientation may say that they *see* what you are saying. (Readers of this book with an *S* in their Myers-Briggs personality type will have particularly appreciated these concrete examples.)

Whatever style of interaction is used, it is essential that it be supplemented with provision of written information. There are too many important pieces of information for a patient to be able to take them all in during a few appointments. Anything that is essential for the patient to know should be provided in written form as well as discussed.

12.13 Structuring Appointments

The following sections list some activities that can usefully be performed in a service protocol nominally comprising three-appointments plus one remote follow-up appointment. This must not be interpreted rigidly. Some patients will need two assessment appointments before they are ready to acquire hearing aids and/or choose a style or performance level. Fittings that do not go smoothly for technical or human reasons may need two fitting appointments. Many people will need additional follow-up appointments because of special problems. Many people will not take in things the first time and the information may have to be repeated. Individual idiosyncrasies will sometimes require variation from the following suggestions. Time constraints and difficulties encountered will often make it impossible to achieve all the items listed, and the clinician

---

Home visits

Brooks (1981) strongly recommends that at least one of the appointments should be carried out in the patient's own home. The advantages of this are:

- Patients are more relaxed and more frank about their difficulties, both before and after fitting.
- The clinician can more precisely assess the needs for assistive listening devices.
- The communication pattern between the patient and others at home can be assessed more easily, with a view to suggesting more effective communication strategies.

Unfortunately, such visits are very time consuming. Home visits may also make measurements (e.g. audiometry, real-ear gain) more difficult or impossible, although the availability of portable equipment has lessened this difficulty.

---

will have to judge what should be deleted, handled solely by providing written take-away information, or deferred to a later appointment.

Furthermore, some clinicians will be more drawn to objective procedures and others will be more drawn to interacting with the patient. If the clinician avoids either type of activity in a pronounced way, however, this is likely to be detrimental to a good outcome.

12.13.1 The assessment appointment(s)

- Take history (family history of loss, etiology of loss, work history, noise exposure, tinnitus, dizziness, asymmetry, brief medical history including medications, referral source, flexibility and manipulation ability, vision).
- Determine hearing needs (e.g. via COSI).
- Perform otoscopic examination.
- Measure hearing, using whichever tests are appropriate to the individual patient.

- Explain test results and implications of loss.
- Determine expectations, and modify as necessary.
- Discuss rehabilitation options, including hcaring aid advantages and limitations.
- Choose hearing aid style and performance features.
- Take ear impressions.
- Provide a written report if appropriate.

12.13.2 The fitting appointment(s)

- Program/adjust the hearing aids if not already done.
- Modify the shell or earmolds for comfort and ease of insertion (if necessary).
- Put hearing aids in, adjust volume for comfort, and leave on.
- Teach patient how to change battery, insert and remove hearing aids, and operate the volume control and on/off switch. Mention the presence of the T-switch (if appropriate).
- Measure real-ear gain, and adjust hearing aids to meet prescription targets.
- Evaluate sound quality (including patient's own voice) and fine-tune if necessary.
- Evaluate maximum output and fine-tune if necessary.
- Teach patient how to care for hearing aids, including cerumen management.
- Demonstrate use of the hearing aid with the telephone, including opcration of the T-switch if appropriate. Listening to a recorded message service is useful.
- Advise patient about graduated use of hearing aids.
- Provide batteries and indicate expected battery life and cost.

The most efficient order for doing these things, particular the timing of the real-ear gain measurement, is debatable. If evaluation of the patient's own voice requires the vent to be enlarged, real-ear gain will be affected and the measurement will have to be repeated

if it has already been done. Conversely, if real-ear measurement is delayed, patients may object to the sound quality *because* the response is far from target. Some clinicians leave the measurement until the follow-up appointment if they think they have adequately adjusted the hearing aid by using a test box or by viewing the simulated response on a computer screen. Deferment of real-ear gain testing is not recommended, however, if time permits.

New hearing aid wearers should not be asked about sound quality until they have had at least a few minutes experience listening with their new hearing aids. It is most efficient for them to hear something useful, like how to operate the hearing aids, while they are listening. A duplicate hearing aid facilitates this.

12.13.3 The follow-up appointment(s)

- Ask the patient about the degree of use, benefits, and problems related to the hearing aids.
- Ask about the volume control setting used (if appropriate), adequacy of loudness, sound quality, and intrusiveness of noise.
- Ask about problems with own voice quality, whistling, and loud noises.
- Fine-tune the amplification characteristics if so indicated.
- Ask the patient to remove the hearing aid, change the battery, insert the hearing aid, switch it on, and adjust the volume control to check on his or her ability to manage the hearing aids. (This can be done without it appearing to be an examination of the patient's ability.)
- Ask about ease of insertion and removal, ease of battery changing, and ease of volume control adjustment unless your observations have already convinced you that there are no problems with these operations.
- Examine ear canals for signs of irritation and ask about physical comfort.

- Ask about battery consumption (to check on reported use), provide information on battery life and battery tester (if appropriate).

- Note hearing aid condition and ask about cleaning.

- Ask how much the hearing aids have helped with the problems that originally led the patient to seek help, and how much difficulty remains (e.g. via COSI).

- Check on the ability of the patient to use the telephone (with or without a T-switch, as appropriate).

- Evaluate the need for assistive listening devices and provide appropriate information.

- Teach appropriate hearing strategies and provide written material for the patient to take away.

- Provide information about repairs, warranty, after-care, service charges, and consumer support groups.

- Evaluate the need for additional follow-up appointments. If success with the hearing aid does not seem assured, schedule another appointment in one to four weeks. Otherwise, advise the patient to make a further appointment at any time in the future.

- At some stage within the period one to three months after the last appointment, perform a mail or telephone follow-up to evaluate benefit, use, satisfaction, and problems.[g] Schedule an additional appointment if any of these indicate there are problems that the clinician could solve.

It is essential to ask patients, on several occasions after fitting, if they are experiencing any problems with their hearing aids or their ease of communication. While one might expect that people experiencing problems would seek help, mostly they do not.[330, 433] In one recent survey conducted three months after fitting, 48% of patients reported having one or more problems with

their hearing aids. Surprisingly, less than a quarter of those reporting a problem indicated in a questionnaire that they would like to make a further appointment with their clinician.[225] In another survey conducted 12 months after fitting, 86% of patients needed help with at least one problem.[682] The people in this study had had an average of four visits to their clinician during the rehabilitation program associated with aid fitting.

One might argue that it is not the responsibility of the clinician to initiate contact to see if there are any problems. This is a dangerous argument unless we know why people so often do not initiate contact, and we do not know. It is also short-sighted: hearing aid owners who are in any way dissatisfied with their hearing aids are walking advertisements for why their friends should not seek rehabilitation, a situation which is to everybody's disadvantage. One large survey indicated that 18% of hearing aid owners do not use their hearing aids at all.[482]

12.13.4 The power of groups

So far, the discussion in this chapter has assumed that the clinician is dealing with one patient at a time. There are many advantages to including one or more group appointments within an overall rehabilitation program for each patient. The group appointments supplement, rather than replace the individual appointments, although some of the things that are usually accomplished in individual appointments can be done just as well, or even better, in group appointments. Patients most likely to benefit from a group, and most likely to be motivated to attend, are people newly fitted with hearing aids, or people with severe or profound hearing loss who are extremely handicapped by their hearing loss. It is beneficial if the regular communication partners of the hearing-impaired participants can also participate.[95] Abrahamson (1997) suggests that groups comprise at least three

---

g   The appointment can, of course, be in person if the patient and the clinician can afford the time and cost.

couples or at least five individuals, but that groups up to 20 are possible if they can be comfortably seated.

Reasons for forming a group

There are many reasons why seeing several patients as a group is a good thing to do:

- Some activities (see panel) can be performed more efficiently in a group, which provides cost savings to the provider or the patient or both. Alternatively, for the same total cost, more rehabilitation activities can be accomplished, thus increasing rehabilitation effectiveness.

- Some patients find that participating in a group of people who are going through similar emotions and experiences to be an extremely positive experience. It is not hard to understand why this might be so.

  –Group discussion can legitimize feelings, including the acceptance of hearing loss. Most people are relieved when they find that others have the same problems, reactions, and emotions when they are confronted with the same circumstances.

  Just knowing this can be liberating; people can then move on to deal with the circumstances and the emotions, instead of worrying about whether they *should* be feeling this way, or having these problems.

  –Other people in a group can sometimes analyze or put into words vague concerns that the patient already feels but does not understand and cannot enunciate. Again, this makes it easier to deal with the concerns.

  –People confronting the same problems often find different solutions. Seeing some alternative means of coping, and hearing first hand that they work, can raise new possibilities in the mind of a patient.

- Consumer groups appreciate the benefits that only groups can provide and have called for them to be available.[761]

- When hearing aids do not provide the clarity of hearing in noise that a patient desires, the patient may attribute the cause

---

Things to do in groups

- *Explaining hearing and hearing loss*: anatomy, frequency, intensity, the audiogram, effects on speech clarity.
- *Consequences of hearing loss*: discussing and sharing the emotional and social consequences of hearing loss.
- *Hearing aids and ALDs*: what a hearing aid is, its effectiveness in different situations (i.e. developing realistic expectations), explanation and demonstration of ALDs, explanation and demonstration of telecoil, care and maintenance, binaural and bilateral advantage.
- *Hearing tactics and strategies:* all of Section 12.6, including collaborative solving of problems volunteered by participants.

The last topic is particularly suitable for groups, because the topic inherently involves interactions between people. This interaction enables participants without specialized knowledge to contribute perspectives that other members of the group will find useful. The first and third topics are more based on the clinician giving information. The emotional benefits of groups are most likely to emerge during discussion on the second and fourth topics.

There are several references available that give further details on how to conduct a group rehabilitation session: Abrahamson (1991, 1997); Kricos (1997); Lesner (1995); Mongomery (1994); Wayner (1990); Williams (1994). Some of these also contain useful handout materials.

of this to the hearing aid, rather than to his or her still-defective hearing mechanism. While the clinician can say that the hearing loss is the problem, having the patient hear other patients relate the same experience reinforces what the clinician is saying.[2] It can also be enlightening for spouses to hear that for other couples, hearing problems did not vanish the day that hearing aids were acquired.

- Because of all this, patients' rehabilitation becomes more successful and they become more satisfied.[494]

- The clinician will appreciate the variation in routine, and will gain greater insight into what it is like to have a hearing problem than is likely to occur in individual appointments.

The value of a group may not be related to the reason the group is formed or to the apparent content of the group session. Ross (1987) recounts his experience at being in a lip-reading class. He concludes in retrospect that while the class did not increase his ability to lip-read, he received many benefits related to the "ancillary and unspoken factors intrinsic to the group experience". Experimental results back this up. In two studies, speech-reading training produced no change in speech-reading ability, but participants reported becoming more confident when conversing with others,[64] and the amount of hearing aid use increased with the extent of the group training[h] administered.[544] This is not to say that the content is necessarily irrelevant. Time spent on hearing strategies, including synthetic communication training tasks seems likely to have more beneficial effects than time spent on analytic communication drills, for example.[495]

Any training aimed at encouraging patients to modify their behavior (including attempting to modify the communication behavior of those around them) is particularly

well suited to group appointments. Groups provide the opportunity for patients to try out new behavior patterns in a safe, supportive, encouraging environment. For example, if several people talk at once, or one person talks while looking away from the intended listener, the listener can practice requesting the talkers to modify their behavior. Polite assertiveness does not come easily to many people, and like any new skill, must be practiced and reinforced.

Groups are most commonly formed after the patients have received their hearing aids. They can, however, be formed before people have actually become patients, at a time when they may have made no commitment to seeking any type of help with their hearing. Many people who participate in such groups are likely to become patients, and apparently such people are extremely unlikely to return their hearing aids once they have obtained them.[241] In pre-fitting groups, there is the potential to involve successful users of hearing aids as "models". The presence of such people may allow those who doubt their ability to manage hearing aids to see that similar people (e.g. of the same age, gender, ethnicity, or socio-economic group) have been able to successfully adapt to hearing aid use. This, and the views of the successful hearing aid wearers, may provide considerable encouragement.

If groups have all these advantages, why are they not more often used? There are several reasons.

Appointment Logistics. It can be difficult to organize times that are mutually convenient for several patients. This is most difficult for a pre-fitting group. Only larger practices would have enough patients undergoing the same stage of rehabilitation at the same time for there to be a reasonable number who can attend. Appointment logistics are less of an issue for post-fitting groups because the

---

h   It is possible that individual post-fitting training would also have been effective, but lengthy individual training is rarely possible, for financial reasons.

group appointment can be organized well in advance, and can be scheduled at the end of the assessment appointment.

Room. Running a group requires the clinic to have (or hire or borrow) a room big enough to hold everyone at once. The room should have good acoustics (i.e. low reverberation), particularly for pre-fitting groups. Even then, some participants may require assistive listening devices, such as FM systems.

Uncertainty. Dealing with a group of people takes different skills (or perhaps just a different sort of confidence) than dealing with one person at a time. Some clinicians are reluctant to try it. A good introduction for uncertain clinicians is to pool patients with another clinician and to jointly run the group. Having two clinicians run the group is actually much easier at first, as there is ample time to gather one's thoughts while the other clinician assumes responsibility.

Perceived unwillingness. Some clinicians report that few of their patients are willing to participate in a group, whereas other clinicians report that most of their patients wish to participate.[i] The willingness of patients to participate thus depends markedly on how the clinician goes about asking each patient. Younger patients (e.g. under 70 years) are more likely to be interested than are older patients.[194] May & Upfold (1984) found that when the invitation was issued with enthusiasm, and the group appointment was presented as a normal part of the service structure, 87% of patients accepted the invitation, despite the median age being close to 80. The attendance rate amongst those who accepted was the same as occurred for individual appointments. Amongst those who would rather not participate will be many that are also reluctant to accept that they have a hearing loss (Hetu, 1996).

Apparent cost. The time required for the group appointment has to be funded in some way. If one takes into account that time that is freed in individual appointments, and the increased satisfaction and decreased device return rate that is reported by those who conduct groups, it seems likely that group appointments save rather than cost money.[3] Consequently, it may even be cost-effective to provide a financial inducement (i.e. a discount) to patients who agree to attend group sessions, rather than consider charging them extra.[3] One study reported a much lower hearing aid return rate amongst those who participated in a post-fitting group than amongst those who did not.[667, j]

Structuring group activities. The topics for group discussion can be highly structured to follow a set curriculum. Alternatively, the group can have the single topic of how to improve difficult communication situations that confront the members of each group. Eventually, this will take in most hearing strategies and probably other topics as well. These alternatives can be combined, so that solving individually proposed difficult situations is just one of the set topics for the group. Unless the sole aim of the group session is to impart knowledge from the clinician to the group members, the participants should sit in a circle to facilitate communication with each other, and to reinforce that exchange of information *among* group members is an essential part of the group's activities.

12.14 Concluding Comments

The approach to counseling described in this book is consistent with a rehabilitative model, rather than a medical model, of service delivery. In a rehabilitative model, patients actively participate in solving their own

---

[i]   In a particular case known to the author, two clinicians with opposite views on whether patients were willing to participate in a group worked in the same clinic seeing patients randomly selected from the same population.
[j]   It is not clear from this study whether people are more satisfied because they participate in group rehabilitation, or whether more highly motivated people are more likely to elect to participate. Both are likely to be true.

problems, rather than having their hearing diagnosed and then having some treatment done to them.[267] In a rehabilitative model, any characteristic of the patient (i.e. not just hearing) is potentially able to affect the type of rehabilitation that the clinician chooses to carry out. In general, treatment via a rehabilitative model is believed to be more effective, and to result in greater patient compliance with treatment recommendations, than a medical model.[267]

This chapter has provided many lists of things to say and do, and even a possible order in which to do them. It is essential, however, for the clinician to be continually tuned into the state of the patient. In counseling, listening is at least as important as instructing. The patient's comments, actions, and reactions (verbal and non-verbal) should dictate the clinician's flow of counseling.[873]

For example, the clinician must be skilled at differentiating between requests for information and requests for acceptance of an emotional reaction, and be able to respond appropriately. This skill can be taught to student clinicians.[264] If the clinician instead works rigidly through a standard, pre-established patter of questions and information giving, patients will assume that they are not being listened to. In such circumstances they may be less than frank, or may appear to the clinician to be making irrelevant and repetitive comments. Competent clinicians must have communication skills that are as excellent as their technical skills if they are to best help their patients.

CHAPTER THIRTEEN

ASSESSING THE OUTCOMES OF HEARING REHABILITATION

Synopsis

Clients and clinicians both benefit when the outcomes of the rehabilitation process are measured in some way. Systematic measurement of outcomes can help clinicians learn which of their practices, procedure, and devices are achieving the intended aims. Some measures can also help determine how the rehabilitation program for individual patients should be structured and when they should be ended. Outcome assessment can be based on an objective speech discrimination test, or on a subjective self-report and/or the report of significant other people. Speech test scores show the increase in listening ability in specific situations, whereas self-report measures more generally reflect the patient's views about the impact of rehabilitation. Many self-report measures, however, do have sub-scales so that outcomes can be separately assessed for different listening environments. Outcome measures can assess the dimension of benefit, defined as a reduction in disability or handicap, the dimension of how often devices are used, or the dimension of how satisfied the patient feels with the rehabilitation process.

Self-report measures that assess benefit can be grouped into various classes. First, patients can be asked to make a direct assessment of the benefit of rehabilitation. Alternatively, patients' views of their disability can be assessed both before and after the rehabilitation program. The change in score provides a measure of the effects of rehabilitation. Measures obtained both before and after rehabilitation provide a more complete view of disability or handicap status and change. These difference measures probably assess change less accurately than those that directly assess benefit because they involve subtracting two scores. The second way in which self-report measures differ is the extent to which the items are the same for all patients or are determined individually for each patient. Results can more easily be compared across patients if a standard set of items is used for all patients. When the items are individually selected for each patient, however, the questionnaires become shorter and can more easily be incorporated within interviews with the patient. There are thus four types of self-report measures: standard questionnaires that directly assess benefit (e.g. HAPI); standard questionnaires that compare handicap or disability before and after rehabilitation (e.g. HHIE, APHAB); individualized questionnaires that directly assess benefit (e.g. COSI); and individualized questionnaires that compare handicap or disability before and after rehabilitation (e.g. GAS).

Self-report measures are the only viable way to assess hearing aid usage and satisfaction. Some measures contain questions that address only one dimension (benefit, use, or satisfaction) whereas others address more than one dimension. One comprehensive questionnaire (GHABP) addresses all three dimensions, contains standard and individualized measures, and assesses benefit both directly and by comparing disability before and after rehabilitation.

While outcomes can be assessed any time after hearing aid fitting, the extent of benefit does not appear to stabilize until about 6 weeks after fitting. Hearing aid use is associated with general improvements in health and quality of life, although generic measures of health outcome are not efficient means by which a clinician can assess the outcomes of rehabilitation.

Lord Raleigh said that if we cannot measure something, we do not know much about it. Measuring the outcomes of a hearing aid fitting can give us invaluable insights into how the services and devices we have provided have affected the life of our patients. As we review methods for measuring the effects of hearing rehabilitation, we should recognize that although hearing aids are the major components of most rehabilitation programs, they are rarely the *entire* program (see Chapter 12). Rehabilitation outcomes are thus likely to be affected by all aspects of the rehabilitation program. There are several reasons why clinicians might choose to measure rehabilitation outcomes:

- A clinician may want to determine if particular rehabilitation procedures, devices, or entire programs are more effective than others in helping their patients. *Rehabilitation procedures* includes things as mundane as the way the clinician instructs a patient to insert an earmold, and as complex as helping a patient comes to terms with the appropriateness of being assertive in a difficult listening situation.

- A clinician may want to determine whether he or she has sufficiently helped a patient. The answer may determine whether further appointments should be scheduled, and whether a change of tactics is required for this patient.

- A third-party provider of funds for health care (government or an insurance company) may make funding conditional on obtaining evidence that rehabilitation is beneficial to patients. Benefit may have to be substantiated for a hearing-impaired population as a whole, or for each individual.

What do we mean by "outcomes"? In general, *an outcome is something that changes in the life of the patient as a consequence of the service and devices provided to that patient by the clinician*. Some specific outcomes that we aim to achieve are:

Decreased disability. We want patients to hear more of the sounds around them, and better understand speech in a range of situations. Using the new World Health Organization terminology, we would describe this as increased communication-related activities.

Decreased handicap. We want patients not to restrict the activities they choose to participate in because of difficulties caused by their hearing loss. Any negative emotions patients feel because of their hearing loss hopefully will also be decreased or eliminated. The new World Health Organization terminology would refer to decreased handicap as increased participation in social, occupational and recreational events.

Use. We want patients to use the devices we provide them in every situation in which they are having trouble hearing.

Satisfaction. Patients have contributed time and money, and have probably undergone some emotional stress from participating in rehabilitation. We hope that they, and any family members involved, will feel satisfied with the process and the results.

We will refer to the first two of these outcomes as ***benefits*** of rehabilitation. Hearing aid ***use*** should be regarded as an important means to an end rather than as a goal in itself. ***Satisfaction*** is affected by benefit, but also involves patient's expectations, monetary and psychological costs, problems encountered, and any communication difficulties that remain. As we shall see, all of these outcomes can be assessed through questionnaires and other self-report techniques. For a recent review of literature on self-assessment of hearing, see Noble (1998). We will return to self-assessment in this chapter after examining how benefit can be assessed through speech identification testing.

13.1 Speech Identification Testing

The major reason hearing-impaired people seek help is to hear speech more clearly.[229] Speech tests are a direct and objective way to measure how much more clearly people can understand speech with their hearing aids than without them. There are many speech tests already developed from which to choose. These vary from tests that are very easy because they include a lot of context or have few highly contrasting response alternatives, through to tests that are very hard because there is little or no context available.

Speech test results can be made as repeatable as is necessary, simply by including enough items in the speech test.[341, 881] Computer-based presentation and scoring techniques enable groups of words to be scored on a phoneme basis (rather than word scoring or sentence scoring) in a reasonable time.[312] Phoneme scoring maximizes the number of scored items per minute of testing time, which therefore maximizes the reliability of the speech score, given the testing time available. Speech tests consequently provide a ready means to assess the benefit of hearing aids. In particular, they assess reduction in disability related to understanding speech.

13.1.1 Limitations of speech tests to assess benefits

Despite these advantages, speech tests are neither *efficient* nor *sufficient* means of demonstrating the overall benefit that hearing aids provide to a patient. There is one major reason for this, which we will consider first, and several minor reasons.

Dependence on measurement conditions. The amount of benefit that hearing aids provide depends hugely on the acoustic environment. The details and reasons for this have been covered in Section 8.1.4, but in brief, hearing aids are most effective when signal levels are low and where consequently, the patients' thresholds limit audibility.

Hearing aids are least effective in noisy places where audibility is limited by background noise.

A hearing aid can thus be shown to provide a large amount of benefit, or very little benefit, depending on the stimuli chosen for the test. The result can not be a general indicator of benefit if the result depends on the measurement condition chosen by the clinician. We can not avoid the problem by measuring in several conditions and simply summing or averaging the results. Two patients with identical hearing losses and auditory processing capabilities, fitted with identical hearing aids, may have vastly different perspectives on how beneficial their hearing aids are. If one of them spends a lot of time in noisy, reverberant places, and the other spends a lot of time in quiet places listening to softly spoken people, both will have excellent reasons for coming to opposite conclusions about the benefit their hearing aids provide. Not surprisingly, there is only moderate correlation between objective measures of benefit and self-reported benefit.

Efficiency relative to other means of measurement. Hearing aids increase speech identification ability primarily by increasing audibility. The amount by which they increase audibility depends on the speech level and spectrum, background noise level and spectrum, the patient's threshold at each frequency, and the real-ear gain of the hearing aid at each frequency. These are all acoustic or electroacoustic variables. The Speech Intelligibility Index method allows us to combine them to predict aided speech intelligibility based on unaided intelligibility.[222] Figure 13.1 shows an example for one subject and one speech test. If we know the unaided speech performance-intensity function, we can predict the aided function based on the patient's thresholds and various electroacoustic measures.

This is not to say that we *should* make such predictions, but that if such predictions *can*

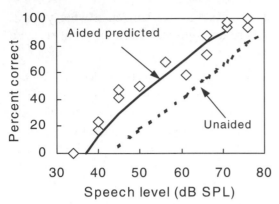

Figure 13.1. Data for one subject showing the aided speech performance (diamonds) and the aided performance that was predicted (solid line). Predictions were based on the insertion gain, the background noise present, and the unaided performance (dotted line).

be made from electroacoustic measures, measurement of aided speech performance is not adding some new type of information. It is faster and easier to measure an insertion gain curve than it is to measure an aided speech performance-intensity function. Furthermore, the insertion gain curve is immediately useful: deficiencies relative to a prescription become evident, as do excessive peaks or troughs, so the corrective action necessary is obvious. Conventional speech tests can indicate that there is little benefit, but they do not indicate how we should change the hearing aid's characteristics to get a better result.

Speech tests presented at a number of levels enable a ***performance-intensity function*** to be visualized (as in Figure 13.1). This enables the clinician to determine the range of speech levels over which speech scores exceed some criterion score. An unduly narrow range would lead the clinician to question whether the hearing aid has enough compression. While the approach has potential, the difficulties are many: What is an acceptable speech score? Over how large a range of levels should this score be achieved or exceeded? If the compression ratio(s) of the

hearing aid are increased, how will the clinician determine when the ratio is so large that speech quality or sound naturalness have deteriorated? When this happens, how will the intelligibility advantages of the larger compression ratio be weighed against its quality disadvantages? In short, measuring a performance intensity function raises many questions, but provides few answers.

Reliance on speech. Speech tests do not measure several potential benefits. Hearing aids can help people detect and recognize environmental sounds, and thus lead to a greater feeling of security by the aid wearer.[272] Hearing aids also help people monitor their own voice level and quality, especially for people with severe and profound hearing loss.

13.1.2 Role of speech testing in evaluating benefit

None of this is to suggest that speech tests have *no* role in assessing benefit. In fact, they are very useful for several things.

- If one can identify and simulate specific acoustic conditions, speech tests provide a clear assessment of how much the hearing aids change the person's ability to understand speech in this situation. The ability to store and quickly access a range of speech and noise materials on CD and computers has increased the feasibility of simulating, in the clinic, environments that are relevant to particular patients. In fact, simulating a known environment is relatively easy. Knowing *what* to simulate is difficult, because the conclusions reached are strongly dependent on having the right speech and noise spectra and levels, appropriate reverberation, and appropriate context in the speech material used.

- Identifying the types of speech sounds that are not well perceived is useful for evaluating the type of benefit that hearing aids provide. A six-sound test /a, i, u, m, sh, and s/ for example, can be used to assess audibility and recognition of these sounds, which each have a relatively high intensity in at least one frequency region. The results apply only to speech presented at the overall level tested.

- Speech tests can provide a convincing demonstration of benefit (in the condition tested) to a patient or to a family member. This can be worthwhile if either of them is not convinced that hearing aids can provide such benefit.

- Speech tests can demonstrate to patients and relatives the importance of visual cues to understanding.

- As we will see in Chapter 14, speech tests can be used to help decide whether a person should wear one or two hearing aids, or in which ear a single hearing aid should be worn.

- Speech tests can be used to predict how much difficulty a patient will have communicating in some specified environment while wearing hearing aids. This information can help the clinician decide if the patient needs some form of communication training or the provision of other devices. An example is using a speech test to see if hearing aid outcomes are sufficiently poor to consider using a cochlear implant (Section 8.2.2).

- If speech perception training is to be provided, speech tests can determine the level of training (speech feature, phonetic, supra-segmental etc) that should be offered.

In summary, speech identification tests are an excellent way to measure the benefit of hearing aids, provided one is interested only in the scores obtained in a specific environment and provided this environment can adequately be simulated in the test room. If one wishes to assess benefit or communication effectiveness across many environments, or in environments that cannot accurately be specified or simulated, other measures of benefit have to be used.

13.2 Self-report Questionnaires for Assessing Benefit

13.2.1 Questionnaire methodology

Another way to assess benefit is to ask the patient, via a questionnaire, how beneficial the hearing aids are. Each item in a questionnaire asks patients to rate something about their hearing in some specific situation. A situation might be described in such a way as: *You are talking to a shop assistant in a busy store.* Additionally, simple pictures can help the patient identify each type of situation being described.[491] For each item there are a number of response alternatives and this number can vary from three (e.g. the Hearing Handicap Inventory of the Elderly)[919] to eleven (e.g. the Gothenburg Profile).[749] There are two ways we can use the information obtained from questionnaires to measure benefit.

Direct assessment of benefit. Patients are asked to directly estimate the degree of benefit their hearing aids provide in each designated situation. Response options are generally a set of words or phrases that vary evenly from some negative rating to some positive rating. Questionnaires that directly assess benefit need be answered only once, and this obviously has to be after the patient has received hearing aids and the associated rehabilitation activities. The *Hearing Aid Performance Inventory* is an example of this approach. Each rating is given a score (e.g. 1 to 5 in this example), and the scores for all the items in the questionnaire are summed or averaged to produce the final measure of benefit. Measures that directly assess the benefit of rehabilitation are referred to as *change measures* (Gatehouse, 1999).

Subtraction of unaided and aided scores. The alternative to direct assessment of benefit is to ask patients how well they can hear, or how much handicap they experience, in the designated situations. In this case, they are asked twice: once for the unaided condition and once for the aided condition.[a] Response options are generally a set of words or phrases that vary evenly from extreme difficulty in hearing to no difficulty in hearing. In the *unaided administration* of the questionnaire, patients state how well they can hear when they are not wearing their hearing aids. This provides a *baseline measure* of hearing disability. Patients then answer all the questions a second time; the questionnaire is the same, but this time they state how well they hear while they are wearing their hearing aids (i.e. the *aided administration*). Each questionnaire is scored and benefit is defined as the difference between the aided and unaided scores. The *Abbreviated Profile of Hearing Aid Benefit* and the *Hearing Handicap Inventory of the Elderly* (see panel) are examples of this approach.

The first administration can be before the patients receive their hearing aids or after they receive them. Both times of administration have pluses and minuses. If the unaided questionnaire is administered before provision of hearing aids, there has to be a delay of weeks or months before the patient has accumulated enough experience with the hearing aid for benefit to be assessed. If the general mood of the patient is more negative or positive on the day of the second administration than on the first, this could affect the difference score markedly. Having the patients complete both questionnaires on the same day can solve this problem. Delayed administration of the unaided questionnaire, however, introduces a new problem: Patients who are full-time hearing aid users in any of the situations addressed may have difficulty remembering how much trouble they had hearing unaided in those situations. Separate measures of unaided and aided hearing are referred to as *state measures*.[304]

Either overall type of assessment method (direct assessment of benefit, or aided versus unaided difference) can be used, but each type has its advantages and disadvantages.

• The aided versus unaided method is probably the least accurate (and hence least sensitive) measure of benefit.[228, 304] When separate unaided and aided questionnaires are administered, the scores for each have to be subtracted to calculate benefit. Unfortunately, the random errors implicit in each score add,[b] so the result can have an error component comparable in size to the benefit measured.

Examples of self-report items and response choices

Abbreviated Profile of Hearing Aid Benefit (APHAB) (Cox & Alexander, 1995)
I have difficulty hearing a conversation when I'm with one of my family at home.
[*Always, Almost always, Generally, Half-the-time, Occasionally, Seldom, Never*]

Hearing Handicap Inventory for the Elderly (HHIE) (Ventry & Weinstein, 1982)
Does a hearing problem cause you to avoid groups of people?
[*Yes, Sometimes, No*]

Hearing Aid Performance Inventory (HAPI) (Walden, Demorest & Hepler, 1984)
You are talking with the bank teller at the bank.
[*Hinders, No help, Very little help, Helpful, Very helpful*]

---

[a]   Although we refer to these conditions as unaided and aided for convenience, the aided condition will probably be affected by things other than wearing hearing aids. The primary example of another difference between the two states is the counseling that the patient will have received prior to the aided administration.

[b]   This statement assumes that the random fluctuations in the unaided answers are not correlated to the random fluctuations in the aided answers.

Understanding the construction and reliability of questionnaires: Factors, subscales, internal consistency, item-total correlation, and test-retest differences

Although items could be grouped into pre-defined *subscales* on the basis of their content, it is more common to analyze the results of a large number of patients and then group items on a statistical basis using either *factor analysis* or *principal components analysis*. These techniques examine how correlated the answers of each item are relative to each other item, and attempt to find some common underlying factors that are highly correlated to a number of items. These items are said to be *loaded* onto this common factor and it is these items that are grouped to form a subscale. Simply expressed, if a patient assigns a high rating to one item, the patient is also likely to assign a high rating for other items in that same subscale. The meaning of the factor, and hence of the subscale, is determined by examining the items that form the subscale and noting what content they have in common.

The reason for using multiple items in each subscale is to increase the accuracy of the subscale, and of the entire scale. One way to express accuracy is via the *internal consistency* of the subscale or scale. This measure is estimated by a statistic called *Cronbach's alpha*. It is equal to the correlation that, on average, would be obtained between two randomly divided sets of items. If half the items in a scale give a very similar total score to that of the other half, we can be confident that neither half is producing random results. Consequently, when the two halves are recombined, the total scale also must produce a repeatable result. A good subscale will contain multiple items that look different, but in fact have a high internal consistency and thus provide multiple estimates of the same underlying phenomenon.

One way to produce such a scale is to weed out items that appear to be measuring something different from the rest of the items. This is achieved by calculating the correlation between the score for one item and the total score for all the remaining items. Items with a low *item-total correlation* are deleted. Generally, their content appears to contain different concepts from those of the remaining items.

Two other desirable statistical properties are *relevance* and *inter-patient variability*. There is no point including an item if a large proportion of patients indicate that the situation described is not relevant to them. Similarly, an item has little predictive value if nearly all patients answer it with the same rating.

As with any measure, the reliability of a questionnaire can be assessed by calculating the correlation between scores obtained with a group of patients versus the scores obtained on a retest using the same questionnaire and the same patients. The people chosen to be tested, however, heavily influence these *test-retest correlations*. The test-retest correlation of an audiometric threshold, for example, would be extremely poor if we only tested people with normal hearing: The apparent variations from test to retest would be comparable to the true variations between people in the sample. By contrast, if our sample included people with a range of threshold sensitivity from normal to profound impairment, the test-retest correlation would be extremely high. The audiometric test, however, is the same! Test-retest correlations of any measure should be treated with great caution as they apply only to the particular population tested.

A more robust and useful measure is the standard deviation of the test-retest differences. This indicates the spread of test-retest differences that can be expected due to chance variations. Two scores are significantly different at the 95% confidence level if they are separated by approximately two test-retest standard deviations or greater. Note that the test-retest differences expected for a questionnaire may depend on the method of administration as well as on the items. For one test, for example, the critical differences are almost twice as large when the client self-administers the test as when the clinician administers it (Weinstein, Spitzer & Ventry, 1986).

Further explanation of the psychometrics of self-report questionnaires can be found in an excellent paper by Demorest & Walden (1984).

- The direct assessment method does not reveal the full picture. A small benefit is not a problem if it occurs in a situation where the patient has little difficulty hearing. Conversely, a small benefit is a serious problem if it occurs in a situation where the patient has a lot of difficulty hearing. The direct assessment method, by itself, does not allow us to distinguish between these two extremely different cases.

- In principle, the best compromise seems to be a combination of two types of questions. The first type directly assesses benefit. The second type assesses either the initial disability or handicap, or else the residual disability or handicap after the rehabilitation program has been completed. This situation can be approximated in the unaided versus aided approach if the patients are allowed, while they are doing the aided questionnaire, to see and change the answers they previously gave for the unaided questionnaire.[166] The intention is that the patients will mark the aided scale in such a way that their ratings, relative to those on the unaided scale, reflect their direct assessment of benefit. The degree to which patients can simultaneously respond in this absolute and relative manner, and the resulting effect on accuracy, has not been quantified.

Irrespective of which approach is used, the items on the questionnaire can be grouped into *subscales* that examine different aspects of benefit (see panel on Understanding Questionnaires). For example, one subscale could relate to listening in quiet situations, and another could relate to listening in noise.

Although this section has discussed the patient's own perception of the changes that occurred following rehabilitation, the concept can easily be generalized to reports by other people who have frequent contact with the patient. Most commonly this is the spouse[148, 687] but can also be a friend, and for a child, it could be a parent or teacher.

13.2.2 Practical self-report measures

Unaided and aided questionnaires

If one wishes to separately measure the aided and unaided states, there are several well-standardized questionnaires from which to choose. With this approach, any questionnaire that assesses disability or handicap can be used to derive a benefit score. It is important, however, that any questionnaire used quantitatively have known psychometric properties (see panel). Some questionnaires that could be answered in a way that relates to either aided or unaided communication ability are shown in Table 13.1. These questionnaires are particularly suitable for adults; Section 15.6 shows some measures that are more suitable for children.

Table 13.1 lists the APHAB measure because one half of the questionnaire assesses unaided ability and the other half assesses aided ability. The two halves are otherwise identical. These same comments apply to its longer parent questionnaire, the PHAB, but the shorter version is more practical for clinical use. The APHAB questionnaire is scored separately for its four subscales: *Ease of Communication (EC)*, *Reverberation (RV)*, *Background Noise (BN)*, and *Aversiveness of Sounds (AV)*. The first three of these assess the increase in speech understanding in various everyday environments, and the last assesses negative reactions to more intense sounds. It is usual for this last measure to reveal a negative benefit. That is, patients find intense sounds more unpleasant when they are wearing their hearing aids than when they are not. A particularly poor score on this subscale indicates that the limiting and/or compression ratio for intense sounds (for a hearing aid with WDRC) should be reviewed.

A dilemma with all questionnaires incorporating subscales is that the most specific information is obtained if one examines each subscale score, whereas the most reliable information is obtained if one examines the total score (because of the greater number of items). Because the first three subscales in

Table 13.1 Questionnaires assessing hearing disability or handicap.

	Questionnaire	Authors	Year	No of items
HHS	Hearing Handicap Scale	High et al.	1964	20
HMS	Hearing Measurement Scale	Noble & Atherley	1970	42
SHI	Social Hearing Handicap Index	Ewertsen & Birk-Nielson	1973	21
DS	Denver Scale of Communication Function	Alpiner et al.	1974	25
WISH	Weighted Index of Social Hearing Handicap	Brooks	1979	19
HPI	Hearing Performance Inventory	Giolas et al	1979	158
HHIE	Hearing Handicap Inventory for the Elderly	Ventry & Weinstein	1982	25
RHPI	Revised Hearing Performance Inventory	Lamb et al.	1983	90
HHIE-S	Hearing Handicap Invent for the Elderly - Screening	Ventry & Weinstein	1983	10
CPHI	Communication Profile for the Hearing Impaired	Demorest & Erdman	1987	145
PIPSL	Performance Inventory for Profound and Severe Loss	Owens & Raggio	1988	74
SAC	Self Assessment of Communication	Schow et al	1989	10
PHAP	Profile of Hearing Aid Performance	Cox & Gilmore	1990	66
OI	Oldenburg Inventory	Holube & Kollmeier	1991	21
PHAB	Profile of Hearing Aid Benefit	Cox et al.	1991	66
HHIA	Hearing Handicap Inventory for Adults	Newman et al.	1990	25
APHAB	Abbreviated profile of Hearing Aid Benefit	Cox & Alexander	1995	24
HCA	Hearing Coping Assessment	Andersson et al.	1995	21
AIADH	Amsterdam Inventory for Auditory Disability & Handicap	Kramer et al.	1995	60
GP	Gothenburg Profile	Ringdahl et al.	1998	20

the APHAB are measuring something very different from the Aversiveness subscale, a good compromise is to combine the scores for the first three subscales into a single global measure of speech understanding benefit, and to keep the final subscale separate.[179] Table 13.2 shows some statistics for the APHAB subscales and for the global benefit combination. The critical difference is defined here as the difference needed between two administrations (e.g. with different devices) for a 10% probability of the difference occurring by chance alone.[c]

The *Hearing Handicap Inventory for the Elderly* (*HHIE*) has been used in numerous studies to quantify the benefit associated with hearing aid fitting. After hearing aid fitting, handicap scores typically decrease by 20 to 30 points (on a 100-point scale). The HHIE has two sub-scales (Emotional and Social/ situational) and each of these subscales contributes approximately equally to the decrease in measured handicap.

Direct assessment of benefit.
If one wishes to use the direct assessment approach, there are fewer choices, as shown in Table 13.3. The *SHAPI* and *SHAPIE* questionnaires are shortened versions of the original HAPI questionnaire. In one evaluation of the sensitivity and reliability of different methods for assessing benefit,[228] scores obtained with the SHAPIE were better

---

[c] Critical differences for the stricter 5% probability level commonly used in research studies are about 1.2 times those shown in Table 13.2.

Table 13.2 Statistics for the APHAB scale and subscales. Large numbers for the unaided and aided scores indicate a lot of difficulty in hearing, whereas large numbers for the benefit scores indicate that the hearing aid provides substantial benefit.

Scale / Subscale	No of items	Median unaided problems	Median aided problems	Median benefit	Critical difference for aided score change (p=0.1)
Ease of Communication	6	65	16	41	22
Reverberation	6	81	33	39	18
Background Noise	6	81	37	35	22
Aversiveness of Sounds	6	17	60	-25	31
Global score (avg of EC+BN+RV)	18	73	31	37	14

Using APHAB

- The APHAB questionnaire can be downloaded (Cox, 2000) as either a printed form, or as a software program that can be used directly by the patient. This program can also be used to score the responses, irrespective of whether the patient uses the paper and pencil version or the computer version.

- Explain to the patient that the *Always* end of the scale sometimes means easy listening and sometimes means extreme difficulty in listening. This makes patients consider each item carefully, but unfortunately makes the questionnaire too difficult for some elderly patients to complete.

- Administer the unaided part of the scale before hearing aids are fitted.

- Administer the aided portion several weeks after fitting. Allow the patient to see, and change if they desire, the answers they previously gave for the unaided scale.

- Explain that it will help you to receive an honest account of how well, or poorly, the patient hears when aided, so that you can be sure the hearing aid is adjusted as well as possible.

The steps in this panel are based upon Cox (1997). Further instructions and applications can be found in that paper and in Cox (2000).

Table 13.3 Questionnaires directly assessing improvement in hearing disability or handicap.

	Questionnaire	Authors	Year	No of items
HAPI	Hearing Aid Performance Inventory	Walden, Demorest & Hepler	1984	64
HAUQ	Hearing Aid Users' Questionnaire	Forster & Tomlin	1988	6
HAR	Hearing Aid Review	Brooks	1990	5
SHAPI	Shortened Hearing Aid Performance Inventory	Schum	1992, 1993	38
SHAPIE	Shortened Hearing Aid Performance Inventory for the Elderly	Dillon	1994	25
GPHAB	Glasgow Hearing Aid Benefit Profile	Gatehouse	1999	28-56

Applications of APHAB

- Some predictions can be made about likely benefit from hearing aids, as detailed in Section 8.1.3.
- Patients can be advised how much benefit they get relative to other users of hearing aids and/or how much difficulty they have, when aided and when unaided, relative to normal-hearing people. If they are in doubt about continuing with hearing aids, this may help them decide whether to keep their hearing aids, try other hearing aids, or discontinue attempts to wear hearing aids.
- The relative benefit provided by different types of hearing aids *could* be assessed using APHAB, but the large differences needed for statistical significance make APHAB (and other self-report measures) fairly insensitive for this purpose, except when averaged over a number of people.
- Particularly poor benefit scores in background noise can indicate the need for directional microphones or wireless transmission of signals.
- Large negative scores on the Aversiveness scale can indicate the need for a lower SSPL and/or a higher compression ratio for medium- to high-level signals.

---

correlated with an overall consensus measure of benefit than were scores obtained using the HHIE or a modified version of the PHAB.[d] This advantage may be because the SHAPIE directly measures change. The two questionnaires in Table 13.3 with a very small number of items measuring benefit (HAUQ and HAR) both contain further questions related to other aspects of hearing aid use, as discussed later in this chapter.

13.3 Meeting Needs and Goals

Self-report questionnaires are extremely useful, and have been much used in recent years, particularly the APHAB. There are, however, four main problems with using them:

- Some patients do not like completing them, particularly if many of the items describe situations that the patients consider are irrelevant to them.
- Some clinicians do not like administering them, and if the questionnaires have been self-administered, some clinicians do not like scoring them.
- If the patients spend time in one or two situations in which they would particularly

like to hear more clearly, standard questionnaires will give no insight as to what those situations are, nor what degree of improvement the rehabilitation has provided in those situations.

- Some patients, especially some elderly ones, have difficulty understanding complex questionnaires.

A solution to all three of these problems is to ask each patient to make up his or her own questionnaire. A patient is asked, in an open-ended manner, to list situations in which he or she is having trouble hearing and in which he or she would like to hear more clearly.[36] At the end of the rehabilitation process, the outcomes are assessed for each of these specific situations. Situations are thus never irrelevant to the patient, and the information obtained from the patient at the commencement of rehabilitation may help guide the way the rehabilitation program is organized, or the type of devices that are fitted.

The disadvantage of this approach is that it is more difficult to compare results across patients or across populations.

---

[d]   Unfortunately, the PHAB was not administered in the manner now recommended for the APHAB, in which patients can see and modify their unaided answers while completing the aided scale. The sensitivity of APHAB administered in this way, relative to SHAPIE or other direct measures of benefit, is unknown.

We can liken this type of evaluation more to a structured interview than to administering a questionnaire. There are, however, some parallels with the questionnaire approach. Patients can be asked to directly estimate how much benefit they receive from their hearing aids (the direct assessment of benefit). Alternatively they can be asked how well they hear in each situation when unaided, and then how well they hear when aided. As with the questionnaire methods, the benefit is the difference between the two scores.

Both of these methods have been used. McKenna (1987) applied a technique known as *Goal Attainment Scaling* (*GAS*), that had previously been used in the area of mental health (see Section 8.1.4).[476] At initial interview, two pieces of information are collected for every listening situation: how well the patient initially hears in that situation, and how well he or she would need to hear in that situation if the rehabilitation is to be considered a success. The desired hearing ability is decided after some negotiation between the patient and the clinician. At the end of the rehabilitation program, the patient is asked how well he or she can now hear in each situation. This answer can be compared to both the initial hearing ability (to assess improvement) and to the desired ability (to assess whether any further rehabilitation should be attempted).

The method has advantages and disadvantages similar to the aided-unaided method for questionnaires: We find out about both initial and final disability, but the benefit measure may not be very accurate because it involves subtracting two potentially similar ratings. There is another disadvantage when it is used routinely. Some clinicians say they do not like administering the GAS at the initial interview, before they have established a good relationship with the patient, because of the tediousness of quantifying difficulty and establishing quantitative goals for each listening situation.[228]

These difficulties were overcome by devising the Client Oriented Scale of Improvement (COSI). The broad idea is the same: To administer the COSI, the clinician identifies important individual listening situations at the initial interview, but does not do any quantifying at this stage. The quantitative part of the administration all occurs at the final appointment (see panel on Administering COSI). If the COSI results are expressed as a number, they can be compared to the scores obtained by a large sample of hearing-impaired people with predominantly mild and moderate hearing loss. Figure 13.2 shows the proportion of patients who obtain different COSI change scores. It is apparent that many patients indicate a rating of "much better" (scored as 5.0) for all the listening situations they nominate. This skewing towards high scores makes the COSI unsuitable for detect-

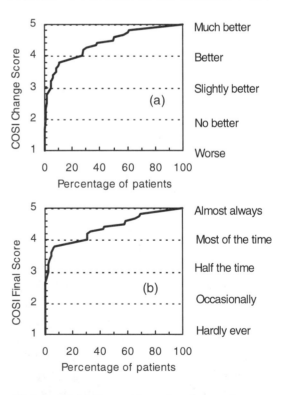

Figure 13. 2 Proportion of patients who obtain less than, or equal to, (a) the COSI change score, and (b) the COSI final score.

Administering COSI

- At the initial interview, identify and write down those specific situations in which the patient would like to hear more clearly. See panel in Section 8.1.4 for more details.

- If some of the listening situations require a different fitting strategy from others, it may be worth finding out what priority or significance the patient places on each of the needs expressed.

- When you believe that the rehabilitation program is completed, read back each of the situations, and for each situation ask the patient (a) how much *more* clearly they now hear in that situation, and (b) how well they can now hear in that situation. The response scales for each of these can be seen in the COSI form reproduced in this section. For indecisive patients, put a check mark on the line midway between the two categories over which they are undecided.

- Evaluate, with the help of the patient, whether the extent of rehabilitation is sufficient for both of you to consider that the program really is completed.

- If you wish to express the results in numerical form, assign 1 point to responses in the left-most column in each section, 2 points for responses in the second column, and so on up to 5 points for the right-most column. Average the number of points across the number of needs listed for that patient. The result will be two scores, each in the range 1 to 5. The first score will describe the benefit of rehabilitation, and the second score will describe the final listening ability of the patient, both averaged across their nominated situations. These can be compared to the normative data shown in Figure 13.2.

- If you wish to compare the results for each listening situation to normative data for that situation (Dillon, Birtles & Lovegrove, 1999), categorise each of the needs into one of the 16 standard categories shown at the foot of the COSI form.

---

ing patients who report scores that are above average, but well suited to detecting patients who report abnormally low benefit.

Having the "items" nominated by the patient only partially solves the problem of some situations being more important than other situations. Although a patient presumably would never nominate a listening need that is irrelevant to that patient, the situations nominated may vary in importance because:

- The patient spends more time in some situations than in others,
- The patient has more difficulty in some situations than in others,
- Understanding everything that is being said is more important in some situations than in others.

Of course, it is possible to ask the patient questions about these things. Dillon, James

and Ginis (1997) asked each subject to rank the importance of the listening situations that each subject nominated, but this did not result in any further increase in the validity of the COSI scores. Gatehouse (1994, 1999) has proposed a method called the *Glasgow Hearing Aid Benefit Profile* (*GHABP*) that measures importance and relevance in a formal way. Patients are asked how often they are in each nominated situation, how difficult each situation is, and how much handicap this difficulty causes. Following rehabilitation they are asked, for each situation, how often they used the hearing aid, how much the hearing aid helps them, how much difficulty they still have, and how satisfied they are with the hearing aid. This obviously provides a lot of information, but quantifying the answers to seven questions for every listening situation makes for a long questionnaire. The seven

NAL
CLIENT ORIENTED SCALE OF IMPROVEMENT

Name :

Audiologist :

Date :   1. Needs Established

2. Outcome Assessed

Category.   New

Return

SPECIFIC NEEDS

Indicate Order of Significance

☐

☐

☐

☐

☐

Categories

1. Conversation with 1 or 2 in quiet
2. Conversation with 1 or 2 in noise
3. Conversation with group in quiet

5. Television/Radio @ normal volume
6. Familiar speaker on phone
7. Unfamiliar speaker on phone

9. Hear front door bell or knock
10. Hear traffic
11. Increased social contact

13. Feeling left out
14. Feeling upset or angry
15. Church or meeting

Degree of Change

					Worse
					No Difference
					Slightly Better
					Better
					Much Better

					CATEGORY

					Hardly Ever
					Occasionally
					Half the Time
					Most of Time
					Almost Always

Final Ability (with hearing aid)

Person can hear

10%   25%   50%   75%   95%

questions are applied to four standard situations and up to an additional four situations nominated by the patient. This gives a total of up to 56 items to be quantified. If the patient indicates that the situation is not experienced, the remaining questions about this situation are not asked, thus decreasing the number of items for that patient. The four standard situations are:

- Listening to television with other people;
- Conversing with one other in quiet;
- Conversing in a busy street or shop;
- Conversing with several people in a group.

The GHABP is based on a longer version that had twelve, and later fourteen, standard situations plus the four individually nominated situations.[303] The research leading to the GHABP showed that including listening situations nominated by individual patients made the questionnaire more sensitive to differences in rehabilitation quality.[304]

13.4 Assessing Usage, Problems, and Satisfaction

Use of hearing aids.
The chapter so far has concentrated on benefits – a reduction in either disability or handicap. As intimated earlier, there are other types of outcomes. Whether a patient wears the hearing aids provided is an outcome, although usage might be regarded as an important means rather than an end. If hearing aids are being worn we cannot deduce how much benefit they provide, but if they are not being worn we can be sure they provide no benefit. Consequently, no use, or much less use than would be expected on the basis of the needs expressed by the patient, are useful indicators that something has gone wrong with the fitting. It is possible, however, for people to report substantial benefit even though they use their hearing aids for only a small amount of time each day or week. Many such people in this category are competent at using their hearing aids, thus supporting their claims that they regularly use and benefit

from their aids, even though they may use them less than one hour per day.[682]

We can most simply determine how much patients use their hearing aid each day or week by asking patients after they have had their hearing aids for a few weeks. We may not get a truthful answer. If patients have been well treated, they may not want to disappoint the clinician by saying they rarely wear their hearing aids. Also, they may see themselves as a failure if they have not learned to use their hearing aids regularly, and may not wish to disclose this fact to the clinician.

Four studies have objectively measured use, based on battery discharge characteristics or electronic timers, and compared the results to subjective estimates of use.[88, 344, 401, 875] These showed that patients overestimated use by an average of 1.4, 0, 4, and 0.3 hours per day, respectively. Some studies show that the extent of the exaggeration is greatest for people who use their hearing aids the least,[86, 88, 344] but the study with the greatest discrepancy had the highest average use.[401]

It may minimize exaggeration if patients are first asked to state in which situations they have found their hearing aids to be useful, and in which situations they have found it not worthwhile to wear them. (This also lets them know that stating they do not wear their hearing aids is an acceptable answer.) Following this they can be asked: *On an average day, for how many hours would you wear your hearing aids?* They can be asked to respond with either their estimate of the number of hours, or can be presented with some categories of use, such as:

- >8 hours per day,
- 4 to 8 hours per day,
- 1 to 4 hours per day,
- less than 1 hour per day,
- more than 1 hour per week, but less than 1 hour per day,
- less than 1 hour per week.

These are, in fact the response choices offered in the *Hearing Aid User's Questionnaire*

(*HAUQ*; Forster & Tomlin, 1988; Dillon, Birtles & Lovegrove, 1999), and are sufficiently differentiated to identify patients who are using their hearing aids so little that the clinician will want to investigate further. The *Hearing Aid Review* questionnaire contains three questions on use, as well as questions on benefit and satisfaction.[92]

Alternatively, for each of a range of situations, patients can be asked what proportion of the time they wear their hearing aids when they are in that situation. This is the approach taken in the GHABP.[304]

Detecting problems with the hearing aids

An absence of problems (e.g. whistling, earmold discomfort) with the hearing aids is obviously desirable. One could argue that a lack of problems caused by the hearing aid hardly qualifies as an outcome of rehabilitation. Avoiding problems is nevertheless an important means to ensuring usage and hence benefit. Not surprisingly, the extent of problems with hearing aids is negatively correlated with the benefits that patients get

---

Problems to specifically ask each patient about

- Own voice quality
- Whistling
- Earmold/earshell discomfort
- Aid insertion and removal
- Operation of controls
- Battery changing
- Loudness discomfort
- Inappropriate loudness of speech
- Inappropriate loudness of background sounds
- Sound quality
- Telephone use
- Internal aid noise
- Loudness balance between ears

When the presence of problems is being assessed in person (as opposed to a phone or mail assessment) some of these problem areas can be assessed by observation of the patient instead of by asking.

---

from hearing aids, and with the satisfaction they express.[225] Chapter 11 discussed methods for solving typical problems, but before problems can be solved, they have to be detected. Detection is most likely if the clinician asks patients specifically about each of the typical problems that occur (see panel).

Questionnaires to assess the presence of problems are reasonably easy to construct. Such questionnaires simply involve asking a series of questions such as: *Do you have any problems getting the hearing aid into your ear?* The precise wording is, however, important if patients are to interpret each question in the way intended by the clinician. One questionnaire addressing problems with the hearing aid is the HAUQ.

Satisfaction with hearing aids

It has become very common to measure how satisfied patients are with their hearing aids and it is easy to see why it is important. Satisfaction probably expresses how happy the patients are with their hearing aids, taking into consideration how much (or little) the hearing aids help in different situations, how easy or hard they are to use, the financial and psychological cost of obtaining and wearing hearing aids, and the expectations that patients had about all of these things.

Considering the complexity of all these factors, it is surprising that it is sensible to ask a simple question: *How satisfied are you with your hearing aids?* The answers to this question are moderately correlated with much more complicated measures of benefit.[228] The accompanying panel shows two simple one-item questionnaires. The Hearing Aid Review includes a similar ten-point scale and was shown to have reasonable test-retest reliability.[92] A four-point scale is used in the HAUQ questionnaire, although the five-point version shown in the panel may be less affected by ceiling effects. There are, however, two problems with measuring *only* satisfaction as a summary of the effectiveness of the hearing aids.

Two simple satisfaction questionnaires

The two questionnaires below provide a simple measure of satisfaction. The second may be more sensitive to small differences in satisfaction[228] but answers to the first may be more interpretable.

1. Overall, how satisfied are you with your hearing aid(s)?
    a) Extremely satisfied
    b) Satisfied
    c) Neither satisfied nor dissatisfied
    d) Dissatisfied
    e) Extremely dissatisfied

2. On a scale of 0 to 100, how satisfied are you, overall, with your hearing aid(s)? A score of 0 means that you are not at all satisfied, and a score of 100 means that you are totally satisfied. Please state any number in between, (or mark the scale at the position) that corresponds to how satisfied you feel.

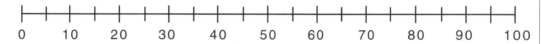

The first problem is one of relativity: The patient does not know what the best available hearing aids would be like, or even what perfect hearing aids would be like. As Ross and Levitt (1997) have expressed the problem: *"Are you satisfied compared to what?"* Their summary succinctly states why achieving satisfaction should not be the major goal of a clinician: *"Hearing aids are still supposed to help people hear better and not just feel better."*

In studies where different hearing aids are compared sequentially, it is not unusual for subjects to say that a hearing aid is "perfect" and far better than anything they previously experienced, but for them subsequently to say that a later hearing aid is even better! By contrast, some patients may have such high expectations of having their hearing restored to normal functioning (or better!) that even the best possible fitting, providing a substantial increase in hearing ability, may not make them very satisfied. The biggest determinant of their satisfaction may be how well the clinician modified their expectations prior to fitting hearing aids. This limitation does not apply when satisfaction is used in a relative way. If we examine which of two different

hearing aid types a patient is more satisfied with, it does not matter what internal scale the patient uses for satisfaction. This is not a viable solution in clinical settings, because we rarely have the luxury of trying several different types of aids or sets of performance characteristics on patients over an extended period.

The second problem is that an overall rating of satisfaction does not tell you anything that is immediately useful! If a patient says that he or she is only slightly satisfied, the answer reveals nothing about the cause of that dissatisfaction. It is, however, worth measuring satisfaction routinely with at least a single item question. Any answer less than *extremely satisfied* (or its equivalent in the questionnaire you use) provides you with the opportunity to ask follow-on questions, the answers to which may reveal some causes of dissatisfaction that you can do something about. The follow-on questions can be open-ended, such as *Which aspects of the hearing aid are you least satisfied with?*, and *Which aspects of the hearing aid are you most satisfied with?*

One study asked subjects to rate overall satisfaction along with satisfaction for each of a large range of factors related to the hearing aids and the way they were dispensed.[478] The factors most related to overall satisfaction were all related to improved hearing in different situations, but many other types of factors (e.g. fit and comfort, dispenser counseling, ease of use, warranty, battery life) were also related to overall satisfaction.

Cox and Alexander (1999) have provided us with a simple questionnaire to better understand the components of satisfaction. Structured interviews with patients indicated that the things affecting satisfaction could be grouped into six domains:

- Cosmetics and self-image,
- Sound quality and acoustics,
- Benefit,
- Comfort and ease of use,
- Cost,
- Service.

Cox & Alexander devised 25 questions addressing these categories, and based on the questions' statistical properties (see panel in Section 13.2.1), they selected 15 items to form the *Satisfaction with Amplification in Daily Life* scale (*SADL*). Items in the SADL are grouped into four sub-scales:

- *Positive effect* – comprising decreased communication disability, improved self-confidence, improved sound quality, and an overall assessment of worth.
- *Service and cost* – comprising reliability, clinician competence, and cost.
- *Negative features* – comprising reaction to background sounds, feedback and the hearing aid's usefulness on the telephone.
- *Personal image* – comprising appearance and the apparent reaction of others.

The SADL thus provides a systematic way in which the reasons for low overall satisfaction can be discerned, with a view to correcting them. Of course, just asking the patient why he or she is dissatisfied is another option. However, Cox & Alexander comment that single negative statements by a patient in response to such open-ended questions might conceal other concerns. When one sub-scale has a much lower score than the other sub-scales, the clinician can be more confident about the reasons for the dissatisfaction.

13.5 Changes in Outcomes with Time after Fitting

When should outcomes be assessed? The answer may look simple: at the end of the last appointment. Even if this is adopted, the timing of this last appointment relative to the fitting is still largely determined by the clinician. On the one hand, we want the outcomes evaluation to be soon after fitting, so that if the evaluation reveals that significant problems remain, these can be addressed as soon as possible. On the other hand, some problems might not emerge until the patients have become sufficiently experienced with their hearing aids. Similarly, patients may not appreciate the full advantages their hearing aids provide until they have become sufficiently experienced with their use.

Experimentally, all types of outcomes scores appear to change during at least the first few weeks after aid fitting. As long as sixty years ago, Berry (1939) referred to increases in speech identification during the months after fitting as a *process of adjustment*. Watson & Knudsen (1940) reported an increase in speech identification of 40 percentage points over the three months following aid fitting for one subject.[e] They refer to this process as *accommodation*. The changes in speech identification ability that occur during the first few months following fitting are now referred to as *acclimatization*.[302, 397] An extensive survey of experimental results indicated, however, that the increase averages

---

e   This subject had a long-standing severe hearing loss, and was receiving a hearing aid for the first time, an unusual combination of circumstances these days. It may be that the magnitude of the acclimatization effect increases with the magnitude of the change in audibility that occurs when a hearing aid is worn.

only a few percentage points, and is therefore usually too small to be significant with individual patients.[894]

Self-reported benefit, measured using APHAB scores, also increases from two weeks post-fitting to three months post-fitting.[168] By contrast, there is *less* handicap (based on HHIE scores) three weeks after fitting than there is three months after fitting.[571, 876] This is particularly true for the emotional subscale of the HHIE. Similarly, there is higher satisfaction two weeks after fitting than twelve months after fitting.[592]

It appears that there may be a halo or honeymoon effect a few weeks after fitting. Noble (1999) hypothesizes that shortly after fitting, tensions at home resulting from poor communication ability have been dissipated by the patient seeking rehabilitation and by the beneficial effects of the hearing aids on communication at home. As more time passes, the patient becomes aware of situations in which the hearing aids provide minimal benefit, so self-reported handicap increases, although not to the level reported prior to rehabilitation. Reduced satisfaction may also result from an increased awareness of the limitations of hearing aids.

Self-assessed outcomes appear to settle down from about six weeks after fitting. Satisfaction, handicap reduction (HHIE scores), attainment of goals (GAS scores), and change in listening ability (COSI scores) all appear to be no different six weeks after fitting than they are three months after fitting.[228, 230] Handicap reduction (HHIE scores) and communication function (Denver Scale of Communication scores) are both little different six weeks after fitting than four months after fitting.[633] Handicap reduction measured at three months is unchanged when it is measured at various later times up to one year after fitting.[571, 635, 876] Similarly, both objectively measured benefit (speech identification ability) and subjectively measured benefit (PHAB scores) appear to be the same

one year after fitting as they were six weeks after fitting.[864] There is conflicting evidence regarding changes in hearing aid usage during the first year. Mulrow, Tuley & Aguilar (1992b) found a decrease in the number of hours per day that hearing aids were worn whereas Brooks (1981) found an increase.

There is slightly conflicting evidence regarding changes over periods longer than a year. Usage may either remain stable four years after fitting,[378] or may decrease slightly.[511] The long-term decrease is small, and is probably caused by patients making more refined decisions about the situations in which hearing aids are helpful.

In any situation where payment for a device and services is linked to demonstrating a favorable outcome, there is great advantage in the patient having a 45 or 60 day trial rather than the commonly offered 30-day trial. The longer trial period, which has apparently been requested by the consumer organization, Self Help for the Hard of Hearing, is consistent with the time needed for benefits to stabilize. There is, however, no reason a single time has to be chosen:

- One measure (e.g. APHAB or COSI) can be administered at the end of the regular appointments, which may well be within the current 30-day period during which patients can return their hearing aids at no cost to themselves.

- Another measure (e.g. HAUQ) can be administered 6 to 12 weeks after fitting to

> **Conclusion: changes in outcomes with time**
>
> Taken together, these studies imply that self-reported use and benefit is reasonably stable by six weeks after fitting, although small changes may occur for many months or years thereafter. The first few weeks following fitting does therefore not seem to be the best time for evaluation, though for practical reasons, it is often the most convenient time.

ensure that any problems subsequently found are discovered and dealt with. HAUQ also provides simple measures of usage, benefit, and satisfaction. The Hearing Aid Review (HAR)[92] is similar except that it does not address specific problems with the hearing aid. The last check can be performed by mail or by telephone to minimize the cost of administering it, and both HAUQ and HAR have been designed with this application in mind.

13.6 Impact of Hearing Aids on General Health and Quality of Life

Untreated hearing loss is associated with a general decrease in physical and psychosocial well being.[61] It is possible that hearing aids can also cause a patient's general health to improve. The logic of this is as follows.

- Hearing impairment decreases a person's ability to communicate.
- Decreased communication with others can lead to a range of negative emotions such as depression, loneliness, anxiety, paranoia, exhaustion, insecurity, loss of group affiliation, loss of intimacy, and anger.[379, 428, 892]
- Negative emotions can affect general health.
- Hearing aids increase a person's ability to communicate, and can therefore partially reverse the above trends.

Various aspects of this reversal have been documented. In a randomized and controlled prospective study, hearing aids have been shown to lessen depression and other negative emotions associated with hearing loss.[635] These benefits were established by four months after hearing aid fitting and were still present 12 months after fitting. Other studies have measured increased psychosocial well-being, including increased social interaction, increased alertness, increased leisure activity, improved mood, decreased paranoia, less

depression, improved memory, and improved ability to learn following hearing aid fitting.[187, 252]

Several studies have found that, on numerous counts, hearing-impaired people with hearing aids fare better than hearing-impaired people without hearing aids. Those who use hearing aids report better mood, less depression, greater participation in social activities, warmer inter-personal relationships, greater self-sufficiency, more positive self-image, less self-perceived discrimination, greater emotional stability, greater control of their lives, better health, less anger, less paranoia, less anxiety, less self-criticism, less introversion (as assessed by others) and a greatly decreased mortality rate.[26, 78, 355, 484]

Of course, significant correlations do not prove that hearing rehabilitation *causes* the improved health outcomes. It is possible that better-adjusted and healthier people are more likely to seek rehabilitation, but it seems unlikely that this is the sole reason for improved quality of life amongst those with hearing aids. Certainly, people report retrospectively that they experienced many of these benefits as a *consequence* of obtaining hearing aids.[484]

Despite the connection between hearing rehabilitation and general mental and physical health, so many other things impact on general health that it is not sensible to assess the outcomes of hearing rehabilitation for an individual patient by measuring general health.[633] When we attempt to describe the outcomes of hearing rehabilitation for a population, however, it would be wise not to overlook the beneficial effects of hearing aids on general health. It would also be appropriate to mention to prospective hearing aid wearers that the benefits of hearing aids extend far beyond simply hearing better.[484] Crandell (1998a) gives a longer review of this topic.

There is a need for well-controlled research studies that enable us to better identify and quantify all the effects of hearing loss on general well-being. Such research may also allow us to compare the general health effects of hearing rehabilitation to the results of treatment for other disabilities and diseases.

13.7 Concluding Comments

Should clinicians routinely measure outcomes? If so, which measurement tools should a clinician routinely use? If a third party (e.g. an insurer) demands proof of benefit, then the clinician must use some formal measurement tool like the ones described in this chapter. What if there is no external demand for a measurement of outcomes? "Outcomes" are multi-faceted, and there are good reasons why a clinician should find out if patients are using their hearing aids, are deriving benefit from them, are satisfied, and have any remaining problems that can be dealt with.

These things *can* all be done to some extent without using any questionnaire or formal procedure. The use of a systematic procedure, however, makes it more likely that a clinician *will* check these things. The use of a formal procedure, whether it be APHAB, COSI, GHABP, HAUQ, HHIE, SADL, SHAPIE or any of the other acronyms may well teach or remind clinicians about the type of questions they should ask. Clinicians may continue to ask these questions even when they are not using a formal procedure. Each of these questionnaires offers a unique perspective:

- APHAB teaches that hearing aids will be more effective in some situations than in others, and may have adverse effects on intense sounds.

- COSI teaches about the importance of identifying and solving the specific hearing problems that caused the patient to seek help in the first place.

- GHABP gives a well-rounded picture of the disability, handicap, benefit, use, and satisfaction that patients experience in a range of situations.

- HAUQ teaches the importance of following up on whether all mechanical

and electroacoustic aspects of the fitting have been adequately dealt with and provides simple, single item measures of usage and satisfaction.

- HHIE shows us how much hearing aids and other rehabilitation have affected the lifestyle and emotions of the patient.

- SHAPIE is a relatively sensitive tool for examining the degree of disability reduction, but is probably more suitable for research studies or comparative evaluations than for routine clinical use.

- SADL enables us to analyze the reasons why a patient may not be fully satisfied.

In summary, whether we use a formal or an informal procedure, it is worth finding out *something* about each of:

- Benefit (e.g. APHAB, COSI, GHABP, HHIE, or SHAPIE),

- Aided performance (e.g. APHAB, COSI, GHABP, HHIE, or speech discrimination tests),

- Usage,

- Problems with the hearing aids (e.g. HAUQ), and

- Satisfaction (an overall rating, and if a low rating is obtained, following up with either informal questioning or the SADL).

Numerous studies have shown that the various types of measures are partially, but imperfectly, correlated with each other.[399] As Brooks (1990) points out, a high rating on one type of outcome in conjunction with a low rating on another alerts the clinician that there may be further work to do on either the fitting, instructions to the patient, or discussion with the patient about his or her expectations relative to the performance achievable with available technology. Furthermore, as self-report measures become more sophisticated and detailed, they teach us what has to be attended to during service provision, and what questions we should ask when we think that service provision is finished.

CHAPTER FOURTEEN

BINAURAL AND BILATERAL CONSIDERATIONS IN HEARING AID FITTING

Synopsis

Sensing sounds in two ears (binaural hearing) makes it possible for a person to locate the source of sounds and increases speech intelligibility in noisy situations. Wearing two hearing aids (a bilateral fitting) instead of one hearing aid (a unilateral fitting) increases the range of sound levels for which binaural hearing is possible. Bilateral fitting is thus increasingly important as hearing loss increases.

Accurate horizontal localization is possible because sounds reaching the two ears differ in level and in arrival time, and hence in phase. These cues are also present, but altered, when people wear hearing aids. Most hearing-impaired people, once they become used to the effect of their hearing aids on these cues, can localize sounds accurately in the horizontal plane. Vertical localization, which is based on very high-frequency cues created by the pinna, is very adversely affected by hearing loss and is not improved by hearing aids.

When speech and noise arrive from different directions, head diffraction causes the signal-to-noise ratio to be greater at one ear than at the other. A person with two hearing aids benefits from this by selectively attending to the ear with the clearer signal. Further, the auditory system can combine the different mixtures of speech and noise arriving at each ear to effectively remove some of the noise. This ability is known as binaural squelch.

Bilateral fitting of hearing aids has several other advantages. These include improved sound quality, suppression of tinnitus in both ears, and greater convenience when one hearing aid breaks down. In addition, a unilateral fitting can lead to decreased speech processing ability in the unaided ear if this ear is deprived of auditory stimulation for too long.

The advantages of bilateral fittings also apply to patients with asymmetrical hearing thresholds. If such patients must receive a unilateral fitting, it may be generally advisable to fit the ear with thresholds closest to about 60 dB HL.

Bilateral fittings also have disadvantages: they cost more, are more susceptible to wind noise, and are more difficult for some elderly people to manage. Also, some people regard two hearing aids as an indication of severe hearing loss, and do not wish to be perceived in this way. For a small proportion of people, inappropriate fusion of the signals presented to the two ears causes speech identification ability to be better when unilaterally aided than when bilaterally aided.

Because of the variability associated with speech intelligibility testing, conditions have to be chosen carefully to reliably demonstrate bilateral advantage on an individual patient. Loudspeaker positions should be chosen to maximize both head diffraction and binaural squelch. Speech tests with steep performance-intensity functions should be used.

There are many advantages to listening with two ears instead of one. Using two ears enables a person to understand more when speech is heard in background noise or when there is reverberation. The ability to localize sounds is highly dependent on being able to perceive sounds simultaneously in both ears. Loss of hearing in one ear will therefore leave a person with a considerable hearing deficit in many listening situations.[155] Similarly, when a person has a moderate or severe loss in both ears but wears a hearing aid in only one ear, a considerable deficit remains. A normal-hearing person can gain some appreciation of this by blocking one ear while trying to listen in a noisy and/or reverberant environment. Noises that were previously not noticed suddenly become apparent. It becomes very difficult to listen to, and understand, one particular signal in the midst of all this noise. Sounds will also be difficult to localize.

Despite the difficulties that arise from listening with only one ear, the question of how many hearing aids a person should have is not as simple as just fitting everybody with two hearing aids.

The purpose of this chapter is to outline the factors underlying the following decisions that the clinician has to make for every patient:

- Should one or two hearing aids be recommended?
- If the patient disagrees with the recommendation, how important is it to attempt to convince the patient to decide otherwise?
- If one hearing aid is provided, in which ear should it be worn?

A hearing aid in each ear is commonly called a *binaural fitting*, as contrasted to a *monaural fitting*. This book, however, will follow the terminology suggested by Noble & Byrne (1991) and refer to these conditions as a *bilateral fitting* and a *unilateral fitting* respectively. Appropriate terminology can help us appreciate the real situation:

- A person with a hearing aid in one ear is still able to hear many sounds in both ears (at least for people with mild and moderate losses) and thus hears many sounds binaurally.
- A person with hearing aids in both ears may not hear some sounds in one ear, and it is possible that sounds heard in one ear will interfere with sounds heard in the other.

These simple examples show that a unilateral fitting does not always imply monaural hearing, and a bilateral fitting does not necessarily imply that sounds in both ears will contribute positively towards perception. Consistent with these definitions, *binaural advantage* will be used in this chapter to mean the advantage of listening with two ears instead of one. *Bilateral advantage* will refer to the advantage of listening through two hearing aids rather than one.

The fitting of two hearing aids is now more common than the fitting of one. One large survey in 1994 indicated that, in the USA, 65% of people who obtained hearing aids in the previous 12 months obtained a bilateral fitting.[482] This average bilateral rate in no way indicates a rate that each clinician should feel obliged to mimic. Indeed, a decade earlier,

---

Some definitions

Binaural stimulation: Sounds are presented to (or perceived in) both ears.

Monaural stimulation: Sounds are presented to (or perceived in) one ear.

Bilateral fitting: Hearing aids are worn in both ears.

Unilateral fitting: A hearing aid is worn in one ear.

Diotic: Identical sounds are presented to both ears.

Dichotic: A different sound is presented to each ear.

the rate was only 25%.[482] The average bilateral fitting rate indicates only what *is* being done, not what *should* be done.

Not everyone who receives two hearing aids wears them. In one survey of over 4000 patients, 48% of patients had been fitted bilaterally. Most of these (94%) reported, three months after the fitting that they used hearing aids regularly. Of the bilaterally fitted, regular hearing aid users, however, 20% reported that they only used one hearing aid.[225]

There is overwhelming evidence that two hearing aids provides better performance than one for most people in most situations, and this evidence has been available for nearly two decades. For excellent reviews see Byrne (1980, 1981) and Ross (1980). Nonetheless, bilateral hearing aids are not the best choice for all hearing-impaired persons, particularly when one takes cost, self-image, listening needs, aid management ability, and some central factors into account. Every clinician must therefore have a clear understanding of the benefits and limitations of two hearing aids relative to one. The first two sections of this chapter will review the advantages and mechanisms of listening with two ears instead of one, for both normal-hearing and hearing-impaired people. We will then apply these concepts to clinical decisions about fitting one versus two hearing aids, and to testing bilateral advantage.

14.1 Binaural Effects in Localization

14.1.1 Localization cues in normal hearing

Localization of sounds can conveniently be discussed under the headings: horizontal localization, vertical localization, front-back differentiation, externalization, and distance perception. The last of these is not as well

understood as the others. Distance perception depends on perception of reverberation, echoes, and overall spectral shape. Hearing impairment adversely affects distance perception.[661] The effect of hearing aids on distance perception has not been studied and will not be further discussed here.

Horizontal localization is made possible by differences in time and intensity between the two ears. As is evident from Figure 14.1, sounds will arrive at the ear closer to the source (the *near ear*) before they arrive at the other ear (the *far ear*). The resulting difference in arrival time at the two ears is called the *interaural time difference*. It depends on the size of the head and the speed of sound. The interaural time difference is zero for frontally incident sound and increases to a maximum of about 0.7 ms for sounds coming from 90° with respect to the front, as shown in Figure 14.2.[a] Because any time delay leads to a phase delay, an interaural time difference results in an *interaural phase difference*.

As frequency increases, this phase cue becomes increasingly ambiguous for sounds that do not have rapid onsets or offsets. Once frequency is high enough for the time differ-

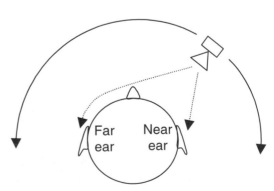

Horizontal localization

Figure 14.1 Variation of the source direction in the horizontal plane.

---

[a]   Interaural time differences for high-frequency sounds are about two-thirds of the value for low-frequency sounds, because of the complexities of sound diffraction around the head (Kuhn, 1977).

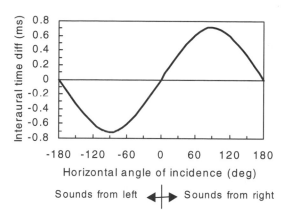

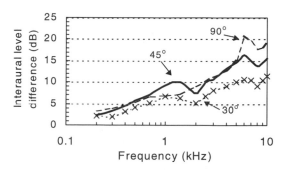

Figure 14.3 Interaural level difference for three source directions in the horizontal plane. Data are calculated from Shaw (1974). Interaural level differences are zero for frontally incident sound.

Figure 14.2 Interaural time difference for low-frequency sounds as a function of direction measured from directly in front. Data are the average of measurements on people and on a manikin (Kuhn, 1982).

ence to cause more than half a cycle of phase shift for sounds coming from the side, multiple source directions will lead to the same interaural phase difference. This occurs for frequencies higher than about 700 Hz. Also, neural responses are highly synchronized to the sound waveform only for low-frequency sounds. Interaural phase difference is thus a useful cue only for low-frequency sounds. Interaural time differences are, however, also present in the **envelope** of sounds, and thus *can* be conveyed across the whole frequency range.[376] Time difference cues are nevertheless carried most efficiently by the low-frequency components of sounds, up to about 1500 Hz.[619, 964, 965, 975]

The head acts as acoustic barrier and causes a level difference between the ears. **Head diffraction** produces an attenuation of sound on the far side of the head and this is usually referred to as **head shadow.** Head diffraction also produces a boost on the near side of the head. Both effects have the greatest magnitude for high-frequency sounds (see Section 1.2.1). The resulting **interaural level differences** are thus much more pronounced at high frequencies.

Figure 14.3 shows how the interaural level difference varies with frequency for three source directions. Level difference cues are most valuable for high frequencies, above about 1500 Hz. Horizontal localization accuracy is in fact, worst at 1500 Hz, presumably because neither the time nor level difference cues are entirely effective around this frequency.[603] Horizontal localization accuracy is most precise for frequencies around 800 Hz and for sources directly in front. Under these conditions, people can detect differences in source direction as small as 1°, corresponding to an interaural time difference of only 10 µs.[603] At 1500 Hz this rises to about 3°.

The relative importance of interaural time and level differences can be deduced from experiments in which signals are presented to the two ears with conflicting time and level difference cues. There is a trading relationship between the cues, which confirms the dominance of time cues for low-frequency sounds, and the dominance of level difference cues for high-frequency sounds. For complex, broadband sounds, the time cues carried in the parts of the signal below 1500 Hz appear to dominate.[770, 959, 975]

In summary, accurate and easy horizontal localization is possible provided the low-frequency components of sounds are clearly audible in both ears.

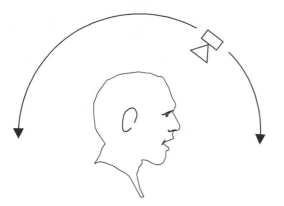

Vertical localization

Figure 14.4 Variation of the source direction in the vertical plane.

Vertical localization in the mid-sagittal (or medial) plane is made possible by reflections and resonances that occur within the pinna prior to sound entering the ear canal.[103, 373, 756, 800, 943] These reflections cause cancellations, and hence spectral peaks and notches, at frequencies that depend on the elevation of the source relative to the head. The resulting cues to localization in the mid-sagittal vertical plane are all above 5 kHz, because it is only in this high-frequency region that the wavelength of sound is small enough, compared to the size of the pinna, for the necessary reflections and resonances to occur. People can detect changes in vertical angle as small as 3°.[698] Sources that are not in the mid-sagittal plane are localized by a combination of pinna effects and interaural time and intensity differences.

Front-back localization is less well understood, but depends in part on spectral balance. The pinna boosts high-frequency sounds when they arrive from the front, but attenuates them when they arrive from the rear.[637, 638] Front-back localization may also depend on fine spectral features below 2 kHz.[29] Sound during the first few milliseconds of a signal has a particularly strong influence on perceived direction.[70]

Externalization refers to the perception that a sound is originating from some point in space outside the head. For sounds to be externalized, there must be appropriate interaural time and level differences at the ears, including those caused by resonances in the pinna.[251] This is achieved if the *head related transfer function (HRTF)*, from the source location to each eardrum, is appropriate to the position of the source.[957] The HRTF, and hence the interaural time and level differences, must also vary appropriately as a person moves his or her head.[b] Reverberation adds to the sense of externalization. Although people become used to their individual HRTFs, it is possible to achieve good externalization with sounds that have been altered by someone else's HRTF.[251] Thus, sounds that have been recorded through a dummy head and played back over headphones with a suitable flat frequency response can be readily externalized.

Mills (1972) and Wightman & Kistler (1993) both give a more detailed review of localization.

14.1.2 Effects of hearing loss on localization

Patients do not often spontaneously complain about poor localization ability. When specifically questioned about localization, however, patients are likely to be aware of difficulties they face because of poor localization, particularly if they have a severe hearing loss.[126] Some researchers consider that impaired localization is one of the two biggest problems caused by hearing loss.[434]

Impaired localization may also contribute to the biggest problem – listening in noise. Difficulty in following a conversation between a group of people may be exacerbated by being unable to quickly locate the person talking, particularly when the conversation switches rapidly between

---

b　Head movements also help with all other aspects of localization, as they can be used to resolve ambiguous cues that can otherwise occur (Perrett & Noble, 1970; Wallach, 1940). Head movement also helps people with unilateral deafness to localize horizontally provided the sound lasts long enough to listen using several head orientations.

speakers.[126] Our sense of localization helps us assign a separate identity to sounds that come from different directions.[39] Without this identification of different sound sources, multiple noises may become a confusing general background, rather than a collection of individual sounds that can be perceived, and ignored if desired. When hearing aids are worn for the first time, localization is likely to be disrupted (see Section 14.3.4), possibly contributing to the common experience that hearing aids seem to amplify noise more than they do speech.

Poor localization ability can create a feeling of being isolated from the environment, potentially contributing to a feeling of anxiety.[270] Difficulty in locating environmental sounds can be inconvenient, or in some situations can put the hearing-impaired person in danger.

As low-frequency sensorineural hearing loss (below 1500 Hz) increases, horizontal localization ability gradually deteriorates.[659, 660] Provided sounds are audible in both ears, however, very little deterioration occurs until low-frequency hearing loss exceeds about 50 dB HL.[128] In the low frequencies, many signals have their most intense components, hearing loss is usually least, and neural responses remain phase locked to stimuli. Consequently, interaural time difference cues presumably remain available. The difficulties in localization reported by people with mild or moderate hearing loss must then primarily be due to some sounds being inaudible (or at a very low sensation level) in at least one ear, rather than an inability to use information that is well above threshold at each ear.[126] Adequate audibility is achieved if the sounds are more than 10 dB above threshold.[575]

When one ear is occluded, localization in the horizontal plane initially deteriorates greatly, as would be expected, because horizontal localization depends primarily on differences between the signals at the two ears. However, the ability to discriminate frontal from backward sources remains, because this distinction can be made based on spectral shape. In addition, individuals can become accustomed, over several days, to sound being softer in one ear than in the other, and can then use interaural level differences to localize sounds.[289] Indeed, when an artificially induced attenuation in one ear is removed, it also takes some days for normal localization ability to return.[289]

Other binaural phenomena also occur for asymmetrical sensation of sound. Binaural beats[c] can be perceived even when the sensation level in one ear is 50 dB greater than the sensation level in the other.[887] Good horizontal localization ability should therefore be possible even for an asymmetrical hearing loss provided the sound is audible in both ears.

Vertical localization, by contrast, deteriorates markedly with hearing loss.[126, 128, 736] In the high frequencies, most sounds have their least intensity, hearing loss is usually greatest, and frequency resolution is often adversely affected. Consequently, high-frequency components of a signal will often not be audible. Even when high-frequency components are audible, listeners with sensorineural hearing loss may not have enough frequency selectivity to identify the frequencies at which the important peaks and troughs occur.[126] Vertical localization ability in the mid-sagittal plane is decreased only slightly by occlusion of one ear, provided the other ear has normal hearing.[372, 673] This is understandable because the necessary spectral cues will be available to the normal-hearing ear.

By contrast with sensorineural hearing loss, conductive hearing loss causes a marked reduction in localization ability.[250, 659] As conductive loss increases, a greater

---

[c]   Binaural beats occur when there is a small frequency difference between the sounds presented to the two ears. See Moore (1989) for a more detailed discussion on this and other aspects of binaural interactions.

proportion of the sound that activates the cochlea is carried by bone conduction rather than by air conduction and middle-ear transmission. Inter-aural attenuation is much lower for bone-conducted sound than for air conducted sound, so interaural time and level differences at the cochlea may be much less than the corresponding differences at the eardrum.[659, 973] Also, phase differences between the bone and air paths can markedly alter inter-aural phase differences when the two paths combine at the cochlea, even when the bone-conducted sound is much weaker than the air-conducted sound.

Section 14.3.4 will outline the advantages of bilateral versus unilateral hearing aids for localization. Byrne & Noble (1998) give an excellent and more detailed review of the effects of hearing loss and hearing aids on localization.

14.2 Binaural Effects in Detection and Recognition

In noisy and/or reverberant environments, people can understand speech much more clearly with two ears than with one. The ability to combine information at the two ears in order to listen to one person talking in the midst of many people talking at similar levels is often called the *cocktail party effect*.

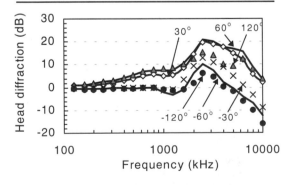

Figure 14.5 Head diffraction effects from the undisturbed field to the eardrum for five source directions in the horizontal plane, with positive angles representing sound arriving from the side of the ear in question. Data are from Shaw (1974).

There are three reasons why people can more easily understand speech with two ears than with one. The first of these arises from *head diffraction* effects and is a purely acoustic phenomenon. The second is referred to as *binaural squelch* and relies on the brain taking advantage of differences between the signals arriving at the two ears.[135] The third, which will be referred to as *binaural redundancy*, also relies on the brain being able to combine signals arriving at the two ears, but does not require the signals at the two ears to be different.[356]

14.2.1 Head diffraction effects

Figure 14.5 shows head diffraction effects to the eardrum for sounds arriving at the head from five directions in the horizontal plane. (Note that around 3 kHz, diffraction effects are positive even for sounds arriving from the far side of the head. This boost occurs because all curves include the effects of the ear canal resonance.)

A person able to listen with both ears can benefit from head diffraction effects just by attending to the ear with the better SNR. The

> **Example: How head diffraction changes SNR**
>
> The following example shows how head diffraction (including head boost and head shadow) alters the SNR at each ear. Suppose that speech was arriving at 30° from the right and that noise was arriving at 60° from the left, as shown in Figure 14.6. At 3 kHz, the ear canal and head will boost the speech in the right ear by 19 dB, but because of head shadow, the noise will be boosted by only 8 dB. The SNR will therefore be 11 dB *greater* at the right eardrum than it would be in the undisturbed field. In the left ear the opposite happens. Speech is boosted by only 11 dB whereas noise is boosted by 20 dB. Consequently, the SNR at the left eardrum is 9 dB *worse* than in the undisturbed field.

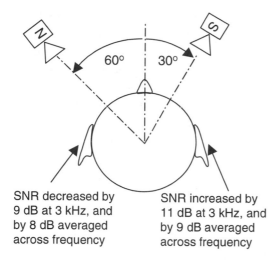

SNR decreased by 9 dB at 3 kHz, and by 8 dB averaged across frequency

SNR increased by 11 dB at 3 kHz, and by 9 dB averaged across frequency

Figure 14.6 Effect of head diffraction on the SNR at each ear, relative to the SNR in the undisturbed field. The SNR at the right ear is thus 20 dB better than at the left ear at 3 kHz, and 17 dB better when averaged across frequency.

effect on speech can be estimated by weighting the improvement in SNR at each frequency by the importance function used in the Speech Intelligibility Index.[331] For the orientations shown in Figure 14.6, the weighted-average SNR will increase at the right ear by 9 dB and will decrease at the left ear by 8 dB. The ear nearer the speech will thus effectively have a SNR 9 dB higher than in the undisturbed field, and 17 dB higher than at the far ear.

By contrast, head diffraction will severely disadvantage a person who can hear in only one ear if the good ear is on the side of the noise and opposite the side of the speech.

The magnitude of these head diffraction effects is very large – enough in some situations to make speech totally understandable at one ear and totally incomprehensible at the other. In many circumstances, the effects of head diffraction will be less than those indicated above. First, reverberation will diminish the differences in speech and noise levels arriving at each ear. This will be especially true when the listener is sufficiently far from the sources of both

speech and noise that diffuse sounds dominate the direct sounds. In the extreme case of a listener in a reverberant room, far from both the speech and noise sources, head diffraction will have no effect on the SNR at either ear. Second, the effects of head diffraction on speech intelligibility will be small if the SNR is already so large over part of the frequency range that further improvements do not help. Nonetheless, head diffraction has a substantial effect on understanding speech in many real-life situations.

Head diffraction effects are a purely physical effect, so in a given situation, the SNR at each frequency will be affected in the same way for a hearing-impaired person as for a normal-hearing person. (There will be minor differences when the hearing-impaired person is aided, because of microphone location effects.) For people with a steeply sloping high-frequency hearing loss, however, the benefit of head diffraction effects will be less than for normal-hearing persons. Individuals with steeply sloping high-frequency losses will usually be more reliant on low-frequency cues, where head diffraction effects are less pronounced. Also, an improved SNR at high frequencies will not benefit a hearing-impaired person if the high-frequency components of speech are below hearing thresholds.[83] This situation will often occur when the hearing-impaired person is unaided.

14.2.2 Binaural squelch in noise

The preceding section discussed how simply attending to the ear that is presented with the more favorable SNR can minimize the effects of noise. The brain and ears can, however, do better than this. The auditory system can combine the waveforms available to each cochlea to produce an internal, central representation of the signal that effectively has a SNR higher than is available at either ear in isolation.

We can think of this process as the auditory system using the noise at the ear with the poorer SNR to partially remove the noise from the ear with the more favorable SNR. While the physiology responsible for this is unclear, the inputs and results are similar to those of the electronic adaptive noise-reduction schemes shown in Figures 7.4 and 7.5.

Suppose, for instance, that the noise were to arrive from directly in front, and thus have the same amplitude and phase at the two ears, as shown in Figure 14.7. The signal, in this case a pure tone, arrives from the right and therefore has a greater amplitude at the right ear than at the left ear. If the brain were to subtract the total waveform at the left ear from the total waveform at the right ear, the resulting waveform would have no noise at all. By contrast, the resulting signal amplitude would be similar to that in the right ear.[d]

The auditory system cannot perfectly subtract the waveform at one ear from the waveform at the other. It can, however, make imperfect combinations of the waveforms at each ear to significantly decrease the effects of noise. Furthermore, the auditory system is very adaptable; it is not essential for either the noise or the signal to be in phase at the two ears for some noise suppression to occur. The amount of noise suppression that occurs when the signal has an interaural amplitude or phase difference that is different from that of the

noise is called the **binaural masking level difference (BMLD or MLD)**. It is also referred to as **binaural release from masking, binaural unmasking, binaural squelch**, and when the signal is speech, it is also referred to as the **binaural intelligibility level difference (BILD).** In an excellent analysis, Zurek (1993a) has shown that the size of the BMLD for pure tones can be used to predict the size of the BILD for speech, thus strongly suggesting that the same mechanism is responsible for both effects.

For two waveforms to be combined centrally, the details of the waveform must be represented within the auditory system. Consequently, it is not surprising that the BMLD is strongest (up to 15 dB) for low-frequency sounds, where neural impulses remain phase-locked to the stimulus.[619]

The magnitude of the BILD for speech in a sound field is much smaller than that observed for low-frequency sounds presented under headphones. One reason is that whereas both low- and high-frequency regions contribute to intelligibility, the BMLD is large only for the low-frequency region.[136, 528] Furthermore, over much of the low-frequency region, the biggest phase differences that can be created by head diffraction are too small to achieve the maximum possible BMLD

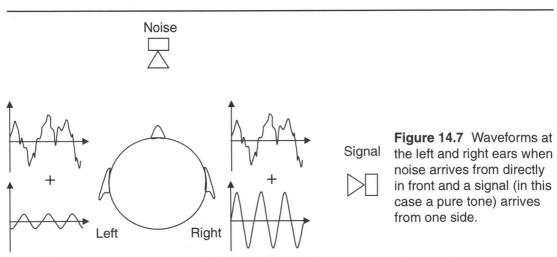

Figure 14.7 Waveforms at the left and right ears when noise arrives from directly in front and a signal (in this case a pure tone) arrives from one side.

[d]   The signal in the resulting waveform may be slightly larger or smaller than the signal at the right ear, depending on the phase relationship between the signals in the right and left ears.

advantage that can be observed when stimuli are artificially delayed and presented by headphones.

The amplitude and phase differences that are necessary for a BILD occur whenever speech and noise come from different directions. The magnitude of the BILD thus varies with the direction of arrival of both speech and noise. Zurek (1993a) estimates that averaged over all directions from which noise can come, the BILD is about 2 dB, compared to simply attending to the ear with the better SNR. He also estimates that the benefits from head diffraction provide a further 3 dB advantage in SNR. The total average binaural advantage, relative to listening with a single, randomly chosen ear, is thus 5 dB. Of course, considerably larger advantages will be found for particular combinations of speech and noise orientation, speech and noise spectral shapes, and overall speech and noise levels.

The BMLD and BILD also exist for hearing-impaired people, but their magnitudes are often decreased.[250, 677] The greatest reduction occurs for people with the greatest hearing loss[350, 417] and for people with the greatest asymmetry of hearing loss.[417] This is primarily caused by an inability to benefit from the SNR improvement offered by head diffraction (if high-frequency sounds fall below threshold) rather than a reduction in the binaural interactions that contribute to binaural squelch.[83] Binaural squelch can thus operate even when loudness is not well balanced between the ears.

Binaural squelch also partially suppresses the adverse effects of reverberation,[485, 609, 641] and the combined effects of reverberation and noise.[368, 609, 641, 642, 643, 718] Such a result is not surprising, as reverberation is similar in nature to background noise. Although reverberation is itself squelched by binaural effects, reverberation will decrease the extent by which noise is squelched, because it diminishes the interaural time and level differences of the speech and noise.[556, 642, 718]

14.2.3 Binaural redundancy

Binaural redundancy refers to the small advantage arising from listening with two ears even though identical combinations of signal and noise are presented to each ear.[203, 206, 625, 835] The phenomenon has also been referred to as **diotic summation,** or **duplication.**

Binaural advantage for diotic listening is not too surprising if one considers that hearing impairment can in many ways be simulated by an additive noise that produces appropriately elevated thresholds. We can think of binaural redundancy as the suppression of internal noise within each ear, or as an improvement in decision-making ability when the brain combines the two ostensibly identical signals sensed by each ear. It is as if the brain gets two "looks" at each sound. Binaural redundancy produces 1 to 2 dB improvement in SNR.[82, 181, 556, 718]

Binaural redundancy results in better speech discrimination in quiet.[432] Even people with severe hearing loss,[206] and people with an apparent central component to the hearing loss[432] benefit from binaural redundancy. Binaural redundancy seems to require a lower level of binaural interactions than binaural squelch. In one experiment, hearing-impaired subjects who obtained a 3 dB binaural advantage could not distinguish a diotically presented stimulus from a dichotically presented stimulus, although normally hearing subjects easily could.[180] Binaural redundancy is one component of binaural squelch if binaural squelch is defined as the improvement relative to monaural stimulation. We can more clearly understand all the components of binaural advantage, however, if the reference condition for binaural squelch is diotic stimulation.

One study with older children, all of whom had a congenital or pre-lingual bilateral profound loss, failed to find any bilateral advantage, even though the experimental conditions would have allowed binaural redundancy and perhaps binaural squelch to operate.[337] The impact of severe and profound congenital loss on the capacity of people to form binaural interactions has not been sufficiently studied to draw any general conclusions about it.

14.2.4 Binaural loudness summation

For a normal-hearing person, the loudness of a sound is greater if is heard in two ears than if it is heard in only one ear. This loudness increase occurs for all levels although not to the same degree.[215, 345, 349, 578, 746]

- Near threshold, binaural summation of loudness is equivalent to increasing the level in one ear by 3 dB.[215, 801]

- At a comfortable level, binaural summation of loudness is equivalent to a level change of 5 to 6 dB,[150] although some studies indicate that the difference is around 10 dB.[345]

- At very high levels, binaural summation of loudness is equivalent to a level change of around 10 dB, although some studies indicate that the difference is only around 6 dB.[412, 773]

Taken together these studies indicate that binaural summation of loudness increases from around 3 dB or lower near threshold to some value in the range 6 to 10 dB at high levels. The change in level when the number of ears is doubled is about the same as the change in level needed to double loudness when listening via one ear.[e] If this is more than a coincidence, and if the same principle applies to hearing-impaired people, then we would expect slightly less loudness summation (when expressed in dB of level change) for hearing-impaired people because of their steeper loudness growth curves. Experimental data suggest that binaural loudness summation is equivalent to a similar or perhaps slightly smaller level change[f] for hearing-impaired people than for normal-hearing people.[215, 349, 365]

Note that the 3 dB change near threshold is the amount expected for the optimal combination of two physical detectors, each of which senses the same signal but which have their own, independent internal noise sources that determine the weakest signal they can detect. This improved ability to detect and rate the loudness of weak sounds is therefore just another aspect of the binaural redundancy advantage described in the previous section.

Although one might expect that binaural loudness summation might also apply to loudness discomfort level (LDL), experimental data suggest otherwise. Depending on the method by which LDL is measured, binaural summation decreases LDL by some amount between 0 and 5 dB.[345, 365, 844] The inescapable conclusion is that with binaural stimulation, sounds can be louder than for monaural stimulation without causing loudness discomfort.

By itself, the binaural summation of loudness leads to neither an increase nor a decrease in the benefits provided by bilateral hearing aids relative to a unilateral aid. There are, however, several implications of loudness summation for fitting procedures, and these will be considered in Section 14.8.

14.3 Advantages of Bilateral Fittings

Various advantages result from wearing two hearing aids rather than one hearing aid. The following sections outline these bilateral advantages.

14.3.1 Speech intelligibility

In many situations, most people can understand speech more clearly with two hearing aids than with one. This occurs for the same

---

[e]   Loudness grows more steeply with level at low SPLs than at high SPLs, so the change in dB needed to double loudness is much less near threshold than at higher SPLs.

[f]   The comparison is affected by whether summation is compared at the same SPL, the same SL, or the same loudness category.

three reasons that listening with two ears is better than listening with one.

Head diffraction effects.

When speech and noise come from different directions, the SNR will be better at one ear than at the other. If the ear with the better SNR is unaided, the patient may be unable to take advantage of this better SNR. The bilateral advantage arising from head diffraction will thus occur for those patients and situations where the high-frequency components of speech fall below unaided threshold. The bilateral advantage arising from head diffraction will be least for those whose high-frequency hearing loss is only mild and for those whose high-frequency hearing loss is so severe that the high frequencies make no contribution to intelligibility. Otherwise, the bilateral advantage for intelligibility caused by head diffraction will occur for all patients, because the SNR variations underlying the advantage depend only on head size.

Binaural squelch

The bilateral advantage arising from binaural squelch occurs for those patients and situations where the low-frequency components of speech and noise are not clearly audible in the unaided ear.[g] The bilateral advantage arising from squelch will thus be small for those whose low-frequency hearing loss is only mild. Binaural squelch can not lead to a significant bilateral advantage if the low-frequency components of speech and noise are already well above threshold in both ears in the unilateral condition.

Binaural redundancy

Binaural redundancy can also only be useful if sounds are audible in each ear. A bilateral advantage will therefore occur if sounds are audible in both ears when a patient is aided bilaterally but not when aided unilaterally.

Experimental evidence

These theoretical expectations arising from diffraction, squelch and redundancy are consistent with experimental evidence. Of 19 laboratory studies reviewed by Ross (1980), 15 showed a bilateral advantage for speech, and four showed no difference. None showed a unilateral advantage. Some studies are unfairly biased in favor of a bilateral advantage by preventing any sound from reaching the unaided ear in the unilateral condition. Such studies really demonstrate the advantage of two ears (binaural advantage) rather than the advantage of two hearing aids (bilateral advantage). Other studies are unfairly biased against a bilateral advantage by using a single loudspeaker for signal and noise.

Despite the bilateral advantage that laboratory studies show for listening in noise, many early surveys of bilateral use found that patients often used one (or no) hearing aid in noisy situations, even if they used two hearing aids in more favorable listening situations.[85, 89, 105, 152, 239, 778] This is not a surprising result when one considers that hearing aids in the 1970s and 1980s were mostly linear and used peak clipping to limit the maximum output. Hearing aids would commonly have been saturated and produced highly distorted sound in noisy places. Consequently, the disadvantages of a hearing aid would be greatest, and because of the high signal levels, the advantages would be least. Removing one or both hearing aids in such situations would seem to be well justified.[644]

Despite this conclusion, one survey of people with symmetric moderate and severe hearing loss showed at least as much bilateral advantage in noisy places as in quiet places.[576] We certainly cannot extrapolate any negative findings in noise to modern hearing aids that have some combination of the following features:

---

[g]   Markides (1982a) estimates that an ear will contribute to squelch if speech is more than 20 dB above the speech detection threshold for that ear.

- Tone controls that offer wide variation in gain-frequency response (to meet prescription targets and so limit upward spread of masking);

- WDRC to maintain the output within the patient's comfort range for a wide range of input levels, and to minimize the amount of limiting necessary;

- Compression limiting to limit the maximum output while minimizing distortion;

- A directional microphone to decrease the incoming noise prior to amplification, or;

- Microphone placement deep within the concha or within the ear canal, so that the hearing aid suppresses noise from the rear to the same degree that the unaided ear does.

With such hearing aids, communication in noisy places should be considerably easier with two hearing aids than with one or none. People more strongly want to use two hearing aids if they are listening through high quality hearing aids than if listening through distorting ones, especially at high signal levels and when noise is present.[644]

Effects of signal processing schemes on bilateral advantage

For those with a moderate hearing loss or greater, the speech advantage provided by bilateral hearing aids over a single aid is robust. It is additive to the advantages provided by directional microphones.[368] This is fortunate as directional microphones considerably alter the phase of sounds.[h] When an FM system provides the input (a monophonic signal) to hearing aids, we would not expect to gain any advantages from head diffraction or binaural squelch. We would, however, expect to retain the very small bilateral advantage arising from binaural redundancy. This is consistent with available evidence.[362]

Summary: Bilateral advantage for speech intelligibility for different degrees of hearing loss

Bilateral advantage for speech intelligibility is greatest for those with severe hearing loss and least for those with mild loss:

- For people with a severe loss in an unaided ear there are unlikely to be any situations in which the unaided ear can contribute useful information at all frequencies (Festen & Plomp, 1986). The bilateral advantage for people with severe hearing loss applies even when there is some asymmetry between the ears (Day, Browning & Gatehouse, 1988).

- For people with a mild loss in the unaided ear, signals are likely to be well above threshold in noisy places. Consequently, the ear will contribute to speech understanding even when it is unaided. When signal levels are low there is the potential for a bilateral advantage. In such circumstances SNR is large, however, so intelligibility with a single hearing aid may be more than adequate. Consequently, there may be few real-life situations in which there is a significant bilateral advantage.

There is a theoretical possibility that compression applied independently at the two ears could disturb the binaural squelch effect. Such disturbance is not too likely because binaural squelch relies mainly on timing or phase differences, and most forms of compression do not affect these. Experimentally, a binaural[i] advantage is found irrespective of whether the hearing aids contain wide dynamic range compression or linear amplification.[625] Nonetheless, it may not be advisable to use compressors with

---

h   Either the phase alterations are equal at each ear (unlikely), or the particular alterations do not adversely affect the bilateral advantage.

i   The term *binaural* is used here rather than *bilateral* because the non-test ear was occluded with a switched-off hearing aid.

attack and release times that differed between the ears, because this could lead to potentially confusing level difference cues. Similarly, it may not advisable to use digital hearing aids with different processing algorithms in each ear. For patients with asymmetrical hearing loss it will usually be necessary to use different compression ratios and possibly compression thresholds in each ear, and there is no reason to refrain from such prescriptions.

14.3.2 Sound quality

Binaural listening provides sound quality superior to that of monaural listening. This advantage is found for a number of attributes, such as clarity, fullness, spaciousness, and overall quality.[33] People can generally make more discriminating judgements about sound when listening binaurally than when listening monaurally. For example, just noticeable differences for intensity are smaller[350, 351, 422, 764] as are just noticeable differences for frequency.[422, 705] The adverse effects of peak clipping are also more evident for binaural listening than for monaural listening.[644] (This could be viewed as a disadvantage of bilateral fitting, but only if one is fitting poor quality hearing aids!)

In these experimental results, however, the monaural results were just that – stimuli were presented to only one ear. Consequently, we can not confidently generalize the finding to the wearing of two hearing aids rather than one, except where the person has a sufficiently severe loss that unilateral aid use will indeed provide monaural stimulation. For people with mild hearing loss, there *may* nonetheless be quality advantages for bilateral aid use, such as the sound being laterally balanced in loudness.

14.3.3 Avoiding late-onset auditory deprivation.

After a person with a symmetrical hearing loss (referring both to pure-tone thresholds and to speech recognition ability) is fitted

with a hearing aid in only one ear, the ability of the other ear to recognize speech may progressively deteriorate over the subsequent few years.[805] The phenomenon is referred to as *late-onset auditory deprivation.* Late-onset auditory deprivation affects a significant minority of unilaterally aided patients.[406] Auditory deprivation in the unaided ear has been demonstrated for children as well as for middle-aged and old adults.[315, 358, 405] In children, the positive effects of maturation offset the negative effects of deprivation in the unaided ear. Consequently, speech scores may actually increase over time in the unaided ear, but to a lesser extent than occurs in the aided ear.[358]

Along with the decrease in speech recognition in the unaided ear, there is sometimes a small increase in speech recognition in the aided ear.[73, 301] This aspect is referred to as acclimatization (see Section 13.5). Both deprivation and acclimatization suggest that there is *plasticity* in the auditory system. Neural reorganization occurs when the inputs to the auditory system are changed. There is physiological evidence for plasticity in animals, as reviewed by Neuman (1996).

The exact time course of auditory deprivation is unknown, but the effect is observable in group data as soon as one year after fitting.[807] It takes from seven months to five years for individual scores to significantly decrease.[313, 406, 407] Although performance decreases with time over the first few years, a further period of unilateral use does not seem to lead to a further decline in speech performance in the unaided ear.[316]

The magnitude of reduction varies across patients. One study using subjects with mild, moderate, and severe hearing losses showed a mean decrease in speech scores of 7% in the unaided ear compared to 3% in the aided ear.[316] By contrast, a case report on one subject with profound loss revealed a decrease of 40%.[73] Another study using subjects with primarily conductive hearing loss with symmetrical hearing thresholds showed a mean difference in speech scores of 30% between the aided and unaided ears.[216]

Auditory deprivation effects are well documented in people with moderate to severe hearing loss.[647] The effects also occur in ears with a three-frequency average loss as small as 35 dB.[316, 407] A comparison across studies suggests that the size of the deprivation effect increases with the degree of pure tone loss.[406]

Although the phenomenon affecting the unaided ear is referred to as *deprivation,* the phenomenon may be more complex than a simple lack of stimulation. When people with a similar degree of loss continue to live without any hearing aids, no effects of deprivation occur.[316] Furthermore, prior to aiding, people with a small threshold difference between the ears often have a marked difference in speech recognition ability.[395] Similarly, speech recognition for the impaired ear in a unilateral loss is likely to be much worse than for an ear with the same pure tone thresholds when the loss is symmetrical.[395] The findings regarding auditory deprivation suggest that an ear may *become* strongly dominant for intelligibility because the other is initially only *marginally* inferior. This initial inferiority may be because of a slightly asymmetrical hearing loss or because only one ear has been aided. *It is as if the brain gives up attending to an ear that transmits a relatively poor signal when it has the option of attending to a better signal coming from the other ear.* [j]

Auditory inferiority, auditory inactivity,[216] or *lazy ear* may perhaps be more accurate descriptions of the process than auditory deprivation. The deprivation term is, however, useful, because the root cause is an inadequate output from the cochlea. The extent of auditory deprivation in the unaided ear may therefore depend on the degree of

loss in the aided ear. Perhaps auditory deprivation occurs only if the aided ear sends a signal sufficiently rich in information to cause the brain to cease to attend to the unaided ear. Note that it is not necessary for the signal from the cochlea of the unaided ear to be distorted. Dieroff (1993) showed that speech recognition scores under headphones in the unaided ears of people with symmetric, essentially conductive hearing loss were on average 33 percentage points lower than scores from the normally aided ears of a matched group of subjects. This finding indicates that a simple attenuation of signals prior to the cochlea, relative to that occurring prior to the other cochlea, is enough to cause auditory deprivation.

Recovery of the unaided ear following bilateral amplification is possible, although it does not always occur.[73, 806, 808] It can also be dramatic. In the case reported by Boothroyd (1993), commencement and later recommencement of bilateral aiding each led to increases in speech recognition performance in the previously unaided ear of around 40 percentage points.

Unfortunately, recovery of the unaided ear is not guaranteed.[313, 647] When recovery does occur it may only be partial.[313, 407] Recovery is possible only after bilateral aiding for many months to several years. Individual case histories suggest that patients who have a rapid onset of deprivation effects also have a more rapid recovery, but this finding requires confirmation.[313] A substantial proportion of people simply give up trying to use the second hearing aid because the composite sound is poorer than when using the unilateral hearing aid to which they have become accustomed.[407]

Differences between the aided and unaided ears have been observed for stimuli other than speech. Intensity discrimination is better in the aided ear than in the unaided ear for

---

j   Even the concept of the relative deprivation of the two ears is overly simplistic: the unaided ear can actually have better speech discrimination when both ears are presented with speech at a low sensation level (Gatehouse, 1989). Presumably the brain is more used to receiving low-level signals from the unaided ear than from the aided ear, and is therefore better at dealing with them.

Minimizing the risk of auditory deprivation
1. Prescribe bilateral hearing aids.
2. If the patient insists on wearing only one hearing aid, encourage the patient to alternate aid use between the ears on a daily or weekly basis (Hattori, 1993).
3. Monitor speech discrimination ability annually for unilaterally aided patients.

All of these methods involve greater cost than a unilateral fitting with no ongoing monitoring. |

intense sounds, but is better in the unaided ear than the aided ear for weak sounds.[754] That is, each ear appears to perform best for the sensation levels that it most commonly receives. This finding reinforces the conclusion that the abilities of the ear and brain to analyze sounds are affected by the nature of the sounds they are used to dealing with.

14.3.4 Localization

The advantages of hearing aids to localization apply principally to people with a flat or gently sloping moderate hearing loss, and to those with a severe or profound loss. Based on our understanding of localization, and the psycho-acoustic characteristics of hearing loss, it is easy to understand, in principle, how hearing aids affect localization.

Horizontal localization

Without audibility there can be no localization. Bilateral hearing aids will enable better localization than a unilateral hearing aid whenever the sound is inaudible in the unaided ear in the case of the unilateral fitting. The localization advantages of bilateral hearing aids are thus greater for patients with a moderate or severe loss than for those with a mild loss.[128] For any degree of loss, the bilateral advantage for localization increases as the stimulus level decreases.[214] Patients with a moderate hearing loss may or may not report improved localization in real world situations when aided bilaterally,[661, 733] though such an advantage *must* be present for soft sounds.

For patients with a mild hearing loss, localization may be worse when aided than when unaided.[126] This may partly be explained by test subjects being unfamiliar with the hearing aids with which they were tested (bilateral when they are used to unilateral or vice versa), and partly explained by the more complex low-frequency response they

Theoretical background: The effect of hearing aids on interaural phase and time.
Hearing aids alter interaural time and intensity cues. Within a hearing aid, tubing, transducers, and filters (i.e. tone controls) all create delays. These delays can be several hundred micro-seconds long, and are thus very significant compared to interaural time difference cues. Digital processing can delay sounds by several milliseconds. In the low-frequency region, sounds often arrive at the eardrum via two paths: an amplified path through the hearing aid and a direct acoustic path through the vent and/or leakage around the mold or shell. Such multi-path transmission can drastically alter the phase response of the combined response at the eardrum, and hence can alter the interaural phase cues,. Furthermore, small changes in the characteristics of either path can cause large changes in the phase response of the combined path. Characteristics of the leakage path vary whenever the aid wearer moves his or her jaw. The amplified path varies its characteristics whenever a compressor or volume control causes the gain to change. It should not be surprising that putting on one or two hearing aids will cause localization to immediately deteriorate. Although the sense of localization is very adaptable (see other panel), it may not be possible to fully adapt to such a changing interaural phase difference.

Acclimatization: When can localization be measured?

Hearing aids almost always alter localization cues. If people are tested with hearing aid type or fitting configuration (e.g. unilateral instead of bilateral) that they have not previously worn, localization performance deteriorates markedly (Noble & Byrne, 1991). There is substantial evidence that people adapt to altered interaural time and intensity cues to localization (Byrne & Dirks, 1996). Significant adaptation commences within a few hours and adaptation continues for a few days and to a lesser extent for a few weeks (Bauer, Matusza & Blackmer, 1966; Florentine, 1976; Heyes & Gazely, 1975; Javer & Schwarz, 1995). Consequently, assessing localization ability (see Section 14.5.5) at a fitting appointment is not feasible; assessment at a follow-up appointment within a typical hearing aid fitting and rehabilitation program is feasible though not usually necessary.

---

experience when aided (see panel). Normal low-frequency cues can be maximally retained by using as open an earmold as possible.[128]

For patients with conductive hearing loss, hearing aids can produce a marked improvement in horizontal localization ability. This presumably occurs because, in addition to increasing audibility, hearing aids increase the proportion of sound delivered by air conduction, and hence increases the interaural time and level differences at the cochlea.[127] The material used in the earmold, or perhaps the tightness of the earmold, also affects the amount by which localization improves. Unfortunately, the mechanisms are not yet understood sufficiently well to say which materials work best for which patients.[127]

Differences in localization accuracy between BTE, ITE or ITC hearing aids appear to be small,[518, 679] especially when subjects have had time to become used to the localization cues their particular hearing aid or hearing aids provide.[128] This should not be surprising, as bilateral fittings of any type are able to preserve inter-aural time and level differences. ITE, ITC, and presumably CIC hearing aids, however, may be better able to preserve front-rear distinctions than BTE hearing aids, because BTE hearing aids are less shielded by the pinna.[893, 952] On the basis of surveys, people are more satisfied with

sound localization when using CIC hearing aids than when using other aid types.[481, 631]

Some advanced digital hearing aids are being designed to restore the normal phase cues, and hence time cues, at the eardrum.[475, 913] This should enable a hearing aid to be inserted with minimal initial loss of localization ability. Intensity cues will, of course, be disrupted because of the amplification provided. The long-term value of ensuring that the normal phase and time cues are unaltered is not yet known.

As processing schemes in hearing aids become more complex, it is possible that some schemes in the future will cause the phase response of hearing aids to vary with the signal, and to vary by different amounts in each ear. Any such schemes would adversely affect horizontal localization.[126]

Vertical localization

Once an ITE or a BTE earmold is inserted, the concha bowl shape that normally gives rise to vertical localization cues is removed. Consequently, vertical localization ability is almost totally destroyed. For a CIC hearing aid, vertical localization cues up to at least 10 kHz are present at the microphone inlet, because they are fully formed just inside the entrance to the ear canal.[594, 600, 798] Whether the aid wearer is able to use these cues to localize sounds vertically is another matter. Because the cues are all above 5 kHz, localization is possible only if the hearing aid makes information audible over enough of the 5 to 12 kHz range, and if the aid wearer has enough frequency resolution to identify spectral shape within this range.

For ITC hearing aids, the situation should be intermediate to that for ITE and CIC hearing aids. Some of the concha remains open, but the sensing point (the hearing aid microphone inlet) will not be in the normal place (the ear canal entrance). Consequently, any vertical localization cues that remain will be drastically different from normal and the user will have to learn to use them, if indeed that is possible.

Experimental evidence confirms that BTE, ITE, and ITC hearing aids do not improve vertical localization, and can even make it worse.[657] Vertical localization with CIC hearing aids has had limited evaluation. It seems that normal-hearing people can localize vertically reasonably well if the CIC has a bandwidth extending up to 8 kHz or higher.[810]

For those few patients who have near-normal high-frequency thresholds, an open earmold can preserve vertical localization, natural-ness, and externalization.[131]

14.3.5 Suppression of tinnitus

The use of hearing aids can mask, or even suppress, tinnitus. Tinnitus is often bilateral. It is not surprising, therefore, that bilateral hearing aids are more effective than unilateral hearing aids at masking tinnitus.[94] In one study, 66% of people with tinnitus reported that two hearing aids lessened the effects of tinnitus, compared to only 13% who found one hearing aid to be effective.[94] Unfortu-nately, and less commonly, hearing aids can sometimes exacerbate tinnitus.

14.3.6 Miscellaneous advantages

One practical advantage to bilateral fittings is particularly important for people with a severe or profound hearing loss: When a hearing aid breaks down, people with two hearing aids still have one working aid.

While a patient can be loaned a hearing aid while the repair takes place, the *loaner aid*:
- can be provided only for BTE hearing aids, or perhaps for modular ITC hearing aids;
- takes clinical time to fit;
- may have unfamiliar amplification characteristics and controls; and
- is available to the patient only after the patient arrives at the clinic.

A permanent, second, individually fitted hearing aid is a much better option.

Bilateral hearing aids need a little less gain than unilateral aids (see Section 14.8). The gain reduction needed to achieve some criterion loudness is less than the reduction (if any) in SSPL needed to avoid loudness discomfort. Consequently, bilateral hearing aids will be less saturated less often than unilateral hearing aids, which should confer some sound quality advantages at high input levels. Also, high presentation levels adversely affect speech intelligibility (Sections 9.2.4 and 9.3.7), so the lower gain of a bilateral hearing aid may confer a slight advantage relative to a unilateral aid. Feedback will also be less of a problem if the hearing aid has less gain. All of these advantages of bilateral hearing aids stemming from a lower gain are relatively minor.

People with chronic drainage problems in their ears who own bilateral hearing aids can alternate use between the ears if a hearing aid in their ear canal exacerbates the problem. For such people, the earmold should be as open a style as possible.

Finally, people who have two hearing aids always have a choice – they can use two hearing aids, or one hearing aid in whichever ear they choose, in any situation they choose. People with only a single hearing aid have a more limited choice.

14.4 Disadvantages of Bilateral Fittings

14.4.1 Cost

Unless hearing aids are free to patients, the cost of the second hearing aid, and the batteries for it, will be a major disadvantage for many patients. In service delivery systems in which the hearing aids are free to patients, the additional costs are borne by government or an insurance provider. The additional cost may be a significant issue for the funds provider, who may require clinicians to justify their actions if bilateral hearing aids are provided to a larger proportion of patients than the funds provider thinks is reasonable.

Expectations as to what is reasonable appear to be rising, in keeping with the growing proportion of people who acquire bilateral hearing aids. (This is, of course, a circular argument.) Fortunately, the trend is also in keeping with the vast amount of research that indicates additional benefits for bilateral compared to unilateral hearing aids. Irrespective of who pays for the provision of hearing aids, costs must always be balanced against the benefits outlined in Section 14.3.

It is unfortunate that in some delivery systems bilateral hearing aids cost patients twice as much as unilateral hearing aids. It does not take twice the work to fit two hearing aids as it does to fit one. Many of the activities are the same whether the patient is provided with one or two hearing aids (assessment, providing information about hearing loss and hearing strategies, and much of the training in how to use the hearing aid or aids). There is therefore no justification for a rehabilitation service incorporating a bilateral fitting to cost twice as much as one incorporating a unilateral fitting.

14.4.2 Binaural interference

A small proportion of elderly people will have poorer speech discrimination when listening binaurally than when listening monaurally.[27, 420, 803] Small sample sizes and uncertain experimental details make it difficult to accurately estimate the proportion, but it may be around 10%.[420] It seems possible that the proportion is higher for people with asymmetrical thresholds than for people with symmetrical thresholds. A binaural deficit is believed to be related to a deterioration in the way that signals from the two ears are fused to form a single auditory percept.[149, 420]

A binaural deficit can be simulated in normal-hearing people. When speech is artificially distorted in a different manner for each ear, to simulate different cochlear distortions, binaural speech scores are lower than monaural scores.[396] Applying the same type of distortion to each ear, however, restores the usual binaural advantage. Subjects reported that when they were listening to the asymmetrically distorted signals, they attempted to attend selectively to the ear with the clearer signal.

One mechanism that might give rise to destructive mixing of information from the two ears is a change in the tuning properties of one cochlea relative to another. Such changes may be caused by a loss of outer hair cell function. Hair cell dysfunction may be exacerbated if the brain's control of the cochlea via efferent nerve fibers is decreased.[521, 735, 774] Diplacusis, in which the person hears a different pitch in each ear, would be one possible psycho-acoustic consequence of differential retuning in the two ears. Diplacusis has indeed been shown to be an indicator of a lack of benefit from bilateral amplification.[574, 575]

Chmiel et al. (1997) give a second reason why bilateral performance may be worse than unilateral performance. They hypothesize:

in aging, there may be a significant loss of efficiency of interhemispheric transfer of auditory information through the corpus callosum. As a result, the left ear is at an increased disadvantage for the processing of verbal tasks. (p. 8)

The supporting evidence for this included:

- Worse phonetically balanced word scores for the left ear than for the right, despite reasonably symmetrical pure tone thresholds and distortion-product otoacoustic emissions;
- Symmetrical ABR wave V latencies and amplitudes;
- Substantially lower speech identification scores for the left ear than for the right ear on several dichotic listening tasks;
- Strongly asymmetrical event-related potentials (P_{300}) for right ear versus left ear targets in response to dichotic PB word pairs. Furthermore, the asymmetry reversed for verbal versus non-verbal targets.

A prolonged period of wearing only one hearing aid may cause or exacerbate interference from the previously unaided ear, when the client subsequently obtains bilateral hearing aids.[420] This idea should be regarded as a hypothesis, rather than as a fact, until it is tested.[k]

In summary:

- A small proportion of patients will perform better with one hearing aid than with two.
- This unilateral advantage may be because the two cochleae generate neural signals sufficiently different that they interfere with each other, or because information is distorted as the brain transfers it between the hemispheres.

14.4.3 Self-image

Even when hearing aids do not cost the patient any money, many patients will choose to obtain one rather than two hearing aids.[867]

Sometimes patients will say something like *I am not that deaf* to justify their choice of a unilateral fitting. (This was very common when only BTE hearing aids were available.) Three different beliefs may underlie this statement:

- If patients associate a hearing aid with being old or deaf, they may associate two hearing aids with being very old or very deaf. In some cases, friends and relatives will reinforce this negative assessment of bilateral hearing aids.[94] People who wear two hearing aids are more likely than those who wear one hearing aid to report that their hearing aids are noticeable to other people.[867] On the positive side, they are also more likely to report that other people have noticed how much more alert they are when they wear their hearing aids.[867] This last finding might be valuable to pass on to patients who do not wish to try two hearing aids because of cosmetic concerns.
- Patients may have an overly optimistic assessment of how well they will be able to hear with just one hearing aid.
- Patients with a mild loss may make an accurate assessment that the second hearing aid will not provide them with significant benefit in the short term.

14.4.4 Miscellaneous disadvantages

Wind noise. Even a light breeze can create noise in a hearing aid that is equivalent to the noise created by a 100-dB SPL sound at the *input* of a hearing aid.[235] The only thing worse than a hearing aid amplifying 100 dB SPL of unpleasant noise is two hearing aids amplifying this noise. Consequently, it is not surprising that for windy situations people

---

[k]   It is interesting to speculate whether there is any relationship between the ear dominance that results from auditory deprivation and the ear dominance found in dichotic speech testing. Even for people with normal hearing in both ears, speech identification ability is not necessarily symmetrical when a different speech stimulus is presented to each ear. When one ear is found to have higher speech scores, the opposite hemisphere is found to have greater event-related brain potentials. Superior speech identification is more common in the right ear than in the left (Ahonniska et al., 1993). The right ear also appears to be more resistant to the effects of auditory deprivation, although confirmation of this is required (Hurley, 1999). The effects and reversibility of unilateral deprivation, and its relationship to the normal differences between the way the left and right hemispheres process verbal and non-verbal signals (Studdert-Kennedy & Shankweiler, 1970; Deutsch, 1975) are exciting areas for future research.

do not rate bilateral hearing aids any more highly than unilateral hearing aids.[89] The problem is less for CIC hearing aids than for other hearing aids, but a substantial problem remains.

Aid management. Managing a hearing aid presents a major difficulty for some people with decreased physical or mental abilities. With two hearing aids, there is more scope for confusion with insertion, on-off control, battery changing, and volume control. For bilateral fittings, volume adjustment has two aspects – overall loudness and balance between the two ears. This is inherently more complex than managing a single volume control. Even some able-bodied and able-minded people report difficulty in balancing the two hearing aids during the first week or so of aid use, although the skill is eventually attained.[268]

14.5 Tests of Bilateral Advantage

There is a long history of failing to demonstrate a significant bilateral advantage in speech identification for any individual, even though there is usually no difficulty in demonstrating benefit for an experimental group as a whole.[119, 374, 418, 534, 786] There have been exceptions: Jerger, Darling & Florin (1994) demonstrated a significant bilateral advantage for seven out of ten subjects, using the Cued Listening Test (Jerger & Jordan, 1992). In this test, patients have to indicate every occurrence of a target word within continuous discourse coming from a loudspeaker on one side of the head, while different continuous discourse comes from a second speaker on the other side of the head.

Two important details in this experiment were that all subjects were experienced at using bilateral hearing aids, and that the test used 100 target words per amplification condition. For regular clinical practice, there does not seem to be much point in administering a lengthy test of bilateral advantage to patients

who are already successfully using bilateral hearing aids.

There are no tests of binaural functioning that can be given under headphones, prior to hearing aid fitting, to establish whether bilateral amplification is likely to be better, the same, or worse than unilateral amplification for that person. The reasons for this include:

- Interactions between the ears may be different if each ear is given a gain-frequency response appropriate to the hearing loss in that ear rather than the flat response that is most easily obtained using an audiometer;

- The nature of binaural interactions may change markedly after some months, weeks, days, or even hours of listening experience with appropriately amplified sound in each ear;

- Headphone testing can most easily create monaural and binaural stimulation. For clinical applications, however, we wish to infer the relative performance of unilateral versus bilateral amplification.

Consequently, the tests to be outlined in this section are tests of bilateral and unilateral aided functioning, for people who have already been provided with two hearing aids, but for whom there is some doubt about the value of bilateral fitting relative to unilateral fitting. Research should urgently be directed to developing tests that can be used *prior* to fitting to determine if a patient is likely to have adverse, rather than helpful, binaural interactions.

Before giving recommendations for when and how aided testing should be performed (Section 14.5.3), two complicating issues will be discussed.

14.5.1 Bias in choosing the reference ear for the unilateral condition

If speech performance ability with two hearing aids is to be compared to a score obtained with one hearing aid, how should the ear be chosen for the unilateral condition? If we choose an ear randomly, or on some practical grounds (like the person being right-handed), or because the ear has less pure-tone loss, there is a possibility that in fact the other ear has superior speech recognition ability. An apparent bilateral advantage may thus occur just because the bilateral condition includes the other (better) ear. This would cause a systematic bias in favor of bilateral hearing aids.

On the other hand, if both ears are measured as "the" unilateral condition, and the higher of the two scores is chosen as the baseline, there is a systematic bias against bilateral hearing aids.[106] This bias occurs because all speech scores have a random component, so the higher of the two unilateral scores is likely to be greater than the bilateral score, even when there is in fact no difference between the conditions. If there *is* a true underlying bilateral advantage, this statistical bias towards a unilateral fitting will decrease the chance of the bilateral advantage emerging during any particular test. The extent of the bias is substantial unless the speech test contains many items. For a 25 item test, for example, the bias towards the unilateral condition can be as high as 6%,[120] which is nearly as large as the expected bilateral advantage in some conditions.

Some methods for reducing bias when testing for bilateral advantage are:

1. Average the two unilateral scores and compare this average to the bilateral score.

2. Test the bilateral condition twice and compare the higher of the two scores to the higher of the two unilateral scores.

3. Subtract, from the higher of the unilateral scores, an amount that on average compensates for the bias.[120]

4. Use a large number of test items in each condition (like 100, but this is rarely possible because of time constraints).

5. Use a high-context test with a steep performance-intensity function, so that the true differences are as large as possible compared to the degree of bias (see Section 14.5.2).

6. Test the unilateral condition for only one ear, but choose the ear for which the patient thinks speech is clearer.

None of these methods is perfect. When it seems likely that the two ears have identical speech performance ability (based on the audiogram and the patient's opinion), method 2 or 3 should be adopted. When there are strong grounds for believing that one ear is better than the other, method 6 should be adopted. Method 5 should always be adopted, but may not by itself decrease bias sufficiently.

14.5.2 The sensitivity of speech tests for assessing bilateral advantage

Is it possible to reliably test for bilateral advantage with individual patients using speech identification tests? Suppose we performed a speech test based on 50 scored items when the patient was bilaterally aided and when he or she was unilaterally aided. For scores in the range 30 to 70% correct, the standard deviation of test-retest differences will be 10%.[341, 881] To achieve a significant difference at the 95% confidence level, the bilateral score will have to exceed the unilateral score by 20%. If the speech test comprises isolated words, the ***performance-intensity (P-I) function*** is likely to have a slope around 3% per dB of SNR. The bilateral advantage will therefore have to be considerably more than 7 dB if it is to be reliably confirmed in the speech test. An advantage this large is possible only if the ear that is unilaterally aided is further from the speech and/or nearer to the noise. Were the unilateral score to be obtained with the hearing aid in the ear that receives the better SNR, the bilateral advantage is most unlikely to be significant.

The situation is slightly more promising for speech tests with high context, and in which the masking noise has a similar spectrum to the speech. For such tests, the P-I function has a slope of at least 10% per dB of intensity or SNR.[625, 651, 722] Consequently, a bilateral advantage as small as 2 dB could sometimes be detected with a list of 50 genuinely independent items.[1] We can hope to detect the presence of binaural squelch only if there are different combinations of signal and noise at the two ears. Such differences can arise only when the speech and noise are spatially separated, in which case the highly predictable head diffraction effects will also be present. If both head diffraction and squelch contribute towards bilateral advantage, we can be confident of an advantage much bigger than 2 dB. If only squelch contributes (i.e. the ear with the better SNR is chosen as the unilateral reference), we could not be so confident.

In summary, it seems that we can easily demonstrate a bilateral advantage for an individual patient if we:

- arrange the test situation so that head diffraction favors the bilateral condition relative to one of the unilateral conditions, and then use this more adverse unilateral condition as the reference unilateral condition; and

- use material with a steep P-I function.[m] Such materials include spondees and high-context sentence tests like the **Bamford-Kowal-Bench (BKB)** sentences,[45] **Hearing In Noise Test (HINT)**,[651] the **Speech In Noise (SIN)** test;[464] equi-intelligible Dutch sentences,[722] Swedish re-mixed sentences.[342]

The SNR has to be chosen so that scores for both the bilateral and unilateral conditions are obtained from the sloping part of the P-I functions. Because of the steepness of the P-I functions, this can most easily be achieved by adaptively varying the SNR after each sentence. If less than half the words in the sentence are correct, increase the SNR; if more than half are correct, decrease the SNR. Increases in SNR should have the same step size as decreases. The average of four or so reversals provides an estimate of the SNR corresponding to 50% words correct. A greater number of reversals increases the accuracy of the estimate. Alternatively, if only recordings with fixed SNRs are available, it will be necessary to obtain and plot scores for a few SNRs so that the position of the sloping part of the P-I curve can be estimated.

To maximize the chance of detecting bilateral advantage, testing level should be as low as is possible but realistic. The higher the test level used, the greater are the chances that the unaided ear will contribute useful information, so that both the unilateral and bilateral conditions will actually involve binaural listening. A speech level of 55 dB SPL seems like a suitable compromise in that it is lower than the level of typical speech, but high enough nonetheless to be encountered reasonably often in real life.

14.5.3 Role for speech tests in assessing bilateral advantage

Most patients receiving their first hearing aids are able to indicate a preference for bilateral hearing aids over a unilateral aid within the first few hours of trying hearing aids. This initial preference is indicative of their long-term acceptance of bilateral hearing aids.[268] Furthermore, we have seen that the reliable detection of bilateral advantage requires head

---

[1] For high-context sentences, there will need to be more than 50 words but less than 50 sentences to obtain the same statistical reliability that is obtained for 50 independent words.

[m] The benefits of using sentence material to evaluate hearing aids was pointed out at least 60 years ago (Fletcher, 1939). The intrinsic relationship between P-I function slope and bilateral advantage (in percent) may explain the observation that individuals with the steepest P-I functions tend to obtain the greatest bilateral advantage (Mueller, Grimes & Jerome, 1981).

diffraction effects to favor the bilateral condition. There is no point in *routinely* testing for the bilateral advantage that arises from the head diffraction component of improved SNR. This advantage will occur, in some real life situations, for every patient who has a head, and aidable hearing up to at least 1 kHz! Detection of a bilateral advantage caused in part by head diffraction effects does not indicate that any true binaural interactions are taking place. It does, however, indicate that the patient will gain more benefit from two hearing aids than from a single aid in at least some situations.[106]

There seems to be two reasons for measuring bilateral advantage when the circumstances of a particular patient so indicate. For the reasons in the preceding paragraph, it does not seem sensible to use clinical time to perform either of these measurements routinely.

Demonstration to skeptics. A speech test can be used to demonstrate bilateral advantage to people (either the patient or influential friends or relatives) who doubt the benefit of the second aid. The physical arrangement for these tests, as depicted in Figure 14.8, is designed to maximize bilateral advantage by capturing the benefits of head diffraction, squelch, and redundancy, but retain face validity by having speech in the frontal quadrant. An angle of 30° rather than 45° can be used if desired, because binaural advantage increases sharply as angle increases from 0° to 30° from the front.[82]

Detection of adverse binaural interactions. A speech test can be used to ensure that the patient is not someone for whom binaural stimulation is worse than monaural stimulation. For this purpose, we should minimize head diffraction effects, as their positive effect on intelligibility may partially cancel the negative binaural interactions that we are aiming to detect. Figure 14.9 shows a suitable test arrangement. Because only a small minority of people will suffer from

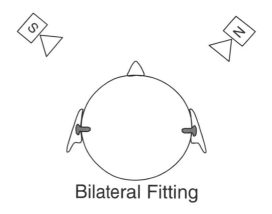

Bilateral Fitting

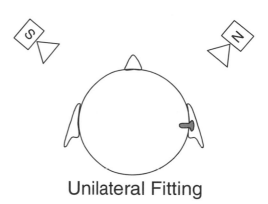

Unilateral Fitting

Figure 14.8 Test arrangement for demonstrating bilateral advantage, showing the location of the speech (S) and noise (N) loudspeakers. Speakers should be 0.5 m or more from the patient. For unilateral fittings to the left ear, the S and N sources should be reversed for both the bilateral and unilateral tests.

adverse binaural interactions,[803] it is not worth performing this test routinely. The test can be performed to confirm complaints from patients who have tried two hearing aids and consider them worse than one aid. Also, if the test shown in Figure 14.8 failed to show the expected advantage, the test in Figure 14.9 could be used to investigate the reason.

Acclimatization effects. The need to confirm bilateral advantage, or to eliminate adverse binaural interactions, is greatest for patients who have become used to unilateral amplification. Unfortunately, the same factors that make initial acceptance of the second aid less

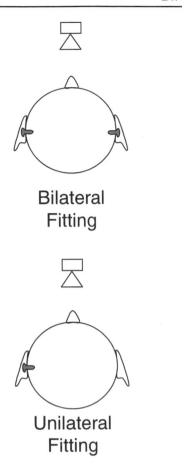

Bilateral Fitting

Unilateral Fitting

Figure 14.9 Test arrangement for detecting negative binaural interactions. Speech and noise both come from the same loudspeaker.

likely also make it less likely that objective benefit can be demonstrated initially. The improvements in speech intelligibility that follow training with bilateral hearing aids illustrate the importance of listening experience.[787]

14.5.4 Localization tests

Localization is not commonly tested in clinical situations, though such testing is simple to do (see panel). If localization testing is performed to compare one versus two hearing aids, it is important that the stimulus presentation level be as low as possible while still being realistic.[214] Otherwise, the patient may in fact be listening binaurally in both the unilateral and bilateral conditions.

Localization ability is important in its own right, but, in principle, can be used to assess whether useful binaural interactions occur for an individual patient.[106] If the binaural interactions necessary for localization can occur, it is possible that the interactions necessary for binaural squelch or binaural redundancy will also be present.[214, 388, 786] So far, however, localization has been shown to be only weakly related to bilateral advantage in speech identification.[660, 786] Self-reported

---

A simple localization test

Ask the patient to point to a (low intensity) noisemaker while wearing a blindfold, or while keeping his or her eyes closed. A correct response would be when the patient points within approximately 20 degrees of the correct direction.

At least ten presentations should be given in each condition tested (e.g. unaided versus unilateral fitting, or unilateral versus bilateral fitting), to improve the reliability of the results. If each trial is scored as correct or incorrect, the significance of a difference in scores between conditions is assessed in the same way as for speech identification tests (Hagerman, 1976; Thornton & Raffin, 1978). Test accuracy and sensitivity therefore increases with the number of trials used.

It is advisable to vary the stimulus from trial to trial, but present each stimulus the same number of times in each amplification condition tested. Otherwise, the patient may be able to localize using the spectral shape at the aided ear. This is a monaural cue, so the test results could not be used to infer anything about binaural interactions or the ability to localize unfamiliar sounds.

localization ability is, however, correlated with ease of understanding speech, even when hearing loss is controlled for.[661]

14.6 Fitting Asymmetrical Hearing Losses

For a patient with hearing thresholds that are asymmetrical by more than about 30 dB, or speech discrimination scores that are asymmetrical by more than about 20%, the clinician will have to make the following decisions:

- Should a bilateral or unilateral fitting be recommended?

- If a unilateral fitting is recommended, should the better or worse ear (based on either pure tone thresholds or speech discrimination scores) be aided?

- Should an alternative such as some variety of CROS hearing aid, or FM system, be recommended?

These three questions are addressed in the following three sections.

14.6.1 Bilateral versus unilateral fittings for asymmetrical losses

Asymmetrical hearing loss may be defined on the basis of thresholds averaged across frequency, threshold shape, speech intelligibility testing, discomfort levels, or dynamic ranges. There have been many suggestions that patients with hearing losses that are asymmetrical by more than a certain degree on any of these criteria will not benefit from bilateral fittings.[55, 80, 203, 574]

It is true that the binaural redundancy component of binaural advantage diminishes as the average hearing thresholds of the two ears become more dissimilar.[374] The decrease is significant for a difference in four-frequency average hearing levels of 15 dB or more.[203, 306, 345]

Binaural squelch, however, occurs even when the poorer ear has thresholds 50 dB worse

than the better ear[889] or when sounds are greatly attenuated in one ear.[556] The ear further from the speech source may thus contribute to binaural squelch even when it is unaided, and this is most likely to happen when it is the better ear. Conversely, when the far ear is the worse ear, aiding it is more likely to be essential if binaural squelch is to occur.

The physical effects of head diffraction on SNR at each ear occur no matter what hearing loss the person has. A bilateral advantage arising from head diffraction should occur whenever the following are all true:

- The ear nearer the speech source and/or further from the noise has enough inherent speech identification ability under ideal conditions;

- The sound arrives from the unaided side in the unilateral reference condition; and,

- The sound is at a level lower than is optimal for the unaided ear.

In some listening conditions, intelligibility has been found to be maximized by either a bilateral fitting or a unilateral fitting to the *worse* ear.[306] In other listening situations, intelligibility has been found to be maximized by either a bilateral fitting or a unilateral fitting to the *better* ear.[306] The only solution common to all situations is therefore a bilateral fitting.

One survey showed that people with an asymmetric loss (defined according to the shape of the audiogram) were *more* likely than people with symmetric audiograms to use two hearing aids.[152] This is particularly understandable for some asymmetrical hearing loss profiles. For the hearing loss shown in Figure 14.10, for example, the patient has less loss for low-frequency sounds in the left ear, but less loss for high-frequency sounds in the right ear. We know that on average the ability to use audible information decreases as the degree of loss increases (see Section 9.2.4). If the person whose audiogram

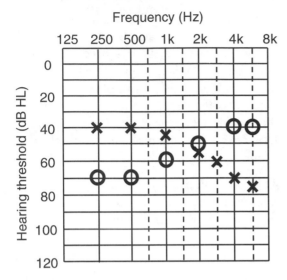

Figure 14.10 An audiogram for a person who is likely to benefit from the hearing aid cross-over effect if a bilateral fitting is provided.

is shown in Figure 14.10 is to make the maximum use of his residual hearing, it is essential that his left ear receive amplified sound in at least the low-frequency region, and that his right ear receive amplified sound in at least the high-frequency region. The brain is able to combine information at different frequencies sent to it by the two ears.[291] This variation of the better ear from frequency to frequency has been called the ***cross-over effect***.[118, n]

The cross-over effect is an extreme example of the binaural redundancy advantage that occurs for normally hearing people – the same acoustical information may be presented to the two ears, but the sum of the information sent to the brain is greater than that which can be sent by either ear alone.

It is *possible* that excessive asymmetry in either thresholds or speech intelligibility precludes bilateral advantage, but it is unclear what constitutes "excessive". As an example,

> **Conclusion: asymmetrical hearing loss and bilateral fittings**
>
> If each ear, considered in isolation, has a loss that could effectively be aided, then in at least some situations, the person is likely to benefit from a bilateral fitting, irrespective of the degree of ear asymmetry. The greater the loss in the better ear, the greater will be the range of situations and sound levels for which a bilateral fitting will be better than a unilateral fitting to the worse ear.

a person with a three-frequency average loss of 30 dB HL in the better ear and 80 dB HL in the poorer ear requires, on average, a SNR 8 dB higher in the poorer ear than in the better ear for the same speech intelligibility.[460] As shown in Section 14.2.1, the SNR at one ear, averaged across frequency, can effectively be 17 dB better than the SNR at the other. When speech is on the side of the poorer ear and noise is on the side of the better ear, the poorer ear is therefore likely to provide considerably higher intelligibility than the better ear.[o] Thus, even for an asymmetry as great as 50 dB, there is a theoretical basis for aiding both ears.

In short, there is no convincing evidence that an asymmetrical hearing loss precludes a patient from benefiting from a bilateral fitting. Furthermore there is much direct and indirect evidence that people with asymmetrical loss *will* benefit from a bilateral fitting in at least some situations.

14.6.2 Better ear versus poorer ear for unilateral fittings

If the patient prefers to have only one hearing aid, but has a hearing loss in both ears, which ear should you fit? Let us first consider two

---

n   This use of the term cross-over effect should not be confused with the transfer of sound from one side of the head to the other by bone conduction that can occur when masking one ear.

o   This analysis overestimates the poorer ear advantage by some amount. A considerable part of the 17 dB advantage arises from high-frequency head diffraction effects. For flat and high-frequency hearing losses, the high-frequency regions contribute relatively little to intelligibility for severe hearing loss, so the poorer ear will not be able to take full advantage of the increase in SNR caused by head diffraction.

extreme examples to illustrate the two principles at work. For the audiogram shown in Figure 14.11, the loss in the left ear is so mild that only very weak sounds will be inaudible in that ear if the ear remains unaided. A hearing aid in the right ear, however, will improve audibility in that ear for many sounds. This will be valuable to the patient whenever head diffraction creates a better SNR in the right ear than in the left ear. Aiding the right (poorer) ear will also increase the likelihood that binaural squelch and binaural redundancy will operate, because many more sounds will be audible in both ears than if the better ear were to be aided.

The situation is very different for the audiogram in Figure 14.12. The right ear is capable of sending some signals to the brain, but the signal quality is likely to be grossly inferior to the quality of the signals sent by the left ear. The left ear can send its higher quality signals only when sounds are audible to it, and hence a hearing aid in the left ear will greatly improve the range of sounds over which it is able to operate. The person will thus be helped more by a hearing aid in the left (better) ear than in the right (worse) ear.

The same three factors are actually operating in the decisions about both audiograms:

1. Aiding the better ear will maximize the range of sounds *audible* to the person.

2. Aiding the poorer ear maximizes the range of sounds that will be audible in both ears. Consequently, aiding the poorer ear will maximize the likelihood of the person being able to use binaural interactions to assist understanding and localization. Depending on the losses in each ear, it may also maximize the likelihood of the sounds being audible at the ear that has the better SNR because of head diffraction effects.

3. The better ear, when aided, is able to send higher quality signals to the brain than the poorer ear, when aided.

For the audiogram shown in Figure 14.11, factor 2 is the most important, whereas for the audiogram shown in Figure 14.12, factor 3 is the most important. Note that for factor 1, "better ear" means the ear with the better pure tone thresholds, whereas for factor 3, "better ear" means the ear with the better aided speech discrimination scores. This is usually, but not necessarily, the ear with the better pure tone thresholds. In factor 2, both

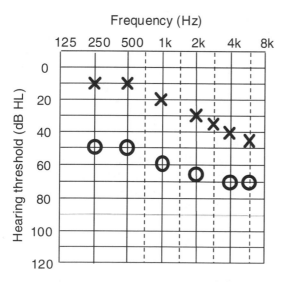

Figure 14.11 An audiogram where the poorer ear should be aided if the person chooses to have a unilateral fitting.

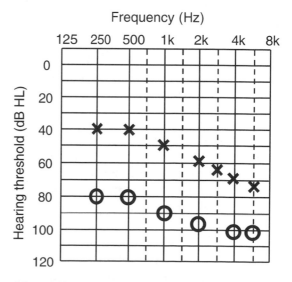

Figure 14.12 An audiogram where the better ear should be aided if the person chooses to have a unilateral fitting.

Counselling suggestion: handling patient preference for unilateral amplification

When a patient wants only one hearing aid, resulting in a difficult decision as to which ear should be aided, advise the patient how a hearing aid in each ear will be advantageous:

- The better ear should be aided because you will then be able to hear a wider range of sounds, and you will be best able to understand speech when it comes from that side of the head.
- The poorer ear should be aided because otherwise speech will be **very** unclear when it comes from your poorer side. Furthermore, aiding that ear will help prevent further deterioration in the speech recognition ability of the poorer ear.

Hopefully, the person will let you off the hook by agreeing to try hearing aids in *both* ears, which is the only way to meet the requirements of all three decision-making factors listed in the text. One possibility is to offer the second hearing aid at no charge for the first 30 days, so that patients can assess the extra benefit before making any financial commitment to the second aid (Harford & Curran, 1997).

---

pure tone thresholds and speech discrimination ability are involved in the definition of the better ear.

For hearing losses where the decision about which ear to aid is less straightforward than these two examples, the same three factors operate. In many cases, it will not be obvious which of the factors should take precedence. Such cases are difficult because in reality, all three factors are important, and the best option is actually to fit both ears.

Swan, Browning & Gatehouse (1987) carried out an extensive study into the preferred side of fitting. They concluded that on the basis of subjects' real-life experience over 20 weeks (comprising 10 weeks with hearing aids on each side), there was a strong overall preference for fitting the poorer ear.

The poorer ear was preferred whether "poorer" was defined in terms of audiometric criteria or speech discrimination criteria. In terms of audiometric thresholds, the favored ear was the one with the poorer 4FA thresholds and/or with the higher degree of slope. In terms of speech recognition ability, the poorer ear was the one with the greater half-peak level elevation (HPLE)[p] and/or with the lesser maximum discrimination score. Of

those subjects who had a preference for hearing-related reasons, the speech-based criteria correctly predicted preferences for 87% of subjects, whereas the audiometric criteria correctly predicted preferences for 77% of subjects. Note that all subjects had 4FA thresholds less than 75 dB HL in both ears. The experimental finding should not be applied to patients with losses greater than this in the poorer ear, as in the example shown in Figure 14.12.

Swan, Browning and Gatehouse (1987) suggest that the reason most subjects preferred the fitting in their poorer ear is because of the large disadvantage they would suffer for speech arriving from the poorer side when they are aided only on the better side. Follow-up studies supported this suggestion.[870, 871] For frontal speech and noise, and for speech from the better side, people understand slightly more when the aid is in the better ear. When the speech comes from the poorer side, however, people understand much less when the aid is in the better ear than when it is in the worse ear. People may thus prefer a fitting on the worse side because it minimizes their disability in the most adverse situations they encounter, even if it is not optimal in other, easier situations.

---

p   The HPLE is the level of speech needed to produce a score equal to half that of the maximum score achievable at any level.

Which ear to fit: a simple practical rule
Fit the ear that has the four-frequency average (4FA) threshold closer to 60 dB HL. Although this rule is simple and practical, and is consistent with the three decision-making factors listed in the text, there is no experimental evidence that directly tests its adequacy.

The possibility of deprivation and acclimatization further complicates the issue of deciding how poor the poorer ear really is. The research into auditory deprivation (see Section 14.3.3) shows that speech discrimination ability in a previously unaided ear can improve markedly some time after a hearing aid is fitted to that ear. It is reasonable to hypothesize that for a person with an asymmetric hearing loss, auditory deprivation may occur in the ear with poorer pure tone thresholds, even when neither ear is aided. If that does happen, unaided speech discrimination ability will be an inaccurate guide to the *potential* speech discrimination ability of the poorer ear. Avoiding further deprivation is another reason for fitting the poorer ear. Indeed, fitting the better ear may exacerbate auditory deprivation effects in the poorer ear. Of course, fitting only the poorer ear may not be best for the patient in the short term, and the patient should be made aware of this.

Finally, it is worth noting that factors other than the inherent speech discrimination capacity of each ear can influence the ear of choice for unilateral fittings, whether the hearing loss is symmetrical or asymmetrical. These factors may include:

- Manipulation difficulties in an arm or hand;

- Ear canal complications including chronic otitis externa, suppurating otitis media, exostoses, and possibly even collapsed ear canals;

- The need for help in situations where the wanted signal, or the noise, is predominantly on one side of the head;

- The need to use a telephone on one side.

14.6.3 Alternatives: FM and CROS

Several options should be considered for people with markedly asymmetrical hearing loss, including those with unilateral loss. Because a major symptom of the loss of full binaural function is the need for a SNR higher than that required by normal hearers, any hearing aid fitting that improves SNR is particularly worthwhile. Chief amongst these is an FM or other type of wireless connection to a remote microphone near the source (see Section 3.5). Directional microphones are another alternative. CROS hearing aids are a third alternative (see Section 16.1), and these can incorporate a directional microphone if desired. Not surprisingly, a wireless connection produces much better speech performance than either of the alternatives.[362, 449, 897] A directional microphone is more effective than a CROS aid, but these solutions are not mutually exclusive.

14.7 Deciding on Bilateral versus Unilateral Fittings

How should a clinician approach the decision of whether to fit bilaterally or unilaterally? The research evidence suggests that almost all hearing-impaired people will be better off in some listening situations with two hearing aids than with one. Unfortunately, many patients do not share this view. Even when there is no cost involved, and the patients have the opportunity to compare a bilateral versus a unilateral fitting, patients will not necessarily choose two hearing aids.

In one study, approximately half the patients preferred a unilateral fitting.[847] Those who opted for a unilateral fitting were less impaired (a four-frequency average loss of 33 dB HL) and reported much less handicap when unaided. The reasons given for adopting a single hearing aid were mixed, and included convenience, comfort, and self-consciousness as well as reasons related to hearing. All the hearing aids were linear/peak-clipping BTEs, and one cannot extrapolate the finding to all hearing aid types. Significantly better localization ability was reported by subjects while they were wearing two hearing aids, and those who eventually chose two hearing aids indicated that superior localization, as well as clarity, were the reasons behind their choice. Other studies, also with linear/peak-clipping hearing aids, have indicated a much higher bilateral take-up rate.[94, 119]

Although one might expect that a recommendation for bilateral versus unilateral fitting could be based on the audiometric profile, this is true only in the extreme cases of normal hearing or profound hearing loss in one of the ears. Studies that have attempted to find differences between the audiometric profiles of those who choose a bilateral fitting compared to those who choose a unilateral fitting have been largely unsuccessful,[268, 868] although on average, those who choose a bilateral fitting have slightly more hearing loss.[847] Ear asymmetry has not emerged as a significant factor.[847, 868] Factors other than hearing thresholds, such as cosmetic concerns and listening needs, apparently influence the choice to a greater degree than does the audiometric profile. Age is also a factor: those over 75 years of age are less likely to accept bilateral hearing aids than those under 75 years.[868] The inadequacy of hearing thresholds to determine bilateral candidacy parallels the considerations of who is a candidate for hearing aid fitting (Chapter 8).

Because the final choice rests with the patient, let us look at the choice from the patient's perspective: what information does the patient need to make the decision that is best for him or her?

First, the patient would like to know which configuration will enable him or her to hear best. Except for a very small proportion of

people with an extremely asymmetrical loss (see Section 14.6.1), and for a small proportion of people who cannot achieve satisfactory binaural fusion (see Section 14.4.2) this will be a bilateral fitting.

Second, the patient would like to know how *much* additional benefit will be obtained if he or she chooses to have two hearing aids rather than one. This is a much harder question because we do not know the answer with any precision. In general terms, we can say that:

- A patient with a moderate or severe hearing loss in both ears will gain *substantially* more benefit from two hearing aids than from one.[88, 152, 206] The advantage in speech understanding, averaged across listening situations, is likely to be equivalent to a 5 dB improvement in SNR.[974] This increase is enough to make the difference between understanding very little of a conversation compared to understanding most of a conversation. Bilateral advantage will be even greater than this when wanted sounds arrive from the unaided side in a unilateral fitting, provided the patient has aidable high-frequency hearing. Conversely, bilateral advantage will be less when wanted sounds arrive from the aided side in a unilateral fitting. Asymmetry in hearing will decrease the degree of bilateral advantage, but some advantage should remain even when thresholds are asymmetrical by 50 dB. Bilateral hearing aids will also significantly increase the patient's ability to localize. This will be valuable in itself and will also indirectly increase speech understanding by helping the patient locate the person speaking in a group conversation.

- A patient with a bilateral loss that is mild in at least one ear will gain only a small benefit from two hearing aids compared to one. Bilateral advantage for intelligibility may be noticeable only in situations where the signal of interest is soft and arrives from the unaided side of the head.

- A patient with a hearing loss between these extremes will experience a degree of benefit somewhere in between.

Many patients will understandably have trouble deciding with certainty whether to acquire one or two hearing aids. A trial with two hearing aids for some weeks is extremely helpful. The following information may also be helpful.

- *There is a reasonable expectation of eventual superiority for two hearing aids.* Even 25 years ago, the vast majority of patients who tried bilateral hearing aids chose to wear both of them in at least some situations.[119] With the improvement in hearing aid quality that has occurred since then, there should now be even more situations in which two hearing aids are more helpful than one.

- *Changing from unilateral to bilateral fitting can be particularly difficult.* Many experienced unilateral aid wearers who acquire a second hearing aid consider that it took them some months to adapt to the second aid, although most eventually find it to be very helpful.[94] They rate their listening ability in a wide range of situations much more highly than when they wore only one aid.[576]

Where both ears are potentially aidable, and where the aided ear will receive sounds with a sensation level higher than that of the unaided ear, the clinician should advise the patient that speech recognition ability in the unaided ear may deteriorate if not aided. The patient should be further advised that there is a reasonable possibility that the unaided ear will not recover any lost ability even if a

---

Should two hearing aids be provided at the same time or sequentially?

A common strategy is to initially provide patients with one hearing aid, and subsequently (some weeks, or months later) fit a second one (Vaughan-Jones et al., 1993). This sequential approach has advantages:

- Patients can make a more gradual commitment to owning hearing aids, which can be useful if they initially associate two hearing aids with being very deaf or very old, or are unsure if the expense will be justified.

- Patients can acquire the necessary manipulation skills on one hearing aid at a time, which some patients may find less daunting.

The sequential approach also has disadvantages:

- The patient has to undergo two successive periods of adjustment. In the first period, the brain may learn to partially ignore the unaided ear (see Section 14.3.3). For this reason, the unilateral period should be as short as possible, and preferably less than six months. In the second period, the brain must learn to use the information provided by the newly fitted ear, and to properly combine the signals coming from both ears.

- The number of visits and time taken to fit two hearing aids sequentially is greater than if they are fitted simultaneously, thus increasing the expense.

- The initial sensation of hearing being unbalanced between the two ears may induce rejection of hearing aids altogether.

There are no data on which approach is more effective, but the arguments for fitting the hearing aids simultaneously seem more compelling. Sequential fitting can be reserved for patients who are totally unwilling to try two hearing aids when they are first aided. When two hearing aids are fitted at the outset, it usually takes only a few hours or a few days for patients who are going to benefit from bilateral hearing aids to appreciate their advantages over a unilateral aid (Erdman & Sedge, 1981).

second hearing aid is subsequently acquired. If a patient rejects a second hearing aid, the clinician should document that it was recommended, and the basis of the recommendation, but that the recommendation was rejected.

The provision of bilateral hearing aids is extremely important for hearing-impaired people with severe visual problems. Even small improvements in localization are likely to be extremely important because of the increased importance to such people of auditory perception.

Similar bilateral considerations also apply to cochlear implants and to bone-anchored hearing aids[910] despite the much smaller interaural attenuation that exists for bone-conducted stimuli. Amazingly, the decision about unilateral versus bilateral fitting has to be made even for tactile aids. Bilateral vibrotactile aids, with head mounted microphones, enable localization of competing talkers, and are anecdotally reported to result in a greater externalization of sound than occurs for a single tactile aid.[747]

14.8 Effect of Bilateral versus Unilateral Fitting on Electro-acoustic Prescriptions

Because of binaural loudness summation (see Section 14.2.4), we would expect that bilaterally aided people will use less gain than unilaterally aided people with the same hearing loss. The gain difference should be about 5 to 6 dB for mid-level inputs. Because the extent of binaural loudness summation depends on level, the gain difference should be slightly greater for high input levels and slightly less for low input levels. This implies that a very slightly higher compression ratio is optimal for bilateral fittings. At any level, the gain difference between bilateral and unilateral prescriptions should decrease as the degree of asymmetry increases. Corrections along these lines are included in the NAL-NL1 software (version 1.2).

Although the decreased gain has been deduced by assuming that the aim of a hearing aid fitting is to produce a certain loudness, similar conclusions would be reached if we aimed to achieve some target speech intelligibility score. In this case, binaural squelch and binaural redundancy allow the gain to be decreased in a bilateral fitting without affecting speech intelligibility.

LDL appears to be only slightly lower, if at all, when people listen binaurally than when they listen monaurally (see Section 14.2.4). From the perspective of avoiding discomfort, we would therefore not adjust SSPL differently for a bilateral fitting compared to a unilateral fitting.[360] Of course, discomfort is not the only thing that determines the target SSPL. We also wish to avoid excessive saturation in the hearing aid. Because we can prescribe about 8 dB less gain for mid-level inputs for a bilateral fitting, we can therefore prescribe SSPL to be 8 dB lower than for a unilateral fitting, without changing the degree of saturation. Alternatively, we can leave SSPL unchanged, and consequently, the hearing aid will be less saturated for mid-level inputs. Looked at differently, a bilateral fitting makes the selection of the correct SSPL less critical than it is for a unilateral fitting. This is particularly valuable for people with a severe or profound hearing loss where it can be difficult to achieve an SSPL low enough to avoid discomfort but high enough to avoid saturation. This is an indirect benefit of bilateral fittings.

It is theoretically possible that the optimum amplification characteristics for one ear depend on what is provided to the other ear. There are however, no compelling reasons why this should be true, and an experimental investigation of it failed to provide any evidence that it is true.[733]

Overall, it seems reasonable to adjust each aid in isolation to obtain the best performance. It seems reasonable to allow for binaural effects by making sure that loudness at the two ears is balanced, and that overall loudness is acceptable. This is likely to require less gain for a bilateral fitting than for a unilateral fitting, especially at high input levels. There does not seem to be strong case for having different SSPL values for bilateral fittings than for unilateral fittings, however.

14.9 Concluding Comments

Despite many years of research, there is much about bilateral hearing aid fitting that we do not yet understand. Part of the problem is that we do not have an adequate understanding of how the auditory system performs the binaural processing that it does. Further, a bilateral fitting does not necessarily imply that sounds will be above threshold in both ears, or that useful binaural interactions must occur. Similarly, many of the advantages of binaural hearing can occur with a unilateral fitting if the sound is sufficiently intense or the hearing loss is sufficiently mild. Head diffraction effects, however, are a reliable source of bilateral advantage in many situations.

Generally, therefore, the clinician should start from the assumption that two hearing aids will be most appropriate and look for reasons why this may not be true for the individual patient, rather than the other way around.

CHAPTER FIFTEEN

SPECIAL HEARING AID ISSUES FOR CHILDREN

Synopsis

When children are born with a hearing loss, early provision of hearing aids is essential if the child is to learn to speak and listen with the greatest possible proficiency. Evidence is accumulating that hearing aids should be provided prior to six months of age. For these hearing aids to be optimally adjusted, hearing thresholds must be determined, as accurately as possible, separately for each ear. No matter what type of transducer is used, the small size of a baby's ear complicates the interpretation of hearing threshold. This difficulty is overcome either by expressing threshold in dB SPL in the ear canal, or by expressing it as equivalent adult hearing threshold in dB HL.

BTE hearing aids are most likely to be provided, in conjunction with a soft earmold, until the child is at least 8 years old (and possibly much older). The hearing aid should contain features that will enable the child to receive the best possible signal. This is likely to include an audio input socket, so that an FM wireless aid can be connected when required. Ideally, the wireless device should be able to automatically attenuate the local microphone whenever the person wearing the transmitter talks.

The amplification prescription that is optimal for children is controversial. There is no doubt that to communicate effectively, children learning language need a better signal-to-noise ratio than do adults. There is, however, uncertainty about how much gain they need relative to adults with the same hearing loss. Compared to adults, they almost certainly do not need any more real-ear gain for high-level sounds, they probably do not need any more gain for medium level sounds, but they possibly need more gain for low-level sounds. There is an even greater need for wide dynamic range compression in hearing aids for infants (who cannot manipulate the volume control) than there is for adults.

To achieve a certain real-ear gain, young children need less coupler gain than do adults, because children have smaller ear canals. An efficient way to allow for small ear canals is to measure the real-ear to coupler difference before prescribing the hearing aid, and to calculate the coupler gain that will result in the target rear-ear aided gain.

Hearing aid fittings can be evaluated by speech testing (for those over three years of age), paired-comparison preference testing (for those over six years of age), and subjective reporting by the child, the parents, or the teachers. The maximum output that has been prescribed should be evaluated by observing the child when intense sounds are made, and for those over approximately six years of age, by assessing the loudness of these sounds.

Effective amplification of young children is not possible without the support and understanding of parents. The audiologist must therefore inform and support the parents in a variety of ways. One way to provide ongoing habilitation is to base the service activities around goals determined jointly by the audiologist and the parents (and by the child when old enough).

Part of the information provided to parents includes safety aspects of amplification and hearing loss. Hazards include battery ingestion, excessive exposure to noise, physical impact, and failure to detect warning sounds if amplification is not functioning correctly.

This chapter gives an overview of amplification for children, and particularly for infants. One chapter can not do justice to the importance of getting fully functioning hearing aids on a child as early as possible. Much of the information about hearing aids in the other chapters, however, is also relevant to children. For additional information specific to hearing-impaired children, the reader should refer to the following excellent sources: Bess, Gravel & Tharpe, 1996; Feigin & Stelmachowicz, 1991; Northern & Downs, 2000; and Seewald, 2000.

15.1 Sensory Experience and Deprivation

There are two reasons why it is important for a child to be fitted with hearing aids as early as possible. The first is to start improving the quality of life of the child and family. A year without hearing aids is a year in which the child has not been able to enjoy those inter-actions that require a sense of hearing. The second reason is similar, but has effects that are more permanent. Neural connections in the brain that allow speech to be understood are formed based on the signals they receive from the cochlea.[500] Although neural connec-tions can form or disappear at any stage of life,[336a] these connections are more effectively formed during the early years of life. The brain's opportunity to form during the first two or three years of life, and even during the first six months,[606, 963] must not be missed if the child is to have the best possible sense of auditory perception for the rest of his or her life.

Providing rehabilitation early in life also maximizes expressive language ability.[737] Children who receive amplification prior to six months of age develop clearer speech than those who first received amplification when they were older.[577, 963] In short, no age is too low to provide amplification, once it is clear that the child has a hearing loss, and once the degree of loss can be estimated.

Early stimulation should be binaural. Some parts of the ascending auditory pathway (e.g. the inferior colliculus) combine and compare signals from the two cochleae, presumably to perform functions like localization and the binaural suppression of noise. These parts of the neural system can only do their job, and presumably learn how to do their job, if both cochleae are sending out signals. For this reason, binaural stimulation that contains inter-aural difference cues appears to be essential during the first few years of life.[44] For people with a severe bilateral hearing loss, bilateral amplification maximizes binaural stimulation (see also Section 14.3.3).

There may, however, be some children who have such differences between the way each ear processes sound that better performance is obtained with a single hearing aid in the better ear only (see Sections 14.4.2 and 14.6.1). How can this dilemma be resolved? The most conservative option is to aid both ears and continue to encourage use in both ears until it is clear that this is counter-productive. Evidence for withdrawing amplification from one ear would include:

- Consistent and prolonged rejection of one hearing aid by the child after the clinician has made every effort to fine-tune the fitting for earmold comfort and loudness comfort.

- Reports from the parent that the child functions better with one hearing aid during trial periods of a few days with only one hearing aid (see Section 15.6 for some subjective report tools to assist with this evaluation).

- Poorer speech test results when fitted bilaterally than when fitted unilaterally.

Although the effects of a unilateral hearing loss are not as devastating as those of a bilateral loss, even unilateral loss can adversely affect educational performance.[62] Such an effect is not surprising, because a unilateral loss will make speech harder to understand whenever there is noise or rever-beration and this applies to many classrooms.

For the future: speech tests for babies

Although speech discrimination tests are usually only given to older children, even babies can do speech tests. Visual reinforcement speech-sound discrimination can be used to determine whether babies can distinguish between the different sounds of speech (Kuhl et al., 1992). It may be possible to apply this technique to determine the effectiveness of amplification in general, and to detect any cases where bilateral amplification should not be provided.

It therefore seems reasonable to aid the impaired ear wherever possible, so that binaural stimulation is as effective as possible. Where hearing thresholds on the impaired side are profound, the only form of device that is likely to be effective is the use of wireless transmission from a microphone worn by the teacher to a receiver worn by the child (see Section 14.6.3).

15.2 Assessment of Hearing Loss

15.2.1 Frequency-specific and ear-specific assessment

Methods for assessing the degree and type of hearing loss are not within the scope of this book. It is, however, essential that hearing loss be assessed as accurately as is possible prior to fitting hearing aids. The accuracy with which hearing loss can be assessed will vary with the age of the child, but the range of techniques now available will allow a reasonable assessment to be made at any age. The minimum requirements are estimated thresholds for one low frequency (preferably 500 Hz) and one high frequency (preferably 2 kHz), separately for each ear. Of course, it is better if thresholds can be estimated at more frequencies. If time and the behavior of the child prevent this, however, an appropriate fitting is more likely to be achieved with two

reasonably accurate thresholds than with a greater number of inaccurate thresholds. As more audiological information is obtained during subsequent appointments, the hearing aid fitting can be fine-tuned.

Although many infants have approximately symmetrical hearing losses, it is unreasonable to assume that they all do. For 180 aided children surveyed at random, the absolute value of the differences between thresholds in the left and right ears (at the same frequency) averaged only 8 dB but varied up to 90 dB.[563] At any frequency, hearing thresholds in the two ears differed by 20 dB or more for approximately 10% of the children. It is thus essential to obtain thresholds separately for each ear. Obtaining separate thresholds for each ear is most easily achieved by using insert earphones, which are more comfortable and more readily tolerated, than supra-aural headphones. Insert earphones can also be calibrated more appropriately for small ears, as explained in the next section. The use of insert earphones is thus strongly recommended.

Frequency-specific assessment techniques that can be used with insert earphones include:

- tone-burst auditory brainstem response (ABR);

- single or multi-frequency steady-state evoked potentials (SSEP);

- distortion-product evoked otoacoustic emissions, or click-evoked otoacoustic emissions, although these currently give only a generalized impression of high-frequency outer hair cell activity, rather than specific hearing thresholds.

- behavioral techniques such as visual reinforcement audiometry (VRA), tangible reinforcement operant conditioning audiometry (TROCA), visual reinforcement operant conditioning audiometry (VROCA), and play audiometry.

The choice of techniques is determined by the age of the child and by the equipment available. To increase the accuracy and surety with which thresholds are known, more than one technique should be applied. For infants, these should preferably include one behavioral measure (when the infant is old enough), at least one electrophysiological measure (usually frequency specific ABR), and otoacoustic emissions to confirm a cochlear abnormality.

15.2.2 Small ears and calibration issues

Hearing thresholds may be determined using stimuli generated by a loudspeaker, by supra-aural headphones, or by insert earphones. In the last case, the insert phones may be connected to the child's ear by the standard foam earplugs, or may be coupled to the child's individual earmold. Even if all these have been calibrated so that an average adult with normal hearing has thresholds of 0 dB HL, there is no guarantee that the same will be true for an infant with normal hearing. For example:

- A baby will have an ear canal resonance nearer to 6 kHz than to 2.7 kHz.[498] If stimuli are presented via a loudspeaker the baby may have better-than-normal hearing at 6 kHz, but an apparent loss at 2 and 3 kHz.

- When an insert earphone or individual earmold is used, an infant will have a much smaller residual ear canal volume (the volume medial to the tip of the earmold) than an adult. Consequently, for the same audiometer setting, a higher SPL will be present in the infant's ear than in the adult's ear. The infant will therefore appear to have less hearing loss than the adult, even if their middle ears and cochleae function equally effectively.

Hearing thresholds (in dB HL) may thus appear to change during the first few years of a child's life, just because of changes in the size of the child's ears.[614] There are two equally effective solutions to this problem. One is to express all thresholds in dB SPL in the ear canal. Expressing threshold in this way simplifies comparisons between threshold and hearing aid output expressed in the same manner.

The second is to express thresholds as **equivalent adult hearing level**. This is the hearing threshold level that an average adult would have if the adult has the same threshold in dB SPL at the eardrum as the child. Comparisons with hearing aid output are less straightforward (unless done within a computer program), but the familiar characterization of hearing loss in dB HL is maintained.[a]

Determining threshold in dB SPL in the ear canal

The best way to determine threshold in the ear canal is to use an individually measured real-ear to coupler difference (RECD; see Section 10.7 and 15.4.3). Thresholds obtained with an insert earphone expressed in dB HL are first converted to dB SPL in a 2 cc coupler by adding the reference equivalent threshold SPLs (RETSPLs) shown in Table 15.1. These coupler SPLs are then converted to real-ear SPL by adding the individually measured RECD values.

Alternatively, the clinician can directly measure the difference between the audiometer setting (in dB HL) and the SPL in the real ear for each patient. This difference is known as the **real-ear to dial difference (REDD)** and can be obtained for any type of headphone.[743, 785]

---

[a]   DSL software uses the first of these solutions to the problem of changing ear geometry, and NAL-NL1 software uses the second.

Table 15.1 Useful correction factors for hearing thresholds. Reference equivalent threshold SPL values are those applicable to insert earphones calibrated in HA1 or HA2 style 2 cc couplers (ISO 389-2; ANSI S3.6 – 1996). Adult average REDD is the eardrum SPL corresponding to 0 dB HL for the average adult.[52] These REDD values can be subtracted from eardrum SPL at threshold if one wishes to convert thresholds from eardrum SPL to equivalent adult-average hearing level.

Correction Factor	Frequency (Hz)						
	250	500	1000	2000	3000	4000	6000
RETSPL HA1 2-cc	14.5	6.0	0.0	2.5	2.5	0.0	-2.5
RETSPL HA2 2-cc	14.0	5.5	0.0	3.0	3.5	5.5	2.0
REDD$_{average\ adult}$	16.0	12.0	10.0	16.0	15.0	13.0	16.0

Both methods require threshold to be expressed in dB SPL in the ear canal. For the first method, no further calculations or conversions are necessary. For the second method, this ear canal threshold is converted to equivalent adult hearing level by subtracting the adult average REDD values shown in Table 15.1. Both methods are most conveniently carried out with the aid of software (e.g. NAL-NL1 or DSL[i/o]) which make the appropriate calculations and contain age-appropriate corrections for those cases where it is not possible to measure RECD or REDD for the individual.

15.3 Hearing Aid and Earmold Features and Styles

15.3.1 Hearing aids

The appearance and size of the hearing aid is likely to be important to teen-aged children, and to parents of children of all ages. When worn by infants, even average-sized hearing aids look very big behind tiny ears. Parents will ultimately make the final decision about the size and style of hearing aids for young children. It is essential that they first understand the likely serious consequences of choosing a hearing aid that has inferior electroacoustic qualities, if such a choice is being considered. For example, the strong link between receiving an adequate signal during the first few years of life, and the development of good language and speech should be impressed on the parents. To achieve an adequate signal, the maximum output must be appropriate to the degree of loss, and this may dictate a large hearing aid.

To maximize information transmitted to the child in noisy or reverberant situations, the child may need a wireless system immediately or within the life of the hearing aid. If so, it is desirable for the hearing aid to have a direct audio input connector. Alternatively, a neck-loop (see Section 3.7.2) used in conjunction with the hearing aid telecoil will decrease the number of cords that a young child can grab and disconnect. A wireless receiver built into, or clipped onto, the hearing aid eliminates these cords. These options may necessitate selecting a larger size hearing aid.

Switchable directional microphones, telecoils, and multiple memories are as useful for older children as they are for adults. For any of these features to be useful, the child has to be old enough to perform the switching necessary, or the child has to be in an environment (such as an early intervention center) where an adult takes responsibility for the hearing aid setting at all times.

Microphones that are permanently directional have the same disadvantages that they do for adults: increased pick-up of wind noise and slightly decreased sensitivity when a wanted sound (such as a warning sound, the noise of an approaching car, or comments by other children in the classroom) comes from behind.

Practical tip: Securing the hearing aids

When children are active enough to lose their hearing aids but not old enough to make sure they do not, hearing aids can be secured by a Huggie™ aid. This is a large loop that encircles the pinnae attached to two small loops that encircle the hearing aid. Alternatively, a fishing line can be tied around each earhook and secured by a safety pin to the collar at the back of the child's clothing. (A tip from the dad of an active child.)

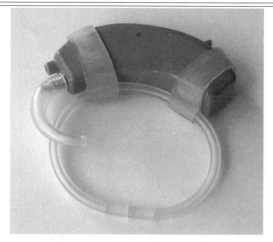

Figure 15.1 A Huggie Aid™ attached to a BTE hearing aid.

For younger children, directional microphones (whether fixed or switchable) will not be as advantageous as they are for adults because very young children will not routinely look at the person to whom they are trying to listen.[837] It is difficult to be definitive about when directional microphones should be provided, but the balance of benefits is less positive than it is for adults. Fixed directional microphones should perhaps be avoided. Individual problems, circumstances, behavior, and the availability of alternative solutions like wireless systems, should all be considered when contemplating switchable directional microphones.

The advantages of digitally programmable hearing aids over fully analog hearing aids are even greater for children of all ages than for adults. Given the greater difficulty of being sure that a child's fitting has been optimally adjusted, the greater range of adjustment of digitally programmable aids is an important advantage. The younger the child, the greater is the likely advantage.

Most hearing-impaired children are fitted with BTE hearing aids. These have the advantage over body aids that sound is picked up at head level instead of being affected by clothing noise and body baffle effects, especially if the infant is prone. Body aids

should be considered for children who have additional disabilities that require their head to be supported if this head support would:
- muffle sound pick-up by the BTE aid;
- frequently bump the BTE aid; or
- induce feedback oscillation in the BTE aid.[880]

There is no fundamental reason why ITE hearing aids (or more generally ITC or CIC hearing aids) can not be used for children of any age, but there are several strong practical disadvantages.
- It may be difficult to fit an ITE within a small ear.
- Small ears grow, rapidly at first, and then more slowly. If an ITE is worn too early, it will have to be replaced frequently as the ear grows. Replacing an ITE aid is much more expensive than replacing an earmold. A pediatric working group[60] considered that ear growth stabilizes sufficiently by the age of 8 to 10 years to consider ITE hearing aids.
- All hearing-impaired children will benefit from the use of an FM or other wireless system in many circumstances. It is not common for ITE hearing aids to have the necessary audio input socket or possibly even telecoil. This deficiency makes it difficult or impossible to combine the

signal-to-noise ratio (SNR) advantages of the wireless system with the individually pre-scribed electroacoustics of the hearing aid.

- There is a small risk factor with ITE hearing aids. Because the shell is a thin layer of hard plastic, breakage of the hearing aid while it is in the ear can cause sharp edges that can lacerate the canal wall. This fracturing can happen to people of any age who receive a blow to the ear. The risk has to be balanced against the cosmetic, social, emotional and acoustic advantages of an ITE aid.

- It is more difficult for a parent or teacher to visually identify whether an ITE is on or off, and where the volume control is set.

- A particularly difficult issue is whether transposition hearing aids should be used for children. On the one hand, many children with high-frequency hearing in the profound and upper severe range will never have access to high-frequency cues without transposition. On the other hand, the efficacy and candidacy for transpos-ition has not definitely been established for adults let alone for children (see Section 7.4). It seems risky to train a young child's auditory system to use modified cues that may turn out to be sub-optimal when further research becomes available. Research is urgently needed to establish guidelines.

15.3.2 Earmolds

Concerns similar to those for ITE shells also exist for the safety of hard earmolds for BTE hearing aids. Soft earmolds are used more commonly than hard earmolds, because soft molds are less likely to cause discomfort, feedback oscillation, or injury to the ear if they are broken.

As with adults, soft materials deteriorate more rapidly with time, but this is less of an issue for young children because their earmolds will have to be replaced more often as the ear grows. In summary, either hard or soft materials can be used for earmolds, but

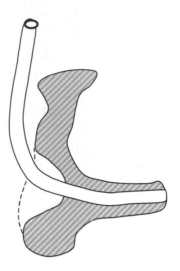

Figure 15.2 Cross section of a hollow-concha earmold.

for younger children, the advantages of soft materials usually outweigh their disadvantages.

The small size of a baby's ear can create three other problems. The angle at which the tubing protrudes from the earmold, combined with the close proximity of the earmold to the tip of the earhook can pull the hearing aid away from the surface of the head. The solution is for the tubing to bend more sharply, but often this can not be done without kinking the tubing. A solution is to hollow out the center of the conchal part of the earmold, prior to inserting the tubing.[665] A cross-section through the earmold is shown in Figure 15.2. (This process is most conveniently done by the earmold laboratory when the earmold is first made.) The hollowed area allows the tubing to commence its upward bend closer to the ear canal.

The second problem created by a small ear is that it can be difficult to achieve even a 2-mm sound bore. The only solutions are careful drilling, plus terminating the sound tubing some distance from the medial tip of the earmold. If the tubing is constricted at any point, decreased high-frequency gain and maximum output are likely to result. Third,

---

FM systems and advanced nonlinear hearing aids

There should be no more problems coupling an FM system to an advanced, nonlinear hearing aid than there are to a linear-peak clipping hearing aid. The hearing aid must be properly adjusted to operate by itself, and the output level from the FM receiver must be properly adjusted (see Section 3.7.3). Once these adjustments are achieved, the signal from the receiver is processed in exactly the same way as a signal picked up by the hearing aid microphone.

As with any non-linear hearing aid, the aid should be measured with a broadband signal with a speech-like spectrum rather than a pure tone (see Section 4.1.3). If the hearing aid contains adaptive noise suppression, this function should be disabled during measurement.

Amplification, compression, noise suppression, output limiting, transposition, and possibly even feedback suppression should all operate normally. They should operate just as they do for acoustic input signals with overall levels around 70 dB SPL (or as they do for acoustic signals of varying input levels if the FM transmitter does not normally operate in compression). Microphone directionality will not be relevant if the FM system is operating in a mode that attenuates the hearing aid microphone.

---

it can be difficult or impossible to use the acoustic modifications (horns and vents) that can be achieved in an adult-sized ear.

15.3.3 FM wireless transmission systems

Frequency modulation (FM) wireless systems improve signal quality and hence intelligibility much more than any signal processing scheme located entirely within the hearing aid.[b] Although FM systems will provide an improved signal for any hearing-impaired person, they are particularly relevant to children. This is partly because children need a higher SNR than adults, and partly because children spend a lot of their day in situations where there is one dominant talker who can conveniently wear the transmitter.

In addition to their use in schools, FM systems can be used at home and elsewhere. FM systems will help a child of any age understand conversation in the car, television, coaches of sports teams, parents on outings, etc.[530] As in schools, a major problem to overcome is ensuring that the child receives a signal from the transmitter only when the

person wearing the transmitter is talking to the child, and that the local microphone has enough sensitivity at all other times.[101, 607] Speech-operated switching is thus just as useful in home or social situations as it is at school. Speech-operated switching is not a complete solution, however. Parents, teachers and care-givers still have to remember to switch the FM transmitter off whenever they are engaging in conversations that are not relevant to the child. The inappropriateness of receiving a transmission from someone in another room could perhaps be demonstrated to parents while they attempt to converse with someone in front of them. This may reinforce the importance of the child always receiving the correct input signal.

In systems with speech-operated switching, switching off the transmitter should enable the local microphone to resume operation, but it is worth checking to ensure that this happens. Systems without either speech-operated switching or squelch are likely to inject high-level noise into the hearing aid when the receiver is not receiving a transmission. This noise must be avoided.

---

[b] The principles of FM wireless transmission systems, and their adjustment methods are covered in Section 3.8.

If the local microphone is located in a body-level FM receiver rather than in the hearing aid, the receiver should be worn at chest level rather than at belt level, as the latter will be shadowed by a desk when the child is seated.[532] At the time of writing, body-level receivers with self-contained hearing aids tend not to have the advanced compression circuitry available in personal BTE hearing aids. On the other hand, the greater separation of the microphone from the ear canal enables the hearing aid to have a higher gain without feedback oscillation. Furthermore, the larger controls are easier for children with fine-motor problems.[530]

15.4 Prescribing Amplification for Children

15.4.1 Speech identification ability and amplification requirements

A fundamental question for which we do not yet have an answer is whether children, and infants in particular, need amplification characteristics different from those needed by adults with the same degree of loss. An easy aspect of this question relates to the small size of infants' ear canals and the implications this has for SPL at the eardrum. In this respect, children's requirements are definitely different. Children need less coupler gain and OSPL90 than adults if they are to receive the same gain and maximum output at the eardrum as adults. Procedures for dealing with this issue are described in Sections 10.7 and 15.4.3.

The more difficult part of the question is whether the *real-ear* gain and maximum output should be different for children than for adults. Unfortunately, few data address this question directly. Let us first examine why children *might* have real-ear amplification requirements different from those of adults. After the theoretical review, we will conclude with an extremely tentative practical recommendation.

When we adults hear speech, we use our knowledge of the language to fill in any sounds that are too weak for us to perceive directly. This occurs so naturally that we are not even aware that we are doing it unless the proportion of information that we can directly perceive is very small. An infant still faces the task of acquiring language and so is unable to fill in gaps. A young child with some knowledge of language can only partially fill in the information that the child cannot perceive directly.[652]

Even when speech material contains no semantic, syntactic, or linguistic context, such as is the case for nonsense syllables, normal-hearing infants need the level to be 26 dB higher than that needed by adults to discriminate between syllables with the same accuracy.[670] Similarly, 5-year old children need levels considerably higher than do older children if they are to achieve the same performance on a monosyllabic word test, even though the words are familiar to them.[110] Does this mean that we should prescribe more gain for hearing-impaired infants than for hearing-impaired adults with the same pure tone hearing loss? Possibly, but the data obtained with normal-hearing infants do not answer this question.

What the data directly tell us is that if we were prescribing amplification on the basis of achieving optimal speech scores, we would fit normal-hearing infants with a hearing aid that had a gain of approximately 26 dB for low-level sounds! There are two problems in applying this to hearing-impaired people. First, the data do not tell us how much gain children need at higher input levels. Second, the optimum gain for a particular input level is a delicate balance between choosing the gain and frequency response that optimizes intelligibility, but subject to the overall loudness of the sensation being acceptable to the listener in that listening situation. The balance *may* swing more towards increased gain for those with little or no knowledge of language than it does for those with well-developed language skills. It seems very likely that *if* there is a difference between what is best for adults and what is best for infants, this difference will be greater for low-level sounds than for high-level sounds. At the high extreme, the loudness discomfort level for hearing-impaired children aged 7 to 14 years has been shown to be the same as for hearing-impaired adults with the same pure tone hearing losses.[439] Consequently, we would not want to prescribe any more high-level gain and OSPL90 for infants than we do for adults.

The previous discussion has been about overall maximum output and gain. Of course, we also have to decide how much gain should be applied at each frequency. That is, it is possible that the *shape* of the frequency response should be different from that which is optimal for adults. Some experts have hypothesized that children need additional high-frequency gain, because high-frequency cues are often the most difficult for children to perceive. Other experts have argued that infants first need additional low-frequency gain because intonation and other supra-segmental cues seem to be important components of communication when language is first developing. Either of these conjectures could be right or wrong.

While it is possible that children need different response shapes as their knowledge of the language develops, we simply do not have the knowledge needed to link stages of language acquisition to optimal response shapes. Because important cues to speech reside in all frequency ranges, it seems unwise to make such an assumption without some evidence that it is true. The question is linked to the previous discussion about gain and loudness: Every gain increase in one frequency region will be at the expense of

amplification for the rest of the frequency range, unless the signal is also made louder overall.

Similarly, infants need a SNR 7 dB higher than that needed by adults to achieve a given speech discrimination score,[671] and pre-school children need a SNR 3 dB higher than that needed by adults.[75] The clearest implication from these findings is that there will be listening situations in which normal-hearing adults can discriminate between sounds, but in which normal-hearing infants cannot. The situation is most unlikely to be different in nature for hearing-impaired adults and infants.

The implication of these findings for the SNR provided by hearing aids is much more straightforward than it is for gain and frequency response. There is often no problem if SNR is improved more than is necessary, whereas if too much gain is applied, the result can be discomfort, decreased intelligibility, or both. (In some circumstances, improving SNR too much is a problem if accomplishing it has deprived the child from hearing his or her own voice or the voices of others nearby.) In practical terms, children will benefit from provision of wireless hearing aids in many situations, and these devices should be provided for every situation in which they can be used. Section 15.3.3 contains more details.

Unfortunately, there have been no studies directly comparing the optimal amplification for infants to that for adults, or to the prescriptions resulting from any selection procedure.[c] This is not surprising, as such studies would be extraordinarily difficult to do.

Several studies[129, 146, 823] have shown that the average gain preferred by children is the same as that preferred by adults with the same

---

[c]   There have been studies comparing prescribed amplification characteristics to what children younger than six years have been fitted with, but this has an illogical circularity if the fittings have been influenced by this fitting procedure or by a similar procedure.

degree of loss, although the youngest age studied was 6 years. These studies also showed that the optimum shape of the frequency response could be predicted from the audiogram using the same rules that are appropriate for adults. On the other hand, Snik and Hombergen (1993) showed that older children prefer gains 7 dB higher than those preferred by adults with the same degree of loss. The gains used by the children were, however, extremely close to those prescribed by the NAL-RP method.

How can we translate the preceding information into practical guidelines for prescribing amplification? The finding that normal-hearing children, hearing-impaired children, and hearing-impaired adults all need a better SNR than normal-hearing adults to achieve the same performance is the easiest, and has already been discussed. Wireless systems, and, to a lesser extent, directional microphones, will help. It may be desirable for children to sometimes receive a noisy signal so that they can develop skills at perceiving speech in noise. Such opportunities are likely to occur without being especially arranged: Use of a wireless system will not be possible in many situations.

The question of how much real-ear gain is needed for children relative to adults is more difficult. We need to consider not just *gain*, but gain for high-level sounds, gain for medium-level sounds, and gain for low-level sounds.

High-level sounds (e.g. a group of children playing at 80 dB SPL). It seems very unlikely that children will benefit from more gain for high-level sounds than that given to adults, given the impact of hearing aid limiting, loudness discomfort, and hearing loss desensitization. (Hearing loss desensitization refers to a person's decreased ability to extract useful information from an audible signal in any frequency region where the loss is severe or profound, as discussed in Section 9.2.4.) The close proximity that infants often have

to the talker, and the consequently increased speech levels[843] further argue against giving additional gain for high input levels. The likely frequent occurrence of high input levels suggests that compression to decrease gain as input level rises above about 70 dB SPL is even more important for infants than it is for adults.

Medium-level sounds (e.g. one person talking at 65 dB SPL). The weight of evidence is that children do not *prefer* more gain than do adults for medium-level sounds. There is no evidence regarding what gain children need, relative to adults, if they are to understand medium-level speech as well as possible. There is no evidence about the gain that hearing-impaired infants prefer or benefit most from. Indirect knowledge lets us say only that they need at least as much gain as do adults.

Low-level sounds (e.g. a person talking quietly, and/or in the distance at 50 dB SPL). There is no doubt that children are less able than adults to make full use of low-level speech signals. A major complication in comparing children's requirements to that of adults is that we do not know how much gain should be prescribed for adults for low-level sounds! As discussed in Section 9.3.9, there is great uncertainty over what the compression threshold should be, and hence what the gain for low-level sounds should be. It does, however, seem likely that the optimum low-level gain for children will be greater than for adults. For low-level sounds, increasing the gain is unlikely to cause a decrease in speech intelligibility in the way it can do for high-level sounds. Increasing the gain for low-level sounds may also increase the distance over which children can hear or overhear comments. Normal-hearing children enrich their language (whether parents approve or not!) by overhearing comments that were not intended for them.[838] Increasing the gain for low-level sounds may, however, increase the risk of feedback oscillation.

It is not clear how quickly compressors should change the gain as input varies. It may be safest for compressors to have release times longer than a few hundred milliseconds to minimize any increase of gain during pauses in a signal of interest.[d] Infants learning speech presumably do not initially have the ability to recognize the amplified noise as being separate from the speech signal they are trying to unravel.

It would also seem desirable for children to have some experience receiving signals that are just above threshold. When adults are amplified in one ear only, their ability to process low-level information in that ear decreases in the months following hearing aid fitting.[301] We would not want to deny children the ability to process low-level signals by amplifying to such an extent that they get no practice listening to such signals. Many low-level signals originate some distance away.

The inability of infants to alter a volume control, their decreased speech understanding at low input levels, and the likelihood of infants frequently receiving above-average input levels, all argue for the inclusion of wide dynamic range compression in hearing aids for infants. If it is true that children need more gain than adults for low-level sounds but not for high-level sounds, the inescapable consequence is that a higher compression ratio or a lower compression threshold (or both) should be prescribed for children than for adults.

The question of how frequency response shape should be altered for an infant or toddler relative to that prescribed for an adult is extremely difficult. There is no evidence to support an intentional variation from the shape prescribed for an adult with the same hearing loss. By contrast, there is no evidence to show that the same response should be prescribed.

The reader should recognize that all the conclusions in this section on gain requirements are highly conjectural. Data to support or refute these conclusions do not exist.

15.4.2 Threshold-based versus loudness-based procedures

The question of whether to base prescription on individually measured hearing thresholds or on individually measured supra-threshold loudness growth is easier to answer for children than it is for adults. Furthermore, the younger the child, the easier the answer. There is no proven way to obtain loudness growth data from an infant, so there is no choice: we must base prescription on hearing thresholds alone. For older children, it is possible to measure loudness growth curves by representing different degrees of loudness pictorially. Unfortunately, children do not always interpret the pictures in the way that we expect.[515]

If children can reliably perform a loudness-rating task, the advantages and disadvantages of loudness scaling become similar to those for adults (see Section 9.3.8). Of course, a loudness scale is no use unless one also has a validated prescription procedure that makes use of it. As discussed in Section 15.4.1, the balance between achieving some target loudness and achieving an output level that maximizes intelligibility may be different for children than it is for adults.

In summary, there are too many uncertainties to justify use of loudness scaling with children at the present time. It may be possible to derive some electrophysiological measures, such as ABR latency, ABR amplitude, or acoustic reflex threshold, as surrogates for loudness measures.[198, 452] For the moment, this is a topic for research rather than clinical practice, and as for adults, there is the problem of what to do with the loudness measure once it has been obtained.

---

d   Hearing aids with an adaptive release time would also fulfil this requirement.

15.4.3 Allowing for small ear canals

As a child grows, so too does the length and volume of his or her ear canal. Ear canal length determines the resonant frequency of the unaided ear, and hence the frequency of the peak of the real-ear unaided gain (REUG) curve. The change in this peak frequency with increasing age is rapid. At birth, the peak of this curve is approximately 5 to 6 kHz, but on average decreases to 3 kHz (only 10% above the average adult value) by the age of 2 to 3 years.[50, 213, 440, 498, 954] The REUG value for a person will affect the insertion gain measured for that person, and it may or may not be appropriate to take these changing values into account during hearing aid prescription (see Section 9.2.4).

The prescription procedure recommended for infants in this book is based on real-ear aided gain (REAG) rather than insertion gain. Consequently, the REUG characteristics of the individual have no effect on the prescription. The frequency of the peak in the REUG curve does, however, allow us to estimate the length of the ear canal of infants, and this is useful

to know when placing probe tubes. Figure 15.3 shows the typical variation of ear canal length inferred from the peaks in REUG curves using a two-cylinder model of the ear canal and concha.[440]

The second change with age relates to the volume of the residual ear canal when aided. This volume, in conjunction with the input impedance of the middle ear, determines the real-ear to coupler difference (RECD). For babies, the impedance of the canal walls also affects RECD,[441] Changes in RECD occur most rapidly during the first year of a baby's life. On average, the RECD approaches adult values when the child is older than approximately five years.

Figure 15.4 shows, for several ages, average values for RECD relative to those for adults. That is, the figure shows how much greater SPL a hearing aid is likely to generate in a child's ear compared to an adult's ear.[e] The greatest difference occurs in the high frequencies for the first few months of life. Values for individual children may be much lower or higher than the average values shown.

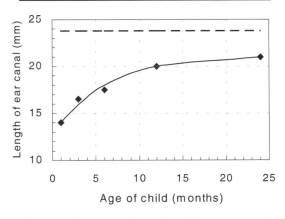

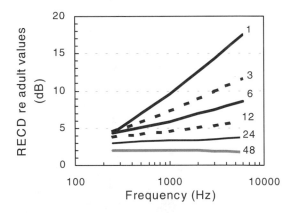

Figure 15.3 Typical length of the ear canal as a function of age (Keefe et al, 1994). Solid line is a smooth curve fitted to the data and dashed line shows the average length of the adult ear canal (Keefe et al., 1994; Salvinelli et al., 1991).

Figure 15.4 The increase in SPL generated by a hearing aid in an average child's ear relative to that in an average adult's ear. Children are aged from 1 to 48 months, as indicated for each curve.

e   The data in Figure 15.4 come from an equation fitted to the value of RECD or residual ear canal impedance for children of different ages relative to the corresponding value in an average adult's ear. The equation was fitted to the data from multiple experiments (Feigin et al., 1989; Keefe et al., 1993; Scollie, Seewald & Jenstad, 1998; Westwood & Bamford, 1995).

As explained in Section 10.7, the RECD values appropriate to an individual affect both the coupler gain and OSPL90 values needed to achieve a target REAG and real-ear saturation response (RESR). The coupler gain and OSPL90 values needed to achieve these real-ear targets can be predicted most accurately if RECD is measured for the individual patient, rather than estimated from the average values shown in Table 15.2. The accompanying panel shows the steps involved in prescribing and adjusting gain and OSPL90. If individual values of RECD have been used in this process, there is no need for any further verification of real-ear gain. Adjustment of the hearing aids to the prescription targets is thus achieved while the hearing aid is in the test box, and only a single real-ear measurement (i.e. of RECD) has to be obtained from the child.

It will sometimes be necessary to fit hearing aids to a child with a ventilation tube (also known as pressure equalization tube) in the eardrum. The ventilation tube has two effects on hearing aid performance. First, for low-frequency sounds, it connects the middle ear cavity directly to the residual ear canal volume, without the intervening effect of the eardrum. This decreases the RECD by 15 dB, averaged across a number of children and the frequencies 125 to 750 Hz.[580] The hearing aid must therefore have additional gain and OSPL90 to achieve the same SPL that would be present at the eardrum with no ventilation tube present. This additional gain is automatically prescribed if the prescription is based on individually measured RECD. No additional gain or OSPL90 is needed at those frequencies where vent-transmitted sound causes the hearing aid to have a gain of 0 dB (see Section 5.3.1).

Individual measurement of RECD does not allow for the second effect of the ventilation tube. Because the ventilation tube allows low-frequency sound to reach both sides of the eardrum, the sensitivity of the eardrum to low-frequency sounds is decreased, even if the SPL achieved in the ear canal is the same as for an intact eardrum. The loss of effective stimulation of the cochlea can be estimated from an acoustic model of a hearing aid and ear. Such modeling indicates even when the

Table 15.2 Average values of RECD for children of different ages. These values apply when the real-ear SPL has been measured using an individual earmold, and the coupler SPL has been measured using a HA2 2-cc coupler. The measurement conditions are shown in Figure 10.3(c) and (d). Data have been derived by applying the relative data in Figure 15.4 to the adult data reported by Scollie, Seewald & Jenstad (1998). These adult data (final row) differ slightly from those in Table 4.1 (row 2) because the data in Table 15.2 contain typical leakage and sound bore constriction effects, and because both sets of data contain independent random measurement errors.

Age (months)	Frequency (Hz)						
	250	500	1000	2000	3000	4000	6000
1	5	12	18	21	19	21	22
3	5	11	15	17	15	16	16
6	5	10	14	15	13	13	13
12	4	9	13	14	10	11	10
24	4	8	11	12	9	9	8
36	3	7	11	11	8	8	7
48	2	7	10	10	7	7	6
60	2	6	10	10	6	6	5
adult	1	5	8	9	5	5	4

Prescribing and adjusting hearing aids for infants

1. Obtain at least one low-frequency threshold and at least one high-frequency threshold for each ear.

2. Prescribe RESR, using the NAL-NL1 or DSL prescription software (prescriptions for RESR are similar). Alternatively, convert thresholds to equivalent adult average dB HL, as shown in Section 15.2.2, and use the RESR prescription shown in Tables 9.4 and 9.5.

3. Prescribe REAG, using the prescription procedure you have chosen (caution: the prescriptions may depend markedly on the procedure you select). For nonlinear hearing aids (definitely recommended), calculate the target gain for at least the input levels of 50 and 80 dB SPL.

4. Measure the RECD of the child, using the method outlined in Section 10.6.3. If the child is too active (most will be) to use the 6 kHz probe tone method of determining insertion depth (Section 4.2.1), insert the probe tube past the inter-tragal notch by 15 mm for babies under 12 months, by 20 mm for children from one to five years, and by 25 mm for older children (Moodie, Seewald & Sinclair, 1994). These distances are approximate guidelines; the location of the probe tip relative to the eardrum during insertion should be observed by otoscopy and a smaller insertion depth should be used when required (Scollie et al., 1998). It is more important to avoid causing pain (and hence fear of the real-ear measurement equipment) than it is to obtain accurate measurements at and above 4 kHz, especially the first time a probe microphone is used (Scollie & Seewald, 1999). Prior to measuring RECD, apply lubricating cream to the mold so that it can easily be inserted without disturbing the probe and so that feedback is minimized (Westwood & Bamford, 1995). Alternatively, if the canal is wide enough, the earmold can be ordered with an extra hole through which the probe tube is inserted. This makes it very easy to control the depth of insertion, and avoids the probe tube increasing leakage around the earmold. If the child is old enough, allow him or her to hold and look into a mirror while you position the probe and earmold. This keeps the child still (Seewald, 2000a). If measurement of RECD is not possible, estimate it from the data in Table 15.2.

5. Calculate the target OSPL90 curve, by subtracting RECD from the target RESR.

6. Calculate the target coupler gain for 50 and 80 dB SPL input levels, by subtracting RECD from the target REAG.
    - Microphone location effects could also be allowed for, but as these are small for the BTE hearing aids that will invariably be fitted to infants, this correction can be overlooked.
    - At any frequency at which the REAG target is 0 dB or less, the coupler gain target can be ignored, as the required gain can be achieved by sound entering via the vent path or possibly even by leakage around the earmold.

7. Adjust the hearing aid in a test box to match the OSPL90 and coupler gain targets.

Although you could easily do steps 2 to 6 manually, prescription is much easier if you use software specially prepared for the task. Both the NAL-NL1 and the DSL[i/o] software will allow you to enter thresholds in a variety of forms. They will also allow you to enter individual values of RECD, but will use age-appropriate values if you do not enter individual RECD values. There the similarities end. The prescriptions the two programs produce are markedly different for people with severe or profound hearing loss and for people with flat or steeply sloping hearing losses.

SPL in the ear canal is held constant, adding a ventilation tube with an internal diameter of 1.3 mm and a length of 1.8 mm causes the input to the cochlea at 500 Hz to decrease by 12 dB.[153] The effects are less than this above 500 Hz, but grow rapidly below 500 Hz.

15.5 Verifying Real-ear Performance

If the individual RECD procedure discussed in the previous section has been carried out, there is no strong necessity to further evaluate real-ear gain. If time permits, and if the child is sufficiently cooperative, the REAG can be measured with probe-tube equipment to check that no errors have been made. Assuming you, or your software has correctly allowed for the effects of any vent or leak in the earmold, the results should be entirely consistent with the test-box adjustment of the hearing aid to the target calculated using the individual RECD measurement.

If, for example, the gain when the aid was adjusted in the text box was deficient at 4 kHz relative to the target, the measured REAG should be deficient to the same degree relative to the REAG target. Any inconsistency indicates that an error was made in the RECD measurement, the test-box adjustment, or the REAG measurement.

In the past, aided thresholds were commonly used to verify a fitting. These measurements should be viewed as a possible supplement to the RECD procedure or direct measurement of real-ear gain, *not* as an alternative to these electroacoustic measurements. As with adult testing, aided threshold determination, is slower, less accurate, less detailed (in that only a few frequencies can realistically be measured), applies to only one input level (for nonlinear hearing aids), and may give invalid results if a threshold is masked by ambient noise (Section 4.5). The following are some arguments that are sometimes made in favor of aided threshold testing. With the exception of the last, they are weak reasons:

- They demonstrate to the parents that the child is capable of reacting to sound (and in some cases, this may be the first time the parents have seen their child react to *any* sound).

- They demonstrate that the hearing aid maximum output exceeds the child's hearing threshold at each frequency tested, although OSPL90 will always exceed threshold if it has been prescribed using either the DSL or NAL procedures.

- An aided threshold at the level expected, given the hearing aid coupler gain and unaided hearing threshold, provides further confirmation of the child's unaided thresholds. Calculating the expected aided thresholds is tricky, however, unless suitable software is available.

- In the case of profound hearing loss, aided thresholds at the expected levels confirm that the unaided thresholds were not based solely on vibratory sensations.

If, for some reason, neither the RECD procedure nor real-ear gain measurement can be carried out (one of them should be!), aided threshold testing provides a greatly inferior fallback means of verifying real-ear performance. The thresholds obtained should be compared to those prescribed by the selection procedure used.

15.6 Evaluating Aided Performance

Simply verifying that the prescribed response has been obtained is not enough (any more than it is for adults). The effectiveness of the hearing aids in providing auditory information to the child also has to be established. The appropriateness of the hearing aids (as well as their continued correct operation) must at first be checked frequently, perhaps every few weeks. The time between checks can increase to perhaps every 6 to 12 months once both audiologist and parents are convinced that everything that can be done, has been done.

There are several methods by which the effectiveness of amplification can be evaluated. Methods based on speech tests are absolute evaluations in that they indicate how well a particular amplification scheme works, against some criterion. These tend to be time consuming to perform, and are therefore not usually suitable for comparing multiple amplification schemes to see which is the most effective. The paired-comparison technique, by contrast, provides no information about how effective any scheme is, but can be used to select which of several schemes is preferred for clarity or other listening criteria.

Speech tests

Hearing aid performance can be assessed with any speech test that has a level of difficulty appropriate to the age and degree of hearing loss of the child. The report of a Pediatric Working Group[60] contains an extensive listing of tests commonly used with children. Features covered include the type of speech material, the number of items and lists available, response choices (open set or

---

Evaluating maximum output in children seven years or older.

The goal of this procedure is to ensure that hearing aid maximum output is sufficiently low that the output never causes loudness discomfort. The following instructions are adapted from Kawell, Kopun & Stelmachowicz (1988):

> "We're going to see how loud this hearing aid makes sounds. You will hear some whistles and I want you to tell me how loud the whistle is. (Go over the descriptor list shown in Figure 15.5, explaining each choice, starting with *Too soft*.) When the sounds are *Too loud*, this is where you want the hearing aid to stop and you do not want the sounds to be this loud. Now, for every whistle, tell me how loud it sounds."

When the child appears to have understood the instructions, and while he or she is wearing hearing aids at their normal volume control setting, present sounds from a loudspeaker, starting from approximately 65 dB SPL and increasing in 5 dB steps. It should be possible to increase level up to the highest level achievable (at least 85 dB SPL and preferably higher) without eliciting a response of *Too loud*. Use two or three successive ascending runs, starting from progressively higher levels. If it is not possible to elicit a response of *Loud* the maximum output may be too low.

As with adults, one never knows how a patient interprets loudness descriptors. If a child gives a response of *Too loud* while appearing to be totally untroubled by a sound's loudness, it is worthwhile re-instructing or quizzing the child about how loud the sound really is (depending on the language ability of the child). Provided the child remains cooperative and attentive, ensure comfort for at least one low-frequency sound, one high-frequency sound, and one broadband sound (see Section 10.9). Evaluation can be done while the child is wearing two hearing aids, though if a response of *Too loud* is obtained it may be necessary to evaluate each hearing aid individually, especially in the case of asymmetrical hearing thresholds.

For children who do not appear to understand the verbal instructions or the pictorial analogy, a tactual analogy can be tried (Pascoe, 1982). Describe each of the degrees of sensation. Along with each description, make an appropriate face and squeeze the child's arm with an appropriate degree of firmness. For example, *Too soft* corresponds to a light squeeze, *Just right* to a comfortable squeeze, *A little bit loud* to a firm squeeze, and *Too loud* to a very firm (but not painful!) squeeze. (If you are charged with assault, re-read these instructions.) Following this training, ask the child to squeeze your arm to show you how loud each sound is.

closed set) the type of response (verbal, picture-pointing, or other action), and the range of ages and hearing losses considered to be appropriate. The difficulties associated with using a speech test to evaluate the effectiveness of a hearing aid are the same as those with adults (Section 13.1.1), plus any associated with retaining the child's cooperation for the duration of the test.

Paired-comparison tests

Just as with adults (Section 11.2), children aged six or older can indicate which of two hearing aid responses they prefer when they are presented with two alternatives in quick succession.[145, 258] It appears that with children aged six to ten, more reliable responses can be obtained if the material is presented via auditory-visual means rather than via auditory alone.[145] It is not clear if this is because the visual component maintains the children's interest or because it makes the continuous discourse easier to follow, thus preventing all the alternatives from being so difficult that the child cannot tell which one is better. The same frequency response shape is optimal in the auditory-visual mode as in the auditory mode.[145]

Evaluation of discomfort

Maximum output must be carefully prescribed,[f] but even so, its suitability for the individual child must be evaluated. The most essential part of this evaluation is to ensure that the hearing aid does not cause loudness discomfort.

Several investigators have recommended the use of face icons to represent different loudness categories when a child's loudness discomfort level (LDL) is measured.[115, 439, 692] The technique appears to be suitable at least down to the age of seven.[439] Although this book does not recommend the routine *measurement* of LDL, even for adults (see Section 9.6.3), loudness can be rated to ensure

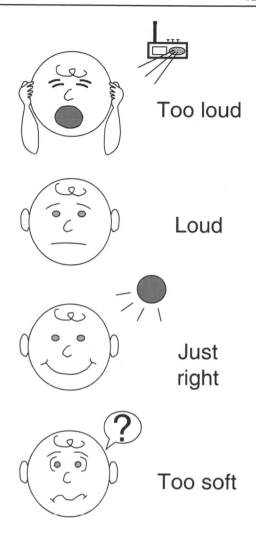

Figure 15.5 Verbal and pictorial loudness categories used for evaluation of loudness comfort and discomfort while wearing hearing aids.

that the hearing aid can never cause loudness discomfort. Details are given in the accompanying panel and in Figure 15.5. The pictures have been adapted from the three pictures used by Byrne (1982) and the five pictures used by Kawell et al. (1988).[g]

By using a different technique, the minimum age (or perhaps language level) at which LDL can be measured can be lowered slightly.[558]

---

[f]   Both the NAL-NL1 and DSL software prescribe maximum output in a way that allows for ear size.

[g]   The top three categories from Kawell et al. (1988) have been combined into two as the distinction between *Too loud* and *Hurts* is a difficult one for young children. This also makes the pictures more distinctly different.

This technique requires the clinician to first train the child to indicate *Stop* when excessive water, excessive weight, or an excessive number of small toys are placed into a container. The child is then asked to indicate *Stop* when the level of sound becomes excessive.

Even for children younger than seven (or five if the tangible-excess method is used), intense noises should be made while the child is looking at the person creating or controlling the noise. The child should be observed for any visible sign of discomfort as the noise is made.

You should not be afraid to generate intense noises in front of the child and observe the child's response while he or she is wearing hearing aids. Outside the clinic, the child will frequently be exposed to intense noises (self-generated or generated by play-mates) and if the hearing aid maximum output is excessive, it is best to discover this as soon as possible.

Subjective report measures

Just as for adults, the performance of hearing aids can be evaluated by asking the child, parent, or teacher how much they help. Several tools are available, and Table 15.3 lists the characteristics of these tools. There is a choice between measures that contain standard items versus measures where the items are created individually for each child, at each stage of development. The advantages of each approach are the same as for adults (see Section 13.3).

As with adults, devising individual assessment items each time the measure is used can be an integral part of structuring a habilitation program. The *Family Expectations Worksheet* (*FEW*)[688] uses the same concept as Goal Attainment Scaling (see Sections 8.1.4 and 13.3). As well as individually defining the item to be measured, the degree of success desired by the child or parent and the degree of success considered likely by the audiologist are discussed, which provides an opportunity to establish realistic expectations. At some subsequent time, the degree to which the goal has been attained is rated.

Another individualized measure for children is the *COSI-C*, which is similar to the adult COSI (Client Oriented Scale of Improvement; see Section 13.3). Differences are that the COSI-C form:

- Includes space to record any strategies that will help achieve each goal;

For the future: objective indicators of discomfort

Because it is difficult to measure LDL reliably (even in some adults) there have been several attempts to estimate LDL on the basis of acoustic reflex threshold (Greenfield, Wiley & Block, 1985), or on the basis of ABR latencies (Thornton, Yardley & Farrell, 1987). Electrically evoked acoustic reflex thresholds have successfully been used to guide the programming of cochlear implants (Hodges et al., 1997). It remains to be experimentally determined whether such objective measures can be used to adjust OSPL90 more accurately than can be achieved based on pure tone thresholds (e.g. Table 9.4). There are two aspects to this question.

- Can the optimum OSPL90 at each frequency be predicted more accurately from objective measures than from pure tone thresholds?
- Can objective measures predict how OSPL90 should vary across frequency, even if the final overall adjustment of OSPL90 is based on subjective assessment?

Note that the question to be answered is how accurately optimum OSPL90 can be predicted, not how accurately LDL can be predicted. The latter question may, however, be more easily answered.

Table 15.3 Subjective outcome-assessment tools suitable for use with children. The *type* column refers to whether the items are standard for all children or are individually devised each time the measure is used.

	Measure	Respondent	Age	Items	Type	Reference
FEW	Family Expectations Worksheet	Parent or child	>0	5	Indiv	Palmer & Mormer (1999)
COSI-C	Client Oriented Scale of Improvement for Children	Parent or Child	>0	5	Indiv	Lovelock (unpublished)
IT-MAIS	Infant-Toddler Meaningful Auditory Integration Scale	Parent	0.5 to 3 years	10	Stand	Zimmerman-Phillips et al (1997)
P-SIFTER	Preschool Screening Instrument for Targeting Educational Risk	Teacher	3-5 years	15	Stand	Anderson & Matkin (1996)
CHILD	Children's Home Inventory of Listening Difficulties	Parent or child	3-12 years	15	Stand	Anderson & Smaldino (2000)
SIFTER	Screening Instrument for Targeting Educational Risk	Teacher	>5 years	15	Stand	Anderson (1989)
TOOL	Teacher Opinion and Observation List	Teacher	>5 years	4	Stand	Smaldino & Anderson (1997)
LIFE	Listening Inventories for Education	Teacher	>6 years	16	Stand	
		Child	>8 years	15	Stand	
HPIC	Hearing Performance Inventory for Children	Child	8-14 years	31	Stand	Kessler et al (1990)
MAIS	Meaningful Auditory Integration Scale	Parent	>5 years, profound loss	10	Stand	Robbins et al. (1991)
APHAP-C	Abbreviated Profile of Hearing Aid Performance for Children	Parent or child	>10 years	24	Stand	Kopun & Stelmachowicz (1998)

- Replaces the *change* and *final ability* five-point scales with a single four-point scale having the following alternatives: *No change, Small change, Significant change, Goal achieved*.

- Specifies review date(s) at which progress towards each of the current goals will be assessed.

For either the FEW or the COSI-C, the actual listening goals can be established in a number of ways. One useful method is to consult the milestones of normal hearing listed in the *Developmental Index of Audition* (*DIAL*) shown in the panel.[688] The ages shown against each listening activity are approximate, even for children with normal hearing. When setting goals, the current abilities of the child must be considered: It is inappropriate to select a goal (e.g. *uses telephone meaningfully*) if a less complex goal (e.g. *listens on telephone*) has not yet been accomplished, no matter how old the child is.[688]

A second method is to ask the parents, at the outset of each interview:[880]

- What are the most important results you hope to get from today's appointment?

- What are the chief problems that your

Age	Milestone
Developmental Index of Audition and Listening (DIAL) From Palmer & Mormer (1999), by permission	
Infant	
0-28 days	Startle response; attends to music and voice; soothed by parent's voice; some will synchronize body movements to speech pattern; enjoys time in *en face* position; hears caregiver before being picked up.
1-4 months	Looks for sound source; associates sound with movement; enjoys parent's voice; attends to noise makers; imitates vowel sounds.
4-8 months	Uses toys/objects to make sounds; recognizes words; responds to verbal commands – bye bye; learning to recognize name; plays with noise makers; enjoys music; enjoys rhythm games.
8-12 months	Attends to TV; localizes to sounds/voices; enjoys rhymes and songs; understands NO; enjoys hiding game; responds to vocal games (e.g. so Big!!)
Toddler	
1 year	Dances to music; sees parent answer telephone/doorbell; answers to name calls; attends to books.
2 years	Listens on telephone; dances to music; listens to story in group; goes with parent to answer door; awakens to smoke detector; attends to travel activities and communication.
Preschool	
3 years	Talks and listens on telephone; sings with music; listens to books on tape; smoke detector means danger; enjoys taped books; attends to verbal warnings for safety.
4 years	Telephone play; attends movie theatre; dance/swim lessons/ watches TV/videos with family; neighborhood play.
Early School Age 6-8 years	Uses telephone meaningfully; enjoys walkman/headphones; uses alarm clock independently; responds to smoke detector independently.
Late Elementary 8-10 years	Uses television for entertainment & socializing; attends to radio; responds to sirens for street safety; participates in clubs and athletics; enjoys privacy in own room; enjoys computer/audio games; plays team sports.
Middle School 10-14 years	Uses telephone as social vehicle; attends movies/plays; develops musical tastes; watches movies/TV with friends.
Older Adolescent	
14-18 years	Goes to dances; begins driving (e.g. needs to hear sirens/turn signal); participates in school groups/clubs; employment/ ADA
18-22 years	Employment/career decisions; travels independently; listens in college halls/classrooms; participates in study groups/extra-curricular activities.

child's hearing loss has caused you or your child?

- What milestones or changes have recently occurred, or are about to occur, in the life of your child (e.g. starting at a new school, joining a sporting team[h])?
- Is there anything that you fear will result from your child's hearing loss?

Parents may be able to give a more considered response if they are advised, in advance of the appointment, that their input into the child's program will be sought in this way. When choosing goals, it may also be useful to review the habilitation goals and strategies discussed in Section 15.8.

If any goals related to responses to sound are

---

[h] Some specific goals for coping with sports activities, and strategies to achieve them, can be found in *Time Out! I didn't hear you* by Palmer, Butts, Lindley & Snyder, and can be downloaded from www.pitt.edu/~cvp.

not achieved, the appropriateness of the prescription, and the correct functioning of the hearing aids should both be reviewed . In experiments examining the appropriateness of different prescription procedures, changes in auditory responsiveness following a change in frequency response have been observed within the first week after the change has been made (Ching, Psarros & Hill, 1999). Unfortunately, it is not possible to give any general guidelines as to how or when the amplification characteristics should be altered if the child has not made the progress expected.

There is a need for further validation of - subjective-report measures, although early indications of correlations between reports by children, reports by teachers and parents, and responses preferred by children in paired comparison tasks are encouraging.[387] Similarly, a correlation of 0.75 between subjective responses on the Meaningful Auditory Integration Scale and monosyllabic word identification scores has been reported for children with cochlear implants.[750] Reports by parents and children are thought to be more reliable if they are obtained through a structured interview rather than simply by asking for ratings of behavior using a questionnaire.[387] Within this structured interview, behavior points are given for each example that can be given by the respondent of a specific type of behavior exhibited by the child.[387] For a more extensive description of parent and teacher report forms, see Stelmachowicz (1999).

Articulation Index

The Articulation Index or Speech Intelligibility Index methods can be used to predict speech intelligibility for a specified type of speech (e.g. sentences) at a specified level in a specified level and spectrum of background noise. The problems with using these methods are the same as apply to adults. First, very high AI values can be achieved simply by applying enough gain at each frequency to make speech at that frequency highly audible. If this results in excessive loudness, or excessive saturation of the hearing aid, the result is not likely to be any more satisfactory for a child than it is for an adult. Second, the conclusion reached about how much gain at each frequency is needed to maximize intelligibility depends strongly on how hearing loss desensitization (see Section 9.2.4) is allowed for in the calculation of AI. Many simple applications of AI make no allowance for hearing loss desensitization. Suppose such a simple AI calculation method were used to evaluate the fitting of a hearing aid to a child with low-frequency thresholds around 60 dB HL and high-frequency thresholds around 115 dB HL. The calculation implies that the best intelligibility would be achieved only when the high-frequency gain was large enough to make all the high-frequency speech components completely audible. This conclusion is not likely to be correct, even if it was technologically achievable.

In short, the AI method is not a reliable way to choose between different amplification options. It has the potential to be useful once we learn more about how hearing loss desensitization should be allowed for when it is applied to children, and how the trade-off between intelligibility and loudness should be optimized. It does, however, provide a crude metric of how much information is likely to be available, and should be reasonably accurate for any child whose thresholds remain in the mild or moderate ranges at all frequencies. The visual display showing how much of the speech spectrum is not audible can also be a useful counseling tool for parents.

15.7 Helping Parents

For a parent, the world changes the day a hearing loss is diagnosed. For a while, a parent's hopes, aspirations, and beliefs about the child's future are overwhelmed by shock, disbelief, fear, and despair. The audiologist is likely to be the first person to bring to the parents the news they least want to hear, and so has a special responsibility for helping the parents through this time. This help may be direct and/or by referring the parents to others who can help. This section reviews some of the ways that the audiologist can help parents. The counseling skills needed by a pediatric audiologist go far beyond the scope of this book, however. Furthermore, the level of skills needed to best help parents at a time of high emotional shock are increasing. The introduction of universal neonatal hearing screening means that more parents than ever are being confronted with an adverse diagnosis of their child's hearing, without having had time to reflect on the possibility that their child might have a hearing loss.[547]

It is essential for the future of the child that the parents receive every help possible. This is true in many ways, but most relevant for this book is that effective amplification for the child will need the active help of a parent. Amongst their many other tasks, parents are the only people on-the-spot to ensure that hearing aids continue to function and provide maximum benefit to the child.

Several researchers have interviewed or surveyed parents some months or years after their children were diagnosed as having hearing loss.[35, 157, 547, 763] The following list of attributes is based on this research into the things that parents found helpful or unhelpful about the way their audiologist assisted them during and after the time their child was identified as having a hearing impairment.

Parents want their audiologist to be:

Empathetic. The number one thing parents want is for their audiologist to be sensitive to the emotional shock they have received, particularly at the diagnosis, but continuing far beyond that as they adjust to their new circumstances. Audiologists need to be great listeners. Audiologists must also be genuinely accepting of any *emotions* that parents reveal, although counter-productive *behavior* by the parents is a valid target for modification.[546] There are no good or bad emotions.

Informative. Parents want to learn about the hearing loss and its implications for what their child will be able to do, what will change in the life of their family, and what hearing aids do. They want unbiased information regarding devices and education, what other services are available and the means by which they can be financed.

Competent. Parents can tell if their audiologist is a competent specialist versus an audiologist who sees only an occasional child. When parents tell their audiologist what the child does and does not appear to be hearing, they want their audiologist to listen, and to advise them expertly about devices and tactics.

Supportive. Parents do not want the audiologist to take over decision-making, but instead want information and help in arriving at decisions. They want the audiologist to support their chosen course after they have taken a well-informed decision. Supportive audiologists will convey information without using any jargon. Jargon either confuses parents, or sends them the message that the audiologist is the sole expert in the room. This may be true of hearing aids, but when it comes to the child, the parents are the experts.

Patient. Parents need time to think through the implications of different management options for the life of the family. They need time to make decisions, time to experience the ramifications of those decisions, and time to change their minds if necessary.

Positive. Parents need some hope and reassurance for the future, and the audiologist, having seen many other families cope well with hearing loss, is able to give that hope.

If parents are to help their child to the greatest degree, they have to acquire a lot of information as quickly as they are able. Even so, there is so much for parents to absorb, the audiologist has to impart knowledge gradually rather than in one or two sessions crammed with information. Apart from basic

---

Essential: meeting other parents

Parents find an introduction to other parents of hearing-impaired children to be extremely helpful. Other parents, especially those with children whose hearing impairment has been diagnosed longer, can provide emotional support, understanding, and hope in a way that no one else can. Parents consider an introduction to other parents to be *the* most helpful thing an audiologist can do (Luterman & Kurtzer-White 1999).

---

limitations on how quickly anyone can absorb new information, the type of information needed by parents changes as their child grows. The audiologist must appropriately combine explanation, demonstration, hands-on skill development with reinforcement, handouts, videos, and group discussion sessions to help the parents learn.[261] Getting the parents to practice a skill, and providing them with feedback, reinforces the importance of the skill as well as teaching the skill itself. Some topics relating to the hearing aids that should be covered include:

Benefits and limitations. In the end, hearing aids can amplify only what comes into them. Background noise, distance, and reverberation greatly decrease the effectiveness of amplification. Audio demonstrations are invaluable, as is a little information about the nature of speech and the types of distortions that may be occurring in their child's hearing (Section 1.1).

Hearing milestones. Expectations of what the child should be able to do, and approximately when these milestones are expected to occur should be explained to the parents. The parents are the people best placed to confirm the achievement of these milestones, or to raise an alarm if the milestones are delayed by an abnormal amount.

Care and use of hearing aids. Parents will need to know about cleaning the earmold and hearing aid, checking batteries, performing listening checks, putting the hearing aids on, setting the controls (if any), carrying out activities (like talking and playing) that promote their use, and avoiding hazards like moisture. They will need to be able easily to do all these things without the hearing aids or the hearing loss becoming the focus of the family.[261]

Troubleshooting. When listening checks reveal a problem, parents need to know how to diagnose common faults like cracked or loose tubing, weak batteries, moisture, and internal noise. They need to know what they can fix themselves and what they need help with. Such skills can be taught by having available a few faulty hearing aids and asking the parents to diagnose the fault in each.

Safety. See Section 15.10 for further various aspects of safety with hearing aids, some of which should be communicated to parents.

The quality and speed of communication, and the ease with which new skills are imparted, depends on the quality of the relationship between the audiologist and the parents.[157, 261] At review appointments, parents may present general concerns that cannot readily be addressed. In many cases, there is a specific underlying problem. When the specific problem is addressed, the general concern may disappear.[261] A general concern about the child *feeling different from his normal-hearing peers*, for example, may be precipitated by either the child or the parent being concerned about the large size of a body-worn FM receiver. Parents should always be encouraged to contact the audiologist if problems or concerns arise between regular review appointments.

Even when parents and teachers conscientiously check hearing aids, there can be a high incidence of non-functioning hearing aids at any given time. As soon as possible, children should be taught to monitor the status of their own hearing aids.[262]

One thing parents want from a health care system is that the services available be seamless. They appreciate it when early and accurate identification is quickly followed by the provision of amplification. They also appreciate information that will help them make a confident decision about how and when their child should be educated. If the services provided are not well integrated with other services needed by the parents, the audiologist has an especially critical role in helping the parents negotiate the system(s).

15.8 Hearing Habilitation Goals

We must not lose sight of the role of hearing aids: they are only a means to an end.[i] The real goal is that the child develops a high-level ability to speak and listen so that he or she will not be handicapped by the hearing loss. Effective hearing aid (or cochlear implant) fitting is one of the essential steps that must be taken to achieve this goal, as summarized in Figure 15.6. For a child to maximize his or her mastery of language, hearing aids must consistently be worn, and they must be functioning correctly. The child

must also be receiving stimulating auditory input. When the child is young, these three essential ingredients are most likely to occur if the parents have a good understanding of the nature of hearing loss and speech and of the importance of good quality auditory input to the development of language. This knowledge motivates parents to maximize effective hearing aid use.

Many of the initial steps in habilitation thus involve the parents more than the child. It is our goal that as the child grows, so too will the child's motivation to hear well along with his or her understanding of hearing and hearing loss.

Although the broad goal of good language development remains unchanged, the detailed goals and strategies that achieve this vary with the age of the child. The following sections list some goals and strategies that are appropriate to different ages, though many goals shown in one age category are also appropriate to later categories. The goals shown are intended as examples.[j] *They are far from comprehensive, and some will not be appropriate for some families.* To

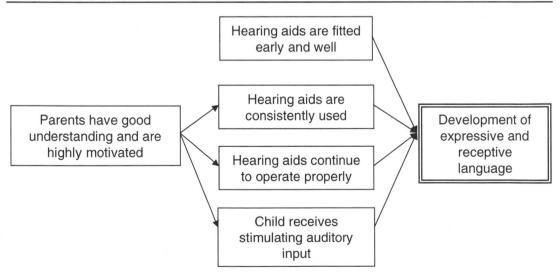

Figure 15.6 Goals of the hearing habilitation process, culminating in maximal development of language.

---

[i] There are other means to hearing habilitation apart from hearing aids, such as participation in an early intervention program, but such things are outside the scope of this book.

maximize the likelihood of goals being achieved, goals should be jointly developed by the audiologist, the parents, and when old enough, the child. Many goals will be prompted by changes facing the child, such as progression to a new school or the commencement of new social or sporting activities.

15.8.1 Goals and strategies for infants

Goal: The child uses the hearing aids consistently

- Assist the parents to accept that their child has a hearing loss.
- Ensure that parents understand the close link between consistent auditory stimulation and language development.
- Explain to parents why this type of hearing aid (nearly always a BTE) has been selected.
- Introduce parents to other parents whose children consistently use hearing aids and/ or to parental support groups.
- Devise a behavior modification plan that links hearing aid use to book reading, food, attention, or some other reward.
- Discuss the child's daily routine to identify when aid use is practical and when it is not.
- Check that the hearing aids appear to be comfortable when the baby is sitting supported or lying down, and that feedback oscillation does not occur in these positions.
- Provide parents with information about hearing aid use in the event of ear infection with suppuration (e.g. earmold disinfecting, use at key listening times only).
- Encourage parents to record hearing aid use, and responses to sound and speech, in a communication diary, over a set period.
- If consistent use is not established, search

for the reasons (e.g. parents not convinced of the need, problems with the hearing aids).

Goal: The hearing aids function properly

- Ensure that parents can operate the controls, can insert and remove the earmolds confidently, and that they understand what the hearing aid does.
- Provide parents with their own earmolds made with 300 mm of tubing, or with a stethoclip, so that they can do listening checks while holding the hearing aid in front of them and manipulating the controls.
- Demonstrate troubleshooting, including battery testing, the use of a puffer to dry earmolds, the causes of feedback oscillation, and the use of feedback oscillation as a quick check of hearing aid functioning. Trouble-shooting can efficiently be taught in small workshops, which if followed by coffee also provides an easy way for parents to meet other parents.

Goal: The child receives high quality auditory stimulation

- Explain to parents the effects of noise, distance, reverberation, and head position on the quality of sound received.
- If possible, demonstrate to parents the effects of noise, distance, reverberation, and hearing loss on sound quality.
- Reinforce to parents the need for regular and interesting auditory stimulation.
- Discuss the use of FM systems and provide if appropriate.

Goal: The parents understand the education options

- Outline the basic education options in an unbiased and factual manner, especially those relating to early intervention. Ensure that parents know where to obtain more detailed information about each option.

---

j   The goals and strategies are heavily based on "Goals for promoting hearing," an unpublished document by Karen Lovelock and Anne-Marie Phillips, (pediatric audiologists in Australian Hearing) and I am grateful for permission to reproduce some of this material.

Direct and continuing liaison between the audiologist and any educational institution may also be necessary.

- Provide written information (this also applies to most other issues discussed).

Goal: *The child reacts to sound*

- Show the comparison of the amplified speech spectrum (measured or calculated from real-ear gain) to hearing thresholds, and explain what sort of sounds should be detectable and what sort should not. Alternatively, the same points can be made using an aided audiogram (see Figure 8.2).

- Ask parents to monitor whether the child reacts to louder environmental sounds, the voice of others, his or her own voice, and whether the child displays any preliminary turn-taking skills.

15.8.2 Goals and strategies for toddlers

Goal: *Child accepts hearing aids*

- Parents reinforce child when he or she indicates that a hearing aid is faulty or is feeding back.

- Parents reinforce child when he or she puts the hearing aids on or asks for them to be put on.

- Hearing aids are put on early each day, as part of the daily routine, such as when getting dressed.

- Parents, rather than toddler, decide when hearing aids are removed.

- Parents encourage child to look after hearing aids by putting them in the same specified place when they are not being worn.

- Parents encourage child to test hearing aids with own voice when they are first put on.

- Parents teach *hearing aids* along with *nose, feet, tummy, etc.*

Goal: *Child develops listening skills and realizes benefits from hearing aids*

- Parents draw attention to environmental sounds and reinforce child when he or she recognizes them.

- Parents and child play games that require the child to respond to sound.

- Parents select toys that have an appropriate auditory reward.

- Parents reward child for appropriate vocalizing and listening.

- Signing (if used) is accompanied by speech.

15.8.3 Goals and strategies for pre-schoolers

Goal: *Child reports when a hearing aid is not working*

- Play a game (with rewards) in which the child has to differentiate between a working and a non-working hearing aid.

Goal: *Child manages hearing aids without help*

- Practice with hearing aid insertion, on/off, and volume control and battery manipulation if appropriate. Reinforce with lots of praise!

Goal: *Child displays appropriate communication skills*

- Reinforce when child uses voice volume appropriate to situation (also useful for normal-hearing children to learn!), displays turn-taking skills, and visually attends to talker.

15.8.4 Goals and strategies for primary school children

Goal: *Child can organize devices or environment to hear well in a range of situations*

- Provide FM hearing aid (if not already provided) and instruct child in its use (battery changing/charging, connectors, use of controls).

- Provide a telephone coupler and TV listening device (if needed and if not already provided) and instruct child in its use. Note that an FM can double as a TV listening device.

- Demonstrate to child the effects of distance, noise, and reverberation.

- Give child practice in identifying the source of communication difficulties and in using age-appropriate hearing strategies to alleviate problems.
- Instruct child in use of FM, T-switch, or listening position (close to source) to solve the problems of distance, noise, and reverberation.
- Show the child how to care for the hearing aids: earmold washing and drying, battery testing.

Goal: Child continues to accept the use of amplification devices

- Demonstrate benefit of device with simple speech test in the clinic.
- Ensure that child knows other hearing-impaired children.

Goal: Child understands about hearing loss in general and his or her hearing loss in particular

- Explain to the child (at an age-appropriate level) the cause of his or her hearing loss.
- Explain to the child the characteristics of his or her loss (e.g. better ear, better frequencies, and difficulty in separating sounds). Achieve an appropriate balance between the difficulties to be overcome and a positive view of what the child *can* do.

The goals and strategies described in this chapter are by no means a complete description of parental and child counseling. Other activities, such as referral for genetic counseling or other medical specialties, referral to speech therapist or occupational therapist, the impact of ear infections, and an explanation of the physiology, type and degree of hearing loss (and its permanency) all go beyond the scope of this book.

15.9 Teenagers and Cosmetic Concerns

Unfortunately (from the perspective of communication ability), children often reject any visible form of prosthetic device early in their teenage years. For them, at that stage of their life, the disadvantages of looking different from their peers presumably outweighs the communication advantages offered by their hearing aids, FM systems, or cochlear implants. Noble (1999) hypothesizes that there may be more to the rejection than simply avoiding a visible device. It may be that using an imperfect device in a world of noise and unpredictable signals, with poor results, poses more of a threat to their self-perceived ability to cope than does not using a device at all. Whatever the reason may be, the audiologist should make sure that the teenager is aware of all the consequences of not using hearing aids. The audiologist should also teach or reinforce alternative strategies to reduce communication breakdown. It may also be important to reinforce the teenager's right to make his or her own decision, and to change that decision at any time. People commonly seek help once more in their late teenage years when the increasing seriousness of education and the demands of the work force, in conjunction with their growing confidence as young adults, changes the balance of the equation for them.

15.10 Safety Issues

Parents should be advised about several aspects relating to the safety of their child, at some suitable time after the child has received his or her hearing aids.

Battery ingestion. Hearing aids are the major source of batteries ingested by children.[538] Parents should be advised that new and used batteries *must* be kept away from young children. This particularly applies to children less than three years of age, but ingestion (deliberate or accidental) occurs in every age group.[k] Loose batteries are not the only danger. In a third of cases of hearing aid battery ingestion, the child removes the battery from his or her own hearing aid. Hearing aids for infants and toddlers *must* have a tamper-resistant battery drawer. This is sometimes achieved by grinding away the ridge that is normally used to open the drawer, thus requiring that a tool be used to open it. The effectiveness of this method depends on the shape and tightness of the battery compartment. Specially designed locks are also available.

Parents should be advised to urgently seek medical attention if they believe a battery has been ingested. The major danger to the child is from chemical burning or choking if the battery becomes lodged in the esophagus, although this is most likely to occur with batteries larger than those used in hearing aids.[538] Common medical practice is to confirm by X-ray that the battery has passed through the esophagus, and then have the parent confirm that the battery has passed through the digestive system. This usually takes 24 to 72 hours, but has been reported to be as short as 12 hours or as long as 14 days.[539] Inducing vomiting is ineffective and potentially harmful as the battery can be ejected from the stomach only to become stuck in the esophagus.[538] Chemical burns can also result from batteries inserted in the nose or ears or under plaster bandages.[529]

Battery explosion. Parents should be advised that hearing aid batteries are not re-chargeable, and that they could explode if they are placed in a recharger. Similarly, they should not be disposed of in a fire or incinerator.

Noise-induced hearing loss. A hearing aid has the potential to exacerbate hearing loss by exposing the ear to high levels of noise. The audiologist can minimize this risk by prescribing gain and OSPL90 appropriate to the loss, and by selecting a hearing aid with low-ratio compression, rather than linear amplification, for at least mid- to high-level sounds (see Section 9.7).

Parents and older children should be advised not to increase the volume control setting above that recommended, except possibly in quiet environments. The need for volume control variation is minimized if a wide dynamic range compression aid is prescribed. For linear hearing aids, the parent and/or child should also be advised that the hearing aid should be removed or turned down if the child is going to be in very noisy places. If the child will be in a very noisy environment for extended periods of time, hearing protection should be worn.

Physical impact. The potential consequences of a blow to the head while wearing a hearing aid have already been discussed in Section 15.3. It is best that the child not wear a hearing aid during sports in which a blow to the head is possible. Such a blanket rule may make it impossible for the child to play sport at all, and if so, parents will have to balance the risks against all the consequences of not participating. The use of headgear that provides some physical protection but that nonetheless provides an open air-path to the hearing aid microphone inlet can be a solution. Soft earmolds should definitely be used.

Warning sounds. Parents should be advised that one of the uses of hearing is to provide warning of imminent danger. (Parents often provide the warning sound, of course.) The child will be best able to hear and understand these warnings if his or her hearing aids are being worn and are adjusted in the usual way. If two hearing aids have been provided, then two hearing aids should be routinely worn, or a child's ability to locate sources of danger may be decreased.

If the hearing aids have switchable directional microphones, the response should be switched to omni-directional in any circumstance where warning sounds are likely to arrive from directions other than the front. (This is really a concern only in outdoors, echo-free situations; indoors, the extent of

---

k   This includes adults who use their mouth as a third hand while changing batteries (Litovitz & Schmitz, 1992). Hearing aid batteries are small and slippery!

directionality is limited by the arrival of echoes from multiple directions.) For infants and toddlers, a gain appropriate to the detection of warning sounds is most likely to be achieved if the volume control is locked or disabled.

15.11 Concluding Comments

Fitting hearing aids to infants is always an ongoing process rather something that is carried out at one point in time. Achieving an optimal fitting, particularly for infants, is likely to remain a considerable challenge for some time. For no one else is it so important that the amplification be just right. Unfortunately, for no one else are we so unsure about what is best in principle. Furthermore, out of all patients, infants are least able to tell us what they like and dislike, and what works and does not work. Improved methods for evaluating the effectiveness of hearing aids for infants are urgently needed.

CHAPTER SIXTEEN

CROS, BONE-CONDUCTION, AND IMPLANTED HEARING AIDS

Synopsis

In the CROS (contralateral routing of signals) family of hearing aids, hearing aid components on opposite sides of the head are electrically linked. Basic CROS aids are most suitable for people with unilateral loss. CROS aids consists of a microphone on the side of the head with a deaf ear, combined with an amplifier, receiver and open earmold or shell, on the side with a normal-hearing ear. Adding a microphone to the side of the good ear converts it to a BICROS hearing aid, which is suitable for patients with loss in both ears. A stereo-CROS aid consists of two CROS aids, such that sounds arriving at each microphone are transferred to the opposite side of the head. This arrangement virtually eliminates feedback problems. A transcranial CROS has all the components in one ear, but sends a signal across the head by bone conduction.

Bone-conduction hearing aids output a mechanical vibration instead of an air-borne sound wave. They are most suited to people who, for medical reasons, cannot wear a hearing aid that occludes the ear in any way. For patients with sensorineural loss, bone-conduction hearing aids can not stimulate the cochlea as effectively as do air-conduction hearing aids because of the relative inefficiency of the bone conduction pathway. For patients with large conductive hearing losses, however, bone-conduction hearing aids can stimulate the cochlea as strongly as air-conduction hearing aids. Prescriptions for air-conduction hearing aids can be converted into bone-conduction prescriptions by using available standards for the thresholds of hearing for air- and bone-conducted sound. Bone-conduction output is specified in terms of output force level instead of output sound pressure level, and in terms of acousto-mechanical sensitivity instead of gain.

An alternative form of bone-conduction hearing aid is the bone-anchored hearing aid, in which the vibrations are transmitted to the skull via an embedded titanium screw. Various experimental devices also enable vibrations to be transmitted directly to the tympanic membrane, to the bones in the middle ear, or to the round window. These devices may have only the output transducers surgically implanted, or may be combined with implanted microphones and batteries to form completely implanted hearing aids.

This chapter discusses several types of non-standard hearing aids that are appropriate for only a small proportion of hearing-impaired people. A good understanding of these hearing aids is important. Otherwise, clinicians will not be able to make an appropriate recommendation when they encounter patients for whom one of these hearing aids will be the most appropriate device.

16.1 CROS Hearing Aids

In the vast majority of cases, people are fit either with a single hearing aid, or with two hearing aids that function independently of each other. In some cases, it is better to fit people with a hearing aid system that has components mounted at each ear, and which thus requires an electrical connection between the hearing aids. This arrangement is known as ***contralateral routing of signals***

(CROS).[352] As the following sections will show, there are several reasons for connecting the two sides, and several variations for how the components on each side of the head are combined.

The major disadvantage of all types of CROS aids is that a connection must be made between the two sides of the head. A cable can be run around the back of the head or along the frame of a spectacle aid. Alternatively, a wireless link can transmit signals from one hearing aid to the other. Cables are a nuisance and are not cosmetically attractive. Spectacle aids are also often unattractive, and are logistically difficult when repairs are made to either the glasses or the hearing aids. These considerable disadvantages have to be weighed against the advantages. The disadvantages of CROS aids are minimized if the connection between the two sides of the head is made by wireless transmission.

16.1.1 Simple CROS aids.

Basic considerations

Figure 16.1 shows the simplest CROS configuration. The microphone, mounted on the ear with the worse hearing, feeds its output to the amplifier and receiver mounted on the opposite side of the head. The

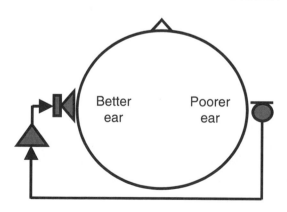

Figure 16.1 Block diagram of a CROS hearing aid system, viewed from above the head.

CROS aids: the essentials.

For patients with a unilateral hearing loss:

- A CROS aid merely *transfers* sound from one side of the head to the other (Courtois et al., 1988; Ericson et al., 1988).

- A CROS fitting should not amplify sound, and if it does, the disadvantages are likely to outweigh the advantages.

---

separated microphone is referred to as a *satellite microphone*. Any signal reaching the side of the head with the poorer ear will be amplified and heard in the better ear. The receiver is coupled to the ear using an open earmold, so that unamplified sound can also directly enter the better ear. The attenuation provided by earmolds with different vent sizes, including maximally open earmolds and shells, is indicated in Figure 5.11.

The major advantage of this arrangement is that sounds can be heard in the ear with the better residual hearing ability no matter which direction they come from. The head acts as a baffle for high-frequency sounds, boosting those sounds that come from the near side of the head and attenuating those that come from the far side. If the signal comes from one side of the listener and the predominant noise comes from the other side, there will thus be a much better signal-to-noise ratio (SNR) at one ear than at the other (see Section 14.2.1). In those cases where signal is arriving from the poorer side, the satellite microphone of the CROS aid will pick up this relatively clear signal. The electrical connection, amplifier, and receiver will transfer the signal to the better ear.

Because of head diffraction effects, a CROS hearing aid will always improve intelligibility in noise (relative to no hearing aid) when speech comes from the side of the poorer ear. These same head diffraction effects will, however, always cause sound amplified by the CROS aid to *decrease* intelligibility when speech comes from the side of the better ear. This disadvantage of a CROS aid when speech is on the normal-hearing side can be minimized by using no more gain than that recommended in the fitting procedure described in this section.

The second advantage of CROS aids is that the microphone and the receiver are well separated. Signal leaking from the receiver back to the microphone is greatly attenuated by having to pass around the head. The gain at which feedback oscillation occurs will therefore be *much* higher than would be the case if the receiver and the microphone were in close proximity.

Candidacy for simple CROS aids

Patients who may benefit from a CROS fitting are those with a **unilateral hearing loss**, where the loss in the poorer ear is so great that aiding it will be of no benefit. The better ear should have normal hearing or at most a mild high-frequency hearing loss. Patients will particularly benefit if they frequently need to listen to signals arriving from the side of the head with the deaf ear. An example would be a taxi driver whose deaf ear is on the passenger side.

Patients who have near-normal low-frequency hearing and moderate or severe high-frequency hearing loss in one ear, combined with an unaidable loss in the other ear, may also benefit from a CROS aid if neither a conventional hearing aid nor a BICROS aid is satisfactory (Section 16.1.2). Such patients require open earmolds to avoid occlusion (Section 5.3.2) but also require substantial high-frequency gain. A CROS hearing aid may be the only way enough gain can be achieved without feedback oscillation occurring. CROS aids for such people should be fit using the method described for Stereo CROS aids (Section 16.1.3) rather than the method described in this section. Patients with bilateral hearing losses that could be aided in both ears are more likely to be satisfied with conventional hearing aids than with CROS aids.[314]

The effect of hearing loss in the better ear on the success of CROS fittings is contentious, probably because CROS aids have mostly been prescribed in an ill-defined manner. Gelfand (1979) found no relationship between loss and degree of use of CROS aids. Many authors have recommended that it is easier to achieve satisfactory sound quality with a CROS aid if the better ear has a mild high-frequency loss rather than normal hearing.[162, 353, 732, 905] This advice should be reviewed in the light of recent technological developments. Flexible tone controls, especially those available in programmable aids, enable the requisite gain, *and no more,* to be obtained in a smooth manner across a wide frequency range. With older hearing aids, one had to compromise between too much gain at some frequencies and inadequate gain at the rest.

If too much gain is used at any frequency, patients will complain about amplified internal noise, will be disadvantaged whenever speech is on the side of the better ear, and overall, will perform more poorly than with no hearing aid.[269, 897] Too much gain in the CROS aid will effectively reverse the better and worse ears.[541, 575] *With a correctly balanced CROS aid, there will be neither a better side nor a poorer side when aided.* Ericson et al. (1988) have shown that a high success rate can be achieved, even for patients whose hearing is within normal limits within the better ear.

It may well be that people with normal hearing in one ear will elect not to use their hearing aid in very quiet environments (which is where internal hearing aid noise is most likely to be a problem). In environments with even moderate noise levels, however, external background noise will easily mask internal hearing aid noise.

Fitting procedure for CROS aids

The better ear receives the sounds that arrive directly at that ear mixed with an amplified version of the sounds that arrive at the poorer ear. When the sound source is on the better ear side, it is advantageous for sounds that enter the better ear directly to dominate this mixture. Conversely, when the sound source is on the poor ear side, it is advantageous for sounds picked up by the satellite microphone to dominate the mixture.

Domination by the side nearer the source is most likely to occur if the CROS aid is adjusted so that a frontally incident sound wave arrives in the ear canal with the same strength no matter which path it takes to the ear canal. That is, for frontally incident sounds, the real-ear aided gain (REAG) from free field input, via the satellite microphone, through the amplifier, to the ear canal of the better ear, should equal the real-ear unaided gain (REUG) of the better ear.[a] The corresponding coupler gain (CG) prescription can be calculated by rearranging Equation 4.4, and equating REAG to REUG:

$$CG = REUG - RECD - MLE - \text{Vent effects} \\ - \text{Tubing effects} \quad ..... \ 16.1,$$

where MLE describes the microphone location effects and RECD is the real-ear to coupler difference.

Figure 16.2 shows coupler gain prescriptions for a BTE and ITE hearing aid coupled to an open earmold or ear shell. These values are appropriate to an average adult. The values used for the terms in Equation 16.1 were taken from Table 4.1 (RECD), Table 4.5 (MLE), Table 4.6 (REUG), and Table 5.1 (Vent effects). The coupler gain allowed for a BTE differs from that for the ITE in the low frequencies principally because there is more room to open the vent path in a BTE fitting than in an ITE fitting. In the high frequencies, the differences arise from the

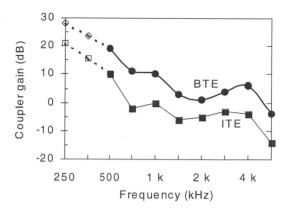

Figure 16.2 Coupler gain prescriptions for BTE and ITE hearing aids at used volume control setting for a CROS hearing aid. For the BTE hearing aid, a tube fitting is assumed. For the ITE hearing aid, a Janssen fitting is assumed. The gains shown are applicable to an average adult with no significant hearing loss in the good ear. The dashed lines below 500 Hz are not coupler gain prescriptions that should be *achieved* but represent upper limits that should not be *exceeded*.

different RECD values for the two hearing aids, which in turn is the result of them being measured in different types of 2-cc couplers.

Over what frequency range should sounds be effectively transferred from one side of the head to the other? Interaural level differences, and hence interaural SNRs, are significant above about 500 Hz (see Figure 14.3). From this perspective, it is desirable to have effective transfer of sounds extending at least as low as 500 Hz. On the other hand, the lower in frequency the transfer extends, the more likely is it that patients will complain about internal hearing aid noise. Internal noise is particularly likely to be a problem if a directional microphone is used. In noisy environments, internal noise is not a problem, and it would be preferable for the transfer of sounds to be effective above 500 Hz. In quiet environments, it may be preferable for the

---

[a]   This derivation of the coupler gain prescription assumes that the mold fitted to the good ear is sufficiently open not to have an appreciable effect on the real-ear unaided gain. The real-ear adjustment procedure shown in the panel does not require this assumption to be true.

Adjusting and verifying the CROS gain-frequency response

After the CROS aid has been pre-adjusted to approximate the coupler response given in Figure 16.2, its response can be more accurately adjusted using a real-ear gain analyzer as follows, and as shown in Figure 16.3.

Step 1 – Good-side response. With the hearing aid turned on, locate the speaker at 45° from the front, on the side of the good ear. Measure the response in the ear canal of the good ear. If the response does not approximate the usual real-ear unaided response of an ear with no mold or hearing aid, the mold is not sufficiently open to achieve a good CROS fitting.

Step 2 – Poor-side response. Move the speaker (or turn the patient) so that the speaker is at 45° on the side of the poor ear. Measure the response in the ear canal of the good ear.

Step 3 – Adjust the hearing aid. If the response measured in Step 2 does not match that measured in Step 1, adjust the hearing aid gain and frequency response, and repeat Step 2, until the poor-side response matches the good-side response. If a large adjustment has to be made, it may be necessary to start again from Step 1, because the good-side response is affected by the gain-frequency response of the hearing aid, although to a lesser degree than is the poor-side response. This interaction can be avoided by holding an earmuff over the ear (including the hearing aid or satellite microphone) on the side of the head away from the loudspeaker.

Step 4 – Check the frontal response. Position the speaker directly in front of the patient. Measure the real-ear aided gain. A smoothly rising response with a low-frequency gain of 0 dB and a maximum gain of 10 to 20 dB somewhere between 2 and 4 kHz should be obtained. If there is a pronounced dip at any frequency, it is possible that the amplified path is out of phase with the direct sound path at that frequency. The position and depth of such notches will vary from aid to aid, and will depend on the settings of the tone control and the polarity with which the receiver is wired.

Note that when performing these measurements, the control (reference) microphone must either be moved to the side of the head nearest the speaker, or be switched off. With many brands of real-ear gain analyzers it is not possible to place the control microphone on the side of the head opposite to the probe microphone, so only the second of these options is a possibility.

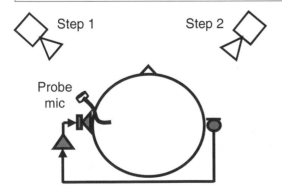

Figure 16.3 Test set-up for verifying and adjusting the gain-frequency response of a CROS hearing aid, showing the two different positions of the single test speaker.

transfer to be effective only for frequencies above 1500 Hz. CROS fittings may therefore be an ideal application for multi-memory hearing aids, although this is an untested proposition.

The coupler gain prescription shown in Figure 16.2 provides a good starting point for a balanced CROS fitting. Unfortunately, one cannot directly verify that for frontally incident sound, the aided path provides the same gain-frequency response as the unaided path. The problem is that while the unaided path can be measured (by turning off the hearing aid) the aided path cannot be measured in isolation because the unaided path is always present. The response can, however, be indirectly verified by measuring the combined gain of the two paths for loudspeaker locations on both sides of the head, as described in the panel.

16.1.2 Bilateral CROS (BICROS) aids

Basic considerations

If the better ear has a hearing loss, the patient is likely to benefit from amplification no matter which side of the head the wanted sound is coming from. The only way to always pick up the clearer signal is to have a microphone mounted on each side of the head. If each of these microphones is connected to the same amplifier and receiver, as shown in Figure 16.4, the result is called a bilateral CROS, or ***BICROS*** hearing aid.[b]

Unfortunately, the less clear signal provided by the microphone on the side of the head further from the signal will always be added to the clearer signal from the closer microphone, thereby reducing the clarity of the clearer signal. Fortunately, some net benefit remains, because the final signal-to-noise ratio will always be better than that provided by a microphone on the head-shadowed side.

The BICROS system also works effectively for signals coming from directly in front of

the listener. In this case, the wanted signal reaches the two microphones simultaneously and so the outputs of the two microphones are added together, in phase, before being amplified. Sounds coming from other directions reach the two microphones out of phase by different degrees. Consequently, the microphone outputs combine less effectively when they are added, and can even cancel each other completely for particular combinations of frequency and direction. Unfortunately, sounds from directly behind the person also arrive at the microphones in phase and are therefore also amplified with maximum gain.

Overall, however, the BICROS hearing aid works as a (weakly) directional microphone. The three-dimensional directivity index (see Section 2.2.4) of a BTE BICROS system, when mounted on the head, increases from 1.5 dB at 500 Hz up to around 3 dB at 4 kHz.[153] The corresponding two-dimensional directivity indices are 2.4 dB at 500 Hz up to around 3 dB at 4 kHz. When each microphone is by itself directional, the combination of the two microphones is even more directional.[727]

The BICROS system confers only a minor advantage in defeating feedback, because one of the two microphones is near the ear canal receiving the amplified sound, just as for a conventional hearing aid. (The maximum frontal high-frequency gain without feedback will be about 5 dB higher than for a conventional hearing aid because the satellite microphone will add to the total gain without increasing the risk of feedback.)

Candidacy for BICROS aids

Patients can benefit from a BICROS hearing aid if they have an asymmetric bilateral hearing loss such that the poorer ear has too great a hearing loss to benefit from a hearing aid, or where amplification of the poorer ear adversely affects speech identification ability (see Section 14.4.2).

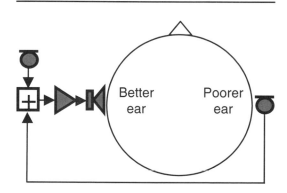

Figure 16.4 Block diagram of a BICROS hearing aid system.

---

[b] BICROS is usually an abbreviation of *Binaural* CROS, but in keeping with the terminology used in this book, *Bilateral* CROS seems more appropriate, as amplified sounds are heard in only one ear.

Fitting procedure for BICROS aids

Fitting a BICROS hearing aid is a combination of fitting a conventional unilateral hearing aid and fitting a CROS hearing aid. Provided the satellite microphone has the same sensitivity as the microphone in the hearing aid (this is usually the case), the necessary balancing of sensitivity between the two sides of the head is achieved without any action by the clinician.

The required gain-frequency response of the hearing aids can be prescribed in the same manner as for a unilateral hearing aid, using the hearing loss of the better ear as the basis of the prescription. No allowance should be made in the prescription for binaural listening. The response should be verified with both microphones in place and the speaker located directly in front of the patient. Averaged across frequency, the BICROS hearing aid has its maximum sensitivity for frontally incident sounds. For other source directions, the real-ear gain may show pronounced peaks and troughs because of the addition and cancellation effects referred to earlier. Real-ear gain should thus be measured only for 0°, and it is particularly important that there be no reflecting surfaces near the patient. If this cannot be achieved, the response should be verified with the satellite microphone disconnected.

16.1.3 Stereo CROS (CRIS-CROS) aids

Basic considerations

What arrangement would enable one to decrease feedback (as with the CROS aid), and be able to receive information arriving at either side of the head (as with the BICROS aid)? The solution, as shown in Figure 16.5, is the *stereo CROS* aid. This arrangement can be thought of as two separate CROS aids. The left microphone feeds the receiver on the right side, and the right microphone feeds the receiver on the left side. Compared to two conventional hearing aids, a much higher gain

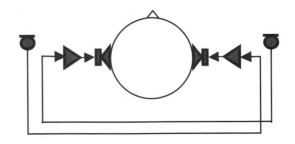

Figure 16.5 Block diagram of the stereo CROS hearing aid.

can be achieved before feedback occurs. As with all CROS aids so far discussed, the major disadvantage is the electrical connection required between the aids. For a stereo CROS aid, there are twice as many connections required: each hearing aid case has to have connections for the signal coming out and for the signal going in.

When first worn, the stereo CROS produces a confusing auditory world. The high-frequency parts of sounds to the left of the person appear to come from the right and vice versa. People apparently adapt to this after some time. The low-frequency parts of sounds arrive at the two ears with the normal inter-aural time and intensity differences, because they enter the ear canal directly through the open earmold or ear shell. Fortunately, these low-frequency components dominate localization perception in the horizontal plane.

Candidacy for Stereo CROS aids

Patients can benefit from a stereo CROS fitting if they have a severe high-frequency loss and near-normal low-frequency hearing in both ears. The only advantage of a stereo CROS hearing aid over two self-contained hearing aids is that the stereo CROS aids are less likely to suffer from feedback oscillation. This advantage has to be weighed against the inconvenience and cosmetic disadvantage of having two cables running between the ears. Advanced signal processing schemes for reducing feedback oscillation will undoubtedly make stereo CROS aids even less commonly used than at present.

Fitting procedure for Stereo CROS aids

A stereo CROS hearing aid is prescribed in just the same way as a conventional hearing aid. For each aid, the hearing loss used as the basis of the prescription is the loss in the ear that contains the receiver. As with a simple CROS aid, when real-ear gain is measured, the control microphone, if used, must be on the side of the head opposite to the probe microphone.

16.1.4 Transcranial CROS aids

A *transcranial CROS* hearing aid (also known as a *power CROS* or *internal CROS* aid) transmits a signal from one side of the head to the other using bone-conducted sound.[601, 861, 905] The arrangement is suitable for a person with no useable hearing in one ear, but who has to listen to sounds arriving from that same side of the head. A hearing aid is fitted to the non-functioning ear. Vibrations induced on that side of the head are coupled through the bones of the head to the cochlea on the opposite side of the head. To achieve the highest possible sensation level in the better ear, use the highest-powered hearing aid possible in the style chosen. Vibrations appear to get into the skull by two paths:[370]

- The hearing aid receiver creates a relatively intense SPL in the residual ear canal volume of the dead ear, and this vibrating air generates vibrations within the temporal bone.

- The hearing aid receiver vibrates the shell of the hearing aid, which in turn vibrates the canal wall. To achieve a high sensation level in the better ear, the hearing aid should be deeply seated so that the case makes close contact with the bony portion of the ear canal (see Section 5.1). It is possible to use a CIC hearing aid in this way.[41]

Candidacy for transcranial CROS aids

The limits of effectiveness of transcranial aids and appropriate fitting methods are still being worked out. If the better ear has too much sensorineural hearing loss, the transcranial CROS fitting will not provide enough excitation to this ear. Also, the transcranial CROS can improve SNR significantly only if the level of sound reaching the better cochlea via the transcranial path is greater than the level that arrives by diffracting around the head to the eardrum of the better ear. Improved localization has been claimed for these devices, but it is difficult to see how this can occur if all sound is being perceived in a single cochlea (see Section 14.1).

As vibrations are coupled from the hearing aid to the ear canal on the dead side in an almost accidental manner, there is presumably good scope for improvement in these devices by using output transducers, transducer mounting methods, and case designs that create a more effective source of vibration.

Fitting procedure for transcranial CROS aids

A transcranial CROS aid has the same fitting goal (i.e. laterally balanced sensitivity) as a conventional CROS aid, but a different method of sound delivery. There is no sound pressure relevant to the fitting goal in either ear canal, so the fitting cannot be verified with a real-ear gain analyzer. The hearing aid should be adjusted so that sounds at all frequencies are as loud when they are presented from 45° on the poor side as when they are presented from 45° on the better side.

The accuracy of the transcranial fitting may be improved by placing a large earmuff over the ear and hearing aid opposite the loudspeaker, but this approach has not been experimentally verified. The extra isolation provided by the earmuff is most valuable at mid-frequencies where interaural level differences are not large enough for the contribution of the far ear to be insignificant compared to the near ear. Balancing can also be accomplished by achieving equal thresholds for presentation from each side, but in this case, the earmuff must not be used.[c]

16.2 Bone-conduction Hearing Aids

Bone-conduction hearing aids vibrate the structures within the cochlea without the sounds passing in the normal way through the middle ear. The output transducer is a vibrator known as a bone conductor (see Section 2.11). Vibrations from the bone conductor have to be effectively coupled to the skull (and hence to the cochlea). To achieve adequate coupling, the bone conductor is usually mounted on one side of a headband, which uses spring tension to push the bone conductor against the head. Alternatively, the bone conductor can be mounted on the arm of a spectacle aid. Apart from the output transducer, the remainder of the hearing aid is no different from a conventional (acoustic output) hearing aid. The hearing aid can be in a spectacle frame, in a BTE case mounted on the transducer headband, or in a body aid.

16.2.1 Applications of bone-conduction hearing aids

Bone-conduction aids are useful for three groups of people, almost all of whom will have a conductive or mixed hearing loss. The first group comprises people who, because of some medical condition, cannot wear a hearing aid that in any way occludes the outer ear. Typically this occurs when occlusion of the ear causes or exacerbates infections of the outer ear, or when the aid wearer has frequent infections of the middle ear combined with missing or perforated eardrums. With a bone-conduction hearing

aid, no part of the hearing aid obstructs the ear. An alternative that could be considered for some of these people is a BTE with a very open earmold, although it may not be possible to achieve enough gain with such open molds (see Section 5.3.3). Also in this first group are some people who have undergone surgery using a canal-wall-down technique, for whom it can be difficult to obtain an adequate earmold.[748]

The second group of candidates for bone-conduction hearing aids comprises those who have a congenitally malformed or absent external or middle ear (atresia or microtia). Vibration of the skull may be the only way to input sound to the cochlea.

The third group of people are those who have an extremely large conductive hearing loss. Because the skull vibrations reach the cochlea without having to pass through the middle ear system in the usual manner, it may be possible to stimulate the cochlea more strongly with a bone-conduction hearing aid than with a conventional, air-conduction hearing aid (but see the next section).

16.2.2 Bone-conduction hearing aid output capabilities

Because the output of a bone-conduction hearing aid is a mechanical vibration rather than a sound wave, these hearing aids can be measured electroacoustically only with equipment that measures vibration (IEC 373, ANSI S3.13). Furthermore, the amount of vibration they cause depends on the characteristics of the surface against which they are held. Consequently, bone-conduction hearing aids can be measured only when coupled to a *mechanical coupler* (which provides a mechanical impedance that matches that of the skull) and an accelerometer (which measures the resulting vibration). The mechanical coupler is commonly called an

[c] At first sight, it might seem that internal aid noise or external noise would invalidate the threshold by masking the signal arriving at the satellite microphone. It can, however, be shown that if the thresholds of the sounds incident from each side of the head are the same, the sensitivity will also be balanced for higher level sounds whether the thresholds were absolute thresholds or thresholds masked by internal noise or ambient noise. For this to be true, both paths must be operating, so an earmuff must not be used.

artificial mastoid, though it actually simulates the skull impedance at locations other than on the mastoid process.

Vibration is expressed in terms of the force (in Newtons or in μN) produced by the vibrator against the artificial mastoid. The vibratory force can be expressed in decibels relative to a reference force of 1 μN. The resulting number, equal to 20 times the logarithm of the actual force divided by the reference force, is then called the *output force level*. Because the input quantity (sound pressure) of a bone-conduction hearing aid is different from the output quantity (force), it is not sensible to talk about the *gain* of a bone-conduction hearing aid. Instead, we can talk about the *acousto-mechanical sensitivity level*. Although this is a mouthful, it is simply equal to the output force level minus the input SPL, and is directly analogous to gain.

Table 16.1 shows the maximum output force levels (*OFL90*) that can be produced at various frequencies by a typical high-powered BTE bone-conduction aid. The table also shows the force levels measured on an artificial mastoid when the same signal produces vibrations at threshold on the human mastoid for an average normal-hearing person (ISO 389-3). The final row of the table shows the sensation level that this bone-conduction hearing aid can therefore produce for a person with no hearing loss. Of course, patients with a sensorineural component to their hearing loss will receive sensation levels even lower than the sensation levels shown in the final row of Table 16.1.

How do these achievable sensation levels compare to those available with an air-conduction hearing aid? The answer depends on how much conductive loss is assumed.

Table 16.1 Maximum output force levels (OFL90) for a particular very high-powered BTE-style bone-conduction hearing aid, Reference Equivalent Threshold Force Levels (RETFL; ISO 389-3) for mastoid placement, and the resulting maximum sensation levels achievable for a person with normal bone-conduction thresholds (i.e. no sensorineural hearing loss). RETFL values given in ANSI S3.26 are very similar.

	Frequency (Hz)				
	250	500	1000	2000	4000
OFL90 (dB re 1μN)	107	122	122	119	104
RETFL (dB re 1μN)	67	58	42	31	35
Sensation level (dB)	40	64	80	88	69

Table 16.2. The first three rows show the maximum output of a sample air-conduction hearing aid (OSPL90), the Reference Equivalent Threshold Sound Pressure Level in a 2 cc coupler (RETSPL; ISO 389-2) and consequently, the sensation levels achievable with the hearing aid for a normal-hearing person. The final row shows the sensation level achievable for a person with the conductive loss shown in row 4.

	Frequency (Hz)				
	250	500	1000	2000	4000
OSPL90 (dB SPL, 2 cc)	128	130	137	132	127
RETSPL (dB SPL, 2cc)	14	5	0	3	5
Sensation level for normal hearing (dB)	114	125	137	129	122
Conductive hearing loss (dB HL)	60	60	60	60	60
Sensation level for maximum conductive loss (dB)	54	65	77	69	62

Table 16.2 shows the maximum acoustic levels that result when the same hearing aid referred to in Table 16.1 drives a receiver (inside the BTE case) rather than a bone conductor. These OSPL90 values can be subtracted from the thresholds of normal hearing referred to a 2-cc coupler (ISO 389-2) as shown in row 2. The resulting maximum sensation levels available to a person with normal hearing are shown in row 3. The sensation level available to someone with a conductive loss depends, of course, on the size of the loss. As an example, row 4 shows a large conductive loss, and the final row shows the resulting maximum sensation levels via air conduction for such a loss.

By comparing these with the values shown in the final row of Table 16.1, we can see that bone conduction provides a greater sensation level above 500 Hz, but air conduction provides a greater sensation level at 250 Hz. Of course, this conclusion depends directly on the degree of conductive loss assumed. As the conductive loss becomes smaller, the sensation level provided by the air-conduction aid increases. For conductive losses of 40 dB or less, this particular hearing aid provides more stimulation as an air-conduction aid than as a bone-conduction aid at all frequencies.

Based on this example, one would not select a bone-conduction hearing aid with the sole aim of maximizing the input to the cochlea unless the patient's hearing loss has a conductive component of approximately 50 dB or greater.

The relative effectiveness of air- and bone-conduction hearing aids is not affected by the degree of any sensorineural loss, but is some-what affected by the particular receivers and bone conductors used. A repeat of the calculations for an extremely powerful body-level bone hearing aid indicated that, for conductive hearing losses of 45 dB HL or less, it provided greater stimulation at all frequencies from 250 Hz to 6 kHz in air-conduction mode than in bone-conduction mode.

These examples also show that for a patient with a large conductive loss, achieving a high sensation level is not possible with either form of output transducer, particularly for low-frequency sounds. This deficiency is exacerbated if the patient also has a sensori-neural loss.

16.2.3 Prescribing electroacoustic characteristics for bone-conduction hearing aids

Few clinicians have access to an artificial mastoid and an accelerometer. Consequently, bone-conduction hearing aids should initially be selected and adjusted based on the hearing aid specifications, followed by measurement of functional gain or the use of other subjective techniques.

Methods for prescribing the electroacoustic performance of air-conduction hearing aids are covered in Chapter 9. This section will describe how any such prescription can be converted into a prescription for a bone-conduction hearing aid. Suppose that some prescription formula has been used to deduce a target insertion gain, IG, for an aid wearer, but that we wish to fit a bone-conduction hearing aid instead of an air-conduction aid. The acousto-mechanical sensitivity level, A, that on average results in a sensation level equal to that provided by an air-conduction hearing aid can be calculated from Equation 16.2:

$$A = IG + (RETFL - MAF) - C \quad .....16.2,$$

where RETFL is the Reference Equivalent Threshold Force Level referred to an artificial mastoid (Table 16.1), MAF is the Minimum Audible Field for normal hearing (ISO 226), and C is the conductive component of the person's hearing loss, as quantified by the air-bone gap. Each of the quantities in Equation 16.2 may be different at different frequencies. The equation is easily understood: the bone conductor acousto-mechanical sensitivity must be different from the insertion gain by the amount that, for normally hearing people, the force level at threshold exceeds the sound pressure level at threshold. In addition, the presence of a conductive component of the hearing loss will have been allowed for in some way in the calculation of insertion gain.[d] The bone-conduction aid does not need such a component in its gain, because the bone-conduction path bypasses the middle ear. Consequently, the term C is subtracted in the equation. For otosclerotic ears, the Carhart correction should be applied to the audiogram prior to prescribing the hearing aid (see Section 9.4).

Alternatively, one may have started from a prescription for real-ear aided gain (REAG) rather than insertion gain. The required acousto-mechanical sensitivity level, A, can be calculated from equation 16.3:

$$A = REAG + (RETFL - MAP) - C \qquad .....16.3,$$

where MAP is the minimum audible pressure for normal threshold of hearing for air-conducted sound, referred to the average ear canal.

An analogous equation can be used to prescribe the maximum output for the bone conductor, OFL90, in terms of the maximum output that would be prescribed for an acoustic hearing aid, OSPL90, for the same person:

$$OFL90 = OSPL90 + (RETFL - RETSPL) - C \qquad .....16.4,$$

where RETSPL is the Reference Equivalent Threshold SPL (for normal hearing) in a 2 cc coupler (see Table 16.2). Table 16.3 gives suitable values for each of the terms in Equations 16.2 to 16.4.

Example of bone-conduction prescription
Suppose a subject with the audiogram shown in the first two rows of Table 16.4 is to be prescribed a bone-conduction aid using the NAL-RP procedure for gain (see Section 9.2.2) and the NAL-SSPL procedure for OSPL90 (see Section 9.6). Note that if this table is used to construct a worksheet or spreadsheet, the correction figures in rows 5 and 8 will be the same for all patients. The acousto-mechanical sensitivity level shown in row 6 equals row 4 plus row 5 minus row 3. Similarly, OFL90 equals row 7 plus row 8 minus row 3.

Table 16.3 Values for MAF (based on ISO 226), MAP (calculated as MAF plus REUG from Table 4.6), RETFL-MAF, RETFL-MAP, and RETFL-RETSPL. Similar computations can be made using the comparable ANSI standards.

	Frequency (Hz)				
	250	500	1000	2000	4000
MAF (dB SPL)	11	6	5	0	-4
MAP (dB SPL)	12	8	8	12	10
RETFL-MAF (dB)	56	52	37	30	39
RETFL-MAP (dB)	55	50	35	19	25
RETFL-RETSPL (dB)	53	52	42	28	30

[d] The derivation (not shown here for reasons of space) of Equation 16.2 does not make any assumption regarding how the insertion gain prescription has compensated for the conductive portion of the hearing loss. Although the equations in this chapter have been independently derived, an equation analogous to Equation 16.2 has been derived and presented for bone-anchored hearing aids (Carlsson & Hakansson 1997).

Table 16.4 Calculation of the prescription for a bone-conduction hearing aid for the person whose air-conduction and bone-conduction thresholds are shown in the first two rows. The insertion gain and OSPL90 prescriptions, if an air-conduction aid were to be used, are shown in rows 4 and 7. A linear hearing aid has been assumed for this example. The correction figures in rows 5 and 8 are used to convert the prescriptions to bone-conduction specifications, in accordance with Equations 16.2 and 16.4.

		Frequency (Hz)				
		250	500	1000	2000	4000
1	AC (dB HL)	60	60	70	80	80
2	BC (dB HL)	10	10	20	30	30
3	Conductive loss (dB)	50	50	50	50	50
4	Insertion gain (dB)	27	36	48	49	48
5	RETFL – MAF (dB)	56	52	37	30	39
6	Acousto-mechanical sensitivity level (dB)	33	38	35	29	37
7	OSPL90 (dB SPL)	137	136	139	143	144
8	RETFL – RETSPL (dB)	53	52	42	28	30
9	OFL90 (dB re 1 μN)	140	138	131	121	124

Note that, with the exception of 2 kHz, the prescription for OFL90 is considerably greater than the OFL90 values that are typically achievable with a high-powered BTE hearing aid (as shown in Table 16.1). Note also that the sensorineural portion of the loss in this example is particularly mild. *Consequently, the maximum output control of bone-conduction hearing aids can routinely be adjusted to give the greatest possible output, rather than being individually prescribed.* The suitability of maximum output should nonetheless be subjectively evaluated (see Section 10.10).

The gain-frequency response selection procedure defined by Equation 16.2 or 16.3, and illustrated in Table 16.4, should, however, be employed for each patient provided with a bone-conduction hearing aid. The target acousto-mechanical sensitivity level should be compared to the published specification for the hearing aid being considered. The appropriate tone control and gain settings can then be deduced.

Two caveats must be applied to the prescription procedure and calculations of sensation level outlined in this chapter. Either of the following aspects of middle-ear function can cause the relationship between air-conducted and bone-conducted sounds to vary from that assumed in this chapter, and hence alter the prescription that is optimum for a patient.

- It has been assumed that the magnitudes of the conductive and sensorineural portions of the loss are known. Although it is common practice to determine these portions based on the air- and bone-conduction thresholds, it is well known that middle-ear disorders can elevate or suppress bone-conduction thresholds.[240] The Carhart notch (see Section 9.4) for an otosclerotic loss is one example of this, but different effects, in both directions, occur for other types of conductive hearing loss.[240]

- High-level sounds from an air-conduction hearing aid pass through the middle ear, and are thus attenuated by the stapedius reflex. Prescriptive formula, to the extent that they are influenced by average discomfort levels, account for the attenuation produced by the stapedius reflex. In a conductive hearing loss, however, the stapedius reflex generally does not affect middle-ear operation.[669] Furthermore, if a reflex is present, it may *increase* the sensitivity for bone-conducted sounds.[138] In practice any effects of the acoustic reflex may be of no consequence, as they are unlikely to change the conclusion that the maximum output of bone-conduction hearing aids should be as high as is technically feasible.

How can the suitability of the electroacoustic performance of a bone-conduction hearing aid be evaluated? Certainly, we cannot directly measure insertion gain as we can with acoustic hearing aid. A worthwhile alternative for linear hearing aids is to measure the aided thresholds of the person and compare these to the target aided thresholds. For non-linear hearing aids, subjective methods of verification, as outlined in Chapter 11, are probably more appropriate.

16.2.4 Disadvantages of bone-conduction hearing aids

Bone-conduction hearing aids have several disadvantages over air-conduction aids. First, the transducer has to be pushed tightly against the head if it is to function well. Continued use can cause hardened skin, permanent depressions in the skin, and pain. Second, the bone vibrator and the means to hold it against the skull are not small or discreet. Third, there is little inter-aural attenuation for bone-conducted sounds. Consequently, although it is possible to pick up different signals on each side of the head, it is not possible to deliver them independently to the respective cochleae. Binaural differences are thus minimal, so localization and the ability to use binaural cues to separate signals and noises coming from different directions are both impaired. Fourth, the cable and plugs between the aid and the transducer can be unreliable. Fifth, the attenuation provided by the skin, and the limitations of the transducer make it difficult to achieve an adequate low-

frequency, and very high-frequency, response. As we have seen, the maximum output of bone-conduction aids is much less than optimal at these same frequencies and is less than optimal at all frequencies. Sixth, the transducer and headband are easily dislodged. Last, the inability to measure the output of the aid electroacoustically (without an artificial mastoid) makes it more difficult to check the functioning of these aids than is the case for air-conduction aids. Despite these considerable limitations, bone-conduction aids remain a better solution than air-conduction hearing aids for a small proportion of people with hearing loss.

16.3 Implanted and Semi-implanted Hearing Aids

16.3.1 Bone-anchored hearing aids

A *bone-anchored hearing aid* (*BAHA*) avoids many of the disadvantages of a bone-conduction aid. Like bone-conduction hearing aids, BAHAs also output a mechanical vibration, but transmit this vibration to the skull via a titanium screw embedded in the mastoid.[884] Because it is titanium, the screw osseointegrates (i.e. bonds) to the bone. The hearing aid, including the vibrator, is attached to a plastic bayonet coupling inserted in a titanium abutment that passes through the skin and is connected to the outer end of the titanium screw fixture, as shown in Figure 16.6. A direct connection through the skin is referred to as *percutaneous coupling*. There appears to be a very low incidence of problems associated with penetrating the skin.[725] The surgery required to fit a BAHA is relatively minor; it is usually done under local anesthesia on an outpatient basis. In some countries, the BAHA is largely replacing traditional bone-conduction hearing aids for patients who have a permanent need for a bone-vibration hearing aid.

The direct mechanical path to the skull enables vibrations to be more effectively and comfortably transmitted, because compres-

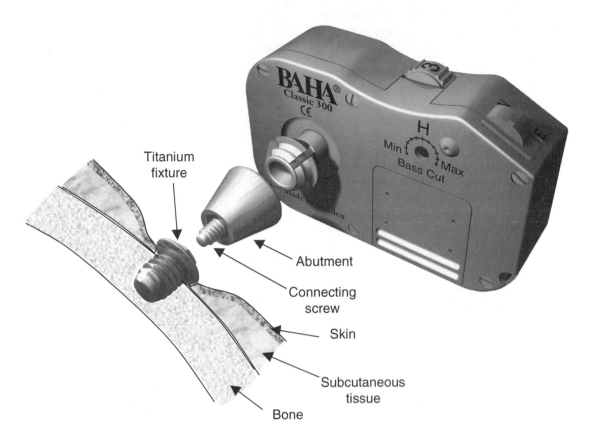

Figure 16.6 Bone-anchored hearing aid, showing its attachment through the skin to the bone. Amended by permission from Entific Medical Systems.

sion of the skin is not necessary.[346] With a conventional bone-conduction hearing aid, most of the vibratory motion of the transducer is absorbed by the skin and subcutaneous soft tissues.[347] BAHAs provide a satisfactory level of stimulation for patients with bone-conduction thresholds (average of 500, 1000, 2000 and 3000 Hz) up to 45 dB HL for the head-worn hearing aid and up to 60 dB HL for the body-worn aid.[5, 909]

Many studies have reported that patients with a suitable hearing loss, and who have a permanent need for a bone-conduction hearing aid, prefer the BAHA to a non-implanted bone-conduction alternative.[72, 96, 348, 822, 825] These preferences apply whether or not the device provides speech discrimination ability better than that provided by a bone-

conduction aid. The BAHA provides markedly greater physical comfort, and is less visible, than a conventional bone conduction hearing aid.[348] The relative effectiveness of the BAHA and air-conduction hearing aids is less certain. The greater the conductive loss of a patient, however, the more likely it is that a BAHA will be more effective than an air-conduction hearing aid.[640]

The effectiveness of a BAHA for a particular patient can be tested without implantation. A test rod is temporarily attached to the BAHA transducer, and the patient grips the test rod between his or her teeth (with the lips closed to prevent feedback). The patient can then assess sound quality and loudness. Coupling to the skull via the permanent screw fixture is slightly more effective than the temporary coupling provided by the teeth, particularly for the high frequencies.

A BAHA on one side of the head transmits vibrations to both cochleae with only 5 to 15 dB interaural attenuation.[653] Bilateral BAHAs can therefore provide some degree of dichotic stimulation. Studies have shown improved localization, as well as speech intelligibility in noise and in quiet, relative to a single BAHA.[821, 910] Some of the advantage for the second BAHA arises because of the bilateral microphones rather than because of the bilateral output vibrators.

It is critical that the patient be instructed in regular but gentle cleaning of the skin and the abutment. It is also essential that patients avoid receiving a blow to the BAHA. In rare cases, fixtures in children have been knocked out by physical trauma.

16.3.2 Middle-ear implants

In the near future, another alternative will be fully or partially *implanted hearing aids*, also referred to as *middle-ear implants*. These devices use either piezoelectric or electromagnetic output transducers, and a variety of means for getting the amplified electrical signal to the transducer.

Piezoelectric transducers are based on a ceramic material that changes its shape when a voltage is applied to it. One end of the transducer is anchored to the skull and the free end connects to some point in the ossicular chain, thus transferring sound vibrations to the cochlea. In one implant system, the free end terminates in a thin plate that is sandwiched between the incus and the stapes by inserting it into the incudo-stapedial joint.[248] In another system the piezoelectric transducer is anchored within a cavity in the mastoid and transmits vibrations to the incus via a coupling link.[520] The link is inserted through a hole cut into the incus by a laser.

Electromagnetic transducers comprise a small permanent magnet mounted within the magnetic field generated by a coil. When a current passes through the coil, the magnet moves. This is the same principle as used in loudspeakers and in receivers for hearing aids (see Section 2.6). With most of the middle-ear implant systems, the magnet is firmly attached to some point in the ossicular chain, enabling vibrations to be transferred from the magnet directly to the middle ear system. Mounting points for the magnet have included the tympanic membrane,[436] the incus,[293, 572, 885] the incudo-stapedial joint,[398] and even the round window.[829] The coil that drives the magnet can either be external to the ear in a hearing aid case or custom shell[436, 829] or in the middle ear cavity.[572]

A different type of electromagnetic transducer works on the same principle as the bone conductor. In the floating-mass transducer, the coil, rather than the magnet, is bonded to the incus.[885] The magnet is loosely suspended inside the coil. When the fluctuating magnetic field vibrates the magnet, the magnet's inertia restrains its motion. Consequently, the inertial forces placed on the coil and casing of the transducer cause them to also move, thus transferring vibrations to the incus.

Microphones for implanted or partially implanted hearing aids can be external to the skin; embedded just under the skin, such as within the posterior wall of the ear canal;[555] or potentially within the middle ear cavity. The major problem to be overcome is the attenuation provided by the skin, and consequently an increase in the level of internal hearing aid noise, caused both by internal microphone noise and by sensing of internal body noises.[211]

A second problem is caused by the desire to keep the ossicular chain intact in case implanted hearing aid use is discontinued. An intact ossicular chain implies that if the output transducer is coupled to the ossicular chain, the microphone cannot be, or feedback oscillation will occur, even for very low gains. This is unfortunate, because the tympanic membrane is perfectly placed to convert air-borne vibrations to mechanical vibrations that could be detected by a suitable sensor.

Batteries can be in an externally worn unit, or can be implanted. If implanted, a minor operation may be needed every 3 to 5 years to replace the battery.

If the microphone and battery are not implanted, then a signal has to be transferred from the external system to the vibrating transducer in some way. Most experimental systems are using a two-stage approach similar to that employed in cochlear implants. An external coil transmits a magnetic field or electromagnetic radiation, which is sensed by an implanted coil or antenna. The signal picked up by the implanted sensing coil is taken by implanted wiring to the piezoelectric transducer or implanted driving coil. Some systems directly transfer the signal: The external coil creates a magnetic field that directly drives an implanted magnet.

Relative to both bone- and air-conduction hearing aids, fully-implanted hearing aids are expected to have advantages related to visibility, convenience, feedback, occlusion, and possibly signal quality. They are, however, still at an experimental or clinical trial stage. Chasin (1997) gives a more extensive review of bone-anchored hearing aids and middle-ear implants.

16.4 Concluding Comments

Hearing aids in the CROS family are not extensively used, even for many patients with hearing losses for whom a CROS fitting would appear to have some advantages. The rapid development of technology may affect this situation in the near future, and there may be some merging of CROS amplification concepts with other signal processing ideas.

For example, when miniature bi-directional wireless links between the ears are widely available, it will be possible for the sound presented to each ear to be a desired combination of the sound picked-up by microphones on each side of the head, without the inconvenience of any cables. Such a combination could range from a simple linear addition of sounds, as in a BICROS fitting, to processing that adaptively reduces noise and reinserts cues to localization, as is done in processing for virtual reality.

Finally, although implanted hearing aids have been presented almost incidentally in this chapter as an alternative to bone-conduction hearing aids, they may prove to have wider appeal. Their potential is greatest if suitable methods for implanting the microphone and (a very long-life) battery can be developed, so that the hearing aid will have no external components needing daily care and attention.

REFERENCES

1. **Abrahamson J. (1997).** Patient education and peer interaction facilitate hearing aid adjustment. *High Performance Hearing Solutions, 1*: 19-22.

2. **Abrahamson J. (1991).** Teaching coping strategies: a client education approach to aural rehabilitation. *J Acad Rehab Audiology, 24*: 43-53.

3. **Abrahamson J, Northern J, Raskind L, Robier T, Warner-Czyz A. (1999).** Contemporary models of real life adult aural rehabilitation. Presented at *Amer Acad Audiol Conv*, Miami.

4. **Abrams H, Hnath CT, Guerreiro S, Ritterman S. (1992).** The effects of intervention strategy on self-perception of hearing handicap. *Ear & Hear, 13*(5): 371-377.

5. **Abramson M, Fay T, Kelly J, Wazen J, Liden G, Tjellstrom A. (1989).** Clinical results with a percutaneous bone-anchored hearing aid. *Laryngoscope, 99*(7): 707-710.

6. **Agnew J. (1996).** Acoustic feedback and other audible artifacts in hearing aids. *Trends in Amplification, 1*(2): 45-82.

7. **Agnew J. (1986).** Ear impression stability. *Hear Instrum, 37*(12): 8, 11-12, 58.

8. **Agnew J. (1997).** Sound quality evaluation of anti-saturation circuitry in a hearing aid. *Scand Audiol, 26*(1): 15-22.

   Ahonniska J, Cantell M, Tolvanen A, Lyytinen H. (1993). Speech perception and brain laterality: the effect of ear advantage on auditory event-related potentials. *Brain & Lang, 45*(2): 127-146.

9. **Ahroon W, Hamernik R, Davis R, Patterson J. (1993).** The relation among postexposure threshold shifts and NIPTS in the chinchilla. In M Vallet (Ed.), *Noise and Man '93, Proceedings of the 6th International Congress on Noise as a Public Health Problem* (Vol 3, Pp 1-4). INRETS.

10. **Alberti PW. (1977).** Hearing aids and aural rehabilitation in a geriatric population. *J Otolaryngol, 6*(Supplement 4).

11. **Alcantara J, Dooley G, Blamey P, Seligman P. (1994).** Preliminary evaluation of a formant enhancement algorithm on the perception of speech in noise for normally hearing listeners. *Audiology, 33*(1): 15-27.

12. **Alcantara J, Whitford L, Blamey P, Cowan R, Clark G. (1990).** Speech feature recognition by profoundly hearing impaired children using a multiple-channel electrotactile speech processor and aided residual hearing. *J Acoust Soc Amer, 88*(3): 1260-1273.

13. **Aleksy W. (1989).** Comparison of benefit from UCH/RNID single-channel extracochlear implant and tactile acoustic monitor. *J Laryngol Otol Suppl, 18*: 55-57.

14. **Allen JB, Berkley DA, Blauert J. (1977).** Multimicrophone signal-processing technique to remove room reverberation from speech signals. *J Acoust Soc Amer, 62*: 912-915.

15. **Allen J, Hall J, Jeng P. (1990).** Loudness growth in 1/2-octave bands (LGOB) - a procedure for the assessment of loudness. *J Acoust Soc Amer, 88*(2): 745-753.

16. **Alpiner JG, Chevrette W, Glascoe G, Metz M, & Olsen B. (1974).** *The Denver Scale of Communication Function.* Denver: University of Denver.

17. **Alvord LS, Farmer BL. (1997).** Anatomy and orientation of the human external ear. *J Amer Acad Audiol, 8*(6): 383-90.

18. **Alvord LS, Morgan R, Cartwright K. (1997).** Anatomy of an earmold: a formal terminology. *J Amer Acad Audiol, 8*(2): 100-3.

19. **Alvord L, Doxey G, Smith D. (1989).** Hearing aids worn with tympanic membrane perforation: complications and solutions. *Amer J Otol, 10*(4): 277-280.

20. **American Speech-Language-Hearing Association. (1994).** Guidelines for fitting and monitoring FM systems. Report of the ad hoc committee on FM systems and auditory trainers. *ASHA, 36*(Suppl 12): 1-9.

21. **Anderson K. (1989).** *Screening instrument for targeting education risk (SIFTER).* Austin, Texas: Pro-Ed.

22. **Anderson K, Matkin N. (1996).** *Screening instrument for targeting educational risk in pre-school children (Age 3-kindergarten) (Pre-school S.I.F.T.E.R).* Tampa, Florida: Educational Audiology Association.

   Anderson K, Smaldino JJ. (2000). *Children's home inventory of listening difficulties (CHILD).* URL www.edaud.org.

23. **Andersson G, Melin L, Lindberg P, Scott B. (1995)**. Development of a short scale for self-assessment of experiences of hearing loss. The hearing coping assessment. *Scand Audiol, 24*(3): 147-154.

24. **Andersson G, Melin L, Scott B, Lindberg P. (1994)**. Behavioral counselling for subjects with acquired hearing loss. A new approach to hearing tactics. *Scand Audiol, 23*(4): 249-256.

25. **Andersson G, Palmkvist A, Melin L, Arlinger S. (1996)**. Predictors of daily assessed hearing aid use and hearing capability using visual analogue scales. *Brit J Audiol, 30*(1): 27-35.

26. **Appollonio I, Carabellese C, Frattola L, Trabucchi M. (1996)**. Effects of sensory aids on the quality of life and mortality of elderly people: a multivariate analysis. *Age & Ageing, 25*(2): 89-96.

27. **Arkebauer HJ, Mencher GT, McCall C. (1971)**. Modification of speech discrimination in patients with binaural asymmetrical hearing loss. *J Speech Hear Disord, 36*(2): 208-212.

28. **Armitage S, Preves D. (1998)**. Microcard: A new hearing aid programming interface. *The Hear J, 51*(9): 37-42.

29. **Asano F, Suzuki Y, Sone T. (1990)**. Role of spectral cues in median plane localization. *J Acoust Soc Amer, 88*(1): 159-168.

30. **Bade P. (1991)**. Hearing impairment and the elderly patient. *Wis Med J, 90*(9): 516-519.

31. **Baer T, Moore BCJ, Gatehouse S. (1993)**. Spectral contrast enhancement of speech in noise for listeners with sensorineural hearing impairment: effects on intelligibility, quality and response times. *J Rehab Res Dev, 30*: 95-109.

32. **Baer T, Moore B. (1994)**. Effects of spectral smearing on the intelligibility of sentences in the presence of interfering speech. *J Acoust Soc Amer, 95*(4): 2277-2280.

33. **Balfour P, Hawkins D. (1992)**. A comparison of sound quality judgments for monaural and binaural hearing aid processed stimuli. *Ear & Hear, 13*(5): 331-339.

34. **Ball V, Faulkner A, Fourcin A. (1990)**. The effects of two different speech-coding strategies on voice fundamental frequency control in deafened adults. *Brit J Audiol, 24*(6): 393-409.

35. **Bamford J, Davis A, Hind S, McCracken W, Reeve K. (2000)**. Evidence on very early service delivery: what parents want and don't always get. In R Seewald (Ed.), *A sound foundation through early amplification* (151-157). Stafa, Switzerland: Phonak.

36. **Barcham LJ, Stephens SD. (1980)**. The use of an open-ended problems questionnaire in auditory rehabilitation. *Brit J Audiol, 14*(2): 49-54.

37. **Barker C, Dillon H. (1999)**. Client preferences for compression threshold in single-channel wide dynamic range compression hearing aids. *Ear & Hear, 20*(2): 127-139.

38. **Barker C, Dillon H, Newall P. (In Press)**. The use of wide dynamic range compression for people with severe and profound hearing loss. *Ear & Hear*.

39. **Barsz K. (1991)**. Auditory pattern perception: the effect of tone location on the discrimination of tonal sequences. *Percept & Psychophys, 50*(3): 290-296.

40. **Bauer RW, Matusza JL, Blackmer RF. (1966)**. Noise localization after unilateral attenuation. *J Acoust Soc Amer, 40*: 441-444.

41. **Bauman N, Braemer M. (1996)**. Using a CIC hearing aid in transcranial CROS fittings. *The Hear J, 49*(3): 27-28, 45-46.

42. **Baumfield A, Dillon H. (Submitted)**. Factors affecting the selection, preference, and perceived benefit of hearing aids.

43. **Beck LB. (1983)**. Assessment of directional hearing aid characteristics. *Audiol Acoust, 22*: 178-190.

44. **Beggs WDA, Foreman DL. (1980)**. Sound localization and early binaural experience in the deaf. *Brit J Audiol, 14*: 41-48.

45. **Bench J, Kowal A, Bamford J. (1979)**. The BKB (Bamford-Kowal-Bench) sentence lists for partially hearing children. *Brit J Audiol, 13*: 108-112.

46. **Bennett C. (1989)**. Hearing aid use with minimal high-frequency hearing loss. *Otolaryngol Head Neck Surg, 100*(2): 154-157.

47. **Bennett D, Byers V. (1967)**. Increased intelligibility in the aypoacousic by slow play frequency transposition. *J Audit Res, 7*(107-118).

48. **Bennett MJSS, Browne LMH. (1980)**. A controlled feedback hearing aid. *Hear Aid J, 33*(5): 12, 42-43.

49. **Bentler R. (1994)**. CICs: Some practical considerations. *The Hear J, 47*(11): 37, 40-43.

50. **Bentler RA. (1989)**. External ear resonance characteristics in children. *J Speech Hear Disord, 54* : 264-268.

51. **Bentler R, Pavlovic C. (1989a)**. Comparison of discomfort levels obtained with pure tones and multitone complexes. *J Acoust Soc Amer, 86*(1): 126-132.

52. **Bentler R, Pavlovic C. (1989b)**. Transfer functions and correction factors used in hearing aid evaluation and research. *Ear & Hear, 10*(1): 58-63.

53. **Beranek LL. (1954)**. *Acoustics*. New York: McGraw-Hill.

54. **Berger K. (1984).** *The hearing aid - its operation and development.* Livonia, MI: National Hearing Aid Society.

55. **Berger KW, Millin JP. (1980).** Choosing the binaural candidate and checking the fitting. In ER Libby (Ed.), *Binaural Hearing and Amplification, Vol 2.* (177-186) Chicago: Zenetron Inc.

56. **Berger RA, Hagberg EN, Rane RL. (1977).** *Prescription of hearing aids: rationale, procedures and results.* Kent, OH: Herald Publishing House.

57. **Bernstein L, Eberhardt S, Demorest M. (1989).** Single-channel vibrotactile supplements to visual perception of intonation and stress. *J Acoust Soc Amer, 85*(1): 397-405.

58. **Berry G. (1939).** The use and effectiveness of hearing aids. *Laryngoscope, 49*: 912-938.

59. **Bess F, Gravel J, Tharpe A. (1996).** *Amplification for children with auditory deficits.* Nashville, TN: Bill Wilkerson Center Press.

60. **Bess FH, Chase PA, Gravel JS, Seewald RC, Stelmachowicz PG, Tharpe AM, Hedley-Williams A. (1996).** Amplification for infants and children with hearing loss. *Amer J Audiol, 5*(1): 53-68.

61. **Bess FH, Lichtenstein MJ, Logan SA. (1991).** Making hearing impairment functionally relevant: Linkages with hearing disability and handicap. *Acta Otolaryngol (Stockh), 476*: 226-231.

62. **Bess F, Klee T, Culbertson J. (1986).** Identification, assessment, and management of children with unilateral sensorineural hearing loss. *Ear & Hear, 7*(1): 43-51.

63. **Bevan MA. (1997).** Matching hearing technology to hearing needs. *High Performance Hearing Solutions (Suppl to Hear Rev), 1*: 32-36.

64. **Binnie CA. (1977).** Attitude changes following speechreading training. *Scand Audiol, 6*: 13-19.

65. **Binnie CA, Montgomery AA, Jackson PL. (1974).** Auditory and visual contributions to the perception of consonants. *J Speech Hear Res, 17*: 619-630.

66. **Blamey P, Arndt P, Bergeron F, Bredberg G, Brimacombe J, Facer G, Larky J, Lindstrom B, Nedzelski J, Peterson A, Shipp D, Staller S, Whitford L. (1996).** Factors affecting auditory performance of postlinguistically deaf adults using cochlear implants. *Audiol & Neuro-Otology, 1*: 293-306.

67. **Blamey PJ, Pymnan BC, Gordon MB, Clark GM, Brown AM, Dowell RC, Hollow RD. (1992).** Factors predicting postoperative sentence scores in postlinguistically deaf adult cochlear implant patients. *Ann Otol Rhinol Laryngol, 101*(4): 342-348.

68. **Blamey P, Cowan R, Alcantara J, Clark G. (1988).** Phonemic information transmitted by a multichannel electrotactile speech processor. *J Speech Hear Res, 31*(4): 620-629.

69. **Blamey P, Dowell R, Brown A, Clark G. (1985).** Clinical results with a hearing aid and a single-channel vibrotactile device for profoundly deaf adults. *Brit J Audiol, 19*(3): 203-210.

70. **Blauert J. (1971).** Localization and the law of the first wavefront in the median plane. *J Acoust Soc Amer, 50*: 466-470.

71. **Bloom PJ. (1982).** Evaluation of a dereverberation technique with normal and impaired listeners. *Brit J Audiol, 16*(3): 167-176.

72. **Bonding P, Jonsson M, Salomon G, Ahlgren P. (1992).** The bone-anchored hearing aid. Osseointegration and audiological effect. *Acta Otolaryngol Suppl Stockh, 492*: 42-45.

73. **Boothroyd A. (1999).** Private communication.

74. **Boothroyd A. (1997).** Auditory capacity of hearing-impaired children using hearing aids and cochlear implants: issues of efficacy and assessment. *Scand Audiol Suppl, 46*: 17-25.

75. **Boothroyd A. (1997).** Auditory development of the hearing child. *Scand Audiol Suppl, 46*: 9-16.

76. **Boothroyd A. (1993).** Recovery of speech perception performance after prolonged auditory deprivation: case study. *J Amer Acad Audiol, 4*(5): 331-337.

77. **Boothroyd A, Iglehart F. (1998).** Experiments with classroom FM amplification. *Ear & Hear, 19*(3): 202-17.

78. **Bridges J, Bentler RA. (1998).** Relating hearing aid use to well-being among older adults. *The Hear J, 51*(7): 39-44.

79. **Brink RHS, van den Wit HP, Kempen GIJM, Heuvelen MGJ. (1996).** Attitude and help-seeking for hearing impairment. *Brit J Audiol, 30*: 313-324.

80. **Briskey RJ. (1980).** Selecting and fitting a hearing aid: binaurally. In ER Libby (Ed.), *Binaural hearing and amplification.* (187-204) Chicago: Zenetron.

81. **British Standard. (1993).** *Code of practice for audio-frequency induction-loop systems (AFILS).* BS7594.

82. **Bronkhorst AW, Plomp R. (1988).** The effect of head-induced interaural time and level differences on speech intelligibility in noise. *J Acoust Soc Amer, 83*(4): 1508-1516.

83. **Bronkhorst A, Plomp R. (1989).** Binaural speech intelligibility in noise for hearing-impaired listeners. *J Acoust Soc Amer, 86*(4): 1374-1383.

84. **Brookhouser P, Auslander M. (1989)**. Aided auditory thresholds in children with postmeningitic deafness. *Laryngoscope, 99*(8 Pt 1): 800-808.

85. **Brooks D. (1980)**. Binaural hearing aid application. In ER Libby (Ed.), *Binaural hearing and amplification.* (159-176) Chicago: Zenetron.

86. **Brooks DN. (1979)**. Counselling and its effect on hearing aid use. *Scand Audiol, 8:* 101-107.

87. **Brooks DN. (1996)**. The time course of adaptation to hearing aid use. *Brit J Audiol, 30*(1): 55-62.

88. **Brooks D. (1984)**. Binaural benefit - when and how much? *Scand Audiol, 13*(4): 237-241.

89. **Brooks D. (1989)**. The effect of attitude on benefit obtained from hearing aids. *Brit J Audiol, 23*(1): 3-11.

90. **Brooks D. (1985)**. Factors relating to the under-use of postaural hearing aids. *Brit J Audiol, 19* (3): 211-217.

91. **Brooks D. (1990)**. Measures for the assessment of hearing aid provision and rehabilitation. *Brit J Audiol, 24*(4): 229-233.

92. **Brooks D. (1994)**. Some factors influencing choice of type of hearing aid in the UK: behind-the-ear or in-the-ear. *Brit J Audiol , 28*(2): 91-98.

93. **Brooks D. (1981)**. Use of post-aural aids by National Health Service patients. *Brit J Audiol, 15*(2): 79-86.

94. **Brooks D, Bulmer D. (1981)**. Survey of binaural hearing aid users. *Ear & Hear, 2*(5): 220-224.

95. **Brooks D, Johnson D. (1981)**. Pre-issue assessment and counselling as a component of hearing-aid provision. *Brit J Audiol, 15*(1): 13-19.

96. **Browning G, Gatehouse S. (1994)**. Estimation of the benefit of bone-anchored hearing aids. *Ann Otol Rhinol Laryngol, 103*(11): 872-878.

97. **Bryant MP, Mueller HG, Northern JL. (1991)**. Minimal contact long canal ITE hearing instruments. *Hear Instrum, 42*(1): 12-15, 48.

98. **Bunnell H. (1990)**. On enhancement of spectral contrast in speech for hearing-impaired listeners. *J Acoust Soc Amer, 88*(6): 2546-56.

99. **Burkhard MD, Sachs RM. (1978)**. Anthropometric manikin for acoustic research. In MD Burkhard (Ed.), *Manikin measurements.* Elk Grove Village, Illinois: Industrial Research Products, Inc.

100. **Burkhard M, Sachs R. (1977)**. Sound Pressure in Insert Earphone Couplers and Real Ears. *J Speech Hear Res, 20*(4): 799-807.

101. **Burnip L, McGuire B. (1995)**. FM amplification in the preschool: An investigation of the FM signal and child attention. *Aust J Audiol, 17*(2): 123-129.

102. **Bustamante D, Braida L. (1987)**. Multiband compression limiting for hearing-impaired listeners. *J Rehabil Res Dev, 24*(4): 149-160.

103. **Butler RA. (1969)**. Monaural and binaural localization of noise bursts vertically in the median sagittal plane. *J Aud Res, 3:* 230-235.

104. **Byrne D. (1982)**. Private communication.

105. **Byrne D. (1999)**. Private communication.

106. **Byrne D. (1980)**. Binaural hearing aid fitting: research findings and clinical application. In ER Libby (Ed.), *Binaural hearing and amplification.* (23-73) Chicago: Zenetron.

107. **Byrne D. (1981)**. Clinical issues and options in binaural hearing aid fitting. *Ear & Hear, 2*(5): 187-193.

108. **Byrne D. (1986)**. Effects of bandwidth and stimulus type on most comfortable loudness levels of hearing-impaired listeners. *J Acoust Soc Amer, 80*(2): 484-493.

109. **Byrne D. (1986)**. Effects of frequency response characteristics on speech discrimination and perceived intelligibility and pleasantness of speech for hearing-impaired listeners. *J Acoust Soc Amer, 80*(2): 494-504.

110. **Byrne D. (1996)**. Hearing aid selection for the 1990s: Where to? *J Amer Acad Audiol, 7*(5): 377-395.

111. **Byrne D. (1999)**. Now that hearing aids can do almost anything, what should they do to be really helpful? Presented at *Hearing Aid Amplification for the New Millenium,* Sydney.

112. **Byrne D. (1978)**. Selection of hearing aids for children with severe deafness. *Brit J Audiol, 12* : 9-22.

113. **Byrne D. (1989)**. Technical aspects of hearing aids. In DN Brooks (Eds.), *Adult aural rehabilitation.* (48-67) London: Chapmand & Hall.

114. **Byrne D. (1982)**. Theoretical approaches for hearing aid selection. In GA Studebaker, FH Bess (Eds.), *The Vanderbilt hearing aid report: state of the art - research needs* (175-179). Upper Darby, Pa.: Monographs in Contemporary Audiology.

115. **Byrne D. (1983)**. Theoretical prescriptive approaches to selecting the gain and frequency response of a hearing aid. *Monographs in Contemporary Audiol, 4*(1).

116. **Byrne D. (1983)**. Word familiarity in speech perception testing of children. *Aust J Audiol, 5*(2): 77-80.

117. **Byrne D, Cotton S. (1988).** Evaluation of the National Acoustic Laboratories' new hearing aid selection procedure. *J Speech Hear Res, 31*(2): 178-186.

118. **Byrne D, Dermody P. (1975).** Binaural hearing aids. *Hear Instrum, 26*(7): 22, 23, 36.

119. **Byrne D, Dermody P. (1974).** An incidental advantage of binaural hearing aid fittings - the "cross-over" effect. *Brit J Audiol, 8*: 109-112.

120. **Byrne D, Dillon H. (1979).** Bias in assessing binaural advantage. *Aust J Audiol, 1*(2): 83-88.

121. **Byrne D, Dillon H. (2000).** Future directions in hearing aid selection and evaluation. In M Valente, H Hosford-Dunn, RJ Roeser *Audiology: Treatment.* New York: Thieme.

122. **Byrne D, Dillon H. (1986).** The National Acoustic Laboratories' (NAL) new procedure for selecting the gain and frequency response of a hearing aid. *Ear & Hear, 7*(4): 257-265.

123. **Byrne D, Dillon H, Tran K, Arlinger S, et al. (1994).** An international comparison of long-term average speech spectra. *J Acoust Soc Amer, 96*(4): 2108-2120.

124. **Byrne D, Dirks D. (1996).** Effect of acclimatization and deprivation on non-speech auditory abilities. *Ear & Hear, 17*: 29S-37S.

125. **Byrne D, Fifield D. (1974).** Evaluation of hearing aid fitting for infants. *Brit J Audiol, 8*: 47-54.

126. **Byrne D, Noble W. (1998).** Optimizing sound localization with hearing aids. *Trends in Amplification, 3*(2): 51-73.

127. **Byrne D, Noble W, Glauerdt B. (1996).** Effects of earmold type on ability to locate sounds when wearing hearing aids. *Ear & Hear, 17*: 218-228.

128. **Byrne D, Noble W, LePage B. (1992).** Effects of long-term bilateral and unilateral fitting of different hearing aid types on the ability to locate sounds. *J Amer Acad Audiol, 3* (6): 369-382.

129. **Byrne D, Parkinson A, Newall P. (1990).** Hearing aid gain and frequency response requirements for the severely/profoundly hearing impaired. *Ear & Hear, 11*(1): 40-49.

130. **Byrne D, Parkinson A, & Newall P. (1991).** Modified hearing aid selection procedures for severe/profound hearing losses. In GA Studebaker, FH Bess, & L Beck (Eds), *The Vanderbilt hearing aid report II* (295-300). Parkton, MD: York Press.

131. **Byrne D, Sinclair S, Noble W. (1998).** Open earmold fittings for improving aided auditory localization for sensorineural hearing losses with good high-frequency hearing. *Ear & Hear, 19*(1): 62-71.

132. **Byrne D, Tonisson W. (1976).** Selecting the gain of hearing aids for persons with sensorineural hearing impairments. *Scand Audiol, 5*: 51-59.

133. **Carhart R. (1950).** The clinical application of bone conduction audiometry. *Arch Otolaryngol, 51* : 798-808.

134. **Carhart R. (1965).** Monaural and binaural discrimination against competing sentences. *Int Audiol, 4*(3): 5-10.

135. **Carhart R. (1946).** Selection of hearing aids. *Archives of Otolaryngology, 44*: 1-18.

136. **Carhart R, Tillman TW, Johnson KF. (1967).** Release of masking for speech through interaural time delay. *J Acoust Soc Amer, 42*: 124-138.

137. **Carlin W, Browning G. (1990).** Hearing disability and hearing aid benefit related to type of hearing impairment. *Clin Otolaryngol, 15*(1): 63-67.

138. **Carlsson PU, Hakansson BE. (1997).** The bone-anchored hearing aid: reference quantities and functional gain. *Ear & Hear, 18*(1): 34-41.

139. **Carney AE, Osberger MJ, Carney E, Robbins AM, Renshaaw J, Miyamoto RT. (1993).** A comparison of speech discrimination with cochlear implants and tactile aids. *J Acoust Soc Amer, 94*(4): 2036-2049.

140. **Carney A, Beachler C. (1986).** Vibrotactile perception of suprasegmental features of speech: a comparison of single-channel and multichannel instruments. *J Acoust Soc Amer, 79* (1): 131-140.

141. **Carter, LF. (1993).** *Smooth real ear aided responses: open ear resonance characteristics and hearing aid selection.* Unpublished dissertation, Macquarie University, Sydney.

142. **Chasin M. (1997).** Current trends in implantable hearing aids. *Trends in Amplification, 2*(3): 84-107.

143. **Cheng AK, Grant GD, Niparko JK. (1999).** Meta-analysis of pediatric implant literature. *Ann Otol Rhinol Laryngol Suppl, 177*: 124-128.

144. **Chermak G, Miller M. (1988).** Shortcomings of a revised feasibility scale for predicting hearing aid use with older adults. *Brit J Audiol, 22*(3): 187-194.

145. **Ching TY, Newall P, Wigney D. (1994).** Audio-visual and auditory paired comparison judgments by severely and profoundly hearing impaired children: reliability and frequency response preferences. *Aust J Audiol, 16*(2): 99-106.

146. **Ching TY, Newall P, Wigney D. (1997).** Comparison of severely and profoundly hearing-impaired children's amplification preferences with the NAL-RP and the DSL 3.0 prescriptions. *Scand Audiol, 26*(4): 219-22.

147. **Ching TYC, Dillon H, Byrne D. (1998).** Speech recognition of hearing-impaired listeners: Predictions from audibility and the limited role of high frequency amplification. *J Acoust Soc Amer, 103*(2): 1128-1140.

Ching T, Psarros C, Hill M. (1999). Optimising hearing aid fittings of children who also use cochlear implants. Presented at *Hearing Aid Amplification for the New Millenium,* Sydney.

148. **Chmiel R, Jerger J. (1993).** Some factors affecting assessment of hearing handicap in the elderly. *J Amer Acad Audiol, 4*(4): 249-257.

149. **Chmiel R, Jerger J, Murphy E, Pirozzolo F, Tooley YC. (1997).** Unsuccessful use of binaural amplification by an elderly person. *J Amer Acad Audiol, 8*(1): 1-10.

150. **Christen R. (1980).** Binaural summation at the most comfortable loudness level (MCL). *Aust J Audiol, 2*(2): 92-98.

151. **Christensen L, Lee L, Humes L. (1994).** Can clinical word-recognition measures predict aided word recognition? *American Auditory Society Bulletin, 19*(1): 11,16.

152. **Chung S, Stephens S. (1986).** Factors influencing binaural hearing aid use. *Brit J Audiol, 20*(2): 129-140.

153. **Coelho J, Dillon H. (2000).** Unpublished calculations.

155. **Colletti V, Fiorino F, Carner M, Rizzi R. (1988).** Investigation of the long-term effects of unilateral hearing loss in adults. *Brit J Audiol, 22*(2): 113-118.

156. **Coogle K.L. (1976).** NAEL's standard terms for earmolds. *Hear Aid J, 3*(5).

157. **Corcoran JA, Stewart M, Glynn M, Woodman D. (2000).** Stories of parents of children with hearing loss: A qualitative analysis of interview narratives. In R Seewald (Ed.), *A sound foundation through early amplification* (167-174). Stafa, Switzerland: Phonak.

158. **Cornelisse L, Gagne J, Seewald R. (1991).** Ear level recordings of the long-term average spectrum of speech. *Ear & Hear, 12*(1): 47-54.

159. **Cornelisse L, Seewald R, Jamieson D. (1995).** The input/output formula: a theoretical approach to the fitting of personal amplification devices. *J Acoust Soc Amer, 97*(3): 1854-1864.

160. **Cotton, SE. (1988).** *Evaluation of FM fittings.* Unpublished dissertation, Macquarie University, Sydney.

161. **Couch LW. (1990).** *Digital and analog communication systems* (Third ed.). New York: Macmillan.

162. **Courtois J, Johansen PA, Larsen BV, Beilin J. (1988).** Hearing aid fitting in asymmetrical hearing loss. In JH Jensen (Ed.), *Hearing aid fitting: theoretical and practical views* (243-256). Copenhagen: Stougaard Jensen.

163. **Cowan R, Barker E, Pegg P, Dettman S, Rennie M, Galvin K, Meskin T, Rance G, Cody K, Sarant J, Larratt M, Latus K, Hollow R, Rehn C, Dowell R, Pyman B, Gibson W, Clark G. (1997).** Speech perception in children: Effects of speech processing strategy and residual hearing. In GM Clark (Ed.), *Cochlear implants* (49-54). Bologna: Monduzzi Editore.

164. **Cowan R, Alcantara J, Whitford L, Blamey P, Clark G. (1989).** Speech perception studies using a multichannel electrotactile speech processor, residual hearing, and lipreading. *J Acoust Soc Amer, 85*(6): 2593-2607.

Cox H, Zeskind RM, Kooij T. (1986). Practical supergain. *IEEE Trans Acoust Speech Sig Proc, ASSP-34*(3): 393-398.

165. **Cox RM. (1979).** Acoustic aspects of hearing aid-ear canal coupling systems. *Monographs in Contemporary Audiology, 1*(3): 1-44.

166. **Cox RM. (1997).** Administration and application of the APHAB. *The Hear J, 50*(4): 32-48.

167. **Cox RM. (2000).** *The APHAB.* URL www.ausp.memphis.edu/harl.

168. **Cox RM, Alexander GC. (1992).** Maturation of hearing aid benefit: subjective and objective measurements. *Ear & Hear, 13*(3): 131-141.

169. **Cox RM, Alexander GC. (1999).** Measuring Satisfaction with Amplification in Daily Life: the SADL scale. *Ear & Hear, 20*(4): 306-20.

170. **Cox RM, Alexander GC, Gray G. (1999).** Personality and the subjective assessment of hearing aids. *J Amer Acad Audiol, 10*(1): 1-13.

171. **Cox RM, Alexander GC, Taylor IM, Gray GA. (1997).** The contour test of loudness perception. *Ear & Hear, 18*(5): 388-400.

172. **Cox R. (1982).** Combined effects of earmold vents and suboscillatory feedback on hearing aid frequency response. *Ear & Hear, 3*(1): 12-17.

173. **Cox R. (1988).** The MSU hearing instrument prescription procedure. *Hear Instrum, 39*(1): 6-10.

174. **Cox R. (1985).** A structured approach to hearing aid selection. *Ear & Hear, 6*(5): 226-239.

175. **Cox R. (1995).** Using loudness data for hearing aid selection: The IHAFF approach. *The Hear J, 48*(2): 10, 39-44.

176. **Cox R. (1983).** Using ULCL measures to find frequency/gain and SSPL90. *Hear Instrum, 7*: 17-21, 39.

177. **Cox R, Alexander G. (1995).** The abbreviated profile of hearing aid benefit. *Ear & Hear, 16*(2): 176-186.

178. **Cox R, Alexander G. (1983).** Acoustic versus electronic modifications of hearing aid low-frequency output. *Ear & Hear, 4*(4): 190-196.

179. **Cox R, Alexander G. (1991).** Hearing aid benefit in everyday environments. *Ear & Hear, 12*(2): 127-139.

180. **Cox R, Bisset J. (1984).** Relationship between two measures of aided binaural advantage. *J Speech Hear Disord, 49*(4): 399-408.

181. **Cox R, DeChicchis A, Wark D. (1981).** Demonstration of binaural advantage in audiometric test rooms. *Ear & Hear, 2*(5): 194-201.

182. **Cox R, Gilmore C. (1990).** Development of the Profile of Hearing Aid Performance (PHAP). *J Speech Hear Res, 33*(2): 343-357.

183. **Cox R, Gilmore C, Alexander G. (1991).** Comparison of two questionnaires for patient-assessed hearing aid benefit. *J Amer Acad Audiol, 2*(3): 134-145.

184. **Cox R, Taylor I. (1994).** Relationship between in-situ distortion and hearing aid benefit. *J Amer Acad Audiol, 5*(5): 317-324.

185. **Crain TR, Van Tasell DJ. (1994).** Effect of peak clipping on speech recognition threshold. *Ear & Hear, 15*(6): 443-453.

186. **Crandell C, & Smaldino JJ. (1995).** Speech perception in the classroom. In C Crandell, JJ Smaldino, & C Flexer (Eds.), *Sound-field FM amplification* (29-48). San Diego: Singular.

   Crandell C. (1998a). Hearing aids and functional health status. *Audiology Today, 10*(4): 20-23.

187. **Crandell CC. (1998b).** Hearing aids: Their effects on functional health status. *The Hear J, 51*(2): 22-30.

188. **Creel LP, Desporte EJ, Juneau RP. (1999).** Soft-solid instruments: a positive solution to the dynamic ear canal. *Hear Rev, 3*(1): 40-43.

189. **Cunningham DR. (1996).** Hearing aid counseling: helping patients make decisions. *The Hear J, 49*(5): 31-34.

190. **Curran JR. (1990a).** Practical modification and adjustments of in-the-ear and in-the-canal hearing aids Part 1. *Audiology Today, 1*(1).

191. **Curran JR. (1990b).** Practical modification and adjustments of in-the-ear and in-the-canal hearing aids Part 2. *Audiology Today, 2*(3).

192. **Curran JR. (1991).** Practical modification and adjustments of in-the-ear and in-the-canal hearing aids Part 3. *Audiology Today, 3*(1).

193. **Curran JR. (1992).** Practical modification and adjustments of in-the-ear and in-the-canal hearing aids Part 4. *Audiology Today, 4*(1).

194. **Dahl B, Vesterager V, Sibelle P, Boisen G. (1998).** Self-reported need of information, counselling and education: needs and interests of re-applicants. *Scand Audiol, 27*(3): 143-51.

195. **Danaher ES, Pickett JM. (1975).** Some masking effects produced by low-frequency vowel formants in persons with sensorineural loss. *J Speech Hear Res, 18*: 79-89.

196. **Danaher ES, Wilson MP, Pickett JM. (1978).** Backward and forward masking in listeners with severe sensorineural hearing loss. *J Speech Hear Res, 17*: 324-338.

197. **Danhauer J, Mulac A, Eve I. (1985).** Health care providers' and peers' impressions of elderly hearing aid wearers. *Amer J Otol, 6*(2): 146-149.

198. **Davidson S, Wall L, Goodman C. (1990).** Preliminary studies on the use of an ABR amplitude projection procedure for hearing aid selection. *Ear & Hear, 11*(5): 332-339.

199. **Davies J, John D, Stephens S. (1991).** Intermediate hearing tests as predictors of hearing aid acceptance. *Clin Otolaryngol, 16*(1): 76-83.

200. **Davis A. (1995).** *Hearing in Adults.* London: Whurr.

201. **Davis A, Stephens D, Rayment A, Thomas K. (1992).** Hearing impairments in middle age: the acceptability, benefit and cost of detection (ABCD). *Brit J Audiol, 26*(1): 1-14.

202. **Davis AC. (1989).** The prevalence of hearing impairment and reported hearing disability among adults in Great Britain. *Int J Epidemiology, 18*(4): 911-917.

203. **Davis A, Haggard M. (1982).** Some implications of audiological measures in the population for binaural aiding strategies. *Scand Audiol Suppl, 15*: 167-179.

204. **Davis-Penn W, Ross M. (1993).** Pediatric experiences with frequency transposing. *Hear Instrum, 44*(4): 26-32.

205. **Dawson P, Dillon H, Battaglia J. (1991).** Output limiting compression for the severely-profoundly deaf. *Aust J Audiol, 13*(1): 1-12.

206. **Day G, Browning G, Gatehouse S. (1988).** Benefit from binaural hearing aids in individuals with a severe hearing impairment. *Brit J Audiol, 22*(4): 273-277.

207. **de Boer B. (1984).** Performance of hearing aids from the pre-electronic era. *Audiological Acoustics, 23*: 34-55.

208. **De Gennaro S, Braida L, Durlach N. (1986)**. Multichannel syllabic compression for severely impaired listeners. *J Rehabil Res Dev, 23*(1): 17-24.

209. **de Jong R. (1996)**. Microcomputer applications for hearing aid selection and fitting. *Trends in Amplification, 1*(3): 86-114.

210. **DeBrunner V, McKinney E. (1995)**. A directional adaptive least-mean-square acoustic array for hearing aid enhancement. *J Acoust Soc Amer, 98*(1): 437-444.

211. **Deddens A, Wilson E, Lesser T, Fredrickson J. (1990)**. Totally implantable hearing aids: the effects of skin thickness on microphone function. *Am J Otolaryngol, 11*(1): 1-4.

212. **Demorest ME, Erdman SA. (1987)**. Development of the Communication Profile for the Hearing Impaired. *J Speech Hear Disord, 52*: 129-143.

   Demorest M, Walden B. (1984). Psychometric principles in the selection, interpretation, and evaluation of communication self-assessment inventories. *J Speech Hear Disord, 49*(3): 226-240.

213. **Dempster J, Mackenzie K. (1990)**. The resonance frequency of the external auditory canal in children. *Ear & Hear, 11*(4): 296-298.

214. **Dermody P, Byrne D. (1975)**. Auditory localization by hearing-impaired persons using binaural in-the-ear hearing aids. *Brit J Audiol, 9*: 93-101.

215. **Dermody P, Byrne D. (1975)**. Loudness summation with binaural hearing aids. *Scand Audiol, 2*(1): 23-28.

   Deutsch D. (1975). Musical illusions. *Scientific American,* 92.

216. **Dieroff H. (1993)**. Late-onset auditory inactivity (deprivation) in persons with bilateral essentially symmetric and conductive hearing impairment. *J Amer Acad Audiol, 4*(5): 347-350.

217. **Dillon H. (1991)**. Allowing for real ear venting effects when selecting the coupler gain of hearing aids. *Ear & Hear, 12*(6): 406-416.

218. **Dillon H. (1996)**. Compression? Yes, but for low or high frequencies, for low or high intensities, and with what response times. *Ear & Hear, 17*(4): 287-307.

219. **Dillon H. (1985)**. Earmolds and high frequency response modification. *Hear Instrum, 36*(12): 8-12.

220. **Dillon H. (1983)**. Earmould modifications for wide-bandwidth, flat response hearing aid coupling systems for use in audiological measurements. *Aust J Audiol, 5*(2): 63-70.

221. **Dillon H. (1993)**. Hearing aid evaluation: predicting speech gain from insertion gain. *J Speech Hear Res, 36*(3): 621-633.

222. **Dillon H. (1999)**. NAL-NL1: A new prescriptive fitting procedure for non-linear hearing aids. *The Hear J, 52*(4): 10-16.

223. **Dillon H. (1985)**. Rules for selecting acoustic modifications of hearing aids. Presented at *NAL Hearing Aid Conference,* Sydney.

224. **Dillon H**. Unpublished data.

225. **Dillon H, Birtles G, Lovegrove R. (1999)**. Measuring the outcomes of a national rehabilitation program: normative data for the Client Oriented Scale of Improvement (COSI) and the Hearing Aid User's Questionnaire (HAUQ). *J Amer Acad Audiol, 10*(2): 67-79.

226. **Dillon H, Byrne D, Upfold L. (1982)**. The reliability of speech discrimination testing in relation to hearing aid candidacy. *J Otolaryng Soc Aust, 5*(2): 81-84.

227. **Dillon H, Chew M, Deans M. (1984)**. Loudness discomfort level measurements and their implications for the design and fitting of hearing aids. *Aust J Audiol, 6*: 73-79.

228. **Dillon H, James A, Ginis J. (1997)**. Client Oriented Scale of Improvement (COSI) and its relationship to several other measures of benefit and satisfaction provided by hearing aids. *J Amer Acad Audiol, 8*(1): 27-43.

229. **Dillon H, Koritschoner E, Battaglia J, Lovegrove R, Ginis J, Mavrias G, Carnie L, Ray P, Forsythe L, Towers E, Goulias H, Macaskill F. (1991)**. Rehabilitation effectiveness I: Assessing the needs of clients entering a national hearing rehabilitation program. *Aust J Audiol, 13*(2): 55-65.

230. **Dillon H, Koritschoner E, Battaglia J, Lovegrove R, Ginis J, Mavrias G, Carnie L, Ray P, Forsythe L, Towers E, Goulias H, Macaskill F. (1991)**. Rehabilitation effectiveness II: Assessing the outcomes for clients of a national hearing rehabilitation program. *Aust J Audiol, 13*(2): 68-82.

231. **Dillon H, Lovegrove R. (1993)**. Single microphone noise reduction systems for hearing aids: A review and an evaluation. In GA Studebaker, I Hochberg (Eds.), *Acoustical factors affecting hearing aid performance.* Boston: Allyn & Bacon.

232. **Dillon H, & Macrae J. (1984)**. *Derivation of design specifications for hearing aids.* Report No. 102. Sydney: Aust Gov Publ Service.

233. **Dillon H, Murray N. (1987)**. Accuracy of twelve methods for estimating the real ear gain of hearing aids. *Ear & Hear, 8*(1): 2-11.

234. **Dillon H, Revoile S, Moore A. (1992).** Perception of consonants amplified by a spectral enhancement amplification scheme. Presented at *Issues in Advanced Hearing Aid Research,* Lake Arrowhead, California.

235. **Dillon H, Roe I, Katsch R. (1999).** Wind noise in hearing aids. *NAL Annual Report.*

236. **Dillon H, Storey L. (1998).** The National Acoustic Laboratories' procedure for selecting the saturation sound pressure level of hearing aids: theoretical derivation. *Ear & Hear, 19*(4): 255-66.

237. **Dillon H, Storey L, Grant F, Phillips AM, Skelt L, Mavrias G, Woytowych W, Walsh M. (1998).** Preferred compression threshold with 2:1 wide dynamic range compression in everyday environments. *Aust J Audiol, 20*(1): 33-44.

238. **Dillon H, Walker G. (1982).** Comparison of stimuli used in sound field audiometric testing. *J Acoust Soc Amer, 71*: 161-172.

DiMatteo MR, DiNicola DD. (1982). *Achieving medical patient compliance. The psychology of the medical practitioner's role.* New York: Pergamon Press.

239. **Dirks D, Carhart R. (1962).** A survey of reactions of users of binaural and monaural hearing aids. *J Speech Hear Disord, 27*: 311-322.

240. **Dirks DD. (1985).** Bone-conduction testing. In J Katz (Ed.), *Handbook of Clinical Audiology.* (Third Edition, 202-223) Baltimore: Williams & Wilkins.

241. **DiSarno NJ. (1997).** Informing the older consumer - a model. *The Hear J, 50*(10): 49,52.

242. **Doggett S, Stein RL, Gans D. (1998).** Hearing aid effect in older females. *J Amer Acad Audiol, 9* (5): 361-6.

243. **Dowell RC, Blamey PJ, Clark GM. (1997).** Factors affecting outcomes in children with cochlear implants. In GM Clark (Ed.), *Cochlear implants* (297-303). Bologna: Monduzzi Editore.

244. **Dreschler W. (1989).** Phoneme perception via hearing aids with and without compression and the role of temporal resolution. *Audiology, 28*(1): 49-60.

245. **Drullman R, Festen J, Plomp R. (1994).** Effect of reducing slow temporal modulations on speech reception. *J Acoust Soc Amer, 95*(5): 2670-2680.

246. **Drullman R, Smoorenburg G. (1997).** Audiovisual perception of compressed speech by profoundly hearing-impaired subjects. *Audiology, 36*(3): 165-177.

247. **Dubno J, Schaefer A. (1991).** Frequency selectivity for hearing-impaired and broadband-noise-masked normal listeners. *Q J Exp Psychol A, 43*(3).

248. **Dumon T, Zennaro O, Aran J, Bebear J. (1995).** Piezoelectric middle ear implant preserving the ossicular chain. *Otolaryngol Clin North Am, 28*(1): 173-187.

249. **Duquesnoy AJ. (1983).** Effect of a single interfering noise or speech source upon the binaural sentence intelligibility of aged persons. *J Acoust Soc Amer, 74*: 739-743.

250. **Durlach NI, Thompson CL, Colburn HS. (1981).** Binaural interaction in impaired listeners: a review of past research. *Audiol, 20*: 181-211.

251. **Durlach N, Rigopulos A, Pang X, Woods W, Kulkarni A, Colburn H, Wenzel E. (1992).** On the externalization of auditory images. *Presence, 1*(2): 251-257.

252. **Dye C, Peak M. (1983).** Influence of amplification on the psychological functioning of older adults with neurosensory hearing loss. *J Acad Rehab Audiol, 16*: 210-220.

253. **Dyrlund O. (1988).** Some relationships between hearing aid frequency response and speech discrimination of profoundly deaf children. Pilot study. *Scand Audiol, 17*(4): 201-205.

254. **Dyrlund O, Bisgaard N. (1991).** Acoustic feedback margin improvements in hearing instruments using a prototype DFS (digital feedback suppression) system. *Scand Audiol, 20*(1): 49-53.

255. **Dyrlund O, Henningsen L, Bisgaard N, Jensen J. (1994) .** Digital feedback suppression (DFS). Characterization of feedback-margin improvements in a DFS hearing instrument. *Scand Audiol, 23*(2): 135-138.

256. **Egolf DP, Carlson EV, Mostardo AF, Madaffari P.L. (1989).** Design evolution of miniature electroacoustic transducers. Presented at *118th Meeting of the Acoust Soc of Amer,* St Louis.

257. **Eisenberg L, Schaefer-Martinez, A., Sennaroghu G. (1998).** Establishing new criteria in selecting children for a cochlear implant: performance of "Platinum" hearing aid users. In *7th Symposium on Cochlear Implants in Children .*

258. **Eisenberg L, Levitt H. (1991).** Paired comparison judgments for hearing aid selection in children. *Ear & Hear, 12*(6): 417-430.

259. **Eiser JR. (1986).** *Social psychology: Attitudes, cognitions and social behaviour.* Cambridge: Cambridge University.

260. **Elberling C. (1999)**. Loudness scaling revisited. *J Amer Acad Audiol, 10*(5): 248-60.

261. **Elfenbein J. (2000)**. Batteries required: Instructing families on the use of hearing instruments. In R Seewald (Ed.), *A sound foundation through early amplification* (141-149). Stafa, Switzerland: Phonak.

262. **Elfenbein J, Bentler R, Davis J, Niebuhr D. (1988)**. Status of school children's hearing aids relative to monitoring practices. *Ear & Hear, 9*(4): 212-217.

263. **Engebretson A, French-St. George M. (1993)**. Properties of an adaptive feedback equalization algorithm. *J Rehabil Res Dev, 30*(1): 8-16.

264. **English K, Mendel LL, Rojeski T, Hornak J. (1999)**. Counseling in audiology, or learning to listen: pre- and post-measures from an audiology counseling course. *Am J Audiol, 8*(1): 34-9.

265. **Erber NP, Wit LH. (1977)**. Effects of stimulus intensity on speech perception by deaf children. *J Speech Hear Disord, 42*: 271-277.

266. **Erdman S, Crowley J. (1984)**. Considerations in counseling for the hearing impaired. *Hear Instrum, 35*(11): 50-58.

267. **Erdman SA, Wark DJ, Montano JJ. (1994)**. Implications of service delivery models in audiology. *J Acad Rehab Audiol, 27*: 45-60.

268. **Erdman S, Sedge R. (1981)**. Subjective comparisons of binaural versus monaural amplification. *Ear & Hear, 2*(5): 225-229.

269. **Ericson H, Svard I, Hogset O, Devert G, Ekstrom L. (1988)**. Contralateral routing of signals in unilateral hearing impairment. A better method of fitting. *Scand Audiol, 17*(2): 111-116.

270. **Eriksson-Mangold M, Carlsson S. (1991)**. Psychological and somatic distress in relation to perceived hearing disability, hearing handicap, and hearing measurements. *J Psychosom Res, 35*(6): 729-740.

271. **Eriksson-Mangold M, Ringdahl A, Bjorklund A, Wahlin B. (1990)**. The active fitting (AF) programme of hearing aids: a psychological perspective. *Brit J Audiol, 24*(4): 277-285.

272. **Eriksson-Mangold M, Erlandsson S. (1984)**. The psychological importance of nonverbal sounds. An experiment with induced hearing deficiency. *Scand Audiol, 13*(4): 243-249.

273. **Ewertsen HW. (1974)**. Use of hearing aids (always, often, rarely, never). *Scand Audiol, 3*: 173-176.

274. **Ewertsen HW, Birk-Nielsen H. (1973)**. Social hearing handicap index. *Audiol, 12*: 180-187.

275. **Fabry D, Leek M, Walden B, Cord M. (1993)**. Do adaptive frequency response (AFR) hearing aids reduce 'upward spread' of masking? *J Rehabil Res Dev, 30*(3): 318-325.

276. **Faulkner A, Ball V, Rosen S, Moore B, Fourcin A. (1992)**. Speech pattern hearing aids for the profoundly hearing impaired: speech perception and auditory abilities. *J Acoust Soc Amer, 91*(4 Part 1): 2136-2155.

277. **Faulkner A, Walliker J, Howard I, Ball V, Fourcin A. (1993)**. New developments in speech pattern element hearing aids for the profoundly deaf. *Scand Audiol Suppl, 38*: 124-135.

Feigin J, Kopun J, Stelmachowicz P, Gorga M. (1989). Probe-tube microphone measures of ear-canal sound pressure levels in infants and children. *Ear & Hear, 10*(4): 254-258.

278. **Feigin J, Stelmachowicz P. (1991)**. *Pediatric amplification: Proceedings of the 1991 National Conference*. Omaha, NE: Boys Town National Research Hospital.

279. **Festen J, Plomp R. (1986)**. Speech-reception threshold in noise with one and two hearing aids. *J Acoust Soc Amer, 79*(2): 465-471.

280. **Festinger L. (1957)**. *A theory of cognitive dissonance*. Stanford: Stanford University Press.

281. **Field DL, Haggard MP. (1989)**. Knowledge of hearing tactics: (I) Assessment by questionnaire and inventory. *Brit J Audiol, 23*: 349-354.

282. **Fifield DB, Earnshaw R, Smither MF. (1980)**. A new impression technique to prevent acoustic feedback with high powered hearing aids. *Volta Rev, 82*: 33-39.

283. **Fikret-Pasa S, Revit LJ. (1992)**. Individualised correction factors in the preselection of hearing aids. *Journal of Speech and Hearing Research, 35*: 384-400.

284. **Fishbein H. (1997)**. Thank you, thank you, thank you, Chester Z. Pirzanski. *The Hear J, 50*(6): 65.

285. **Fisher M, Dillon H, Storey L. (In preparation)**. Two-band spectral contrast enhanement.

286. **Flack L, White R, Tweed J, Gregory D, Qureshi M. (1995)**. An investigation into sound attenuation by earmould tubing. *Brit J Audiol, 29*(4): 237-245.

Fletcher H. (1929). *Speech and Hearing*. New York: Van Nostrand.

Fletcher H. (1939). Discussion to article by G Berry. *Laryngoscope, 49*: 939-940.

287. **Flexer C. (1995)**. Rationale for the use of soundfield FM amplification systems in classrooms.

In C Crandell, JJ Smaldino, & C Flexer (Eds.), *Sound-field FM amplification* (3-16). San Diego: Singular.

288. **Flexer C, Crandell C, & Smaldino JJ. (1995).** Considerations and strategies for amplifying the classroom. In C Crandell, JJ Smaldino, & C Flexer (Eds.), *Sound-field FM amplification* (49-143). San Diego: Singular.

289. **Florentine M. (1976).** Relation between lateralization and loudness in asymmetrical hearing loss. *J Amer Audiol Soc, 1*: 243-251.

290. **Flynn MC, Dowell RC, Clark GM. (1998).** Aided speech recognition abilities of adults with a severe or severe-to-profound hearing loss. *J Speech Lang Hear Res, 41*(2): 285-99.

Forster S, Tomlin A. (1988). Hearing aid usage in Queensland. Presented at *Audiol Soc Australia Conf*, Perth.

291. **Franklin B. (1975).** The effect of combining low and high frequency passbands on consonant recognition in the hearing-impaired. *J Speech Hear Res, 18*(4): 719-727.

292. **Franks J, Beckmann N. (1985).** Rejection of hearing aids: attitudes of a geriatric sample. *Ear & Hear, 6*(3): 161-166.

293. **Fredrickson J, Coticchia J, Khosla S. (1995).** Ongoing investigations into an implantable electromagnetic hearing aid for moderate to severe sensorineural hearing loss. *Otolaryngol Clin North Am, 28*(1): 107-120.

294. **Freyman RL, Nerbonne GP. (1989).** The importance of consonant-vowel intensity ratio in the intelligibility of voiceless consonants. *J Speech Hear Res, 32*: 524-535.

295. **Fujikawa S, Cunningham J. (1989).** Practices and attitudes related to hearing: a survey of executives. *Ear & Hear, 10*(6): 357-360.

296. **Gagne J, Dinon D, Parsons J. (1991).** An evaluation of CAST: a Computer-Aided Speechreading Training program. *J Speech Hear Res, 34*(1): 213-221.

297. **Galvin K, Cowan R, Sarant J, Tobey E, Blamey P, Clark G. (1995).** Articulation accuracy of children using an electrotactile speech processor. *Ear & Hear, 16*(2): 209-219.

298. **Gantz BJ, Tyler RS, Woodworth GG, Tye-Murray N, Fryauf-Bertschy H. (1994).** Results of multichannel cochlear implants in congenital and acquired prelingual deafness in children: five-year follow-up. *Am J Otol, 15 Suppl 2*: 1-7.

299. **Garstecki DC, Erler SF. (1998).** Hearing loss, control, and demographic factors influencing hearing aid use among older adults. *J Speech Lang Hear Res, 41*(3): 527-37.

300. **Garstecki D. (1982).** Rehabilitation of hearing-handicapped elderly adults. *Ear & Hear, 3*(3): 167-172.

Gatehouse S. (1989). Limitations on insertion gains with vented earmoulds imposed by oscillatory feedback. *Brit J Audiol, 23*(2): 133-136.

301. **Gatehouse S. (1989).** Apparent auditory deprivation effects of late onset: the role of presentation level. *J Acoust Soc Amer, 86*(6): 2103-2106.

302. **Gatehouse S. (1994).** Components and determinants of hearing aid benefit. *Ear & Hear, 15*(1): 30-49.

303. **Gatehouse S. (1999).** Glasgow Hearing Aid Benefit Profile: derivation and validation of a client-centered outcome measure for hearing aid services. *J Amer Acad Audiol, 10*(2): 80-103.

304. **Gatehouse S. (1993).** Role of perceptual acclimatization in the selection of frequency responses for hearing aids. *J Amer Acad Audiol, 4*(5): 296-306.

305. **Gatehouse S, Browning GG. (1982).** A re-examination of the Carhart effect. *Brit J Audiol, 16*(4): 215-20.

306. **Gatehouse S, Haggard M. (1986).** The influence of hearing asymmetries on benefits from binaural amplification. *The Hear J, 39*(11): 15-20.

307. **Gatehouse S, Killion M. (1993).** HABRAT: Hearing aid brain rewiring accommodation time. *Hear Instrum, 44*(10): 29-32.

308. **Geers A, Brenner C. (1994).** Speech perception results: Audition and lipreading enhancement. *Volta Review, 96*(5): 97-108.

309. **Geers AE, Tobey EA. (1995).** Longitudinal comparison of the benefits of cochlear implants and tactile aids in a controlled educational setting. *Ann Otol Rhinol Laryngol Suppl, 166*: 328-329.

310. **Geers A, Moog J. (1991).** Evaluating the benefits of cochlear implants in an education setting. *Amer J Otol, 12 Suppl*: 116-125.

311. **Gelfand SA. (1998).** Optimizing the reliability of speech recognition scores. *J Speech Lang and Hear Res, 41*: 1088-1102.

312. **Gelfand SA. (1979).** Use of CROS hearing aids by unilaterally deaf patients. *Arch Otolaryngol, 105*: 328-332.

313. **Gelfand S. (1995).** Long-term recovery and no recovery from the auditory deprivation effect with binaural amplification: six cases. *J Amer Acad Audiol, 6*(2): 141-149.

314. **Gelfand S, Silman S. (1993)**. Apparent auditory deprivation in children: implications of monaural versus binaural amplification. *J Amer Acad Audiol, 4*(5): 313-318.

315. **Gelfand S, Silman S. (1982)**. Usage of CROS and IROS hearing aids by patients with bilateral high-frequency hearing loss. *Ear & Hear, 3*(1): 24-29.

316. **Gelfand S, Silman S, Ross L. (1987)**. Long-term effects of monaural, binaural and no amplification in subjects with bilateral hearing loss. *Scand Audiol, 16*(4): 201-207.

317. **Gerling IJ. (1998)**. *Hearing Aid Museum and Archives*. URL http://www.educ.kent.edu/elsa/berger.

318. **Gerling IJ, Taylor M. (1997)**. Quest for quality and consumer appeal shaped history of the hearing aid. *The Hear J, 50*(11): 39-44.

319. **Gerling I, Roeser R. (1981)**. A modified polymer foam earplug for the hearing aid evaluation. *Ear & Hear, 2*(2): 82-87.

320. **Getty L, Hetu R. (1991)**. Development of a rehabilitation program for people affected with occupational hearing loss. 2. Results from group intervention with 48 workers and their spouses. *Audiology, 30*(6): 3117-329.

321. **Geurts L, Wouters J. (1999)**. Enhancing the speech envelope of continuous interleaved sampling processors for cochlear implants. *J Acoust Soc Amer, 105*(4): 2476-2484.

322. **Gilhome Herbst K. (1983)**. Psycho-social consequences of disorders of hearing in the elderly. In R Hinchcliffe (ed.), *Hearing and balance in the elderly*. Edinburgh: Churchill Livingstone.

323. **Gioannini L, Franzen R. (1978)**. Comparison of the effects of hearing aid harmonic distortion on performance scores for the MRHT and a PB-50 test. *J Auditory Res, 18*: 203-208.

324. **Giolos T, Owens E, Lamb S, Schubert E. (1979)**. Hearing performance inventory. *J Speech Hear Disord, 44*: 169-195.

325. **Glasberg B, Moore B. (1989)**. Psychoacoustic abilities of subjects with unilateral and bilateral cochlear hearing impairments and their relationship to the ability to understand speech. *Scand Audiol Suppl, 32*: 1-25.

326. **Golabek W, Nowakowska M, Siwiec H, Stephens S. (1988)**. Self-reported benefits of hearing aids by the hearing impaired. *Brit J Audiol, 22*(3): 183-186.

327. **Goldstein D, Stephens S. (1981)**. Audiological rehabilitation: management Model I. *Audiology, 20*(5): 432-452.

328. **Goldstein M. (1933)**. *Problems of the deaf*. St Louis: The Laryngoscope press.

Gordon-Salant S. (1986). Recognition of natural and time/intensity altered CVs by young and elderly subjects with normal hearing. *J Acoust Soc Amer, 80*(6): 1599-1607.

Gordon-Salant S. (1987). Effects of acoustic modification on consonant recognition by elderly hearing-impaired subjects. *J Acoust Soc Amer, 81*(4): 1199-1202.

329. **Gordon-Salant S, Lantz J, Fitzgibbons P. (1994)**. Age effects on measures of hearing disability. *Ear & Hear, 15*(3): 262-265.

330. **Green AC, Byrne DJ. (1972)**. The pensioner hearing aid scheme: a survey in South Australia. *Med J Aust, 2*: 1113-1116.

331. **Greenberg J, Peterson P, Zurek P. (1993)**. Intelligibility-weighted measures of speech-to-interference ratio and speech system performance. *J Acoust Soc Amer, 94*(5): 3009-3010.

332. **Greenberg J, Zurek P. (1992)**. Evaluation of an adaptive beamforming method for hearing aids. *J Acoust Soc Amer, 91*(3): 1662-1676.

333. **Greenfield DG, Wiley TL, Block MG. (1985)**. Acoustic-reflex dynamics and the loudness-discomfort level. *J Speech Hear Disord, 50*(1): 14-20.

334. **Griffing TS, Giles GE, Romriell D. (1998)**. Relationship of TMJ and TMD to successful CIC fittings. *Hear Rev, 5*(4): 14-18.

335. **Griffing T, Heide J. (1983)**. Custom canal and mini in-the-ear hearing aids. *Hear Instrum, 34*: 31-32.

336. **Griffiths LJ, Jim CW. (1982)**. An alternative approach to linearly constrained adaptive beamforming. *IEEE Trans Antennas Propagation, AP-30*: 27-34.

336a **Grimault N, Garnier S, Collet L. (2000)**. Relationship between amplification fitting age and speech perception performance in school-age children. In R Seewald (Ed.), *A Sound Foundation through Early Amplification* (191-197). Stafa, Switzerland: Phonak.

337. **Grimes A, Mueller H, Malley J. (1981)**. Examination of binaural amplification in children. *Ear & Hear, 2*(5): 208-210.

338. **Groth J. (1999)**. Digital signal processing has made active feedback suppression a reality. *The Hear J, 52*(5): 32-36.

339. **Gudmundsen G. (1994)**. Fitting CIC hearing aids- some practical pointers. *The Hear J, 47*(6): 10, 45-48.

Guelke R. (1987). Consonant burst enhancement: a possible means to improve intelligibility for the hard of hearing. *J Rehabil Res Dev, 24*(4): 217-220.

340. **Guilford F, Haug C. (1955)**. The otologist and the hearing aid. *Arch Otolaryngol, 61*: 9-15.

341. **Hagerman B. (1976).** Reliability in the determination of speech discrimination. *Scand Audiol, 5*: 219-228.

342. **Hagerman B. (1982).** Sentences for testing speech intelligibility in noise. *Scand Audiol, 11*(2): 79-87.

343. **Haggard M, Gatehouse S. (1993).** Candidature for hearing aids: justification for the concept and a two-part audiometric criterion. *Brit J Audiol, 27*(5): 303-318.

344. **Haggard M, Foster J, Iredale F. (1981).** Use and benefit of postaural aid in sensory hearing loss. *Scand Audiol, 10*(1): 45-52.

345. **Haggard M, Hall J. (1982).** Forms of binaural summation and the implications of individual variability for binaural hearing aids. *Scand Audiol Suppl, 15*: 47-63.

346. **Hakansson B, Carlsson P, Tjellstrom A. (1986).** The mechanical point impedance of the human head, with and without skin penetration. *J Acoust Soc Amer, 80*(4): 1065-1075.

347. **Hakansson B, Tjellstrom A, Rosenhall U. (1985).** Acceleration levels at hearing threshold with direct bone conduction versus conventional bone conduction. *Acta Otolaryngol Stockh, 100*(3-4): 240-252.

348. **Hakansson B, Carlsson P, Tjellstrom A, Liden G. (1994).** The bone-anchored hearing aid: principal design and audiometric results. *Ear Nose Throat J, 73*(9): 670-675.

349. **Hall J, Harvey A. (1985).** Diotic loudness summation in normal and impaired hearing. *J Speech Hear Res, 28*: 445-448.

350. **Hall JW, Tyler RS, Fernandes MA. (1984).** Factors influencing the masking level difference in cochlear hearing-impaired and normal-hearing listeners. *J Speech Hear Res, 27*: 145-154.

351. **Hall J, Fernandes M. (1983).** Monaural and binaural intensity discrimination in normal and cochlear-impaired listeners. *Audiology, 22*: 364-371.

352. **Harford E, Barry J. (1965).** A rehabilitative approach to the problem of unilateral hearing impairment: Contralateral routing of signals (CROS). *J Speech Hear Disord, 30*: 121-138.

353. **Harford E, Dodds E. (1966).** The clinical application of CROS. *Arch Otolaryngol, 83*: 73-82.

354. **Harford ER, Curran JR. (1997).** Managing patients with precipitous high frequency hearing loss. *High Performance Hearing Solutions, 1*(1): 8-13.

355. **Harless E, McConnell F. (1982).** Effects of hearing aid use on self concept in older persons. *J Speech Hear Disord, 47*(3): 305-309.

356. **Harris JD. (1965).** Monaural and binaural speech intelligibility and the stereophonic effect based upon temporal cues. *Laryngoscope, 75*: 428-446.

357. **Harrison WA, Lim JS, Singer E. (1986).** A new application of adaptive noise cancellation. *IEEE Trans ASSP, 34*(1): 21-27.

358. **Hattori H. (1993).** Ear dominance for nonsense-syllable recognition ability in sensorineural hearing-impaired children: monaural versus binaural amplification. *J Amer Acad Audiol, 4*(5): 319-330.

359. **Hawkins D. (1984).** Selection of a critical electroacoustic characteristic: SSPL90. *Hear Instrum, 35*(11).

360. **Hawkins DB. (1994).** A historical perspective on hearing aid selection. *Hear Rev, 1*(10): 9-12.

361. **Hawkins DB. (1986).** Selection of SSPL90 for binaural hearing aid fittings. *The Hear J, 39*(11): 23-24.

362. **Hawkins D. (1987).** Clinical ear canal probe tube measurements. *Ear & Hear, 8*(5 Suppl): 74S-81S.

363. **Hawkins D. (1984).** Comparisons of speech recognition in noise by mildly-to-moderately hearing-impaired children using hearing aids and FM systems. *J Speech Hear Disord, 49*(4): 409-418.

364. **Hawkins D, Naidoo S. (1993).** Comparison of sound quality and clarity with asymmetrical peak clipping and output limiting compression. *J Amer Acad Audiol, 4*(4): 221-228.

365. **Hawkins D, Prosek R, Walden B, Montgomery A. (1987).** Binaural loudness summation in the hearing impaired. *J Speech Hear Res, 30*(1): 37-43.

366. **Hawkins D, Schum D. (1985).** Some effects of FM-system coupling on hearing aid characteristics. *J Speech Hear Disord, 50*(2): 132-141.

367. **Hawkins D, Walden B, Montgomery A, Prosek R. (1987).** Description and validation of an LDL procedure designed to select SSPL90. *Ear & Hear, 8*(3): 162-169.

368. **Hawkins D, Yacullo W. (1984).** Signal-to-noise ratio advantage of binaural hearing aids and directional microphones under different levels of reverberation. *J Speech Hear Disord, 49*(3): 278-286.

369. **Hayes D, Jerger J. (1979).** Aging and the use of hearing aids. *Scand Audiol, 8*: 33-40.

370. **Hayes DE, Chen JM. (1998).** Bone-conduction amplification with completely-in-the-canal hearing aids. *J Amer Acad Audiol, 9*(1): 59-66.

371. **Hazell J, Wood S, Cooper H, Stephens S, Corcoran A, Coles R, Baskill J, Sheldrake J. (1985).** A clinical study of tinnitus maskers. *Brit J Audiol, 19*(2): 65-146.

372. **Hebrank J, Wright D. (1974).** Sound localization on the median plane. *J Acoust Soc Amer, 56*: 935-938.

373. **Hebrank J, Wright D. (1974).** Spectral cues used in the localization of sound sources on the median plane. *J Acoust Soc Amer, 56*: 1829-1834.

374. **Hedgecock LD, Sheets BV. (1958).** A comparison of monaural and binaural hearing aids for listening to speech. *Arch Otolaryngol, 68*: 624-629.

375. **Hellgren J, Lunner T, Arlinger S. (1999).** System identification of feedback in hearing aids. *J Acoust Soc Amer, 105*(6): 3481-96.

376. **Henning GB. (1974).** Detectability of interaural delay with high-frequency complex waveforms. *J Acoust Soc Amer, 55*: 84-90.

377. **Henrichsen J, Noring E, Christensen B, Pedersen F, Parving A. (1988).** In-the-ear hearing aids. The use and benefit in the elderly hearing-impaired. *Scand Audiol, 17*(4): 209-212.

378. **Henrichsen J, Noring E, Lindemann L, Christensen B, Parving A. (1991).** The use and benefit of in-the-ear hearing aids. A four-year follow-up examination. *Scand Audiol, 20*(1): 55-59.

379. **Herbst KG, Humphrey C. (1980).** Hearing impairment and mental state in the elderly living at home. *Brit Med J, 281*: 903-905.

380. **Hetu R. (1996).** The stigma attached to hearing impairment. *Scand Audiol Suppl, 43*: 12-24.

381. **Hetu R, Jones L, Getty L. (1993).** The impact of acquired hearing impairment on intimate relationships: implications for rehabilitation. *Audiology, 32*(6): 363-381.

382. **Heyes AD, Gazely DJ. (1975).** The effects of training on the accuracy of auditory localization using binaural hearing aid systems. *Brit J Audiol, 9*: 61-70.

383. **Hickson L, Byrne D. (1995).** Acoustic analysis of speech through a hearing aid: effects of linear vs compression amplification. *Aust J Audiol, 17*(1): 1-13.

384. **Hickson L, Hamilton L, Orange SP. (1986).** Factors associated with hearing aid use. *Aust J Audiol, 8*(2): 37-41.

385. **Hickson L, Timm M, Worrall L, Bishop K. (1999).** Hearing aid fitting: outcomes for older adults. *Aust J Audiol, 21*(1): 9-21.

386. **High WS, Fairbanks G, Glorig A. (1964).** Scale for self-assessment of hearing handicap. *J Speech Hear Disord, 29*: 215-230.

387. **Hill M, Ching TYC, Tomkinson D. (1999).** Functional assessment of auditory performance for hearing aid evaluation. Presented at *Hearing Aid Amplification for the New Millenium,* Sydney.

388. **Hirsh IJ. (1950).** The relationship between localization and intelligibility. *J Acoust Soc Amer, 22*: 196-200.

389. **Hodges AV, Balkany TJ, Ruth RA, Lambert PR, Dolan-Ash S, Schloffman JJ. (1997).** Electrical middle ear muscle reflex: use in cochlear implant programming. *Otolaryngol Head Neck Surg, 117*(3 Pt 1): 255-61.

390. **Hodgson WR. (1986).** Hearing aid evaluation. In WR Hodgson (Ed.), *Hearing aid asessment and use in audiological habilitation.* (152-169) Baltimore: Williams & Wilkins.

391. **Hoffman M, Trine T, Buckley K, Van Tasell D. (1994).** Robust adaptive microphone array processing for hearing aids: realistic speech enhancement. *J Acoust Soc Amer, 96*(2 Pt 1): 759-770.

392. **Hogan CA, Turner CW. (1998).** High-frequency audibility: benefits for hearing-impaired listeners. *J Acoust Soc Amer, 104*(1): 432-41.

393. **Hohmann V, Kollmeier B. (1995).** The effect of multichannel dynamic compression on speech intelligibility. *J Acoust Soc Amer, 97*(2): 1191-1195.

394. **Holube I, Kollmeier B. (1991).** Ein fragebogen zur erfassung des subjectiven horvermogens: Erstellung der fragen und beziehung zum tonschwellenaudiogramm [A questionnaire to assess the subjective hearing handicap: Composition of the questions and their relation to the tone audiogram]. *Audiologische Akustik, 30*(2): 48-64.

395. **Hood J. (1984).** Speech discrimination in bilateral and unilateral hearing loss due to Meniere's disease. *Brit J Audiol, 18*(3): 173-177.

396. **Hood J, Prasher D. (1990).** Effect of simulated bilateral cochlear distortion on speech discrimination in normal subjects. *Scand Audiol, 19*(1): 37-41.

397. **Horwitz AR, Turner CW. (1997).** The time course of hearing aid benefit. *Ear & Hear, 18*(1): 1-11.

398. **Hough J, Neely, Fredrickson J, Green JD, Telischi FF. (1999).** Implantable hearing aids. Presented at *Amer Acad Audiol Conv,* Miami.

399. **Humes LE. (1999)**. Dimensions of hearing aid outcome. *J Amer Acad Audiol, 10*(1): 26-39.

400. **Humes LE, Christensen L, Thomas T, Bess FH, Hedley-Williams A, Bentler R. (1999)**. A comparison of the aided performance and benefit provided by a linear and a two-channel wide dynamic range compression hearing aid. *J Speech Lang Hear Res, 42*(1): 65-79.

401. **Humes LE, Halling D, Coughlin M. (1996)**. Reliability and stability of various hearing-aid outcome measures in a group of elderly hearing-aid wearers. *J Speech Hear Res, 39*(5): 923-935.

Humes L, Jesteadt W. (1991). Modeling the interactions between noise exposure and other variables. *J Acoust Soc Amer, 90*: 182-188.

402. **Humes LE, Pavlovic C, Bray V, Barr M. (1996)**. Real-ear measurement of hearing threshold and loudness. *Trends in Amplification, 1*(4): 121-135.

403. **Humes L. (1986)**. An evaluation of several rationales for selecting hearing aid gain. *J Speech Hear Disord, 51*(3): 272-281.

404. **Humphrey C, Herbst K, Faurqi S. (1981)**. Some characteristics of the hearing-impaired elderly who do not present themselves for rehabilitation. *Brit J Audiol, 15*(1): 25-30.

405. **Hurley RM. (1998)**. Is the unaided ear effect independent of auditory aging? *J Amer Acad Audiol, 9*(1): 20-4.

406. **Hurley RM. (1999)**. Onset of auditory deprivation. *J Amer Acad Audiol, 10*(10): 529-34.

407. **Hurley R. (1993)**. Monaural hearing aid effect: case presentations. *J Amer Acad Audiol, 4*(5): 285-295.

408. **Hutton C. (1985)**. The effect of type of hearing loss on hearing aid use. *Scand Audiol, 14*(1): 15-21.

409. **Hvidt C. (1972)**. Features of the history of audiology. *Scand Audiol, 1*(3): 103-109.

410. **Hygge S, Ronnberg J, Larsby B, Arlinger S. (1992)**. Normal-hearing and hearing-impaired subjects' ability to just follow conversation in competing speech, reversed speech, and noise backgrounds. *J Speech Hear Res, 35*: 208-215.

411. **IEC. (1996)**. *Primary batteries. International Electrotechnical Comission, Standard 60086.*

412. **Irwin RJ. (1965)**. Binaural summation of thermal noises of equal and unequal power in each ear. *Amer J Psychol, 78*: 57-65.

413. **Javer A, Schwarz D. (1995)**. Plasticity in human directional hearing. *J Otolaryngol. 24*(2): 111-117.

414. **Jenstad, LM, Cornelisse, LE, Seewald, RC.** (1997). Effects of test procedure on individual loudness functions. *Ear & Hear, 18*(5): 401-8.

415. **Jenstad LM, Pumford J, Seewald RC, Cornelisse LE. (2000)**. Comparison of linear gain and wide dynamic range compression hearing aid circuits II: aided loudness measures. *Ear & Hear, 21*(1): 32-44.

416. **Jenstad LM, Seewald RC, Cornelisse LE, Shantz J. (1999)**. Comparison of linear gain and wide dynamic range compression hearing aid circuits: aided speech perception measures. *Ear & Hear, 20*(2): 117-26.

417. **Jerger J, Brown D, Smith S. (1984)**. Effect of peripheral hearing loss on the MLD. *Arch Otolaryngol, 110*: 290-296.

418. **Jerger J, Carhart R, Dirks D. (1961)**. Binaural hearing aids and speech intelligibility. *J Speech Hear Res, 4*(2): 137-148.

419. **Jerger J, Darling R, Florin E. (1994)**. Efficacy of the cued-listening task in the evaluation of binaural hearing aids. *J Amer Acad Audiol, 5*(5): 279-285.

420. **Jerger J, Silman S, Lew H, Chmiel R. (1993)**. Case studies in binaural interference: converging evidence from behavioral and electrophysiologic measures. *J Amer Acad Audiol, 4*(2): 122-131.

421. **Jerger J, Thelin J. (1968)**. Effects of electro-acoustic characteristics of hearing aids on speech understanding. *Bull Prosth Res, 9*: 159-197.

422. **Jesteadt W, Weir CC. (1977)**. Comparison of monaural and binaural discrimination of intensity and frequency. *J Acoust Soc Amer, 61*: 1599-1603.

423. **Jirsa R, Norris T. (1982)**. Effects of intermodulation distortion on speech intelligibility. *Ear & Hear, 3*(5): 251-256.

424. **Johansen PA. (1975)**. Measurement of the human ear canal. *Acustica, 33*: 349-351.

425. **Johansson B. (1961)**. A new coding amplifier system for the severely hard of hearing. In *Proceedings 3rd Internat Congress on Acoustics* (655-657).

Johns, DM. (2000). *The effects of taking an open jaw ear impression on feedback and comfort for hearing aid users.* Unpublished dissertation, University of Melbourne, Melbourne.

426. **Johnson D, Kelly SW. (1993)**. Survey of radio and personal hearing aid systems. *J Brit Assn Teachers of the Deaf, 17*(4): 92-98.

427. **Johnston RL. (1997)**. Remember the carbon ball hearing aid? *The Hear J, 50*(4): 50-52.

428. **Jones DA, Victor CR, Ve Hev NJ. (1984)**. Hearing difficulty and its psychological implications for the elderly. *J Epidemiol Community Health, 38*: 75-78.

429. **Juneau RP. (1983)**. NAEL: Fitting facts. Part II: Earmold style and selection. *Hear Instrum, 34* (6): 9-10.

430. **Jutten C, Herault J. (1991)**. Blind separation of sources, Part I: An adaptive algorithm based on neuromimetic architecture. *Signal Processing, 24*: 1-10.

431. **Kamm C, Dirks DD, Mickey MR. (1978)**. Effect of sensorineural hearing loss on loudness discomfort level and most comfortable level judgements. *J Speech Hear Disord, 21*: 668-681.

432. **Kaplan H, Pickett J. (1981)**. Effects of dichotic/diotic versus monotic presentation on speech understanding in noise in elderly hearing-impaired listeners. *Ear & Hear, 2*(5): 202-207.

433. **Kapteyn TS. (1998)**. [Rehabilitation possibilities for hearing-impaired subjects]. *Ned Tijdschr Geneeskd, 142*(2): 63-7.

434. **Kapteyn. T.S. (1977)**. Satisfaction with fitted hearing aids II. An investigation into the influence of psycho-social factors. *Scand Audiol, 6*: 171-177.

435. **Kapteyn TS, Wijkel D, Hackenitz E. (1997)**. The effects of involvement of the general practitioner and guidance of the hearing impaired on hearing-aid use. *Brit J Audiol, 31*(6): 399-407.

436. **Kartush J, Tos M. (1995)**. Electromagnetic ossicular augmentation device. *Otolaryngol Clin North Am, 28*(1): 155-172.

437. **Kates J. (1988)**. A computer simulation of hearing aid response and the effects of ear canal size. *J Acoust Soc Amer, 83*(5): 1952-1963.

Kates J. (1994). Speech enhancement based on a sinusoidal model. *J Speech Hear Res, 37*(2): 449-464.

438. **Kates J, Kozma-Spytek L. (1994)**. Quality ratings for frequency-shaped peak-clipped speech. *J Acoust Soc Amer, 95*(6): 3586-3594.

Kates J, Weiss M. (1996). A comparison of hearing-aid array processing techniques. *J Acoust Soc Amer, 99*(5): 3138-3148.

439. **Kawell M, Kopun J, Stelmachowicz P. (1988)**. Loudness discomfort levels in children. *Ear & Hear, 9*(3): 133-136.

440. **Keefe DH, Bulen JC, Campbell SL, Burns EM. (1994)**. Pressure transfer function and absorption cross section from the diffuse field to the human ear canal. *J Acoust Soc Amer, 95* (1): 355-371.

441. **Keefe D, Bulen J, Arehart K, Burns EM. (1993)**. Ear-canal impedance and reflection coefficient in human infants and adults. *J Acoust Soc Amer, 94*(5): 2617-2638.

442. **Keidser G. (1995)**. The relationship between listening conditions and alternative amplification schemes for multiple memory hearing aids. *Ear & Hear, 16*(6): 575-586.

443. **Keidser G. (1996)**. Selecting different amplification for different listening conditions. *J Amer Acad Audiol, 7*(2): 92-104.

444. **Keidser G, Dillon H, Byrne D. (1995)**. Candidates for multiple frequency response characteristics. *Ear & Hear, 16*(6): 562-74.

445. **Keidser G, Dillon H, Byrne D. (1996)**. Guidelines for fitting multiple memory hearing aids. *J Amer Acad Audiol, 7*: 406-418.

446. **Keidser G, Grant F. (1999)**. Evaluation of loudness equalisation versus loudness normalisation. Presented at *Hearing Aid Amplification for the New Millenium*, Sydney.

447. **Keidser G, Pellegrino A, Delifotis A, Ridgway J, Clarke M. (1997)**. The use of different frequency response characteristics in everyday environments. *Aust J Audiol, 19*(1): 9-22.

448. **Kennedy E, Levitt H, Neuman AC, Weiss M. (1998)**. Consonant-vowel intensity ratios for maximizing consonant recognition by hearing-impaired listeners. *J Acoust Soc Amer, 103*(2): 1098-1114.

Kent RD, Wiley TJ, Strennen MJ. (1979). Consonant discrimination as a function of presentation level. *Audiol, 18*: 212-224.

449. **Kenworthy O, Klee T, Tharpe A. (1990)**. Speech recognition ability of children with unilateral sensorineural hearing loss as a function of amplification, speech stimuli and listening condition. *Ear & Hear, 11*(4): 264-270.

450. **Kessler AR, Giolas TG, Maxon AB. (1990)**. The Hearing Performance Inventory for Children (HPIC): Reliability and validity. Presented at *American Speech-Language-Hearing Association*, Seattle, Washington.

451. **Kessler DK, Loeb GE, Barker MJ. (1995)**. Distribution of speech recognition results with the Clarion cochlear prosthesis. *Annals of Otol Rhinol & Laryngol, 104 (Suppl)*: 283-285.

452. **Kiessling J. (1983)**. Clinical experience in hearing-aid adjustment by means of BER amplitudes. *Arch Otorhinolaryngol, 238*(3): 233-240.

453. **Kiessling J, Dyrlund O, Christiansen C. (1995)**. Loudness scaling - towards a generally accepted clinical method. Presented at *European Conference on Audiology*, Noordwijkerhout, The Netherlands.

454. **Kiessling J, Pfreimer C, Dyrlund O. (1997)**. Clinical evaluation of three different loudness scaling protocols. *Scand Audiol, 26*(2): 117-21.

455. **Kiessling J, Schubert M, Archut A. (1996)**. Adaptive fitting of hearing instruments by category loudness scaling (ScalAdapt). *Scand Audiol, 25*(3): 153-160.

456. **Kiessling J, Steffens T. (1991)**. Clinical evaluation of a programmable three-channel automatic gain control amplification system. *Audiology, 30*(2): 70-81.

Killion M. (1976). Noise of ears and microphones. *J Acoust Soc Amer, 59*(2): 424-433.

457. **Killion MC. (2000)**. Private communication.

458. **Killion MC. (1988)**. Earmold design: theory and practice. In JH Jensen (Ed.), *Hearing aid fitting: theoretical and practical views* (155-174). Copenhagen: Stougaard Jensen.

459. **Killion MC. (1993)**. The K-Amp hearing aid: An attempt to present high fidelity for the hearing impaired. *Amer J Audiol, 2*(2): 52-74.

460. **Killion MC. (1988)**. Principles of high fidelity hearing aid amplification. In RE Sandlin (Ed.), *Handbook of hearing aid amplification, Volume I.* (First edition, 45-80) San Diego: Singular .

461. **Killion MC. (1997)**. The SIN report: Circuits haven't solved the hearing-in-noise problem. *The Hear J, 50*(10): 28-32.

462. **Killion MC, Fikret-Pasa S. (1993)**. The 3 types of sensorineural hearing loss: loudness and intelligibility considerations. *The Hear J, 46*(11): 31-36.

463. **Killion MC, Monser EL. (1980)**. Corfig coupler response for flat insertion gain. In GA Studebaker, I Hochberg (Eds.), *Acoustical factors affecting hearing aid performance.* (147-168) Baltimore, MD: University Park Press.

464. **Killion MC, Villchur E. (1993)**. Kessler was right - partly: But SIN test shows some aids improve hearing in noise. *Hear J, 46*(9): 31-35.

465. **Killion MC, Wilber LA, Gudmundsen G. (1988)**. Zwislocki was right ... a potential solution to the "hollow voice" problem. *Hear Instrum, 39*(1): 14-17.

466. **Killion MC, Wilson D. (1985)**. Response modifying earhooks for special fitting problems. *Audecibel, Fall*: 28-30.

467. **Killion M. (1981)**. Earmold options for wideband hearing aids. *J Speech Hear Disord, 46*(1): 10-20.

468. **Killion M. (1995)**. Talking hair cells: what they have to say about hearing aids. In C Berlin (Ed.), *Hair cells & hearing aids* (3-19). San Diego: Singular Publishing Group.

469. **Killion M, Carlson E. (1974)**. A sub-miniature electret-condenser microphone. *J Audio Engineering Society, 22*: 237-243.

470. **Killion M, Carlson E. (1970)**. A wide-band miniature microphone. *J Audio Engineering Society, 18*: 631-635.

471. **Killion M, Revit L. (1987)**. Insertion gain repeatability versus loudspeaker location: you want me to put my loudspeaker where? *Ear & Hear, 8*(5 Suppl): 68S-73S.

472. **Killion M, Schulein R, Christensen L, Fabry D, Revit L, Niquette P, Chung K. (1998)**. Real-world performance of an ITE directional microphone. *The Hear J, 51*(4): 1-6.

473. **Killion M, Staab W, Preves D. (1990)**. Classifying automatic signal processors. *Hear Instrum, 41* (8): 24-26.

474. **Killion M, Tillman T. (1982)**. Evaluation of high-fidelity hearing aids. *J Speech Hear Res, 25*(1): 15-25.

475. **Kimberley B, Dymond R, Gamer A. (1994)**. Bilateral digital hearing aids for binaural hearing. *Ear Nose Throat J, 73*(3): 176-179.

476. **Kiresuk T, Sherman R. (1968)**. Goal attainment scaling: a general method of evaluating comprehensive mental health programs. *Community Mental Health Journal, 4*: 443-453.

477. **Knebel SB, Bentler RA. (1998)**. Comparison of two digital hearing aids. *Ear & Hear, 19*(4): 280-9.

478. **Kochkin S. (1996)**. Customer satisfaction and subjective benefit with high performance hearing aids. *Hear Rev, 3*(12): 16-26.

479. **Kochkin S. (1992)**. Marke Trak III identifies key factors in determining consumer satisfaction. *The Hear J, 45*(8).

480. **Kochkin S. (1993)**. Marke Trak III: Why 20 million in US don't use hearing aids for their hearing loss. *The Hear J, 46*(1): 20-27.

481. **Kochkin S. (1996).** Marke Trak IV: 10 year trends in the hearing aid market - has anything changed? *The Hear J, 49*(1): 23-34.

482. **Kochkin S. (1994).** Marke Trak IV: Impact on purchase intent of cosmetics, stigma, and style of hearing instrument. *The Hear J, 47*(9): 29-36.

483. **Kochkin S. (1997).** Marke Trak IV: What is the viable market for hearing aids? *The Hear J, 50*(1): 31-39.

484. **Kochkin S, Rogin CM. (2000).** Quantifying the obvious: the impact of hearing instruments on quality of life. *Hear Rev, 7*(1): 6-34.

485. **Koenig W. (1950).** Subjective effects in binaural hearing. *J Acoust Soc Amer, 22*(1): 61-62.

486. **Kollmeier B. (1990).** Speech enhancement by filtering in the loudness domain. *Acta Otolaryngol Suppl Stockh, 469*: 207-214.

487. **Kollmeier B, Peissig J, Hohmann V. (1993).** Real-time multiband dynamic compression and noise reduction for binaural hearing aids. *J Rehabil Res Dev, 30*(1): 82-94.

488. **Kompis M, Dillier N. (1994).** Noise reduction for hearing aids: combining directional microphones with an adaptive beamformer. *J Acoust Soc Amer, 96*(3): 1910-1913.

489. **Kopun JG, Stelmachowicz PG. (1998).** Perceived communication difficulties of children with hearing loss. *Amer J Audiol, 7*(30-38).

490. **Kopun J, Stelmachowicz P, Carney E, Schulte L. (1992).** Coupling of FM systems to individuals with unilateral hearing loss. *J Speech Hear Res, 35*(1): 201-207.

491. **Kramer SE, Kapteyn TS, Festen JM, Tobi H. (1995).** Factors in subjective hearing disability. *Audiology, 34*(6): 311-20.

492. **Kricos P. (1999).** Personal communication.

493. **Kricos P, Holmes A, Doyle D. (1992).** Efficacy of a communication training program for hearing-impaired elderly adults. *J Acad Rehab Audiol, 25*: 69-80.

494. **Kricos PB. (1997).** Audiologic rehabilitation for the elderly: a collaborative approach. *The Hear J., 50*(2): 10-19.

495. **Kricos PB, Holmes AE. (1996).** Efficacy of audiologic rehabilitation for older adults. *J Amer Acad Audiol, 7*(4): 219-29.

496. **Kricos P, Lesner S, Sandridge S. (1991).** Expectations of older adults regarding the use of hearing aids. *J Amer Acad Audiol, 2*(3): 129-133.

497. **Kricos P, Lesner S, Sandridge S, Yanke R. (1987).** Perceived benefits of amplification as a function of central auditory status in the elderly. *Ear & Hear, 8*(6): 337-342.

498. **Kruger B. (1987).** An update on the external ear resonance in infants and young children. *Ear & Hear, 8*(6): 333-336.

499. **Kryter K. (1985).** *The effects of noise on man, 2nd ed, (238-239).* New York: Academic Press.

500. **Kuhl PK, Williams KA, Lacerda F, Stevens KN, Lindnlom B. (1992).** Linguistic experiences alter phonetic perception in infants by 6 months of age. *Science, 255*: 606-608.

Kuhn GF. (1977). Model for the interaural time differences in the azimuthal plane. *J Acoust Soc Amer, 62*(1): 157-167.

501. **Kuhn GF. (1982).** Towards a model for sound localization. In RW Gatehouse (Ed.), *Localization of sound: theory and applications.* (51-64) Connecticut: Aphora Press.

502. **Kuhn GF, Guernsey RM. (1983).** Sound pressure distribution about the human head and torso. *J Acoust Soc Amer, 73*(1): 95-105.

503. **Kuk FK. (1997).** Open or closed? Let's weigh the evidence. *The Hear J, 50*(10): 54, 56, 60.

504. **Kuk F. (1994).** Maximum usable real-ear insertion gain with ten earmold designs. *J Amer Acad Audiol, 5*(1): 44-51.

505. **Kuk F. (1991).** Perceptual consequence of vents in hearing aids. *Brit J Audiol, 25*(3): 163-169.

506. **Kuk F. (1990).** Preferred insertion gain of hearing aids in listening and reading-aloud situations. *J Speech Hear Res, 33*(3): 520-529.

507. **Kuk F, Pape N. (1993).** Relative satisfaction for frequency responses selected with a simplex procedure in different listening conditions. *J Speech Hear Res, 36*(1): 168-177.

508. **Kuk F, Pape N. (1992).** The reliability of a modified simplex procedure in hearing aid frequency-response selection. *J Speech Hear Res, 35*(2): 418-429.

509. **Kuk F, Plager A, Pape N. (1992).** Hollowness perception with noise-reduction hearing aids. *J Amer Acad Audiol, 3*(1): 39-45.

510. **Kuk F, Tyler R, Mims L. (1990).** Subjective ratings of noise-reduction hearing aids. *Scand Audiol, 19*(4): 237-244.

511. **Kyle J, Wood P. (1984).** Changing patterns of hearing-aid use and level of support. *Brit J Audiol, 18*(4): 211-216.

512. **Lalande N, Riverin L, Lambert J. (1988).** Occupational hearing loss: an aural rehabilitation program for workers and their spouses, characteristics of the program and target group (participants and nonparticipants). *Ear & Hear, 9*(5): 248-255.

513. **Lamb SH, Owens E, Schubert ED. (1983).** The revised form of the hearing performance inventory. *Ear & Hear, 4*: 152-157.

514. **Larson V, Nelson J, Cooper WJ, Egolf D. (1993).** Measurements of acoustic impedance at the input to the occluded ear canal. *J Rehabil Res Dev, 30*(1): 129-136.

515. **Launer S. (2000).** Loudness scaling: should we predict it from threshold or can children do it? Presented at *A Sound Foundation through Early Amplification,* Chicago.

516. **Lawson GD, Chial MR. (1982).** Magnitude estimation of degraded speech quality by normal- and impaired-hearing listeners. *J Acoust Soc Amer, 72*: 1781-1787.

517. **Lawton BL, & Cafarelli DL. (1978).** *The effects of hearing aid frequency response modification upon speech reception.* ISVR Memorandum No 588. Southampton: Univ Southampton.

518. **Leeuw A, Dreschler W. (1991).** Advantages of directional hearing aid microphones related to room acoustics. *Audiol, 30*(6): 330-344.

519. **Leeuw A, Dreschler W. (1987).** Speech understanding and directional hearing for hearing-impaired subjects with in-the-ear and behind-the-ear hearing aids. *Scand Audiol, 16*(1): 31-36.

520. **Lehner, R, Maassen, MM, Leysieffer, H, Plester, D, Zenner, HP.** (1998). [Cold deformation elements for attaching an implantable hearing aid transducer to ear ossicles or perilymph]. *HNO, 46*(1): 27-37.

521. **LePage EL. (1989).** Functional role of the olivo-cochlear bundle: a motor unit control system in the mammalian cochlea. *Hear Res, 38*(3): 177-198.

522. **Lesner S. (1995).** Group hearing care for older adults. In P Kricos, S Lesner (Eds.), *Hearing care for the older adult.* (203-227) Boston: Butterworth-Heinemann.

523. **LeStrange RE, Burwood E, Byrne D, Joyner KH, Wood M, & Symonds GL. (1995).** *Interference to hearing aids by the digital mobile telephone system.* NAL Report 131. Sydney: National Acoustic Laboratories.

524. **Levitt H. (1987).** Digital hearing aids: a tutorial review. *J Rehabil Res Dev, 24*(4): 7-20.

525. **Levitt H. (1997).** Digital hearing aids: past, present, and future. In H Tobin (Ed), *Practical hearing aid selection and fitting.* (Monograph 001xi-xxiii) Washington, D.C.: Dept of Veterans Affairs.

526. **Levitt H, Bakke M, Kates J, Neuman A, Schwander T, Weiss M. (1993).** Signal processing for hearing impairment. *Scand Audiol Suppl, 38*: 7-19.

527. **Levitt H, Neuman A, Sullivan J. (1990).** Studies with digital hearing aids. *Acta Otolaryngol Suppl Stockh, 469*: 57-69.

528. **Levitt H, Rabiner LR. (1967).** Predicting binaural gain in intelligibility and release from masking for speech. *J Acoust Soc Amer, 42*: 820-829.

529. **Lewandowski R, Leditschke J. (1991).** Cutaneous button battery injury: a new paediatric hazard. *Aust N Z J Surg, 61*(7): 535-537.

530. **Lewis D. (2000).** Personal communication.

531. **Lewis D. (2000).** One size does not fit all: Rationale and procedures for FM system fitting. In R Seewald (Ed.), *A Sound Foundation through Early Amplification: Proceedings of an International Conference* Stafa, Switzerland: Phonak.

532. **Lewis DE. (1999).** Selecting and evaluating FM systems. *The Hear J, 52*(8): 10-16.

533. **Libby ER. (1982).** A new acoustic horn for small ear canals. *Hear Instrum, 33*(9): 48.

534. **Libby E. (1981).** Editorial: binaural amplification—state of the art. *Ear & Hear, 2*(5): 183-186.

535. **Lim JS, Oppenheim AV. (1979).** Enhancement and bandwidth compression of noisy speech. *Proc IEEE, 67*(12): 1586-1604.

536. **Lindholm J, Dorman M, Taylor B, Hannley M. (1988).** Stimulus factors influencing the identification of voiced stop consonants by normal-hearing and hearing-impaired adults. *J Acoust Soc Amer, 83*(4): 1608-1614.

537. **Lippmann R, Braida L, Durlach N. (1981).** Study of multichannel amplitude compression and linear amplification for persons with sensorineural hearing loss. *J Acoust Soc Amer, 69*(2): 524-534.

538. **Litovitz T, Schmitz B. (1992).** Ingestion of cylindrical and button batteries: an analysis of 2382 cases. *Pediatrics, 89*(4 Pt 2): 747-757.

539. **Litovitz T. (1985).** Battery ingestions: product accessibility and clinical course. *Pediatrics, 75*(3): 469-476.

540. **Liu C, Rosenhouse J, Sideman S. (1997).** A targeting-and-extracting technique to enhance hearing in the presence of competing speech. *J Acoust Soc Amer, 101*(5 Pt 1): 2877-2891.

541. **Lotterman S, Kasten R. (1971).** Examination of the CROS type hearing aid. *J Speech Hear Res, 14*: 416-420.

542. **Loven F, Collins M. (1988)**. Reverberation, masking, filtering, and level effects on speech recognition performance. *J Speech Hear Res, 31*(4): 681-695.

543. **Lundberg G, Ovegard A, Hagerman B, Gabrielsson A, Brandstrom U. (1992)**. Perceived sound quality in a hearing aid with vented and closed earmould equalized in frequency response. *Scand Audiol, 21*(2): 87-92.

544. **Lundborg T, Risberg A, Holmqvist C, Lindstrom B, Svard I. (1982)**. Rehabilitative procedures in sensorineural hearing loss. Studies on the routine used. *Scand Audiol, 11*(3): 161-170.

545. **Lunner T, Hellgren J, Arlinger S, Elberling C. (1997)** . A digital filterbank hearing aid: predicting user preference and performance for two signal processing algorithms. *Ear & Hear, 18*(1): 12-25.

546. **Luterman D. (1999)**. Counseling families with a hearing-impaired child. *Otolaryngol Clin North Am, 32*(6): 1037-50.

547. **Luterman D, Kurtzer-White E. (1999)**. Identifying hearing loss: parents' needs. *Am J Audiol, 8*(1): 13-8.

548. **Luterman DA. (1997)**. The dispensing audiologist: Business person or professional? Presented at *Oticon's 2nd Annual Human Link Conference*, Atlanta.

549. **Lutman ME, Brown EJ, Coles RRA. (1987)**. Self-reported disability and handicap in the population in relation to pure-tone threshold, age, sex and type of hearing loss. *Brit J Audiol, 21*: 45-58.

550. **Lybarger S. (1963)**. *Simplified fitting system for hearing aids*. Cantonsburg, Pa: Radioear Co.

551. **Lybarger SF. (1988)**. A historical overview. In RE Sandlin (Ed), *Handbook of hearing aid amplification, Volume I.* (1-29) Boston: College Hill Press.

552. **Lybarger, S. F. (Inventor). (1944)**. US Patent application. SN 543,278).

553. **Lyregaard PE. (1988)**. POGO and the theory behind. In J Jensen (Ed.), *Hearing aid fitting: Theoretical and practical views. Proceedings of the 13th Danavox Symposium.* (81-96). Copenhagen: Danavox.

554. **Lyxell B, Ronnberg J, Andersson J, Linderoth E. (1993)**. Vibrotactile support - initial effects on visual speech perception. *Scandinavian Audiology, 22*(3): 179-183.

555. **Maassen MM, Lehner RL, Muller G, Reischl G, Ludtke R, Leysieffer H, Zenner HP. (1997)**. [Adjusting the geometry of implantable hearing aid components to human temporal bone. II: Microphone]. *HNO, 45*(10): 847-54.

556. **MacKeith NW, Coles RRA. (1971)**. Binaural advantages in hearing of speech. *J Laryngol, 75*: 213-232.

557. **MacKenzie K, Browning G, McClymont L. (1989)**. Relationship between earmould venting, comfort and feedback. *Brit J Audiol, 23*(4): 335-337.

558. **Macpherson B, Elfenbein J, Schum R, Bentler R. (1991)** . Thresholds of discomfort in young children. *Ear & Hearing, 12*(3): 184-190.

559. **Macrae J. (1982)**. Acoustic notch filters for hearing aids. *Aust J Audiol, 4*(2): 71-76.

560. **Macrae J. (1990)**. Static pressure seal of earmolds. *J Rehabil Res Dev, 27*(4): 397-410.

561. **Macrae JH. (1981)**. An improved form of the high-cut cavity vent. *Aust J Audiol, 3*(2): 36-39.

562. **Macrae JH, Dillon H. (1996)**. An equivalent noise level criterion for hearing aids. *J Rehab Res Dev, 33*(4): 355-362.

563. **Macrae JH, Dillon H. (1996)**. Gain, frequency response and maximum output requirements for hearing aids. *J Rehab Res Dev, 33*(4): 363-376.

564. **Macrae JH, Frazier G. (1980)**. An investigation of variables affecting aided thresholds. *Aust J Audiol, 2*(2): 56-62.

Macrae J. (1991a). Permanent threshold shift associated with overamplification by hearing aids. *J Speech Hear Res, 34*(2): 403-414.

565. **Macrae J. (1991b)**. Prediction of deterioration in hearing due to hearing aid use. *J Speech Hear Res, 34*(3): 661-670.

566. **Macrae J. (1994a)**. A review of research into safety limits for amplification by hearing aids. *Aust J Audiol, 16*(2): 67-77.

567. **Macrae J. (1994b)**. An investigation of temporary threshold shift caused by hearing aid use. *J Speech Hear Res, 37*(1): 227-237.

568. **Macrae J. (1994c)**. Prediction of asymptotic threshold shift caused by hearing aid use. *J Speech Hear Res, 37*(6): 1450-1458.

569. **Macrae J. (1995)**. Temporary and permanent threshold shift caused by hearing aid use. *J Speech Hear Res, 38*(4): 949-959.

570. **Madaffari PL. (1983)**. *Directional matrix technical bulletin*. No. 10554-1. Chicago: Industrial Research Products Inc.

571. **Malinoff RL, Weinstein BE. (1989)**. Changes in self-assessment of hearing handicap over the first year of hearing aid use by older adults. *J Acad Rehab Audiol, 22*: 54-60.

572. **Maniglia AJ, Ko WH, Garverick SL, Abbass H, Kane M, Rosenbaum M, Murray G. (1997)**. Semi-implantable middle ear electromagnetic hearing device for sensorineural hearing loss. *Ear Nose Throat J, 76*(5): 333-341.

573. **Manrique M, Huarte A, Cervera-Paz FJ, Espinosa JM, Molina M, Garcia-Tapia R. (1998)**. Indications and counterindications for cochlear implantation in children. *Am J Otol, 19*(3): 332-6.

574. **Markides A. (1986)**. Age at fitting of hearing aids and speech intelligibility. *Brit J Audiol, 20*(2): 165-167.

575. **Markides A. (1977)**. *Binaural hearing aids*. London: Academic Press.

576. **Markides A. (1982a)**. The effectiveness of binaural hearing aids. *Scand Audiol Suppl, 15*: 181-196.

577. **Markides A. (1982b)**. Reactions to binaural hearing aid fitting. *Scand Audiol Suppl, 15*: 197-205.

578. **Marks LE. (1978)**. Binaural summation of the loudness of pure tones. *J Acoust Soc Amer, 64*: 107-113.

579. **Martin ES, Pickett JM. (1970)**. Sensorineural hearing loss and upward spread of masking. *J Speech Hear Res, 13*: 426-237.

580. **Martin HC, Munro KJ, Langer DH. (1997)**. Real-ear to coupler differences in children with grommets. *Brit J Audiol, 31*(1): 63-9.

581. **Martin MC, Grover BC, Worrall JJ, Williams V. (1976)**. The effectiveness of hearing aids in a school population. *Brit J Audiol, 10*: 33-40.

582. **Martin RL, Oltman J, Killion MC. (1997)**. The new high-power batteries are great, if you know how to use them. *The Hear J, 50*(10): 62-65.

583. **Martin RL, Pirzanski CZ. (1998)**. Techniques for successful CIC fittings. *The Hear J, 51*(7): 72,74.

584. **Mason D, Popelka G. (1986)**. Comparison of hearing-aid gain using functional, coupler, and probe-tube measurements. *J Speech Hear Res, 29*(2): 218-226.

May AE, Dillon H. (1992). A comparison of physical measurements of the hearing aid occlusion effect with subjective reports. Presented at *Audiol Soc of Aust Conf*, Adelaide.

585. **May AE, Upfold LJ. (1984)**. The organisation of group hearing aid orientation programs in non-permanent facilities. Presented at *6th National Conf, Audiol Soc Aust*, Coolangatta.

586. **May A, Upfold L, Battaglia J. (1990)**. The advantages and disadvantages of ITC, ITE and BTE hearing aids: diary and interview reports from elderly users. *Brit J Audiol, 24*(5): 301-309.

587. **McCandless GA, Lyregaard PE. (1983)**. Prescription of gain/output (POGO) for hearing aids. *Hear Instrum, 34*(1): 16-21.

588. **McDermott HJ, Dorkos VP, Dean MR, Ching TY. (1999)**. Improvements in speech perception with use of the AVR TranSonic frequency-transposing hearing aid. *J Speech Lang Hear Res, 42*(6): 1323-35.

589. **McGrath M, Summerfield Q. (1985)**. Intermodal timing relations and audio-visual speech recognition by normal-hearing adults. *J Acoust Soc Amer, 77*(2): 678-85.

590. **McKee GJ, Stephens SD. (1992)**. An investigation of normally hearing subjects with tinnitus. *Audiol, 31*(6): 313-317.

591. **McKenna L. (1987)**. Goal planning in audiological rehabilitation. *Brit J Audiol, 21*(1): 5-11.

592. **McLeod B, Upfold LJ. (2000)**. Back in the SADL agin. Presented at *Conference of the Audiol Soc Aust*, Adelaide.

593. **Meding B, Ringdahl A. (1992)**. Allergic contact dermatitis from the earmolds of hearing aids. *Ear & Hear, 13*(2): 122-124.

594. **Mehrgardt S, Mellert V. (1977)**. Transformation characteristics of the external human ear. *J Acoust Soc Amer, 61*(6): 1567-1576.

595. **Mekata T, Yoshizumi Y, Kato Y, Noguchi E, Yamada Y. (1994)**. Development of a portable multi-function digital hearing aid. Presented at *Int Conf Spoken Lang Processing*, Japan.

596. **Melin L, Scott B, Lindberg P, Lyttkens L. (1987)**. Hearing aids and tinnitus—an experimental group study. *Brit J Audiol, 21*(2): 91-97.

597. **Meredith R, Stephens D. (1993)**. In-the-ear and behind-the-ear hearing aids in the elderly. *Scand Audiol, 22*(4): 211-216.

598. **Meredith R, Thomas K, Callaghan D, Stephens S, Rayment A. (1989)**. A comparison of three types of earmoulds in elderly users of post-aural hearing aids. *Brit J Audiol, 23*(3): 239-244.

599. **Meyer TA, Svirsky MA, Kirk KI, Miyamoto RT. (1998).** Improvements in speech perception by children with profound prelingual hearing loss: effects of device, communication mode, and chronological age. *J Speech Lang Hear Res, 41*(4): 846-58.

600. **Middlebrooks JC, Makous JC, Green DM. (1989).** Directional sensitivity of sound-pressure levels in the human ear canal. *J Acoust Soc Amer, 86*(1): 89-108.

601. **Miller AJ. (1989).** An alternative approach to CROS and BI-CROS hearing aids: An internal CROS. *Audecibel, 38*(1): 20-21.

602. **Mills A. (1972).** Auditory localization. In JV Tobias (Ed.), *Foundations of modern auditory theory, Volume 2.* (303-348) New York: Academic Press.

603. **Mills AW. (1958).** On the minimum audible angle. *J Acoust Soc Amer, 30*: 237-246.

Mills J, Gilbert R, Adkins W. (1979). Temporary threshold shifts in humans exposed to octave bands of noise for 16 to 24 hours. *J Acoust Soc Amer, 65*: 1238-1248.

604. **Miyamoto RT, Kirk KI, Robbins AM, Todd S, Riley A. (1996).** Speech perception and speech production skills of children with multichannel cochlear implants. *Acta Otolaryngol, 116*(2): 240-3.

605. **Miyamoto R, Robbins A, Osberger M, Todd S, Riley A, Kirk K. (1995).** Comparison of multichannel tactile aids and multichannel cochlear implants in children with profound hearing impairments. *Amer J Otol, 16*(1): 8-13.

606. **Moeller MP. (1998).** Early intervention of hearing loss in children. In FH Bess (Ed.), *Fourth International Symposium on Childhood Deafness* (305-310). Nashville, Tn.: Bill Wilkerson Center Press.

607. **Moeller MP, Donaghy K, Beauchaine K, Lewis DE, Stelmachowicz PG. (1996).** Longitudinal study of FM system use in non-academic settings: Effects on language development. *Ear & Hear, 17*(1): 28-41.

608. **Moir J. (1976).** On differential time delay. *J Audio Eng Soc, 24*(9): 752.

609. **Moncur JP, Dirks D. (1967).** Binaural and monaural speech intelligibility in reverberation. *J Speech Hear Res, 10*(2): 186-195.

610. **Montgomery A. (1994).** WATCH: A practical approach to brief auditory rehabilitation. *Hear J, 47*(10): 10, 53-55.

611. **Montgomery A, Edge R. (1988).** Evaluation of two speech enhancement techniques to improve intelligibility for hearing-impaired adults. *J Speech Hear Res, 31*(3): 386-393.

612. **Montgomery A, Prosek R, Walden B, Cord M. (1987).** The effects of increasing consonant/vowel intensity ratio on speech loudness. *J Rehabil Res Dev, 24*(4): 221-228.

613. **Moodie KS, Seewald RC, Sinclair ST. (1994).** Procedure for predicting real-ear hearing aid performance in young children. *Amer J Audiol, 3*: 23-31.

614. **Moodie S. (2000).** Individualized hearing instrument fitting for infants. In R Seewald (Ed.), *A Sound Foundation through Early Amplification* (213-217). Stafa, Switzerland: Phonak.

615. **Moore BC. (1997).** A compact disc containing simulations of hearing impairment. *Brit J Audiol, 31*(5): 353-7.

616. **Moore BC, Alcantara JI, Glasberg BR. (1998).** Development and evaluation of a procedure for fitting multi-channel compression hearing aids. *Brit J Audiol, 32*(3): 177-95.

617. **Moore BC, Glasberg BR. (1998).** Use of a loudness model for hearing-aid fitting. I. Linear hearing aids. *Brit J Audiol, 32*(5): 317-35.

618. **Moore BC, Glasberg BR, Vickers DA. (1999).** Further evaluation of a model of loudness perception applied to cochlear hearing loss. *J Acoust Soc Amer, 106*(2): 898-907.

619. **Moore BCJ. (1989).** *An Introduction to the Psychology of Hearing.* London: Academic Press.

620. **Moore BCJ, Glasberg BR. (1997).** A model of loudness perception applied to cochlear hearing loss. *Auditory Neurosci, 3*: 289-311.

621. **Moore BCJ, Peters RW, Stone MA. (1998).** Benefits of linear amplification and multi-channel compression for speech comprehension in backgrounds with spectral and temporal dips. *J Acoust Soc Amer, 105*(1): 400-411.

622. **Moore B, Glasberg B. (1988).** A comparison of four methods of implementing automatic gain control (AGC) in hearing aids. *Brit J Audiol, 22*(2): 93-104.

623. **Moore B, Glasberg B. (1986).** A comparison of two-channel and single-channel compression hearing aids. *Audiology, 25*(4-5): 210-226.

624. **Moore B, Glasberg B, Stone M. (1991).** Optimization of a slow-acting automatic gain control system for use in hearing aids. *Brit J Audiol, 25*(3): 171-182.

625. **Moore B, Johnson J, Clark T, Pluvinage V. (1992).** Evaluation of a dual-channel full dynamic range compression system for people with sensorineural hearing loss. *Ear & Hear, 13* (5): 349-370.

626. **Moore B, Lynch C, Stone M. (1992)**. Effects of the fitting parameters of a two-channel compression system on the intelligibility of speech in quiet and in noise. *Brit J Audiol, 26*(6): 369-379.

627. **Morgan R. (1994)**. The art of making a good impression. *The Hear Rev, 1*(3): 10-24.

628. **Moryl C, Danhauer J, DiBartolomeo J. (1992)**. Real ear unaided responses in ears with tympanic membrane perforations. *J Amer Acad Audiol, 3*(1): 60-65.

629. **Mueller HG. (1994)**. CIC hearing aids: what is their impact on the occlusion effect? *The Hear J, 47*(11): 29-35.

Mueller H, Grimes A, Jerome J. (1981). Performance-intensity functions as a predictor for binaural amplification. *Ear & Hear, 2*(5): 211-214.

630. **Mueller HG, Hawkins DB, Northern JL. (1992)**. *Probe microphone measurements: Hearing aid selection and assessment.* San Diego: Singular Press.

631. **Mueller HG, Holland SA, Ebinger KA. (1995)**. The CIC: more than just another pretty face. *Audiology Today, 7*(5): 19-20.

632. **Mulac A, Danhauer JL, Johnson CE. (1983)**. Young adults' and peers' attitudes towards elderly hearing aid wearers. *Aust J Audiol, 5*(2): 57-62.

633. **Mulrow C, Aguilar C, Endicott J, Tuley M, Velez R, Charlip W, Rhodes M, Hill J, DeNino L. (1990)**. Quality-of-life changes and hearing impairment. A randomized trial. *Ann Intern Med, 113*(3): 188-194.

634. **Mulrow C, Tuley M, Aguilar C. (1992a)**. Correlates of successful hearing aid use in older adults. *Ear & Hear, 13*(2): 108-113.

635. **Mulrow C, Tuley M, Aguilar C. (1992b)**. Sustained benefits of hearing aids. *J Speech Hear Res, 35*(6): 1401-1405.

636. **Murray N, Byrne D. (1986)**. Performance of hearing-impaired and normal hearing listeners with various high frequency cut-offs in hearing aids. *Aust J Audiol, 8*(1): 21-28.

637. **Musicant A, Butler R. (1985)**. Influence of monaural spectral cues on binaural localization. *J Acoust Soc Amer, 77*(1): 202-208.

638. **Musicant A, Butler R. (1984)**. The influence of pinnae-based spectral cues on sound localization. *J Acoust Soc Amer, 75*(4): 1195-2000.

639. **Myers IB, Kirby LK, Myers KD. (1993)**. *Introduction to type.* Palo Alto, Ca.: Consulting Psychologists Press.

640. **Mylanus EA, van der Pouw KC, Snik AF, Cremers CW. (1998)**. Intraindividual comparison of the bone-anchored hearing aid and air- conduction hearing aids. *Arch Otolaryngol Head Neck Surg, 124*(3): 271-6.

641. **Nabelek AK, Pickett JM. (1974)**. Monaural and binaural speech perception through hearing aids under noise and reverberation. *J Speech Hear Res, 17*: 724-739.

642. **Nabelek AK, Pickett JM. (1974)**. Reception of consonants in a classroom as affected by monaural and binaural listening, noise, reverberation and hearing aids. *J Acoust Soc Amer, 56*(2): 628-639.

643. **Nabelek A, Mason D. (1981)**. Effect of noise and reverberation on binaural and monaural word identification by subjects with various audiograms. *J Speech Hear Res, 24*(3): 375-383.

644. **Naidoo SV, Hawkins DB. (1997)**. Monaural/binaural preferences: effect of hearing aid circuit on speech intelligibility and sound quality. *J Amer Acad Audiol, 8*(3): 188-202.

645. **Nejime Y, Aritsuka T, Ifukube T, Matsushima J. (1996)** . A portable digital speech-rate converter for hearing impairment. *IEEE Trans Rehab Eng, 4*: 73-83.

646. **Nejime Y, Moore B. (1998)**. Evaluation of the effect of speech-rate slowing on speech intelligibility in noise using a simulation of cochlear hearing loss. *J Acoust Soc Amer, 103*(1): 572-576.

647. **Neuman AC. (1996)**. Late-onset auditory deprivation: A review of past research and an assessment of future research needs. *Ear & Hear, 17*(3 Suppl): 3S-13S.

648. **Neuman A, Levitt H, Mills R, Schwander T. (1987)**. An evaluation of three adaptive hearing aid selection strategies. *J Acoust Soc Amer, 82*(6): 1967-1976.

649. **Neuman A, Schwander T. (1987)**. The effect of filtering on the intelligibility and quality of speech in noise. *J Rehabil Res Dev, 24*(4): 127-134.

650. **Nielsen C. (1999)**. Private communication.

651. **Nilsson M, Soli S, Sullivan JA. (1994)**. Development of the Hearing in Noise Test for the measurement of speech reception thresholds in quiet and in noise. *J Acoust Soc Amer, 95*(2): 1085-1099.

652. **Nittrouer S, Boothroyd A. (1990)**. Context effects in phonemes and word recognition by young children and older adults. *J Acoust Soc Amer, 87*: 2705-2715.

653. **Nobel Biocare. (1997)**. *The BAHA.*

654. **Noble W. (1999).** Hearing loss and hearing aids in the family. Presented at *Hearing Aid Amplification for the New Millenium,* Sydney.

655. **Noble W. (1998).** *Self-assessment of hearing and related functions.* London: Whurr.

656. **Noble W, Atherly GRC. (1970).** The Hearing Measurement Scale: a questionnaire for the assessment of auditory disability. *J Aud Res, 10:* 229-250.

657. **Noble W, Byrne D. (1991).** Auditory localization under conditions of unilateral fitting of different hearing aid systems. *Brit J Audiol, 25*(4): 237-250.

658. **Noble W, Byrne D. (1990).** A comparison of different binaural hearing aid systems for sound localization in the horizontal and vertical planes. *Brit J Audiol, 24*(5): 335-346.

659. **Noble W, Byrne D, LePage B. (1994).** Effects on sound localization of configuration and type of hearing impairment. *J Acoust Soc Amer, 95*(2): 992-1005.

660. **Noble W, Byrne D, Ter-Horst K. (1997).** Auditory localization, detection of spatial separateness, and speech hearing in noise by hearing impaired listeners. *J Acoust Soc Amer, 102*(4): 2343-2352.

661. **Noble W, Ter-Horst K, Byrne D. (1995).** Disabilities and handicaps associated with impaired auditory localization. *J Amer Acad Audiol, 6*(2): 129-140.

662. **Nolan M, Combe E. (1989).** In vitro considerations in the production of dimensionally accurate earmoulds. I. The ear impression. *Scand Audiol, 18*(1): 35-41.

663. **Nolan M, Combe E. (1985).** Silicone materials for ear impressions. *Scand Audiol, 14*(1): 35-39.

664. **Nolan M, Elzemety S, Tucker IG, McDonough DF. (1978).** An investigation into the problems involved in producing efficient ear moulds for children. *Scand Audiol, 7:* 231-237.

665. **Nolan M, Hostler M, Taylor I, Cash A. (1986).** Practical considerations in the fabrication of earmoulds for young babies. *Scand Audiol, 15*(1): 21-27.

666. **Norman M, George C, McCarthy D. (1994).** The effect of pre-fitting counselling on the outcome of hearing aid fittings. *Scand Audiol, 23*(4): 257-263.

667. **Northern J, Beyer CM. (1999).** Reducing hearing aid returns through patient education. *Audiol Today, 22*(2): 10-11.

668. **Northern JL, Downs MP. (2000).** *Hearing in children* (Fifth Edition). Baltimore, MD: Williams & Wilkins.

669. **Northern JL, Gabbard SA, & Kinder DL. (1985).** The acoustic reflex. In J Katz (Ed.), *Handbook of clinical audiology.* (Third ed., 476-495) Baltimore: Williams & Wilkins.

670. **Nozza JN, Rossman RNF, Bond LC. (1991).** Infant-adult differences in unmasked thresholds for the discrimination of consonant-vowel syllable pairs. *Audiology, 30:* 102-112.

671. **Nozza RJ, Miller SL, Rossman RN, Bond LC. (1991).** Reliability and validity of infant speech-sound discrimination-in-noise thresholds. *J Speech Hear Res, 34*(3): 643-50.

672. **O'Mahoney CF, Stephens SDG, Cadge BA. (1996).** Who prompts patients to consult about hearing loss? *Brit J Audiol, 30:* 153-158.

673. **Oldfield S, Parker S. (1986).** Acuity of sound localisation: a topography of auditory space. III. Monaural hearing conditions. *Perception, 15*(1): 67-81.

674. **Oliveira RJ. (1997).** The active earcanal. *J Amer Acad Audiol, 8*(6): 401-410.

675. **Oliveira RJ. (1995).** The dynamic ear canal. In BB Ballachanda (Ed.), *The human ear canal.* San Diego: Singular.

676. **Oliveira RJ, Hawkinson R, Stockton M. (1992).** Instant foam vs. traditional BTE earmolds. *Hear Instrum, 43*(12): 22.

677. **Olsen W, Noffsinger D, Carhart R. (1976).** Masking level differences encountered in clinical populations. *Audiology, 15:* 287-301.

678. **Ono H, Kanzaki J, Mizoi K. (1983).** Clinical results of hearing aid with noise-level-controlled selective amplification. *Audiology, 22*(5): 494-515.

679. **Orton JF, Preves DA. (1979).** Localization ability as a function of hearing aid microphone placement. *Hear Instrum, 30*(1): 18-21.

680. **Osberger M, Maso M, Sam L. (1993).** Speech intelligibility of children with cochlear implants, tactile aids, or hearing aids. *J Speech Hear Res, 36*(1): 186-203.

681. **Osberger M, Miyamoto R, Robbins A, Renshaw J, Berry S, Myres W, Kessler K, Pope M. (1990).** Performance of deaf children with cochlear implants and vibrotactile aids. *J Amer Acad Audiol, 1*(1): 7-10.

682. **Ovegard A, Ramstrom A. (1994).** Individual follow-up of hearing aid fitting. *Scand Audiol, 23*(1): 57-63.

683. **Owens E, Raggio M. (1988).** Performance inventory for profound and severe loss (PIPSL). *J Speech Hear Disord, 53*(1): 42-56.

684. **Page S. (1996)**. Dual FM sound field amplification: a flexible integrated classroom amplification system for mild to moderate conductive hearing loss. In D Moore, D Stokes (Ed.), *Second National Conference on Childhood Fluctuating Deafness / Otitis Media* (161-172). Melbourne: Australian Conductive Deafness Association.

685. **Page, S. (1998)**. *Twin FM soundfield amplification system.* Instruction Manual and Video. Sydney: Australian Hearing.

686. **Palmer, CV. (1991)**. *The influence of individual ear canal and eardrum characteristics on speech intelligibility and sound quality judgments.* Unpublished dissertation, Northwestern University, Chicago.

687. **Palmer CV, Adams SW, Durrant JD, Bourgeois M, Rossi M. (1998)**. Managing hearing loss in a patient with Alzheimer disease. *J Amer Acad Audiol, 9*(4): 275-84.

688. **Palmer CV, Mormer EA. (1999)**. Goals and expectations of the hearing aid fitting. *Trends in Amplification, 4*(2): 61-71.

689. **Parent TC, Chmiel R, Jerger J. (1998)**. Comparison of performance with frequency transposition hearing aids and conventional hearing aids. *J Amer Acad Audiol, 9*(1): 67-77.

690. **Parving A, Boisen G. (1990)**. In-the-canal hearing aids. Their use by and benefit for the younger and elderly hearing-impaired. *Scand Audiol, 19*(1): 25-30.

691. **Parving A, Philip B. (1991)**. Use and benefit of hearing aids in the tenth decade—and beyond. *Audiol, 30*(2): 61-69.

692. **Pascoe DP. (1982)**. Private communication.

693. **Pascoe D. (1978)**. An approach to hearing aid selection. *Hear Instrum, 29*(6): 12-16,36.

694. **Pascoe D. (1988)**. Clinical measurements of the auditory dynamic range and their relation to formula for hearing aid gain. In J Jensen (Ed.), *Hearing aid fitting: Theoretical and practical views. Proceedings of the 13th Danavox Symposium.* (129-152). Copenhagen: Danavox.

695. **Pavlovic C, Bisgaard N, Melanson J. (1997)**. The next step: "Open" digital hearing aids. *The Hear J, 50*(5): 65-66.

696. **Pavlovic CV, Studebaker GA, Sherbecoe RL. (1986)**. An articulation index based procedure for predicting the speech recognition performance of hearing-impaired individuals. *J Acoust Soc Amer, 80*(1): 50-57.

697. **Payton K, Uchanski R, Braida L. (1994)**. Intelligibility of conversational and clear speech in noise and reverberation for listeners with normal and impaired hearing. *J Acoust Soc Amer, 95*(3): 1581-1592.

Perrett S, Noble W. (1997). The effect of head rotations on vertical plane localization. *J Acoust Soc Amer, 102*(4): 2325-2332.

698. **Perrott D, Saberi K. (1990)**. Minimum audible angle thresholds for sources varying in both elevation and azimuth. *J Acoust Soc Amer, 87*(4): 1728-1731.

699. **Peters RW, Moore BC, Baer T. (1998)**. Speech reception thresholds in noise with and without spectral and temporal dips for hearing-impaired and normally hearing people. *J Acoust Soc Amer, 103*(1): 577-87.

700. **Peterson P, Durlach N, Rabinowitz W, Zurek P. (1987)**. Multimicrophone adaptive beamforming for interference reduction in hearing aids. *J Rehabil Res Dev, 24*(4): 103-110.

701. **Pettersson E. (1987)**. Speech discrimination tests with hearing aids in tele-coil listening mode. A comparative study in school children. *Scand Audiol, 16*(1): 13-19.

702. **Philbrick RL. (1982)**. Audio induction loop systems for the hearing impaired. Presented at *Audio Engineering Society Convention*, California.

703. **Picheny M, Durlach N, Braida L. (1985)**. Speaking clearly for the hard of hearing. I: Intelligibility differences between clear and conversational speech. *J Speech Hear Res, 28* : 96-103.

704. **Picheny M, Durlach N, Braida L. (1986)**. Speaking clearly for the hard of hearing. II: Acoustic characteristics of clear and conversational speech. *J Speech Hear Res, 29*(4): 434-446.

705. **Pickler AG, Harris JD. (1955)**. Channels of reception in pitch discrimination. *J Acoust Soc Amer, 27*: 124-131.

706. **Pirzanski CZ. (1996)**. An alternative impression-taking technique: The open jaw impression. *The Hear J, 49*(11): 30-35.

707. **Pirzanski CZ. (1997a)**. Critical factors in taking an anatomically accurate impression. *The Hear J, 50*(10): 41-48.

708. **Pirzanski CZ. (1998)**. Diminishing the occlusion effect: Clinician/manufacturer-related factors. *The Hear J, 66*(4): 66-78.

709. **Pirzanski CZ. (1997b)**. In taking ear impressions, longer is better. *The Hear J, 50*(7): 32-36.

710. **Plant G. (1994)**. *Analytica: Analytic testing and training lists.* Somerville: Audiological Engineering Corporation.

711. **Plant G. (1989)**. A comparison of five commercially available tactile aids. *Aust J Audiol, 11*(1): 11-19.

712. **Plant G. (1996)**. *Syntrex: Synthetic training exercises for hearing impaired adults (Revised Edition)*. Somerville: Hearing Rehabilitation Foundation.

713. **Plant G, Horan M, Reed H. (1997)**. Speech teaching for deaf children in the age of bilingual/bicultural programs: the role of tactile aids. *Scand Audiol Suppl, 47*: 19-23.

714. **Plant G, Macrae J, Dillon H, Pentecost F. (1984)**. A single-channel vibrotactile aid to lipreading: preliminary results with an experienced subject. *Aust J Audiol, 8*(2): 55-64.

715. **Plant G, Spens KE. (1995)**. *Profound deafness and speech communication*. London: Whurr.

716. **Plant GL. (1979)**. The use of tactile supplements in the rehabilitation of the deafened: a case study. *Aust J Audiol, 1*(2): 76-82.

717. **Plant GL, Macrae JH. (1977)**. Visual identification of Australian consonants, vowels and dipthongs. *Aust Teach Deaf, 18*: 45-50.

718. **Plomp R. (1978)**. Auditory handicap of hearing impairment and the limited benefit of hearing aids. *J Acoust Soc Amer, 63*(2): 533-49.

719. **Plomp R. (1988)**. The negative effect of amplitude compression in multichannel hearing aids in the light of the modulation-transfer function. *J Acoust Soc Amer, 83*(6): 2322-2327.

720. **Plomp R. (1994)**. Noise, amplification, and compression: considerations of three main issues in hearing aid design. *Ear & Hearing, 15*(1): 2-12.

721. **Plomp R. (1976)**. Speech intelligibility in reverberation. *Acustica, 34*: 201-211.

722. **Plomp R, Mimpen AM. (1979)**. Improving the reliability of testing the speech reception threshold for sentences. *Audiology, 18*: 43-52.

723. **Pluvinage V. (1989)**. Clinical measurement of loudness growth. *Hear Instrum, 40*(3): 28-34.

724. **Popelka MM, Cruickshanks KJ, Wiley TL, Tweed TS, Klein BE, Klein R. (1998)**. Low prevalence of hearing aid use among older adults with hearing loss: the Epidemiology of Hearing Loss Study. *J Am Geriatr Soc, 46*(9): 1075-1078.

725. **Portmann D, Boudard P, Herman D. (1997)**. Anatomical results with titanium implants in the mastoid region. *Ear Nose Throat J, 76*(4): 231-236.

726. **Posen MP, Reed CM, Braida LD. (1993)**. Intelligibility of frequency-lowered speech produced by a channel vocoder. *J Rehab Res Dev, 30*(1): 26-38.

727. **Preves DA. (1976)**. Directivity of in-the-ear aids with non-directional and directional microphones. *Hear Aid J, 29*: 7, 32-33.

728. **Preves DA. (1996)**. Revised ANSI standard for measurement of hearing instrument performance. *The Hear J, 49*(10): 49-57.

729. **Preves DA, Sammeth CA, Wynne MK. (1999)**. Field trial evaluations of a switched directional/omnidirectional in-the-ear hearing instrument. *J Amer Acad Audiol, 10*(5): 273-284.

730. **Preves D. (1990)**. Expressing hearing aid noise and distortion with coherence measurements. *ASHA, 32*(6-7): 56-59.

731. **Preves D, Fortune T, Woodruff B, Newton J. (1991)**. Strategies for enhancing the consonant to vowel intensity ratio with in the ear hearing aids. *Ear & Hear, 12*(6 Suppl): 139S-153S.

732. **Punch J. (1988)**. CROS revisited. *ASHA, 30*(2): 35-37.

733. **Punch J, Jenison R, Allan J, Durrant J. (1991)**. Evaluation of three strategies for fitting hearing aids binaurally. *Ear & Hear, 12*(3): 205-215.

734. **Raicevich, G. (1996)**. *Speech intelligibility enhancement technique: multi-microphone array*. Unpublished dissertation, University of Technology, Sydney.

735. **Rajan R. (1995)**. Involvement of cochlear efferent pathways in protective effects elicited with binaural loud sound exposure in cats. *J Neurophysiol, 74*(2): 582-597.

736. **Rakerd B, Vander Velde TJ, Hartmann WM. (1998)**. Sound localization in the median sagittal plane by listeners with presbyacusis. *J Amer Acad Audiol, 9*(6): 466-79.

737. **Ramkalawan T, Davis A. (1992)**. The effects of hearing loss and age of intervention on some language metrics in young hearing-impaired children. *Brit J Audiol, 26*(2): 97-107.

738. **Rankovic C. (1991)**. An application of the articulation index to hearing aid fitting. *J Speech Hear Res, 34*(2): 391-402.

739. **Rankovic C, Freyman R, Zurek P. (1992)**. Potential benefits of adaptive frequency-gain characteristics for speech reception in noise. *J Acoust Soc Amer, 91*(1): 354-362.

740. **Rees R, Velmans M. (1993)**. The effect of frequency transposition on the untrained auditory discrimination of congenitally deaf children. *Brit J Audiol, 27*(1): 53-60.

741. **Revit L. (1997)**. The circle of decibels: relating the hearing test, to the hearing instrument, to the real ear response. *The Hear Rev, 4*(11): 35-38.

742. **Revit L. (1991)**. New tests for signal-processing and multichannel hearing instruments. *The Hear J, 44*(5): 20-23.

743. **Revit L. (1993)**. *The tip of the probe*. URL http://www.frye.com/aud_resources/application/larry16.html.

744. **Revit LJ. (1992)**. Two techniques for dealing with the occlusion effect. *Hear Instrum, 43*(12): 16-18.

Revoile S, Holden-Pitt L, Edward D, Pickett J. (1986). Some rehabilitative considerations for future speech-processing hearing aids. *J Rehabil Res Dev, 23*(1): 89-94.

745. **Revoile S, Holden-Pitt L, Edward D, Pickett JM, Brandt F. (1987)**. Speech cue enhancement for the hearing impaired: Amplification of burst/murmur cues for improved perception of final stop voicing. *J Rehab Res Dev, 24*(4): 207-216.

Revoile S, Holden-Pitt L, Pickett J. (1985). Perceptual cues to the voiced-voiceless distinction of final fricatives for listeners with impaired or with normal hearing. *J Acoust Soc Amer, 77*(3): 1263-1265.

746. **Reynolds GS, Stevens SS. (1960)**. Binaural summation of loudness. *J Acoust Soc Amer, 32*: 1337-1344.

747. **Richardson B. (1990)**. Separating signal and noise in vibrotactile devices for the deaf. *Brit J Audiol, 24*(2): 105-109.

748. **Ringdahl A. (2000)**. Private communication.

749. **Ringdahl A, Eriksson-Mangold M, Andersson G. (1998)**. Psychometric evaluation of the Gothenburg Profile for measurement of experienced hearing disability and handicap: applications with new hearing aid candidates and experienced hearing aid users. *Brit J Audiol, 32*: 375-385.

750. **Robbins AM, Svirsky M, Osberger MJ, & Pisoni DB. (In press)**. Beyond the audiogram: The role of functional assessments. In F Bess, J Gravel (Eds.), *Children with hearing impairments: Contemporary trends*.

751. **Robbins A, Renshaw J, Berry S. (1991)**. Evaluating meaningful auditory integration in profoundly hearing-impaired children. *Amer J Otol, 12 Suppl*: 144-150.

752. **Robertson P. (1996)**. A guide to NOAH-compatible programmable fitting software. *Hear Rev, 3*(2): 12,14,16,19,28-30.

753. **Robinson CE, Huntington DA. (1973)**. The intelligibility of speech processed by delayed long-term averaged compression amplification. *J Acoust Soc Amer, 54*: 314.

754. **Robinson K, Gatehouse S. (1995)**. Changes in intensity discrimination following monaural long-term use of a hearing aid. *J Acoust Soc Amer, 97*(2): 1183-1190.

755. **Robinson S, Cane M, Lutman M. (1989)**. Relative benefits of stepped and constant bore earmoulds: a crossover trial. *Brit J Audiol, 23*(3): 221-228.

756. **Rodgers CAP. (1981)**. Pinna transformations and sound reproduction. *J Audio Eng Soc, 29*(4): 226-234.

757. **Romanow FF. (1942)**. Methods of measuring the performance of hearing aids. *J Acoust Soc Amer, 13* (1): 294-304.

758. **Rosen S, Fourcin A, Moore B. (1981)**. Voice pitch as an aid to lipreading. *Nature, 14*(291(5811)): 150-152.

759. **Ross M. (1987)**. Aural rehabilitation revisited. *J Acad Rehab Audiol, 20*: 13-23.

760. **Ross M. (1980)**. Binaural versus monaural hearing aid amplification for hearing impaired individuals. In ER Libby (Ed.), *Binaural hearing and amplification*. (1-21) Chicago: Zenetron.

761. **Ross M. (1997)**. A retrospective look at the future of aural rehabilitation. *J Acad Rehab Audiol, 30*: 11-28.

762. **Ross M, Levitt H. (1997)**. Consumer satisfaction is not enough: Hearing aids are still about hearing. *Seminars in Hearing, 18*(1): 7-10.

763. **Roush J. (2000)**. Implementing parent-infant services: advice from families. In R Seewald (Ed.), *A Sound Foundation through Early Amplification* (159-165). Stafa, Switzerland: Phonak.

764. **Rowland RC, Tobias JV. (1967)**. Interaural intensity difference limens. *J Speech Hear Res, 10*: 745-756.

765. **Rubinstein A, Boothroyd A. (1987)**. Effect of two approaches to auditory training on speech recognition by hearing-impaired adults. *J Speech Hear Res, 30*(2): 153-160.

766. **Rupp R, Higgins J, Maurer J. (1977)**. A feasibility scale for predicting hearing aid use (FSPHAU) with older individuals. *J Acad Rehab Audiol, 10*: 81-104.

767. **Sachs RM, & Burkhard MD. (1972)**. *Zwislocki coupler evaluation with insert earphones*. Project 20022. Industrial Research Products.

768. **Salvinelli F, Maurizi M, Calamita S, D'Alatri L, Capelli A, Carbone A. (1991)**. The external ear and the tympanic membrane. A three-dimensional study. *Scand Audiol, 20*(4): 253-256.

769. **Sammeth CA, Dorman MF, Stearns CJ. (1999)**. The role of consonant-vowel amplitude ratio in the recognition of voiceless stop consonants by listeners with hearing impairment. *J Speech Lang Hear Res, 42*(1): 42-55.

770. **Sandel TT, Teas DC, Feddersen WE, Jeffress LA. (1955)**. Localization of sound from single and paired sources. *J Acoust Soc Amer, 27*: 842-852.

771. **Saunders G. (1997)**. Other evaluative approaches. In H Tobin (Ed.), *Practical hearing aid selection and fitting*. (Monograph 001103-119) Washington, D.C.: Dept of Veterans Affairs.

772. **Scharf B. (1970)**. Critical bands. In JV Tobias (Ed.), *Foundations of modern auditory theory*. (Vol 1) New York: Academic Press.

773. **Scharf B, Fishken D. (1970)**. Binaural summation of loudness reconsidered. *J Exp Psychol, 86*: 374-379.

774. **Scharf B, Magnan J, Collet L, Ulmer E, Chays A. (1994)**. On the role of the olivocochlear bundle in hearing: a case study. *Hear Res, 75*(1-2): 11-26.

775. **Schilling JR, Miller RL, Sachs MB, Young ED. (1998)**. Frequency-shaped amplification changes the neural representation of speech with noise-induced hearing loss. *Hear Res, 117*(1-2): 57-70.

776. **Schimanski G. (1992)**. [Silicone foreign body in the middle ear caused by auditory canal impression in hearing aid fitting]. *HNO, 40*(2): 67-68.

777. **Schow R, Brockett J, Sturmak M, Longhurst T. (1989)**. Self-assessment of hearing in rehabilitative audiology: developments in the USA. *Brit J Audiol, 23*(1): 13-24.

778. **Schreurs K, Olsen W. (1985)**. Comparison of monaural and binaural hearing aid use on a trial period basis. *Ear & Hear, 6*(4): 198-202.

779. **Schroeder MR. (1959)**. Improvement of acoustic feedback stability in public address systems. In L Cremer (Ed.), *Proc Third Int Cong on Acoust* (771-775). N.Y.: Elsevier Publishing Co.

780. **Schum DJ. (1997)**. Beyond hearing aids: Clear speech training as an intervention strategy. *The Hear J, 50*(10): 36-38.

781. **Schum DJ. (1999)**. Perceived hearing aid benefit in relation to perceived needs. *J Amer Acad Audiol, 10*(1): 40-5.

782. **Schwartz D, Lyregaard P, Lundh P. (1988)**. Hearing aid selection for severe-to-profound hearing loss. *The Hear J, 41*(2): 13-17.

783. **Scollie S, Seewald R. (1999)**. Private communication.

784. **Scollie S, Seewald R, Jenstad L. (1998)**. DSL questions & answers: Age-appropriate norms for RECDs with earmolds. *DSL Newsletter, 3*(1): 2.

785. **Scollie SD, Seewald RC, Cornelisse LE, Jenstad LM. (1998)**. Validity and repeatability of level-independent HL to SPL transforms. *Ear & Hear, 19*(5): 407-13.

786. **Sebkova J, Bamford J. (1981)**. Evaluation of binaural hearing aids in children using localization and speech intelligibility tasks. *Brit J Audiol, 15*(2): 125-132.

787. **Sebkova J, Bamford J. (1981)**. Some effects of training and experience for children using one and two hearing aids. *Brit J Audiol, 15*(2): 133-141.

788. **Seewald R. (1998)**. Private communication.

789. **Seewald R. (2000a)**. Infants are not average adults: Clinical procedures for individualizing the fitting of amplification in infants and toddlers. Presented at *A Sound Foundation through Early Amplification*, Chicago.

790. **Seewald R. (2000)**. *A Sound Foundation through Early Amplification*. Stafa, Switzerland: Phonak.

791. **Seewald RC, Cornelisse LE, Black SL, Block MG. (1996)** . Verifying the real-ear-gain in CIC instruments. *The Hear J, 49*(6): 25-33.

792. **Seewald R, Ramji K, Sinclair S, Moodie K, Jamieson D. (1993)**. *Computer-assisted implementation of the desired sensation level method for electroacoustic selection and fitting in children: Version 3.1. Users Manual*. London, Ontario: The University of Western Ontario.

793. **Seewald R, Ross M, Spiro M. (1985)**. Selecting amplification characteristics for young hearing-impaired children. *Ear & Hear, 6*(1): 48-53.

794. **Sessler GM, West JE. (1962)**. Self-biased condenser microphone with high capacitance. *J Acoust Soc Amer, 34*: 1787-1788.

795. **Shapiro I. (1979)**. Evaluation of relationship between hearing threshold and loudness discomfort level in sensorineural hearing loss. *J Speech Hear Disord, 64*: 31-36.

796. **Shapiro I. (1976)**. Hearing aid fitting by prescription. *Audiology, 15*: 163-173.

797. **Shaw DW. (1999)**. Allergic contact dermatitis to benzyl alcohol in a hearing aid impression material. *Am J Contact Dermat, 10*(4): 228-32.

798. **Shaw EAG. (1974)**. Acoustic response of external ear replica at various angles of incidence. *J Acoust Soc Amer, 55*: 432(A).

Shaw EAG. (1975). The external ear: new knowledge. *Scand Audiol, Suppl 5*: 24-50.

799. **Shaw EAG. (1980)**. Acoustics of the external ear. In GA Studebaker, I Hochberg (Eds.), *Acoustical factors affecting hearing aid performance*. (First edition, 109-125) Baltimore: University Park.

800. **Shaw EAG. (1974)**. Transformation of sound pressure level from the free field to the eardrum in the horizontal plane. *J Acoust Soc Amer, 56*: 1848-1861.

801. **Shaw WA, Newman EB, Hirsh IL. (1947)**. The difference between monaural and binaural thresholds. *J Exp Psychol, 37*: 229-242.

802. **Shorter DEL, Manson WI, & Stebbings DW. (1967)**. *The dynamic characteristics of limiters for sound programme circuits*. BBC Engineering Monograph No. 70. British Broadcasting Corporation.

803. **Siegenthaler B, Craig C. (1981)**. Monaural vs binaural speech reception threshold and word discrimination scores in the hearing impaired. *J Aud Res, 21*(2): 133-135.

804. **Silman S. (1995)**. Binaural interference in multiple sclerosis: case study. *J Amer Acad Audiol, 6*(3): 193-196.

805. **Silman S, Gelfand S, Silverman C. (1984)**. Late-onset auditory deprivation: effects of monaural versus binaural hearing aids. *J Acoust Soc Amer, 76*(5): 1357-1362.

806. **Silman S, Silverman C, Emmer M, Gelfand S. (1992)**. Adult-onset auditory deprivation. *J Amer Acad Audiol, 3*(6): 390-396.

807. **Silman S, Silverman C, Emmer M, Gelfand S. (1993)**. Effects of prolonged lack of amplification on speech-recognition performance: preliminary findings. *J Rehabil Res Dev, 30*(3): 326-332.

808. **Silverman C, Silman S. (1990)**. Apparent auditory deprivation from monaural amplification and recovery with binaural amplification: two case studies. *J Amer Acad Audiol, 1*(4): 175-180.

809. **Simpson AM, Moore BCJ, Glasberg BR. (1990)**. Spectral enhancement to improve the intelligibility of speech in noise for hearing-impaired listeners. *Acta Otolaryngol (Stock) Suppl, 469*: 101-107.

810. **Sinclair S, Noble W, Byrne D. (1999)**. The feasibility of improving auditory localization with a high-fidelity, completely-in-the-canal hearing aid. *Aust J Audiol, 21*: 83-92.

811. **Singer J, Healey J, Preece J. (1997)**. Hearing instruments: A psychologic and behavioral perspective. *High Performance Hearing Solutions, 1*: 23-27.

812. **Skafte MD. (1990)**. Commemorative 50 years of hearing health care 1940-1990. *Hear Instrum, 41*(9 Part 2): 8-127.

813. **Skinner MW. (1980)**. Speech intelligibility in noise-induced hearing loss: Effects of high-frequency compensation. *J Acoust Soc Amer, 67*: 306-317.

814. **Skinner MW, Clark GM, Whitford LA, Seligman PM, Staller SJ, Shipp DB, Shallop JK, Everingham C, Menapace CM, Arndt PL et al. (1994)**. Evaluation of a new spectral peak coding strategy for the Nucleus 22 Channel Cochlear Implant System. *Am J Otol, 15 Suppl 2*: 15-27.

815. **Skinner M, Binzer S, Fredrickson J, Smith P, Holden T, Holden L, Juelich M, Turner B. (1988)**. Comparison of benefit from vibrotactile aid and cochlear implant for postlinguistically deaf adults. *Laryngoscope, 98*(10): 1092-1099.

816. **Skinner M, Karstaedt M, Miller J. (1982)**. Amplification bandwidth and speech intelligibility for two listeners with sensorineural hearing loss. *Audiology, 21*(3): 251-268.

817. **Skinner M, Pascoe D, Miller J, & Popelka G. (1982)**. Measurements to determine the optimal placement of speech energy within the listener's auditory area: A basis for selecting amplification characteristics. In G Studebaker, F Bess (Eds.), *The Vanderbilt hearing-aid report*. (161-169) Upper Darby, PA: Monographs in Contemporary Audiology.

818. **Smaldino J, Anderson K. (1997)**. Development of the Listening Inventory for Education. Presented at *Second Biennial Hearing Aid Research and Development Conference*, Bethsesda, Maryland.

819. **Smaldino S, Smaldino J. (1988)**. The influence of aural rehabilitation and cognitive style disclosure on the perception of hearing handicap. *J Acad Rehab Audiol, 21*: 57-64.

820. **Smith LZ, Boothroyd A. (1989)**. Performance intensity function and speech perception in hearing impaired children. Presented at *Annual Conv American Speech-Language-Hearing Association*, St Louis.

821. **Snik AF, Beynon AJ, Mylanus EA, van der Pouw CT, Cremers CW. (1998)**. Binaural application of the bone-anchored hearing aid. *Ann Otol Rhinol Laryngol, 107*(3): 187-93.

822. **Snik AF, Dreschler WA, Tange RA, Cremers CW. (1998)**. Short- and long-term results with implantable transcutaneous and percutaneous bone-conduction devices. *Arch Otolaryngol Head Neck Surg, 124*(3): 265-8.

823. **Snik AF, van den Borne P, Brokx JP, Hoekstra C. (1995)**. Hearing aid fitting in profoundly hearing-impaired children: comparison of prescription rules. *Scand Audiol, 24*: 225-230.

824. **Snik A, Hombergen G. (1993)**. Hearing aid fitting of preschool and primary school children. An evaluation using the insertion gain measurement. *Scand Audiol, 22*(4): 245-250.

825. **Snik A, Mylanus E, Cremers C. (1995)**. The bone-anchored hearing aid compared with conventional hearing aids. Audiologic results and the patients' opinions. *Otolaryngol Clin North Am, 28*(1): 73-83.

826. **Soede W, Berkhout A, Bilsen F. (1993)**. Development of a directional hearing instrument based on array technology. *J Acoust Soc Amer, 94*(2 Part 1): 785-798.

827. **Soede W, Bilsen F, Berkhout A. (1993)**. Assessment of a directional microphone array for hearing-impaired listeners. *J Acoust Soc Amer, 94*(2 Pt 1): 799-808.

828. **Sorri M, Luotonen M, Laitakari K. (1984)**. Use and non-use of hearing aids. *Brit J Audiol, 18*(3): 169-172.

829. **Spindel J, Lambert P, Ruth R. (1995)**. The round window electromagnetic implantable hearing aid approach. *Otolaryngol Clin North Am, 28*(1): 189-205.

Staab WJ. (1999). Private communication.

830. **Staab WJ, Martin RL. (1995)**. Mixed-media impressions: A two-layer approach to taking ear impressions. *The Hear J, 48*(5): 23-27.

831. **Stach B. (1990)**. Hearing aid amplification and central processing disorders. In RE Sandlin (Ed.), *Handbook of hearing aid amplification. Volume II: clinical considerations and fitting practices*. (87-111) Boston: College-Hill Press.

832. **Stach BA, Loiselle LH, Jerger JF, Mintz SL, Taylor CD. (1987)**. Clinical experience with personal FM assistive listening devices. *Hear J, 10*(5): 24-30.

833. **Stach B, Loiselle L, Jerger J. (1991)**. Special hearing aid considerations in elderly patients with auditory processing disorders. *Ear & Hear, 12*(6 Suppl): 131S-138S.

834. **Stadler RW, Rabinowitz WM. (1993)**. On the potential of fixed arrays for hearing aids. *J Acoust Soc Amer, 94*(3): 1332-1342.

835. **Stearns WP, Lawrence DW. (1977)**. Binaural fitting of hearing aids. *Hear Aid J, 30*(4): 12, 51-53.

836. **Steinberg JC, Gardner MB. (1937)**. The dependence of hearing impairment on sound intensity. *J Acoust Soc Amer, 9*: 11-23.

837. **Stelmachowicz PG. (1999)**. Personal communication.

838. **Stelmachowicz PG. (1996)**. Current issues in pediatric amplification. *The Hear J, 49*(10): 10-20.

839. **Stelmachowicz PG. (1999)**. Hearing aid outcome measures for children. *J Amer Acad Audiol, 10*(1): 14-25.

840. **Stelmachowicz PG, Dalzell S, Peterson D, Kopun J, Lewis DL, Hoover BE. (1998)**. A comparison of threshold-based fitting strategies for nonlinear hearing aids. *Ear & Hear, 19*(2): 131-8.

841. **Stelmachowicz P, Lewis D. (1988)**. Some theoretical considerations concerning the relation between functional gain and insertion gain. *J Speech Hear Res, 31*(3): 491-496.

842. **Stelmachowicz P, Lewis D, Seewald R, Hawkins D. (1990)**. Complex and pure-tone signals in the evaluation of hearing-aid characteristics. *J Speech Hear Res, 33*(2): 380-385.

843. **Stelmachowicz P, Mace A, Kopun J, Carney E. (1993)**. Long-term and short-term characteristics of speech: implications for hearing aid selection for young children. *J Speech Hear Res, 36*(3): 609-620.

844. **Stephens S, Anderson C. (1971)**. Experimental studies on the uncomfortable loudness level. *J Speech Hear Res, 14*: 262-270.

845. **Stephens SD. (1999)**. Private communication.

846. **Stephens SD, Hetu R. (1991)**. Impairment, disability, and handicap in audiology: towards a consensus. *Audiology, 30*: 185-200.

847. **Stephens S, Callaghan D, Hogan S, Meredith R, Rayment A, Davis A. (1991)**. Acceptability of binaural hearing aids: a cross-over study. *J R Soc Med , 84*(5): 267-269.

848. **Stephens S, Callaghan D, Hogan S, Meredith R, Rayment A, Davis A. (1990)**. Hearing disability in people aged 50-65: effectiveness and acceptability of rehabilitative intervention. *Brit Med J, 300*(6723): 508-511.

849. **Stephens S, Meredith R. (1990)**. Physical handling of hearing aids by the elderly. *Acta Otolaryngol Suppl Stockh, 476*: 281-285.

850. **Stephens S, Meredith R, Callaghan D, Hogan S, Rayment A. (1990)**. Early intervention and rehabilitation: factors influencing outcome. *Acta Otolaryngol Suppl Stockh, 476*: 221-225.

851. **Stone MA, Moore BC. (1999)**. Tolerable hearing aid delays. I. Estimation of limits imposed by the auditory path alone using simulated hearing losses. *Ear & Hear, 20*(3): 182-92.

852. **Stone MA, Moore B. (1992)**. Spectral feature enhancement for people with sensorineural hearing impairment: Effects on speech intelligibility and quality. *J Rehab Res Dev, 29*(2): 39-56.

853. **Stone M, Moore B. (1992)**. Syllabic compression: effective compression ratios for signals modulated at different rates. *Brit J Audiol, 26*(6): 351-361.

854. **Storey L, Dillon H**. Real ear unaided responses with and without a control microphone. Unpublished data.

855. **Storey L, Dillon H. (In preparation)**. Self-consistent correction figures for hearing aids.

856. **Storey L, Dillon H, Yeend I, Wigney D. (1998)**. The National Acoustic Laboratories' procedure for selecting the saturation sound pressure level of hearing aids: experimental validation. *Ear & Hear, 19*(4): 267-79.

Studdert-Kennedy M, Shankweiler D. (1970). Hemispheric specialization for speech perception. *J Acoust Soc Amer, 48*(2): 579-594.

857. **Studebaker GA, Sherbecoe RL, McDaniel DM, Gray GA. (1997)**. Age-related changes in monosyllabic word recognition performance when audibility is held constant. *J Amer Acad Audiol, 8*(3): 150-162.

858. **Studebaker G, Bisset J, Van OD, Hoffnung S. (1982)**. Paired comparison judgments of relative intelligibility in noise. *J Acoust Soc Amer, 72*(1): 80-92.

859. **Sullivan J, Allsman C, Nielsen L, Mobley J. (1992)**. Amplification for listeners with steeply sloping, high-frequency hearing loss. *Ear & Hear, 13*(1): 35-45.

860. **Sullivan R. (1988)**. Probe tube microphone placement near the tympanic membrane. *Hear Instrum, 39*(7): 43-44, 60.

861. **Sullivan RF. (1995)**. *Ear impression-taking in modified radical, intact wall, and radical mastoidectomy and fenestration cases*. URL http://www.li.net/~sullivan/rmastimp.htm.

862. **Sullivan RF. (1988)**. Transcranial ITE CROS. *Hear Instrum, 39*(1): 11-12, 54.

863. **Summerfield Q. (1992)**. Lipreading and audio-visual speech perception. *Philos Trans R Soc Lond Biol. 335*(1273): 71-78.

864. **Surr RK, Cord MT, Walden BE. (1998)**. Long-term versus short-term hearing aid benefit. *J Amer Acad Audiol, 9*(3): 165-71.

865. **Surr RK, Montgomery AA, Mueller HG. (1985)**. Effect of amplification on tinnitus among new hearing aid users. *Ear & Hear, 6*(2): 71-75.

866. **Surr RK, Schuchman GI, Montgomery AA. (1978)**. Factors influencing use of hearing aids. *Arch Otolaryngol, 104*: 732-736.

867. **Surr R, Hawkins D. (1988)**. New hearing aid users' perception of the "hearing aid effect". *Ear & Hear, 9*(3): 113-118.

868. **Swan IRC. (1989)**. The acceptability of binaural hearing aids by first time hearing aid users. *Brit J Audiol, 23*: 360.

869. **Swan I, Browning G, Gatehouse S. (1987)**. Optimum side for fitting a monaural hearing aid. 1. Patients' preference. *Brit J Audiol, 21*(1): 59-65.

870. **Swan I, Gatehouse S. (1987)**. Optimum side for fitting a monaural hearing aid. 2. Measured benefit. *Brit J Audiol, 21*(1): 67-71.

871. **Swan I, Gatehouse S. (1987)**. Optimum side for fitting a monaural hearing aid. 3. Preference and benefit. *Brit J Audiol, 21*(3): 205-208.

872. **Sweetow RW. (1999a)**. *Counseling for hearing aid fittings*. San Diego, Ca: Singular Publishing Group.

873. **Sweetow RW. (1999b)**. Counseling: Its the key to successful hearing aid fitting. *The Hear J, 52*(3): 10-17.

874. **Sweetow RW, Valla AF. (1997)**. Effect of electroacoustic parameters on ampclusion in CIC hearing instruments. *The Hear Rev, 4*(9): 8-22.

875. **Taubman LB, Palmer CV, Durrant JD, Pratt S. (1999)**. Accuracy of hearing aid use time as reported by experienced hearing aid wearers. *Ear & Hear, 20*(4): 299-305.

876. **Taylor K. (1993)**. Self-perceived and audiometric evaluations of hearing aid benefit in the elderly. *Ear & Hear, 14*(6): 390-394.

877. **Tecca JE. (1992)**. Further investigation of ITE vent effects. *Hear Instrum, 43*(12): 8-10.

878. **ter Keurs M, Festen JM, Plomp R. (1992)**. Effect of spectral envelope smearing on speech reception. *J Acoust Soc Amer, 91*: 2872-2880.

879. **ter Keurs M, Festen JM, Plomp R. (1993)**. Effect of spectral envelope smearing on speech reception II. *J Acoust Soc Amer, 93*(3): 1547-1552.

880. **Tharpe AM. (2000)**. Service delivery for children with multiple involvements: How are we going. In R Seewald (Ed.), *A Sound Foundation through Early Amplification* (175-190). Switzerland: Phonak.

881. **Thornton AR, Raffin MJM. (1978)**. Speech discrimination scores modeled as a binomial variable. *J Speech Hear Res, 23*: 507-518.

882. **Thornton A, Bell I, Goodsell S, Whiles P. (1987)**. The use of flexible probe tubes in insertion gain measurement. *Brit J Audiol, 21*(4): 295-300.

883. **Thornton A, Yardley L, Farrell G. (1987)**. The objective estimation of loudness discomfort level using auditory brainstem evoked responses. *Scand Audiol, 16*(4): 219-225.

884. **Tjellstrom A, Hakansson B. (1995)**. The bone-anchored hearing aid. Design principles, indications, and long-term clinical results. *Otolaryngol Clin North Am, 28*(1): 53-72.

885. **Tjellstrom A, Luetje CM, Hough JV, Arthur B, Hertzmann P, Katz B, Wallace P. (1997)**. Acute human trial of the floating mass transducer. *Ear Nose Throat J, 76*(4): 204-6, 209-10.

886. **Tobey E, Geers A, Brenner C. (1994)**. Speech production results: Speech feature acquisition. *Volta Review, 96*(5): 109-129.

887. **Tobias JV. (1963)**. Application of a 'relative' procedure to a problem in binaural-beat perception. *J Acoust Soc Amer, 35*: 1442-1447.

888. **Tonning F, Warland A, Tonning K. (1991)**. Hearing instruments for the elderly hearing impaired. A comparison of in-the-canal and behind-the-ear hearing instruments in first-time users. *Scand Audiol, 20*(1): 69-74.

889. **Tonning FM. (1971)**. Directional audiometry III. *Acta Otolaryngol, 72*: 404-412.

890. **Traynor RBK. (1997)**. Personality typings: Audiology's new crystal ball. *High Performance Hearing Solutions, 3*(1): 28-31.

891. **Traynor RM. (1997)**. The missing link for success in hearing aid fittings. *The Hear J, 50*(9): 10-15.

892. **Trychin S. (1991)**. *Manual for mental health professionals, Part II: Psycho-social challenges faced by hard of hearing people*. Bethseda, MD: SHHH Press.

893. **Turk R. (1986)**. A clinical comparison between behind-the-ear and in-the-ear hearing aids. *Audiol Acoustics, 25*(3): 78-86.

Turner CW, Horwitz AR, Souza PE. (1992). Identification and discrimination of stop consonants: formants versus spectral peaks. *Advances in the Biosciences, 83*: 463-469.

894. **Turner CW, Humes LE, Bentler RA, Cox RM. (1996)**. A review of past research on changes in hearing aid benefit over time. *Ear & Hear, 17*(3 Suppl): 14S-28S.

895. **Turner CW, Hurtig RR. (1999)**. Proportional frequency compression of speech for listeners with sensorineural hearing loss. *J Acoust Soc Amer, 106*(2): 877-886.

896. **Tyler R, Parkinson AJ, Fryauf-Bertchy H, Lowder MW, Parkinson WS, Gantz BJ, Kelsay DM. (1997)**. Speech perception by prelingually deaf children and postlingually deaf adults with cochlear implant. *Scand Audiol Suppl, 46*: 65-71.

897. **Updike C. (1994)**. Comparison of FM auditory trainers, CROS aids, and personal amplification in unilaterally hearing impaired children. *J Amer Acad Audiol, 5*(3): 204-209.

898. **Upfold G, Dillon H. (1992)**. Gain and feedback effects in vented ITE and ITC hearing aids. Presented at *Audiol Soc Aust Conf,* Adelaide.

899. **Upfold L, May A, Battaglia J. (1990)**. Hearing aid manipulation skills in an elderly population: a comparison of ITE, BTE, and ITC aids. *Brit J Audiol, 24*(5): 311-318.

900. **Upfold L, Wilson D. (1983)**. Factors associated with hearing aid use. *Aust J Audiol, 5*(1): 20-26.

901. **Upfold L, Wilson D. (1982)**. Hearing-aid use and available aid ranges. *Brit J Audiol, 16*(3): 195-201.

902. **Valente M, Fabry DA, Potts LG, Sandlin RE. (1998)**. Comparing the performance of the Widex SENSO digital hearing aid with analog hearing aids. *J Amer Acad Audiol, 9*(5): 342-60.

903. **Valente M, Fabry D, Potts L. (1995)**. Recognition of speech in noise with hearing aids using dual microphones. *J Amer Acad Audiol, 6*(6): 440-449.

904. **Valente M, Potts L, & Valente M. (1997)**. Clinical procedures to improve user satisfaction with hearing aids. In *Practical hearing aid selection and fitting.* (Monograph 001, 75-93) Washington, D.C.: Department of Veterans Affairs.

905. **Valente M, Valente M, Meister M, Macauley K, & Vass W. (1994)**. Selecting and verifying hearing aid fittings for unilateral hearing loss. In M Valente (Ed.), *Strategies for selecting and verifying hearing aid fittings.* (228-248) New York: Thieme.

906. **Valente M, Van Vliet D. (1997)**. The independent hearing aid fitting forum (IHAFF) protocol. *Trends in Amplification, 2*(1): 6-35.

907. **van Buuren R, Festen J, Plomp R. (1995)**. Evaluation of a wide range of amplitude-frequency responses for the hearing impaired. *J Speech Hear Res, 38*(2): 211-221.

908. **Van Compernolle D, Ma W, Xie F, Van Diest M. (1990)**. Speech recognition in noisy environments with the aid of microphone arrays. *Speech Communication, 9*: 433-442.

909. **van der Pouw CT, Carlsson P, Cremers CW, Snik AF. (1998)**. A new more powerful bone-anchored hearing aid: first results. *Scand Audiol, 27*(3): 179-82.

910. **van der Pouw KT, Snik AF, Cremers CW. (1998)**. Audiometric results of bilateral bone-anchored hearing aid application in patients with bilateral congenital aural atresia. *Laryngoscope, 108*(4 Pt 1): 548-53.

911. **van Dijkhuizen J, Festen J, Plomp R. (1991)**. The effect of frequency-selective attenuation on the speech-reception threshold of sentences in conditions of low-frequency noise. *J Acoust Soc Amer, 90*(2 Pt 1): 885-894.

912. **van Harten-de Bruijn H, van Kreveld-Bos C, Dreschler W, Verschuure H. (1997)**. Design of two syllabic nonlinear multichannel signal processors and the results of speech tests in noise. *Ear & Hear, 18*(1): 26-33.

913. **Van Tasell DJ. (1998)**. New DSP instrument designed to maximize binaural benefits. *The Hear J, 51*(4).

914. **Van Vliet D. (1997)**. Demonstration: Consumer education or just a sales tool? *Hear J, 50*(3): 80.

915. **Van Vliet D. (1996)**. What's that red thing down in my hearing aid? *The Hear J, 49*(10): 84.

916. **Vanden Berghe J, Wouters J. (1998)**. An adaptive noise canceller for hearing aids using two nearby microphones. *J Acoust Soc Amer, 103*(6): 3621-6.

917. **Vaughan-Jones R, Padgham N, Christmas H, Irwin J, Doig M. (1993)**. One aid or two?—more visits please! *J Laryngol Otol, 107*(4): 329-332.

918. **Velmans M, Marcuson M. (1983)**. The acceptability of spectrum-preserving and spectrum-destroying transposition to severely hearing-impaired listeners. *Brit J Audiol, 17*(1): 17-26.

919. **Ventry I, Weinstein B. (1982)**. The hearing handicap inventory for adults: a new tool. *Ear & Hear, 3*(3): 128-134.

920. **Ventry I, Weinstein B. (1983)**. Identification of elderly people with hearing problems. *ASHA,* (July): 37-42.

921. **Verschuure H, Goedegebure A, Dreschler WA. (1999)**. Comfort and speech intelligibility with fast compression. Presented at *Hearing Aid Amplification for the New Millenium,* Sydney.

922. **Verschuure H, Prinsen T, Dreschler W. (1994)**. The effects of syllabic compression and frequency shaping on speech intelligibility in hearing impaired people. *Ear & Hear, 15*(1): 13-21.

923. **Verschuure J, Maas AJ, Stikvoort E, de Jong RM, Goedegebure A, Dreschler WA. (1996)**. Compression and its effect on the speech signal. *Ear & Hear, 17*(2): 162-75.

924. **Villchur E. (1973)**. Signal processing to improve speech intelligibility in perceptive deafness. *J Acoust Soc Amer, 53*: 1646-1657.

925. **von Bekesy G. (1960)**. *Experiments in hearing.* New York: McGraw-Hill.

926. **von der Lieth L. (1972)**. Hearing tactics. *Scand Audiol, 1*: 155-160.

927. **von der Lieth L. (1973)**. Hearing tactics II. *Scand Audiol, 2*: 209-213.

928. **Vonlanthen A. (1995)**. *Hearing instrument technology for the hearing healthcare professional.* Zurich: Singular Press.

    Voss SE, Allen JB. (1994). Measurement of acoustic impedance and reflectance in the human ear canal. *J Acoust Soc Amer, 95*(1): 372-84.

929. **Walden BE, Demorest ME, Hepler EL. (1984)**. Self-report approach to assessing benefit derived from amplification. *J. Speech. Hear. Res., 27*(1): 49-56.

930. **Walden B, Erdman S, Montgomery A, Schwartz D, Prosek R. (1981)**. Some effects of training on speech recognition by hearing-impaired adults. *J Speech Hear Res, 24*(2): 207-216.

    Walden B, Schwartz D, Williams D, Holum HL, Crowley J. (1983). Test of the assumptions underlying comparative hearing aid evaluations. *J Speech Hear Disord, 48(3): 264-73.*

931. **Walker G. (1997)**. Conductive hearing impairment and preferred hearing aid gain. *Aust J Audiol, 19*(2): 81-89.

932. **Walker G. (1997)**. Conductive hearing impairment: The relationship between hearing loss, MCLs and LDLs. *Aust J Audiol, 19*(2): 71-80.

933. **Walker G. (1997)**. The preferred speech spectrum of people with normal hearing and its relevance to hearing aid fitting. *Aust J Audiol, 19*(1): 1-8.

934. **Walker G. (1988)**. The size and spectral distribution of conductive hearing loss in an adult population. *Aust J Audiol, 10*(1): 25-29.

935. **Walker G, Byrne D, Dillon H. (1984)**. The effects of multichannel compression/expansion amplification on the intelligibility of nonsense syllables in noise. *J Acoust Soc Amer, 76*(3): 746-757.

936. **Walker G, Dillon H, Byrne D, Christen C. (1984)**. The use of loudness discomfort levels for selecting the maximum output of hearing aids. *Aust J Audiol, 6*(1): 23-32.

Wallach H. (1940). The role of head movements and vestibular and visual cues in sound localization. *J Exp Psychol, 27*: 339-368.

937. **Wallenfels HG. (1967)**. *Hearing aids on prescription*. Springfield: CC Thomas.

938. **Ward P. (1981)**. Effectiveness of aftercare for older people prescribed a hearing aid for the first time. *Scand Audiol, 10*(2): 99-106.

939. **Ward P, Gowers J. (1981)**. Hearing tactics: the long-term effects of instruction. *Brit J Audiol, 15*(4): 261-262.

940. **Ward P, Gowers J. (1981)**. Teaching hearing-aid skills to elderly people: hearing tactics. *Brit J Audiol, 15*(4): 257-259.

941. **Ward W. (1960)**. Recovery from high values of temporary threshold shift. *J Acoust Soc Amer, 32*: 497-500.

942. **Warland A, Tonning F. (1991)**. In-the-canal hearing instruments. Benefits and problems for inexperienced users given minimal instruction. *Scand Audiol, 20*(2): 101-108.

943. **Watkins AJ. (1978)**. Psychoacoustical aspects of sythesized vertical locale cues. *J Acoust Soc Amer, 63*: 1152-1165.

944. **Watson N, Knudsen V. (1940)**. Selective amplification in hearing aids. *J Acoust Soc Amer, 11*: 406-419.

945. **Wayner DS. (1990)**. *The hearing aid handbook: clinician's guide to client orientation*. Washington, D.C.: Gallaudet University Press.

946. **Wayner DS. (1996)**. Using the hearing aid. In RA Goldenberg (Ed.), *Hearing aids: a manual for clinicians*. (193-214) Philadelphia: Lipincott-Raven.

947. **Weinstein BE, Spitzer JB, Ventry IM. (1986)**. Test-retest reliability of the hearing handicap inventory for the elderly. *Ear & Hear, 7*(5): 295-299.

948. **Weinstein E., Feder M, Oppenheim AV. (1993)**. Multi-channel signal separation by decorrelation. *IEEE Trans Speech Audio Proc, 1*(4): 405-413.

949. **Weisenberger JM. (1989)**. Evaluation of the Siemens Minifonator vibrotactile aid. *J Speech Hear Res, 32*(1): 24-32.

950. **Weisenberger JM, Kozma-Spytek L. (1991)**. Evaluating tactile aids for speech perception and production by hearing-impaired adults and children. *Amer J Otol, 12 Suppl*: 188-200.

951. **Weiss M. (1987)**. Use of an adaptive noise canceler as an input preprocessor for a hearing aid. *J Rehabil Res Dev, 24*(4): 93-102.

952. **Westerman S, Topholm J. (1985)**. Comparing BTEs and ITEs for localizing speech. *Hear Instrum, 36*(2): 20-24, 36.

953. **Westone. (1996)**. *The whole Westone catalog*. Colorado Springs: Westone.

954. **Westwood G, Bamford J. (1995)**. Probe-tube microphone measures with very young infants: real ear to coupler differences and longitudinal changes in real ear unaided response. *Ear & Hear, 16*(3): 263-273.

955. **Wexler M, Miller LW, Berliner KI, Crary WG. (1982)**. Psychological effects of cochlear implant: Patient and 'index relative' comparisons. *Annals of Otology, Rhinology and Laryngology, Suppl 91*: 59-61.

956. **Widrow B, Stearns DS. (1985)**. *Adaptive signal processing*. Englewood Cliffs, NJ: Prentice Hall.

957. **Wightman FL, Kistler DJ. (1989)**. Headphone simulation of free-field listening. II: Psychophysical validation. *J Acoust Soc Amer, 85*(2): 868-878.

958. **Wightman FL, Kistler DJ. (1993)**. Sound localization. In R Fay, A Popper, W Yost (Eds.), *Springer series in auditory research: Human psychophysics.* (155-192) New York: Springer-Verlag.

959. **Wightman F, Kistler D. (1992)**. The dominant role of low-frequency interaural time differences in sound localization. *J Acoust Soc Amer, 91*(3): 1648-1661.

960. **Williams C. (1994)**. *See/hear: An aural rehabilitation training manual*. Washington, D.C.: A.G. Bell Association for the Deaf.

961. **Wilson D, Walsh PG, Sanchez L, & Read L. (1998)**. *Hearing impairment in an Australian population*. Adelaide: Dept of Human Services Centre for Population Studies in Epidemiology.

962. **Wouters J, Litiere L, van Wieringen A. (1999)**. Speech intelligibility in noisy environments with one- and two- microphone hearing aids. *Audiology, 38*(2): 91-8.

963. **Yoshinaga-Itano C, Sedey AL, Coulter DK, Mehl AL. (1998)**. Language of early- and later-identified children with hearing loss. *Pediatrics, 102*(5): 1161-1171.

964. **Yost WA. (1977).** Lateralization of pulsed sinusoids based on interaural onset, ongoing, and offset temporal differences. *J Acoust Soc Amer, 61*: 190-194.

965. **Yost WA, Wightman FL, Green DM. (1971).** Lateralization of filtered clicks. *J Acoust Soc Amer, 50*: 1526-1531.

966. **Yund EW, Buckles KM. (1995).** Discrimination of multichannel-compressed speech in noise: long-term learning in hearing-impaired subjects. *Ear & Hear, 16*(4): 417-427.

967. **Yund E, Buckles K. (1995).** Enhanced speech perception at low signal-to-noise ratios with multichannel compression hearing aids. *J Acoust Soc Amer, 97*(2): 1224-1240.

968. **Yund E, Buckles K. (1995).** Multichannel compression hearing aids: effect of number of channels on speech discrimination in noise. *J Acoust Soc Amer, 97*(2): 1206-1223.

969. **Zabel H, Tabor M. (1993).** Effects of classroom amplification on spelling performance of elementary school children. *Educational Audiology Monograph, 3*: 5-9.

970. **Zelisko D, Seewald R, Gagne J. (1992).** Signal delivery/real ear measurement system for hearing aid selection and fitting. *Ear & Hear, 13*(6): 460-463.

971. **Ziecheck, J . (1993).** *Expectations and experience with amplification.* Unpublished dissertation, University of Florida, Gainesville, FL.

972. **Zimmerman-Phillips S, Osberger MJ, Robbins AM. (1997).** *Infant toddler: Meaningful Auditory Integration Scale (IT-MAIS).* Symlar: Advanced Bionics Corporation.

973. **Zurek PM. (1993a).** Binaural advantages and directional effects in speech intelligibility. In GA Studebaker, I Hochberg (Eds.), *Acoustical factors affecting hearing aid performance.* (Second ed., 255-276) Boston: Allyn & Bacon.

974. **Zurek PM. (1986).** Consequences of conductive auditory impairment for binaural hearing. *J Acoust Soc Amer, 80*(2): 466-472.

975. **Zurek PM. (1993b).** A note on onset effects in binaural hearing. *J Acoust Soc Amer, 93*(2): 1200-1201.

976. **Zwicker E, Schorn K. (1978).** Psychoacoustical tuning curves in audiology. *Audiology, 17*: 120-140.

977. **Zwicker E, Schorn K. (1982).** Temporal resolution in hard-of-hearing patients. *Audiology, 21*: 474-494.

978. **Zwislocki J. (1957).** Some impedance measurements on normal and pathological ears. *J Acoust Soc Amer, 29*(12): 1312-1317.

979. **Zwolan TA, Kileny PR, Telian SA. (1996).** Self-report of cochlear implant use and satisfaction by prelingually deafened adults. *Ear & Hear, 17*(3): 198-210.

980. **Zwolan T, Zimmerman PS, Ashbaugh C, Hieber S, Kileny P, Telian S. (1997).** Cochlear implantation of children with minimal open-set speech recognition skills. *Ear & Hear, 18*(3): 240-251.

INDEX AND GLOSSARY OF ACRONYMS

A

A-B testing, 313
Abbreviated Profile of Hearing Aid Benefit, 354
ABR latency, 415
AC/DC converter, 20
Accelerometer, 442
Acceptance of loss, 224–226
Acclimatization, 308, 331, 366, 383
  affecting tests of bilateral advantage, 393
  for localization, 386
Acoustic hearing aids, 13
Acoustic horns, 137–142
Acoustic mass, 124
Acoustic reflex
  effect on loudness, 446
  estimating loudness, 415
Acousto-mechanical sensitivity level, 443
Acquiring hearing aids, 325–327
Active filters, 38
Active listening training, 339
Adaptive microphone arrays, 191–195
Adaptive noise suppression
  selecting, 288
Adaptive parameter adjustment, 316
Adaptive release time, 164
ADC (analog-to-digital converter), 34
Adder, 20
Additive arrays, 190–191
Adjusting hearing aids, 289–290
  children, 418
Adjustment to amplification, 366
AGC (automatic gain control), 33
AGCi (automatic gain control - input), 168
AGCo (automatic gain control - output), 168
Age, effect on candidacy, 220–221
AI-DI (articulation index directivity index), 28
Aided thresholds, 106–107, 419
Air-bone gap, allowing for in prescription, 262
ALD (assistive listening device), 72–73
Allergic reaction, 153
Alternation between ears, 387
Amplifiers, 28–33
  buffer, 22
  microphone, 22
Amplitude modulation, 64
Analog hearing aids, 50
Analog technology, 34
Analog-to-digital converter, 34
Analytic training, 339
Anger, 368

Angle vent, 136–137
ANSI standards, 89–91
Anti-aliasing filter, 34
Anxiety, 368
Aperture, 120
Aperturic seal, 120
APHAB (Abbreviated Profile of Hearing Aid Benefit), 354, 356
  administering, 358
  applications, 359
  to determine candidacy, 215–216
Appearance, effect on candidacy, 219
Appointment frequency for children, 419
Arithmetic processor, general, 54
Array microphones, 188–195
Articulation Index, 28. See also Speech Intelligibility Index
Artificial mastoid, 443
ASP (automatic signal processing), 178
Assessment of hearing loss in children, 406–408
Assistive listening devices, 72–73
  history, 14
  need for, 340
Asymmetrical loss, 395–399
  better ear versus poorer ear, 396–399
  bilateral versus unilateral aid fitting, 395–396
  binaural beats, 375
  children, 406
  CROS aids, 399
  FM systems, 399
Asymptotic TTS, 277
Atresia, 442
Attack time, 161
Attitude
  effect of listening program, 330
  effect on candidacy, 212–213
  of clinician, 330
Audibility
  determining candidacy, 216–217
  effects on intelligibility, 5
  formants, 2
Audio input, 42–43
  children, 409
  children and aid style, 408
  FM systems, 66–68
  selection, 285
Audiogram mirroring, 235
Auditory deprivation, 383
  avoiding, 385
  children, 405–406
  conductive loss, 383

profound loss, 383
    recovery from, 384
Auditory inferiority, 384
Aural rehabilitation
    communication training, 338–339
    groups, 344–345
    hearing strategies, 332–337
Automatic gain control, 33
Automatic signal processing, 178
Automatic volume control, 33, 172–173
AVC (automatic volume control), 33
Awareness of loss, 211
Azimuth for loudspeaker placement, 104–105

B

Background noise. *See* Noise
BAHA (bone-anchored hearing aid), 447–450
    bilateral, 449
    test rod, 448
Bands, 38
Bandwidth of digital aids, 56
Barrette hearing aids, 15
Baseline measure, self-report, 354
Baseline response, 265
Battery, 45–47
    capacity, 46–47
    changing, 304
    disposal, 432
    implanted, 450
    ingestion, 431
    operating principles, 45
    size and aid style selection, 284
    voltage, 45–46
Battery consumption
    digital versus analog, 57
    effect of prescriptive approach, 278
Beamforming array, 188–195. *See also* Directional microphone array
Behind-the-ear aid, 10
Belling to make horns, 140
Benefit of rehabilitation. *See also* Candidacy
    aided minus unaided scores, 353
    direct assessment, 353
    outcomes measurement, 350
Better ear versus poorer ear in unilateral fitting, 396–399
BICROS (Bilateral CROS), 439–440
    candidacy, 439
    directional microphone, 439
    fitting procedure, 440
Bilateral
    microphone arrays, 194
Bilateral advantage
    bone-anchored hearing aids, 402
    definition, 371

demonstration of advantage, 393
    experimental evidence, 381
    preferences, 392
    test bias, 390
    test sensitivity, 391–392
    tests, 390–395
Bilateral amplification, 371–403
    advantages, 380–387
    disadvantages, 388–390
    effect on prescription, 402–403
    infants and children, 405
    self image, 389
    tinnitus masking, 387
    versus unilateral, 399–402
    vibrotactile aids, 402
    volume control adjustment, 390
Bilateral CROS, 439–440
Bilateral fitting rate, 371
BILD (binaural intelligibility level difference), 378
BILL (bass increase at low levels), 169
    noise reduction, 179
Binaural. *See* Bilateral
    advantage, 371
    beats, 375
    deficit, 371
    interference, 388–389
    interference, detecting, 393
    loudness summation, 380
    loudness summation, effect on gain prescribed, 402
    perception, detection and recognition, 376–380
    redundancy, 381
    squelch, 377–379, 381
Binaural CROS, 439–440
Binaural intelligibility level difference, 378
Binaural masking level difference, 378
Binaural redundancy, 379
Bisection of dynamic range, 236
Bits, in digital aids, 34, 57
BKB (Bamford-Kowal-Bench) test, 392
Blind channel separation, 194–195
Blind source separation, 194–195
Block diagrams, 19–21
BMLD (binaural masking level difference), 378
Body aid, 10
Bone conduction
    binaural cues, 447
    middle-ear function, 446
Bone conductors, 44–45
Bone-anchored hearing aids, 447–450
    bilateral fitting, 402
Bone-conduction hearing aids, 442–447
    candidacy, 442
    disadvantages, 447

evaluation, 447
maximum output adjustment, 446
prescription example, 445
prescription procedure, 444–447
sensation level, 443
Bony canal
comfort, 133
physiology, 120
Brain
development in infancy, 405
plasticity, 383
plasticity and rewiring, 331
Broadband signals, 81
Broadside array, 190
BTE (behind-the-ear) aid, 10

C

Calibration
pressure method, 79
substitution method, 79
test box, 80
Cambridge formula, 240
Canal block, 147
Candidacy
age, 220–221
aid management, 220
APHAB, 215–216
appearance, 219
audibility, 216–217
central auditory processing disorder, 221–222
cochlear implants, 228–232
cosmetics, 219–220
disability, 215
handicap, 215
HHIE, 215–216
listening environment, 216
manipulation ability, 220
medical contraindications, 233
motivation, 212–213
needs, 216, 216–219
personality, 221
profound loss, 228–233
speech intelligibility, 215
tactile aids, 232–233
tinnitus, effect on, 222
visibility, 219
Capture effect, FM systems, 65
Carbon hearing aid, 13–14
Care of hearing aids, 331–332, 427
Carhart
correction, 263
notch, 446
procedure, 235
Carrier wave, 64
Cartilaginous canal, 120

Categorical loudness scaling, 175
CDMA (code division multiple access), 112
Central auditory processing disorder
effect on candidacy, 221–222
Cerumen, effect on real-ear gain, 102
CFA (continuous flow adapter), 121
Change measures of outcomes, 353
Channels, 38
Children, 405–433
amplification requirements, 412–419
assessment of hearing, 406–408
directional microphones, 409
hearing aids, 408–410
injury, 410
REAG versus REIG targets, 248
speech identification ability, 412–415
temporary threshold shift, 277
Choosing hearing aids, 325–327
CIC (Completely-in-the-canal) aids, 10
definition, 122
functional gain measurement, 107
impression technique, 150
Circuit boards, 29
Clarity
improving, 308–312
Class A amplifiers, 31–32
Class B amplifiers, 32
Class D amplifiers, 32
Classroom amplification, 69–70
Cleaning, effect on style selection, 283
Clear speech, 334
Client Oriented Scale of Improvement, 360
Cochlear
distortion, 388
implant candidacy, 228–232
tuning, 388
Cocktail party effect, 376
Coherence, 86
Comb filter, 198
Comfort, in bony canal, 133
Comfort-control compression, 173–175
Communication training, 338–339
analytic, 339
synthetic, 339
Completely-in-the-canal aid, 10
Compliance, acoustic, 23
Compression
advantages and disadvantages, 181–186
amplifier, 33
attack time, 161
automatic volume control, 172–173
bilateral advantage, 382
combinations of compressors, 180–181
comfort control, 173–174
curvilinear, 166

distortion, 162
dual front-end, 164
dynamic characteristics, 161
dynamic range reduction, 160–161
effect on noise, 171
effect on SNR, 178
effects of vents, 130
feedback oscillation, 164, 182
feedforward, 164
for children, 415
history, 15
I-O curve, 85, 161
input-controlled, 167–169
intelligibility maximization, 177
look-ahead, 164
loudness normalization, 175–177
low-level, 176
noise reduction, 177
output-controlled, 167–169
overshoot, 163
phonemic, 170–180
pumping, 172
purpose, 4
range, 166
ratio, 165
rationales, 169–180
release time, 162
static characteristics, 164–166
syllabic, 170–180
threshold, 165
Compression limiting, 161, 165, 182
control of maximum output, 169–170
distortion, 170
parameters, 170
versus peak clipping, 268–269, 287
Compression ratio, 165
effect on speech scores, 352
effective, 166
severe & profound loss, 261
severe loss, 279
Compression threshold, 165, 251
children, 414
effect of microphone location, 295
NAL-NL1 prescription, 256
prescription, 260–262
Conductive loss
aiding and localization, 386
auditory deprivation, 383
bone conduction aids, 442
characteristics, 6
localization, 375
NAL-NL1 prescription, 256
nonlinear prescription, 264
OSPL90 prescription, 275–276
prescription of gain, 262

speech intelligibility, 214
Consonant-to-vowel ratio, 206
Constriction in tubing
effect on gain, 141
infants, 410
Construction of hearing aids, 48–50
Continuous discourse
use in paired comparisons, 313
Continuous flow adapter, 121
Contra-indications to fitting, 233
Contralateral routing of signals, 434–442
Control microphone, 79
insertion gain, 100
REAG, 90
test box, 79
Controls, 51, 303
CORFIG (coupler response for flat insertion gain), 99
Corner frequency
filter, 37
induction loops, 62
Corpus callosum, 388
COSI (Client Oriented Scale of Improvement), 360
administering, 218, 361
determining needs, 218
normative data, 360
teaching hearing strategies, 337
use with children, 422
Cosmetics
effect on candidacy, 219–220, 225
style selection, 283
Cost of hearing aids, 325
bilateral fittings, 388
digital hearing aids, 73
style selection, 284
Counseling
avoiding jargon, 426
definition, 322
explaining hearing loss, 323
group rehabilitation, 226
of parents, 426–428
styles, 340
types, 322
unwilling patients, 223–226
Coupler, 75–79
definition, 9
mechanical, 442
Coupler gain
converting from real-ear gain, 295
customizing, 298
pre-adjustment of aid, 297
relationship to insertion gain, 99–100
relationship to REAG, 93–95
Crest factor, 82

Critical bands, 7
Critical distance, 58
    selection of directional microphones, 286
CROS (contralateral routing of signals), 434–442
    adjustment and verification, 438
    asymmetrical loss, 399
    basic, 435–439
    BICROS, 439
    candidacy, 436
    effect on feedback, 436
    head baffle effects, 435
    mold, 120
    prescription, 437
    stereo, 440–441
    transcranial, 441–442
    wireless connection, 435
Cross-over effect, 396
Cross-over frequencies, NAL-NL1, 256
Current consumption, 57
Current, quiescent, 31
Curvilinear compression, 166
Custom hearing aids, 49
Customizing coupler response, 297
Cut-off frequency, 37

D

DAC (digital-to-analog converter), 36
Damaging hearing
    children, 432
    through aid use, 276–278
Damper, 41–42
    effect on frequency response, 123
    effect on gain, 143–144
    effect on maximum output, 301
    impedance, 42
    ITE/ITC/CIC, 144
    selecting, 146
    to reduce feedback, 199
Decibels, 8
Deeply seated hearing aids, venting, 132
Deficit, binaural, 371
Dehumidifier, 332
Delay, digital aids, 56
Demodulation, 64
Depression, 368
Deprivation, 383, 383–385
    children, 405–406
Deterioration of unaided ear, 401. *See also*
        Deprivation
Developmental Index of Audition, 424
Diagonal vent, 136
DIAL (Developmental Index of Audition), 424
Diaphragm, 21, 39
Dichotic
    definition, 372

speech tests, 389
Diffraction, 6
Digital hearing aids
    advantages, 58
    bandwidth, 56
    basic technology, 53–58
    cost, 73
    hard wired, 54
    history, 16
    open platform, 54
Digital signal processing
    block processing, 55
    group delay, 55
    sequential processing, 55
    windowing, 55
Digital technology, 34–36
    arithmetic processor, 54
    bits, 57
    MIPS, 57
    quantization noise, 57
Digital-to-analog converter, 36
Digitally programmable aids, 51
    adjusting, 290–293
    for children, 409
Digitizing, 34
Diotic
    definition, 372
    summation, 379
Diplacusis, 388
Direct assessment of benefit, 353
Direct audio input, 42–43, 285
    selection, 285
Directional microphone arrays, 188–195
    adaptive arrays, 191–195
    additive array, 190–191
    basic mechanism, 25
    binaural arrays, 194
    blind source separation, 194–195
    broadside array, 190
    end-fire arrays, 190
    fixed arrays, 188–191
    frequency response, 189
    Griffiths-Jim beamformer, 192
    relative effectiveness, 208
    reverberation, effect of, 193
    subtractive arrays, 188–190
    Widrow LMS array, 192
Directional microphones, 25–28
    BICROS, 439
    cardioid pattern, 25
    children, 409
    directivity index, 26
    dual-microphone, 27
    effect of reverberation, 28
    front-to-back ratio, 26

hand held, 285
internal noise, 189
low-cut, 27
measurement, 80
real-ear gain measurement, 105
selection, 286
signal-to-noise ratio improvement, 28
style selection, 283
warning sounds, 432
Directivity
effect of vents, 130
index, 26
style selection, 283
Disability, 211, 323–324
effect on candidacy, 215
outcomes measurement, 350
relationship to pure tone audiogram, 213
Discomfort
avoiding, 270
earmold and earshell, avoiding, 304, 330
evaluation for children, 421–422
loudness, evaluating, 301
Disposable hearing aids, 50, 73
Distance perception, 372
Distortion, 85–87, 112, 269
beneficial effects, 269
compression limiting, 170
definition, 30
in cochlea, 388
own-voice, 306
Downward spread of masking, 245
Dropouts, FM systems, 72
DSL (Desired Sensation Level), 242–243
DSL[i/o], 254–255
experimental evaluation, 258
Dual-microphone, 27
Duration enhancement, 205
Dynamic range
bisection, 236
sensorineural loss, 3

E

Ear canal
bony, 120
cartilaginous, 120
first bend, 120
infants, 416–419
length in children, 416
resonance in infants, 407
second bend, 120
thresholds in SPL, 407
volume, 75
Ear dams, 147
Ear dominance, 389
Ear impression, removal, 148

Ear impression technique, syringing, 148
Ear impressions, 146–152. *See also* Impressions
Ear simulator, 75–79
Ear simulator targets
converting from real-ear ta, 295
Ear trumpet, 13
Ear wax
effect on feedback oscillation, 113
effect on real-ear gain, 102
Eardrum perforation, 248
Earhooks, 142–143
Early intervention, 405, 405–406
Earmold
basic functions, 117–118
discomfort, 304, 330
for babies, 410
instant, 155
materials, 152
re-tubing, 156–157
repairing, 155–157
retention, 122, 305
safety for children, 410
selection of acoustics, 144
simulator, 76
stock, 155
styles, 120–121
temporary, 155
Earshell
basic functions, 117–118
discomfort, 304
materials, 152
modifying, 155–157
retention, 305
selecting acoustics, 144
Educational performance, 405
Effective compression ratio, 166
Efferent control of cochlea, 388
EIN (equivalent input noise), 87
Electret microphone, 21
Electrical input, 42–43
selection, 285
Emotions, impact of hearing loss, 368
End-fire arrays, 190
Envelope, 162
localization cues, 373
Environment
determining candidacy, 216
Equivalent adult hearing level, 407
Equivalent input noise, 87
Evaluating performance
children, 419–425
Evaluation. *See* Outcomes measurement
effectiveness of processing, 207–208
speech tests, 351
Evaluative selection procedure, 235

Event-related potentials, 389
Expansion, 85, 165
Expectations, 212
    affecting candidacy, 216
    hearing low-level sounds, 331
Extended dynamic range, 254
External vent, 118
Externalization, 374
Eyeglass aid, 11

F

Faceplate, 49
Factor analysis, 355
Family influence, 212, 219
Far ear, 372
Fast Fourier transform, 56
Fast-acting compression, 171–172
    selecting, 287
Fault finding
    by parents, 427
    symptoms and causes, 112–113
Feedback management, selecting, 288
Feedback oscillation, 107, 307
    body-level devices, 412
    cause, *107–109*, 200
    effect of compression, 182
    effect of probe tube, 110–111
    effect of venting, 134–136
    feedback loop response, 200
    internal, 24
    maximum achievable gain, 136
    mechanical, 23
    negative feedback, 109
    positive feedback, 109
    preventing, 307
    sound quality, 109
    style selection, 284
Feedback reduction, 198–202
    cancellation, 201–202
    damping, 199
    frequency shifting, 202
    multichannel hearing aids, 199
    notch filters, 200
    peak shifting, 199
    phase control, 200–201
    search and destroy, 200
Feedback suppression, selecting, 288
FET (field effect transistor), 22
FFT (fast Fourier transform), 56
Field reference point, 90
FIG6, 253
Figure-8 pattern, 25
Filters, 37
    active, 38
    passive, 38

switched-capacitor, 39
Fine tuning
    paired comparisons, 312
Fine-tuning, 303–321
    at home, 320
    quality rating, 314–321
Finite impulse response, 39
FIR (finite impulse response), 39
First bend, 120
Flux, magnetic, 42
FM (frequency modulation) systems, 64–66
    adjustment of level, 67
    asymmetrical loss, 399
    capture effect, 65
    central auditory processing disorders, 222
    combined mode, 68
    comparative advantages, 71–72
    coupled to non-linear aids, 411
    coupling to aid, 66–68
    demodulation, 64
    dropouts, 66, 72
    environmental microphone, 68
    FM precedence, 68
    FM priority, 68
    frequency modulation, 64
    interference, 72
    inverse square law, 65
    local microphone, 68
    muting, 66
    receiver, 64
    relative effectiveness, 208
    speech-operated switching, 68
    squelch, 66
    transmission channel, 65
    transmitter, 64
    use with children, 411–412
    voice-operated switching, 68
Follow-up frequency for children, 419
Formants, audibility, 2
Fourier transform, 55
    definition, 7
Frequency, 6
    compression, 204
    domain processing, 55
    modulation, 64. *See also* FM transmission
    range, 81
    resolution, 4
    response, children versus adults, 413
    response curve, 83
    transposition, 202
Front-back localization, 374
Front-to-back ratio, 26
Full-concha ITE, 122
Full-on gain, 83
Functional gain, 106–107, 419

Fundamental frequency, 7
Fundamental frequency aid, 206

G

Gain, 7, 91
Gain-frequency response, 8
  accuracy requirements, 293
  low-level sounds, 309
  prescription, linear, 239
  prescription, nonlinear, 249–262
Gap detection, 6
GAS (Goal Attainment Scaling), 360
GHABP (Glasgow Hearing Aid Benefit Profile),
  361
Glasgow Hearing Aid Benefit Profile, 361
Goal Attainment Scaling, 360
Goals
  for children, 428–431
  negotiation, 360
  strategies for infants, 429
  strategies for pre-schoolers, 430
  strategies for school children, 430
  strategies for toddlers, 430
Graduated exposure to amplification, 327–331
Griffiths-Jim beamformer, 192
Grommet, effect on real-ear gain, 417
Group delay, digital aids, 56
Groups
  for parents, 427, 429
  rehabilitation, 226
  teaching hearing strategies, 337
GSM (global system mobile), 112
Guessing, 333
Guilt, 224, 233

H

HA1 coupler, 76
HA2 coupler, 76
Habilitation goals for children, 428–431
Half-concha ITE, 10, 122
Half-gain rule, 236
Half-tubing, 140
Handicap, 212, 324
  candidacy, 215
  outcomes measurement, 350
  pure tone loss, relationship, 213
HAPI (Hearing Aid Performance Inventory), 354
Hardening against interference, 112
Harmonic distortion, 30, 86
Harmonics, 7
Head diffraction, 93, 373
  effect on SNR, 376, 381
Head related transfer function, 374
Head shadow, 373

Headband, bone conduction aids, 442
Headphones, use with real-ear gain analyzers, 111
Health, impact of hearing aids, 368–369
Hearing
  assessment in children, 406–408
  disability, 211
  handicap, 212
Hearing Aid Performance Inventory, 354
Hearing Handicap Inventory for the Elderly, 354
Hearing loss
  acceptance, 224–226
  awareness of loss, 211
  conductive, 6
  desensitization, 246, 255, 425
  explaining, 323
  incidence, 210
  sensorineural, 2–6
Hearing strategies, 332–337
  clear speech, 334
  COSI, 337
  group appointments, 337
  guessing, 333
  lighting, 335
  non-verbal signals, 333
  observing the talker, 332
  repair strategies, 335
  speech-reading, 333
  teaching, 337
  topic of conversation, 335
Helix lock, 121, 282
Helmholtz resonance
  in microphones, 23
  in receivers, 40
  in vents, 128
Hemisphere differences, 389
HFA (high-frequency average), 81
HHIE, 357
  candidacy, determining, 215–216
HHIE (Hearing Handicap Inventory for the
  Elderly), 354
High-frequency average gain, 81
High-frequency gain
  acclimatization, 247
  differences between formulae, 245–246
  for children, 413
HINT (Hearing In Noise Test), 392
HiPro, 53, 292
History of hearing aids, 12–17
Hollow voice, 305
Horizontal localization, 372
  bilaterally aided advantage, 385
  effect of hearing loss, 375
Horns, 137–142
  belling, 140
  BTE, 139

cut-off frequency, 138
effect on gain, 141
ITE, 139
Libby, 139
Lybarger high-pass, 140
theory, 138
HRTF (head related transfer function), 374
Hybrids, 29
Hyper-cardioid response, 25

I

I-O (input-output) curve, 84–85
I-O diagram, 8
IC (integrated circuit), 29
IEC standards, 89–91
IHAFF (independent hearing aid fitting forum), 250–251
IIR (infinite impulse response), 39
Impedance, 7
of dampers, 42
of microphones, 43
Implantable hearing aids, 449–450
Impression materials
release force, 152
stability, 151
viscosity, 151
Impression technique, 146–149
CICs, 149–150
high gain aids, 149–150
mastoidectomy, 147
open-jaw, 149
three-stage impressions, 150
In-situ gain, 90–91
In-the-canal aid, 10
In-the-ear aid, 10
Incidence of hearing loss, 210
Individual ear characteristics, 297
Individualized questionnaires, 359, 363
Induction, 42
Induction loops, 59–64
comparative advantages, 71–72
corner frequency, 62
designing, 63
field strength, 61
frequency response, 61–62
inductance, 62
installing, 60
resistance, 62
spillover, 64
Infants, speech identification ability, 412–415
Infections, style selection, 283
Inferior colliculus, 405
Infinite impulse response, 39
Information for parents, 426
Infrared transmission, 69

comparative advantages, 71–72
remote controls, 43
Injury, children, 410
Input-controlled compression, 167–169
Input-output diagram, 8
Input-output function, 84–85
Insert earphones
children, 406
RECD measurement, 299
Insertion, ease, 282, 303
Insertion gain, 96–101
accuracy, 101
converting to REAG, 294
probe placement, 98–99
validity, 101
versus real-ear aided gain, 248
Instant earmolds, 155
Integrated circuit, 29
history, 15
Integrated microphone, 22
Intelligibility
compression vs linear, 184
effect of compression ratio, 185
Intelligibility maximization, 177
Intensity enhancement, 206
Interaural attenuation for bone conduction, 447
Interaural level differences, 373
Interaural phase differences, 372
effect of hearing aids, 385
Interaural time difference, 372
Interface, for programmer, 52
Interference, 112
by mobile hearing aids, 112
Interference, binaural, 388–389
Interhemispheric transfer, 388
Intermodulation distortion, 30
Internal CROS. See Transcranial CROS
Internal feedback, 24
Internal noise, 87–88
directional microphones, 189
microphones, 23
Inverse square law, 65
Investment of impression, 152
Isolation, effects of poor localization, 375
ITC (in-the-canal) aids, 10
ITE (in-the-ear) aids, 10
children, 409
half-concha, 10
low profile, 10
shell styles, 122
Item-total correlation, 355

J

Janssen mold, 118, 120

L

Late-onset auditory deprivation, 383
Lazy ear, 384
LDL (loudness discomfort level)
  binaural, 380
  calibration, 271
  children, 421–422
  for children, 420
  measurement, 271
  OSPL90 prescription, 270
  prediction, 270
Leakage of sound, 119, 125
Legislation for rights, 327
Level detector, 20
LGOB (loudness growth in octave bands), 249–250
Libby horn, 139
Lighting, 335
Lights, flashing, 73
Limiting, 85
  compression or peak clipping, 268–269
Linear amplification, 7
Lip-reading, 332–333
  demonstrating benefit, 353
  place of articulation, 333
Lip-reading, digital aids, 56
Listening criterion, 265
Listening program, 327–331
LMS (least mean squares), 192
Loaner aid, 387
Localization
  acclimatization, 386
  adaptation time, 386
  bilaterally aided advantage, 385–387
  effect of aid style, 386
  effect of signal processing, 386
  effects of hearing loss, 374–376
  front-back, 374
  group communication, 334
  horizontal, 372
  normal hearing cues, 372–374
  relation to speech intelligibility, 395
  testing, 394–395
  vertical, 374
Look-ahead compression, 164
Loop, 42. *See also* Induction loops
Loop gain for feedback, 108
Loop response, test box measurement, 88
Loudness
  discomfort, evaluating, 301
  effect on speech intelligibility, 240
  equalization, 239, 256
  excessive, 309
  growth, 175

normalization, 175–177
  scales for evaluating discomfort, 301
  scaling, 175, 259
  scaling, children, 415
  versus speech intelligibility, 412
Loudness discomfort level, sensorineural loss, 3
Loudness normalization, 249, 253, 254
  compression threshold, 262
  efficiency, 260
  speech versus pure tone, 260
Loudness summation
  across frequency, 252
  binaural, 380
  OSPL90 prescription, 273
Loudspeaker orientation, real-ear gain testing, 104–105
Low-frequency gain for children, 413
Low-level compression, 176
Low-level sounds
  expectations of audibility, 331
Low-profile ITE, 10, 122
LTASS (long-term average speech spectrum), 240
Lybarger high-pass tubing, 140

M

Magnetic
  field strength, 61
  flux, 59
  response measurement, 88–89
Magnetic induction, 42. *See also* Induction loops
  remote controls, 44
Mail-order hearing aids, 50, 73
Maintenance by patient, 332
Management ability, 282
  candidacy, effect on, 220
  style selection, 284
  teaching and troubleshooting, 303
Manikin, 76
Manipulation ability, 282
  bilateral fittings, 399
  candidacy, 220
  style selection, 284
Manufacturers, choosing, 291
Masking curves, 4
Mass, acoustic, 23
Mastoid, artificial, 443
Mastoidectomy, 248
  effect on target gains, 300
  impression technique, 147
Maximum achievable gain, limited by feedback oscil, 136
Maximum output
  bilateral corrections, 402
  bone conduction aids, 446
  children, 412, 413, 418

control by compression limiting, 170
effect of dampers, 301
effect of sound bore, 301
effect of vents, 129, 301
evaluation, 300
evaluation for children, 420
prescription, 270
verifying, 300
Maximum power output, 9
MBTI (Myers-Briggs Type Indicator), 340
MCL (most comfortable level), 236
Measurement signals
broadband, 81
for real-ear gain testing, 105–106
pure tone, 80–82
Mechanical coupler, 442
Mechanical feedback, 23
Medical contra-indications to fitting, 233
Ménière's disease, 264
Mercury batteries, 45
Microphone, 21–28
arrays, 188–195
electret, 21
frequency response, 22
implanted, 449
internal noise, 23
low cut, 22
omni-directional, 26
operating principles, 21
piezoelectric, 15
purpose, 10
satellite, 435
silicon, 22
vibration sensitivity, 23
Microphone location effects, 93–95
Microtia, 442
Middle-ear function, bone conduction, 446
Middle-ear implants, 449–450
Milestones
children, 424, 428–431
Mini-canal aids, 122
MIPS (million instruction per seconds), 57
Mirroring of the audiogram, 235
Mixed loss
gain prescription, 262
OSPL90 prescription, 275–276
MLD (masking level difference), 378
MLE (microphone location effects), 93–95
Modified power law, 276
Modular hearing aids, 49–50
Modulation, 64
Mold. See Earmold
Motivation, 212–213
determining, 216
Motor-boating, 45

MPO (Maximum Power Output), 9
MT (microphone-telecoil) switch, 42
Multi-band. See Multichannel
Multi-memory hearing aids, 264–267
baseline response, 265
candidates, 266
crockery noise, 266
listening criterion, 265
purpose, 53
response alternatives, 265–266
selecting, 288
technology, 53
vent, effect of, 267
Multichannel compression, 169
benefits re single channel, 184–186
compression, 184
compression threshold, 262
selecting, 287
Multichannel hearing aids, 38, 169
feedback reduction, 199
venting, 181
Mute, in FM systems, 66

N

NAL (National Acoustic Laboratories), 239
NAL-NL1, 255–256
binaural corrections, 402
experimental evaluation, 258
selecting, 289
NAL-R, 240
NAL-RP
evidence, 246
formula, 239–242
likelihood of TTS, 278
prescription for children, 414
selecting, 289
NAL-SSPL, 270
Naturalness, 279
Near ear, 372
Neck loop, 66. See also Induction loop
Needs, determining candidacy, 216–219
Negative feedback, 109
Negotiated goals, 360
Neural connections, 405
NOAH, 52, 290
Node of standing wave, 92
Noise
bilateral advantage, 381
effect of compression on, 171
effect of poor localization, 375
effect on aided intelligibility, 216–217
effect on intelligibility, 6
effect on real-ear gain, 102
in microphones, 23
internal, 309

low-frequency, 266
low-level, 309
minimizing, 336
minimizing effect on intelligibility, 311
out of hearing aid, 112
traffic, 266
Noise reduction, 177. *See also* Directional
  microphone arrays
  comb filter, 198
  single microphone systems, 195–198
  spectral subtraction, 196–198
  speech detector, 196
  Wiener filter, 196–198
Noise-induced loss
  children, 432
  hearing aid induced, 276–278
Non-occluding molds and shells, 118, 119
Non-programmable aids, adjusting and selecting,
  293–297
Nonlinear hearing aids, coupled to FM systems,
  411
Nonlinear prescription
  comparisons, 256
  experimental comparisons, 257–258
  OSPL90, 275
Notch filters for feedback reduction, 200
Notch frequency, use in probe positioning, 94
Notch in frequency response, 129

O

Occluding molds and shells, 118
Occlusion
  skin reaction, 153
  style selection, 284
Occlusion effect, 130–134
  fixing, 305–306
  mechanism, 131
  real-ear gain analyzers, 134
Octave bands, 7
OFL90 (output force level for 90 dB input), 443
Omni-directional microphone, 26
Open platform, digital, 54
Open-ended questionnaire, 359
Open-jaw impressions, 149
Optical isolation, 73
Ordering hearing aids, 291–292, 296
Orientation in real-ear gain testing, 104
OSPL90 (output SPL for 90 dB input)
  children, 418
  definition, 9
  evaluation, 300
  fine-tuning, 300
  for conductive loss, 275
  for nonlinear hearing aids, 275
  frequency dependent prescription, 272

measurement, 82–83
prescribing, 267–276
verifying, 300
OSPL90 output SPL for 90 dB input). *See*
  maximum output
Osseointegration, 447
Ossicular chain implants, 449
Otitis media
  alternation between ears, 387
  bilateral fittings, 399
Oto-blocks, 147
Otoplastics, 152
Otosclerosis, 263
Outcomes measurement, 350–369
  applications, 350
  correlations, 369
  definition, 350
  speech identification testing, 351–353
  variation with time, 366–368
Output force level, 443
Output-controlled compression, 167–169
Over-amplification, 276–278
Own-voice, 130–134, 305
Ownership of hearing aids, 210

P

Pacemakers, 44
Paired comparisons
  procedures, 312–313
  round-robin strategy, 315
  technology, 53
  tournament strategy, 315
Parallel vents, 136–137
Parental support, 425–428
Passive filter, 38
Peak clipping, 30
  distortion, 85, 170
  in receiver, 39
  profound loss, 182
  versus compression limiting, 287
Peak shifting for feedback reduction, 199
Peaks
  feedback oscillation, 109
  in gain-frequency response, 41
  in OSPL90 response, 41
Percutaneous coupling, 447
Perforated eardrum, 248
Performance-intensity function, 352
  testing bilateral advantage, 391
Peri-tympanic aid, 11, 122
Period, 6
Permanent threshold shift, 276–278
Personality, effect on candidacy, 221
Phase shift, determining oscillation frequency,
  108

Phase shifting, to reduce feedback, 200–201
Phonemic compression, 170–180
Piezoelectric microphones, 15
Piezoelectric transducers, 449
PILL (programmable increase at low levels), 169
Place of articulation, lip-reading, 333
Plasticity, 383. *See also* Acclimatization
Pleasantness of sound, 279
POGO (prescription of gain and output), 239
POGO II, 239
Positive feedback, 109
Potentiometer, 51
Power CROS, 441–442
Pre-adjustment in coupler, 297
Prescriptive procedures
   at medium input levels, 249
   Cambridge formula, 240
   children, threshold- versus loudness-based, 415
   choosing, 288
   comparison of prescriptions, 256
   comparisons, linear, 243–247
   comparisons, nonlinear, 257–258
   compression threshold, 251
   conductive loss, 262
   effect on children's functioning, 425
   effect on usage, 278
   for children, 412, 414
   formula calculation, 238
   half-gain rule, 236
   history, 235–236
   I-O curves, 249
   linear, 239–247
   loudness equalization, 239
   loudness-based, 236
   mixed loss, 262
   nonlinear, 249–262
   OSPL90, 237
   profound hearing loss, 241–242
   reserve gain, 240
   supra-threshold measurements, 258
   threshold-based, 236, 258
Pressure, 7
Pressure equalization tube, real ear gain, 417
Probe insertion depth, children, 418
Probe microphone
   calibration, 101–102
   effect on feedback, 110–111
   positioning for insertion gain, 98
   positioning for REAG, 91–93, 94
Profound loss
   auditory deprivation, 383
   compression, use of, 261
   excessive amplification, 278
   OSPL90 prescription, 272
   peak clipping, 268

prescriptive procedures, 241
   unilateral, children, 406
Programmable hearing aids. *See* Digitally
   programmable hearing aids
Programmers, 52
Programs, for multiple memories, 53
Proprietary prescriptions, 279
PTS (permanent threshold shift), 276–278
Pumping, 172
Pure tone audiogram
   candidacy determination, 213
   disability, relationship, 213
   handicap, relationship, 213
Push-pull amplifiers, 32

Q

Quality
   binaural listening, 383
   troubleshooting complaints, 308
Quantization noise, 57
Quarter-wavelength resonances, in horns, 138
Questionnaires. *See also* Self-report measures
   factor analysis, 355
   individualized, 359
   item-total correlation, 355
   open-ended, 359
   psychometric properties, 355
   subscales, 355, 356
   test-retest correlations, 355
   unaided versus aided, 356
Quiescent current, 31

R

Radio-frequency transmission, 64–68. *See also*
   FM transmission
   remote controls, 44
REAG (real-ear aided gain), 89–96
   converting to insertion gain, 294
   coupler gain, relationship, 93–95
   DSL prescription, 242
   NAL-NL1 prescription, 255
   probe microphone positioning, 94
   use with children, 416
   validity, 95–96
   versus insertion gain, 248
Real-ear aided gain, 89–96
Real-ear aided response, 90
Real-ear gain, 89
   analyzers and occlusion effect, 134
   requirements, children versus adults, 412–415
   verification in children, 417, 419
   viewing results, 292
Real-ear insertion gain, 96–101. *See also*
   Insertion gain

Real-ear occluded gain, 96, 127

Real-ear response
    verifying, 300

Real-ear to coupler difference, 78

Real-ear to dial difference, 407

Real-ear unaided gain, 97

REAR (real-ear aided response), 90

RECD (real ear to coupler difference), 78
    age appropriate values, 416–419
    LDL measurement, 271
    measurement, 297
    reasons for measuring, 297

Receiver, 39–41
    FM, 64
    frequency response, 39–41
    mold, 121
    operating principle, 39
    purpose, 10
    tubing, 40

Recovery from deprivation, 384

REDD (real-ear to dial difference), 407, 408

Redundancy, binaural, 379, 381

Reference equivalent threshold SPL, insert
        phones, 407

Reference frequency, 83

Reference microphone, 79, 90

Reference plane, 76

Reference point, 90

Reference test gain, 83

Reflective listening, 339

REIG (real-ear insertion gain), 96–101. *See also*
        Insertion gain

Rejection of hearing aids by teenagers, 431

Release force, 152

Release time, 162
    adaptive, 164

Reliability, impact on style selection, 283

Reluctance to acknowledge loss, 233

Remote controls, 43–44, 52

Remote sensing and transmission, 58–59
    comparative advantages, 70–72

Removal, ease, 282, 304

REOG (real-ear occluded gain), 96, 127

Repair strategies for communication, 335

Repairs, 111–113

Reserve gain, 100, 240

Residual ear canal volume, 75, 118
    infants, 407

Resonance
    ear canal, 92
    ear canal, children, 416
    ear canal, replacing, 41
    mechanical, 40
    quarter-wave, 138
    wavelength, 40

Response, 91

RESR (real-ear saturation response)
    children, 418
    prescribing, 267–276

RETFL (Reference Equivalent Threshold Force
        Level), 444

RETSPL (reference equivalent threshold SPL)
    insert earphones, 407

REUG (real-ear unaided gain), 97
    infants, 416–433
    preserving individual characteristics, 248

Reverberation
    effect on directionality, 193
    minimizing, 336
    overcoming effects of, 58–59
    selection of directional microphones, 286

Right-ear advantage, 388–389

Ringing, caused by feedback, 110

rms (root-mean-square), 7

Room loops, 60. *See also* Induction loops

Round-robin testing, 315

S

SADL (Satisfaction with Amplification in Daily
        Life), 366

Safety
    issues for children, 431–433
    laceration, 410

Safety limit, excessive amplification, 277

Sampling frequency, 34

Sampling rate, 56

Satellite microphone, 435

Satisfaction
    outcomes measurement, 350
    trends, 17

Satisfaction with Amplification in Daily Life, 366

Saturation, during real-ear measurement, 103

Saturation sound pressure level, 9

ScalAdapt, 252–253

Search and destroy, 200

Second bend, 120

Selecting hearing aids, 295
    children, 291

Self-image, 212
    bilateral hearing aids, 389

Self-report, 353–359. *See also* Questionnaires
    accuracy, 354
    change measures, 353
    children, 422–425
    direct assessment, 353
    state measures, 354
    unaided versus aided, 353
    validity for children, 425

Semi-custom hearing aids, 50

Semi-modular hearing aids, 50

Senility, 212
Sensation level, obtained with bone conduction aid, 443
Sensitivity, microphone, 21
Sensorineural loss
  characteristics, 2–6
  dynamic range, 3
  frequency resolution, 4
  loudness discomfort, 3
  temporal resolution, 5
Severe loss
  compression ratio, 279
  compression, use of, 261
Shame, 224–225, 233
SHAPI (Shortened Hearing Aid Inventory), 357
SHAPIE (Shortened Hearing Aid Inventory for the Elderly), 357
Shouting, 334
Signal processing schemes
  advanced, 188–208
  effect on bilateral advantage, 382
  selecting, 287–288
Signal-to-noise ratio
  deficit in hearing loss, 6
  directional microphones, 28
Signals
  for real-ear gain testing, 105
Significant other person, 337–338
SII (Speech Intelligibility Index), 240, 246
  children, 425
Silicon microphone, 22
Simulated environments, for speech identification, 353
Simulated telephone sensitivity, 89
SIN (Speech In Noise) test, 392
Sine-wave speech, 205, 206
Situations To Experience and Practice, 327–330
Skeleton mold, 120
Ski-slope hearing loss, 214
Sliding Class A amplifier, 33
Slope, of gain-frequency response, 296
Slow-acting compression, 173
  parameters, 173
  selecting, 287
Small ears, 410
Smoothing, in real-ear gain testing, 106
SNR (signal-to-noise ratio), 28
  needed by children, 413
SOP (significant other person), 337–338, 356
Sound bore, 137
  effect on maximum output, 301
  frequency response, 123
  selecting, 145
Sound pressure level, 7
Sound quality

binaural listening, 383
  effect of venting, 130
  in feedback oscillation, *109*
Sound-field amplification, 69–70
  comparative advantages, 71
SOX (speech-operated switching), 68
Speaker direction, in real-ear gain testing, 104
Speaking tube, 13
Spectacle aid, 11
Spectral enhancement, 205
Spectral flattening, 185
Spectral sharpening, 205
Spectral subtraction, 196–198
Spectrum, 7
Speech cue enhancement, 204–207
Speech detector, 196
Speech intelligibility
  bilateral advantages, 380–383
  candidacy, guide to, 215, 227–228
  children versus adults, 412–415
  conductive loss, 214
  downward spread of masking, 245
  hearing loss desensitization, 246
  loudness, 240
  maximization, 256
Speech Intelligibility Index, 240, 255
  predicting aided benefit, 351
Speech intelligibility testing
  babies, 406
  children, 420
  for bilateral advantage, 392
  limitations, 351–352
  phoneme scoring, 351
  relative efficiency, 351
  role in outcomes assessment, 352–353
  simulated environments, 353
Speech pattern processing, 206
Speech re-synthesis aid, 207
Speech simplification, 206
Speech test sensitivity
  bilateral advantage, 391–392
Speech-operated switching, 68, 411
Speech-reading, 333
Speech/non-speech detector, 179
SPLITS (SSPL for inductive telephone simulator), 88
SPLIV (SPL for vertical inductive field), 88
Sport, and hearing aid use, 432
Squelch, 85
  binaural, 377, 381
  in FM transmission, 66
SSPL (saturation sound pressure level), 9, 402
  bilateral corrections, 402
  prescribing, 267–276
Stability, of impression materials, 151

Standard mold, 121

Standards, 89–91

Standing waves
    ear canal, 92
    in real-ear gain testing, 105

Stapedius reflex, 446

State measures, 354

STEP (Situations To Experience and Practice),
    327–330

Stereo CROS
    candidacy, 440
    fitting procedure, 441

Stethoclip, 111

Stigma, 219–220

Stock molds, 155

Structured interviews, for children, 425

STS (simulated telephone sensitivity), 89

Style of hearing aids, 325
    children, selection, 408–410
    selection, 282–284

Sub-oscillatory feedback, 109–110

Subjective report
    children, 422–425

Subscales, 356
    questionnaires, 355

Substitution method, 79

Substrates, 29

Subtractive arrays, 188–190

Summer, 20

Super-cardioid response, 25

Support groups, 340
    for parents, 427

Supra-threshold measurements, 258

Surgically altered ear canals, 300

Swallowing of batteries, 431

Switched-capacitor filters, 39

Switching amplifier, 32

Syllabic compression, 170–180
    parameters, 172

Synthetic communication training, 339

Synthetic speech aid, 207

Syringing, impressions, 148

T

Tactile aids, 233

Target matching, 235
    accuracy requirements, 293

Technology
    choice of type, 325
    relative advantages, 325

Teenagers, 431

Tele-medicine, 320

Telecoils, 42. *See also* Induction loops
    selection, 285
    sensitivity, 61, 88–89

style selection, 283

Telephones
    amplifier, 73
    hearing aid style selection, 283
    magnetic coupler, 62
    magnetic field strength, 61, 62

Temporal resolution, in sensorineural loss, 5

Temporary aid, 387

Temporary threshold shift, 276–278

Test bias, in bilateral advantage, 391

Test box, 79
    calibration, 80

Test level
    avoiding saturation, 104–105
    testing bilateral advantage, 392

Test loop sensitivity, 89

Test signals
    for real-ear gain testing, 105–106

THD (total harmonic distortion), 30, 86

Thick wall tubing, 137

Third-party funds provider, outcomes measure-
    ment, 350

Three-stage impressions, 150

Threshold determination, in infants, 406–407

TILL (treble increase at low levels)
    definition, 169
    for loudness normalization, 176

Time modification, 205

Tinnitus
    effect on candidacy, 222
    masking by bilateral hearing aids, 387

TLS (test loop sensitivity), 89

Tonal quality, 308–312

Tone controls, 37
    treble boost, 336

Top lock. *See* Helix lock

Topic of conversation, 335

Total harmonic distortion, 30, 86

Tournament strategy, 315

Traffic noise, 266

Transcranial CROS, 441–442
    candidacy, 441
    fitting procedure, 441

Transducers, 21
    definition, 10
    for implanted hearing aids, 449

Transistor hearing aids, 15–16

Transistors, 29

Transmission gain, 91

Transmitter, 64

Transposition, 202–204, 269
    children, 410

Trench vent, 118

Trimpot, 51

Troubleshooting, 111–113

by parents, 427
symptoms and causes, 111–113
two-step, 310
using a stethoclip, 111
using headphones, 111
TTS (temporary threshold shift), 276–278
Tubing, 137
  damping, 41
  leakage, 137
  Lybarger high-pass, 140
Tuning curves, 4
TV listening
  direct audio input, 285
2-cc coupler, 9, 75–79

U

UCL (uncomfortable loudness level)
  OSPL90 prescription, 270
Ultrasonic remote controls, 44
Unilateral amplification, 371, 399
  practical considerations, 399
  versus bilateral, 399–402
Unilateral loss
  children, 405
  CROS aids, 399
  FM systems, 399
Unwilling patients, counselling, 223–226
Upward spread of masking, 5, 239, 253
  noise reduction, 177
Use of hearing aids, 363
  by children, 429
  during sport, 432
  outcomes measurement, 350

V

Vacuum tube hearing aids, 14–15
Value for money, 326
Vent-associated resonance, 128
Vent-cavity resonance, 128
Vent-transmitted sound path, 127
Ventilation tube, effect on real ear gain, 417
Vents, 123–137
  deeply seated hearing aids, 132
  definition, 118
  diagonal, 136–137
  effect on amplified sound path, 126
  effect on compressor action, 130
  effect on directivity, 130
  effect on internal noise, 130
  effect on maximum output, 129, 301
  effect on sound quality, 130
  external, 118
  feedback oscillation, 134–136
  frequency response, 123

Helmholtz resonance, 128
  inserts, 125
  low-cut, 126
  molded, 156
  multi-memory candidature, 267
  occlusion effect, 130
  poured, 156
  selecting, 144–146
  shape and feedback, 136
  slit leak, 118
  tree, 125
  trench, 118
Verifying real-ear gain, 300
  children, 417, 419
Vertical localization, 374
  effect of hearing aids, 386–387
  effect of hearing loss, 375
Vibrotactile aids, 232–233
  bilateral fitting, 402
VIOLA (visual input/output locator algorithm), 250, 251
Viscosity, of impression materials, 151
Visibility of aid
  candidacy, 219
  counseling, 225
  style selection, 283
Visual impairment, 402
Voice-operated switching, 68
Voltage, 45
Volume control, 282
  bilateral fittings, 390
  selection, 285
Volume velocity, 7
VOX (voice-operated switching), 68

W

Warning sounds, and directional microphones, 432
Warranty and repairs, 111
Waveform, 7
Wavelength, 6
  resonance, 40
Wax
  effect on feedback, 113
  effect on real-ear gain, 102
WDRC (wide dynamic range compression), 161
  for children, 415
Whistling, 108, 109. *See also* Feedback oscillation
Wide dynamic range compression, 161
  selecting, 287
Widrow LMS array, 192
Wiener filter, 178, 196–198
Wind noise, 24, 283
  bilateral hearing aids, 389

Wireless links
　bilateral, 450
Wireless, remote controls, 44
Wireless systems. *See* FM systems
　use with children, 411–412

Y

Y-vent, 136

Z

Zinc-air batteries, 45
Zwislocki coupler, 76